HealthScape: Intersections of Health, Environment, and GIS&T

HealthScape: Intersections of Health, Environment, and GIS&T

Guest Editors

Lan Mu
Jue Yang

MDPI

Basel • Beijing • Wuhan • Barcelona • Belgrade • Novi Sad • Cluj • Manchester

Guest Editors
Lan Mu
Department of Geography
University of Georgia
Athens
USA

Jue Yang
School of Public Health
Brown University
Providence
USA

Editorial Office
MDPI AG
Grossspeteranlage 5
4052 Basel, Switzerland

This is a reprint of the Special Issue, published open access by the journal *ISPRS International Journal of Geo-Information* (ISSN 2220-9964), freely accessible at: https://www.mdpi.com/journal/ijgi/special_issues/G9YU275HD5.

For citation purposes, cite each article independently as indicated on the article page online and as indicated below:

Lastname, A.A.; Lastname, B.B. Article Title. *Journal Name* **Year**, *Volume Number*, Page Range.

ISBN 978-3-7258-8013-3 (Hbk)
ISBN 978-3-7258-8014-0 (PDF)
https://doi.org/10.3390/books978-3-7258-8014-0

Contents

International Journal of
Geo-Information

MDPI

Article

Capturing Built Environment and Automated External Defibrillator Resource Interplay in Tianjin Downtown

Sara Grigoryan *, Yike Hu and Nadeem Ullah

School of Architecture, Tianjin University, Tianjin 300272, China; huyike11@tju.edu.cn (Y.H.); 6120000154@tju.edu.cn (N.U.)
* Correspondence: 6121000169@tju.edu.cn

Abstract

Automated external defibrillator resources (AEDRs) are the crux of out-of-hospital cardiac arrest (OHCA) responses, enhancing safe and sustainable urban environments. However, existing studies failed to consider the nexus between built environment (BE) features and AEDRs. Can explainable machine-learning (ML) methods reveal the BE-AEDR nexus? This study applied an Optuna-based extreme gradient boosting (OP_XGBoost) decision tree model with SHapely Additive exPlanations (SHAP) and partial dependence plots (PDPs) aiming to scrutinize the spatial effects, relative importance, and non-linear impact of BE features on AEDR intensity across grid and block urban patterns in Tianjin Downtown, China. The results indicated, that (1) marginally, the AEDR intensity was most influenced by the service coverage (SC) at grid scale and nearby public service facility density (NPSF_D) at block scale, while synergistically, it was shaped by comprehensive accessibility and land-use interactions with the prioritized block pattern; (2) block-level granularity and (3) non-linear interdependencies between BE features and AEDR intensity existed as game-changers. The findings suggested an effective and generalizable approach to capture the complex interplay of the BE-AEDR and boost the AED deployment by setting health at the heart of the urban development framework.

Keywords: built environment; automated external defibrillator; machine learning; pattern dependency; non-linear interplay

1. Introduction

Out-of-hospital cardiac arrest (OHCA), defined as a critical state of sudden cessation of cardiac activity, resulting in collapse, loss of consciousness, spontaneous breathing, and blood circulation, remains a global health issue and a major contributor to global mortality [1,2]. OHCA accounts for a considerable proportion of global sudden cardiac arrest (SCA) incidents, with approximately 75% occurring in prehospital residential settings [3]. Due to this context, the United Nations (UN) Sustainable Development Goals prioritize the urgency of addressing non-communicable diseases (NCDs), such as cardiovascular diseases (CVDs), with the aim of promoting universal public health and well-being by 2030 [4,5]. Automated external defibrillators (AEDs) typically refer to life-saving devices that automatically detect ventricular fibrillation (VF) and pulseless ventricular tachycardia (pVT) and restore normal heart rhythm via electrical shock [1]. AEDs are considered the crux and key contributors to OHCA response, improving survival rates to as high as 70% when administered within the first 3–5 min of a collapse-to-shock interval [6]. However, the overall utilization of AEDs remains alarmingly low (<3%) [7], largely due to the fragmented placement and limited public accessibility of AEDs.

China's statistics estimated approximately 330 million CVD patients and 544,000 annual OHCA deaths, with a survival rate of less than 1% [8,9]. The rapid urbanization and population growth in China (from 17.9% of the total population in 1978 to 60.6% in 2019) [10] have boosted public awareness of health and well-being, promoting initiatives such as China's Healthy China 2030 (HC 2030) blueprint, which seeks to improve healthcare services [11]. While the HC 2030 initiative has driven notable healthcare advancements, systemic gaps persist. These include the need to promote a more comprehensive prehospital emergency service system, particularly developing a more adequate approach for AED placement in public areas. In China, the development of AEDs remains fragmented, concentrated in megacities such as Hangzhou (950 units), Shenzhen (6888 units), Guangzhou (1006 units), and Shanghai (283 units) [9,12–14], while most cities lack well-developed and cohesive AED networks. Characterized by considerable regional disparities, China's AED coverage lags behind global benchmarks (e.g., the US, Japan, and Singapore) [12], reflecting insufficient integration of evidence-based placement strategies. In recent years, Tianjin Municipality has taken a series of legislative steps to promote AED development strategies. On 10 September, 2019, the Tianjin Municipal Government announced "Action Plan for the Healthy Tianjin Initiative" to strengthen pre-hospital emergency response systems by targeting cardiovascular emergencies. (https://wsjk.tj.gov.cn/ZWGK3158/GSGG247/202008/t20200803_3355011.html (accessed on 26 June 2025)). Aligned with the objectives of the 14th Five-Year Plan, Tianjin Municipality has initiated a multi-stakeholder collaboration involving the Municipal Health Commission, Municipal Red Cross Society, and district-level governments to promote AED installations across the city to achieve the maximum coverage. Despite the progress, persistent challenges, including geographically uneven AED distribution and underdeveloped maintenance protocols, underscore the need for enhanced regulations and iterative refinements (https://www.tjrd.gov.cn/dbyd/system/2023/12/18/030029705.shtml (accessed on 26 June 2025)).

Over the past years, numerous scholars have attempted to address AED development, proposing different measurements and techniques, particularly in terms of location, accessibility, effectiveness, and equity. Existing studies predominantly analyzed the relationship between built environment (BE) features and automated external defibrillator resources (AEDRs) from the perspective of the following three approaches: population-based (guideline-based), street network-based, and land-use-based techniques. The international AED location guidelines, particularly the European Resuscitation Council (ERC) and the American Heart Association (AHA), recommend placing AEDs in areas with cardiac arrest incidents every 2–5 years [15]. Population-based techniques employ historical OHCA incidence and socioeconomic indicators (e.g., population density, age, gender, education, income) to identify high-risk zones and guide AED placement [15–17]. Street network-based techniques focus on network-oriented developments, prioritizing pedestrian accessibility and visibility, as well as accounting for psychological barriers to improve AED effectiveness in urban areas [18]. Land-use-based techniques integrate facilities (e.g., local businesses, restaurants, train stations, or public buildings) and land-use classifications (e.g., residential, commercial, park/open space, and other public places) to maximize AED geographical coverage in urban–rural environments [6,19,20]. Methodological advancements, including GIS spatial analysis [19,21] and mathematical models [22,23], have refined these techniques, yet critical challenges persist. Prior AED development studies relied on population-based, street network-based, and land-use-based techniques, leading to current AED placement limitations: (1) dependence on location-allocation models; (2) insufficient consideration of how the BE features, such as urban design, service coverage, facility diversity, temperature, etc., affect AED distribution patterns; and (3) lack of multi-scale validation (e.g., block vs. grid scale). For instance, even in areas with similar population densities but varying facility diversity or accessibility, they may exhibit variations in AED availability, highlighting BE impact. By quantifying BE–AEDR interaction, this study aims to uncover the gaps in current frameworks, underscoring the need to integrate BE features to guide future studies of spatially advanced public health resource development.

The impact of the BE factors on the public space is inherently a complex process, involving nonlinear interactions that traditional models often fail to capture. While ML techniques have successfully modeled nonlinear BE–health behavior relationships, such as physical activity [24], urban vitality [25], walking [26], well-being [27], and health-seeking behavior [28], its application to healthcare resource development remains limited. Recent advances in ML, such as variational graph autoencoder (VGAE) with a random forest (RF) model for emergency shelter placement [29] and SHAP-interpreted XGBoost for health equity analysis [30], demonstrate the potential of these tools to address spatial disparities.

To conclude, regardless of the effectiveness of the AED location strategies, most studies neglect the nonlinear interplay between BE features and AEDR intensity. Moreover, the existing studies predominantly rely on single-scale frameworks, overlooking how spatial resolution impacts development outcomes. In addition, while population, street network, and land-use indicators inform AED placement, other BE factors remain underexplored. To avoid scale mismatches and enhance analytical stability for management practices, two basic analytical units were adopted: hexagonal grids (210 m in diameter, bystander maximum distance) in Scenario I (SI), generated with Tessellation tool with a total of 5925 grids and existing blocks in Scenario II (SII). The Zonal Statistics and Join tools were obtained to calculate the values within the hexagons and blocks. This study represents the first application of decision tree-based ML models in AEDR research, wherein we evaluated the performance of the following algorithms: extreme gradient boosting (XGBoost), Light Gradient Boosting Machine (LightGBM), Gradient Boosting Decision Tree (GBDT), AdaBoost, and Random Forest (RF). To ensure a fair and robust evaluation, we applied Optuna hyperparameter optimization uniformly across all the models (OP_XGBoost, OP_LightGBM, OP_GBDT, OP_ AdaBoost, OP_RF). This methodological approach strengthens the rigor and comparability of our experiments, enabling the identification of the most effective model for analyzing the BE_AEDR nexus. To address the aforementioned research gaps, we opted for the best ML model combined with SHapely Additive exPlanations (SHAP) and partial dependence plots (PDPs) to scrutinize the spatial effects, relative importance, and non-linear linkages between BE features and AEDR intensity across grid- and block-scale urban patterns in Tianjin Downtown, China. This study makes contributions by answering the following research questions (RQs): (RQ1) Can ML-based models unveil the BE–AEDR nexus? (RQ2) Which are the most critical BE features affecting AEDR intensity marginally and synergistically? (RQ3) Should spatial resolution disparities be considered in BE–AEDR analysis? (RQ4) Do non-linear effects exist in the BE–AEDR nexus?

The remainder of this paper is organized as follows. We will first present materials and methods, including the study area, analytical framework, database setup, and measurements in Section 2. Then, we will display the results in Section 3 and discuss the related outcomes in Section 4, seeking to interpret the experimental outcomes. Finally, we will conclude the findings and the limitations of the study, proposing future development recommendations for further improvements in Section 5.

2. Methodology

2.1. Study Area

Tianjin (38°34′ N to 40°15′ N, 116°43′ E to 118°04′ E), a coastal megacity in Northern China, is one of the four municipalities directly under the Central Government of China and a pivotal economic hub in the Bohai Rim region [31,32]. The city's rapid urbanization has intensified challenges in healthcare resource development, particularly in Tianjin Downtown (Figure 1). Spanning 1.73 km^2 with a population of 4.0572 million (29.26% of Tianjin's population within 1.54% of its total land area) [33], this hyper-dense urban core encompasses six administrative districts (Heping, Hedong, Hexi, Nankai, Hebei, and Hongqiao) [31]. We target Tianjin Downtown as the study area for three reasons: (1) The extreme population–land disparity demonstrates significant supply–demand mismatches. (2) Despite 2017 healthcare reforms prioritizing prehospital care optimization [34], Tianjin's OHCA response system remains underdeveloped, partly driven by inadequate AED placement. (3) The dense built environment and data availability make it an ideal case to model the BE–AEDR nexus in high-density urban cores.

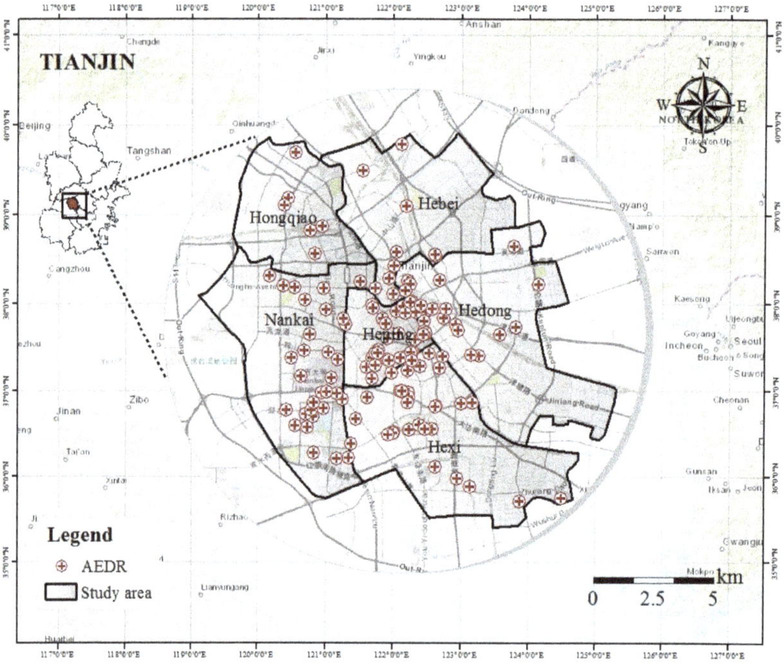

Figure 1. Location of the study area.

2.2. Framework

Our study develops an analytical framework to explore the non-linear BE–AEDR spatial nexus in Tianjin Downtown, China (Figure 2). The framework comprises three main phases. (P1) The first phase is related to database setup and preprocessing, including AEDR and BE feature data collection, screening, calculation, and transformation into spatial layers to ensure the elimination of redundancy. (P2) The second phase is related to BE feature selection. Specifically, the potential indicators were identified via extensive literature review, multicollinearity, and Pearson correlation analysis, ensuring the robustness of model input. (P3) The third phase constructs and evaluates the AEDR prediction models. Then, model training, hyper-parameter tuning, and validation were performed step by step. In this study, all procedures run in ArcGIS 10.8 (with a projected coordinate system: WGS_1984_UTM_Zone_50N) and Python 3.9. Finally, we identified limitations of this study and proposed recommendations for AEDR development. To the best of our knowledge, this is the first study to have conducted such a refined analysis of this nature.

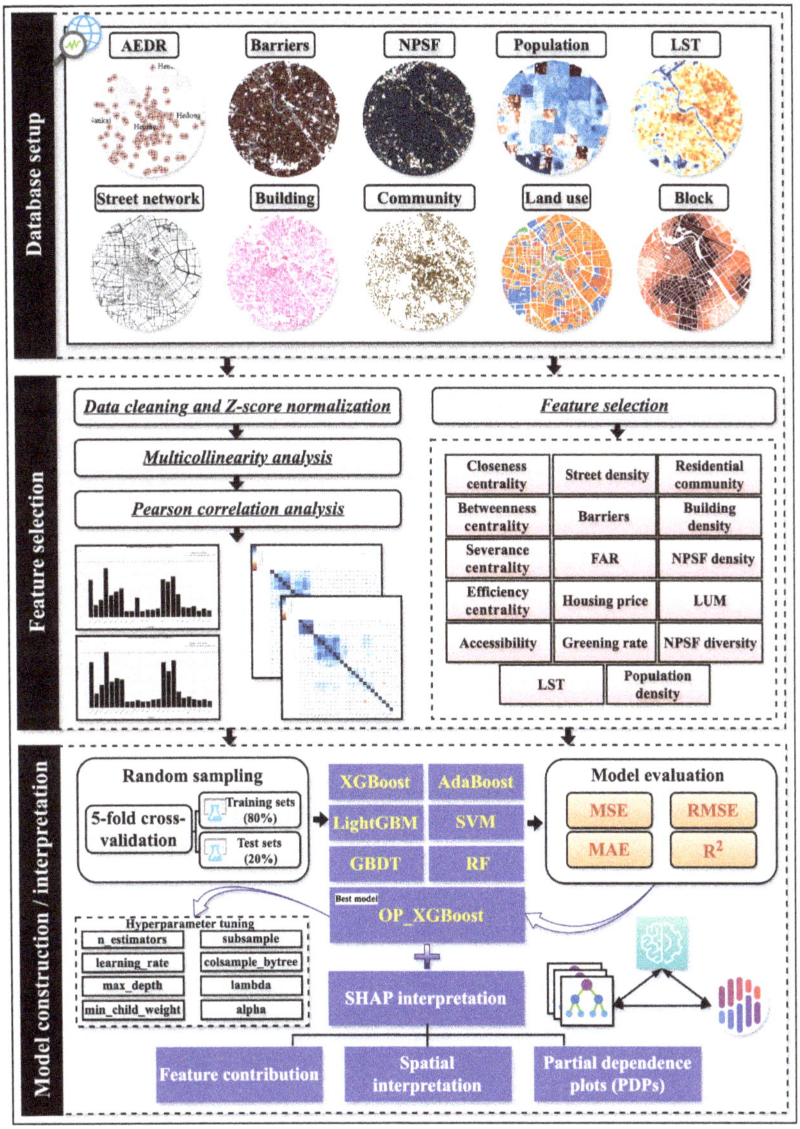

Figure 2. Framework.

2.3. Database Setup

This study utilized three multi-source datasets: AEDR, BE features, and administrative boundaries (Table 1). The first-hand AEDR data, provided by the Tianjin Red Cross Society and supplemented by the geospatial data sourced from the Tianjin EMS and RESCOND WeChat applets, underwent rigorous cleaning of duplicates, errors, and inaccuracies, resulting in 82 valid AEDRs within Tianjin Downtown, which were geocoded and saved into shapefiles. Additionally, the street network data, including crossing and river barriers, were extracted from the OpenStreetMap (OSM) and processed through topological screening: orphan streets were removed, double-line streets were converted into single-line streets, and overlaps were resolved, resulting in 20,708 valid pedestrian-accessible street segments. Furthermore, 3456 residential communities were obtained from Anjuke, China's largest real estate platform, including attributes such as geographic coordinates, community age, floor area ratio, housing price, greening rate, etc. In parallel, the land-use data were sourced from Gong et al. and classified into residential, commercial, industrial, transportation, and public management types by referring to the Essential Urban Land Use Categories in China (EULUC-China) [35] aligned with the national planning standards (Ministry of Housing and Urban-Rural Development of the People's Republic of China, 2018; the Ministry of Natural Resources of the People's Republic of China, 2021). Simultaneously, the buildings, points of interest (POIs), and signage data were crawled via the application program interface (API) provided by AutoNavi one of the largest search engine providers in China. POIs were harmonized with land-use classification to minimize discrepancies (Table A1). Moreover, the land-surface temperature (LST) data were acquired from the USGS Landsat 8 satellite with a spatial resolution of 30 m, while population data were obtained from WorldPop with a spatial resolution of 1 km. The block data were derived from Beiing City Lab (http://www.beijingcitylab.org (accessed on 1 July 2024)), and the national administrative boundaries were obtained from the Chinese Academy of Sciences' Resource and Environment Science and Data Center.

Table 1. Data sources.

Data Type	Data Source
AEDR	Tianjin Red Cross Society (accessed on April 2023), WeChat RESCOND and EMS applet (accessed on December 2023, on August 2024)
Street	https://www.openstreetmap.org
Crossing, river, signage	https://www.openstreetmap.org, https://lbs.amap.com
Community	https://tianjin.anjuke.com
Building	https://lbs.amap.com
Land use	http://www.beijingcitylab.org
NPSF	https://lbs.amap.com
LST	USGS/https://earthexplorer.usgs.gov Landsat-8/
Population	https://www.worldpop.org
Block	http://www.beijingcitylab.com DOI: 10.11982/j.supr.20190302
Administrative boundaries of Tianjin City	https://bzdt.ch.mnr.gov.cn

2.4. Variable Definitions

2.4.1. Dependent Variable: AEDR Intensity Calculation

By referring to previous studies, AEDR density was selected as the dependent variable to capture the spatial heterogeneity attributes. In our paper, Kernel density estimation (KDE) analysis was applied to reflect AEDR intensity in Tianjin Downtown, with 30 m × 30 m cell size and default bandwidth (Table 2) [36]. AEDR intensity (AEDR_D) dependent variable was calculated via KDE analysis, which can be formulated as follows (Equation (1)).

$$f(x,y) = \frac{1}{nr^2}\sum_{i=1}^{n} k\left(\frac{d_i}{r}\right) \quad (1)$$

where $f(x,y)$ is the kernel density function of point (x,y); d_i is the distance between point (x,y), and the i is the observation point; n is the number of observation points, (i.e., AEDRs) within the radius r; k is the kernel function.

Table 2. Variable definitions.

Independent Variables	Description	Scenario I		Scenario II	
		Mean	Std.	Mean	Std.
	Built environment—Comprehensive accessibility				
Closeness centrality	Mean Angular distance (MAD)	1.23	1.25	1.19	1.20
	Network quantity penalized by distance (NQPDA)	0.00	0.00	0.00	0.00
Betweenness centrality	Betweenness (BtA)	0.42	1.58	0.33	0.84
	Two phase betweenness (TPBtA)	0.02	0.01	0.02	0.01
Severance centrality	Mean Crow Flight (MCF) distance	1.44	0.81	1.41	0.71
	Diversion Ratio, Angular (DivA)	0.02	0.01	0.02	0.01
Efficiency centrality	Convex Hull Maximum Radius (HullR)	3.94	2.85	3.59	2.17
	Convex hull shape index (HullSI)	8.51	114.43	8.24	118.33
Service coverage (SC)	Gaussian 2-step Floating Catchment Area (GA2SFCA)	15.92	207.77	5.58	46.50
Street density (ST_D)	Sum street length/unit area	0.01	0.01	0.00	0.01
	Built environment—Psychological barriers				
River (RI_D)	Sum river length/unit area	0.00	0.00	2.40	0.00
Crossing (CR_D)	CR kernel density average value in the unit	5.08	6.01	5.76	6.25
Signage (SI_D)	SI kernel density average value in the unit	0.00	0.00	0.00	0.00
	Built environment—Land use				
Floor area ratio (FAR_A)	Community FAR average value in the unit	0.65	1.00	0.46	0.88
Greening rate (GR_A)	GR average value in the unit	0.08	0.12	0.06	0.11
Residential community (RC_C)	The number of RCs in the unit	0.57	1.12	0.56	1.48
Building density (BU_D)	Building kernel density average value in the unit	0.00	0.00	0.00	0.00
Density of the nearby public service facilities (NPSF_D)	NPSF kernel density average value in the unit	0.00	0.00	0.00	0.00
Shannon's evenness index (SHEI) of land use	SHEI is Shannon evenness index of land use	0.49	0.36	0.27	0.32
Shannon's diversity index (SHDI) of the nearby public service facilities (NPSFs)	SHDI is Shannon's diversity index of NPSF	0.95	0.22	0.90	0.21
	Built environment—Temperature				
Land surface temperature (LST_A)	Temperature average value in the unit	42.05	2.61	41.89	6.54
	Built environment—Demographics				
Housing price (HP_A)	Housing price average value in the unit	12,065.58	18,791.37	9140.96	17,837.80
Average population density (POP_D)	Population average value in the unit	211.41	207.06	178.33	205.25

2.4.2. Independent Variable: BE Feature Calculation

By referring to existing studies, this study delineated BE factors from five dimensions, including comprehensive accessibility, psychological barriers, land use, temperature, and demographics.

(1) Comprehensive accessibility. The comprehensive accessibility was measured by three variables, i.e., street network configuration, service coverage (SC), and street density (ST_D). Street network configuration, a critical determinant of public facility access, was analyzed via the Spatial Network Analysis (sDNA 4.1/https://sdna.cardiff.ac.uk/

sdna/ (accessed on 1 May 2024)) technique in the context of space syntax (SS) theory [37, 38]. OHCA resuscitation requires AED delivery within 3.5 min [12]. Thus, by referring to Kwon's formula MD = (f × 2) × f′/2, where f = 1.0 m/s is the maximum walking speed ("Standard for Urban Pedestrian and Bicycle Transport System Planning") and f′ = 210 s (3.5 min delivery in seconds), the angular choice and integration measures [39], which account for directional influence on route choices, were calculated within a 210 m maximum distance of a bystander. To capture the different dimensions of the street configuration, we computed four indices: closeness (Mean Angular Distance (MAD), network quantity penalized by distance (NQPDA)), betweenness (Betweenness (BtA), Two-phase Betweenness (TPBtA)), severance (Mean Crow Flight (MCF) distance, Diversion Ratio (DivA)), and efficiency (Convex Hull Maximum Radius (HullR), Convex Hull Shape Index (HullSI)) to capture the centrality rate of the street segments [40]. Furthermore, KDE analysis with 30 m × 30 m cell size and default bandwidth was applied to spatially smooth the discrete polylines [41]. SC was evaluated via the Gaussian 2-step Floating Catchment Area (GA2SFCA) method to assess AEDR supply–demand dynamics [42], a widely used approach facility accessibility analysis. Street density (ST_D), a proven EMS accessibility predictor [43], was calculated in ArcGIS through the Intersect tool and length calculation.

(2) Psychological barrier. The psychological barriers, that might delay pedestrian movement, were determined by river density (RI_D), crossing density (CR_D), and signage density (SI_D) [18,44].

(3) Land use. The dimension of land use was assessed by the average floor area ratio (FAR_A) [45], average greening rate (GR_A) [46], residential community count (RC_C), building density (BU_D) [45], nearby public service facility density (NPSF_D) [45], land-use mixture (LUM_SHEI) [47], and nearby public service facility diversity (NPSF_SHDI) [47] as land-use indicators.

(4) Temperature. Existing studies have discovered that BE factors, such as weather conditions, are significantly correlated with EMS response times [45]. The average land surface temperature (LST_A) was used to assess urban heat island effects.

(5) Demographics. Two indicators, average population (POP_A) and average housing price (HP_A), were chosen to reflect demographics and economic activity concentration [17,20].

The KDE cell size of 30 × 30 m was chosen to balance spatial resolution and computational efficiency, consistent with the resolution of ancillary datasets (e.g., LST from Landsat 8) and prior urban spatial analysis literature. All these variables are fundamental BE indicators that reflect the concentration and intensity aspect of residential and commercial endeavors. The driving factor formulas and descriptions are reflected in Table 2, Figures A1 and A2.

2.5. Prediction Model Construction and Performance Evaluation

2.5.1. Data Standardization and Multicollinearity

Ensuring the reliability of the dataset, the z-score standardization method was used, and the missing values were removed. Furthermore, the multicollinearity was assessed via the variance inflation factor (VIF), eliminating the driving factors with VIF > 10 value according to the collinearity verification requirement [48]. The calculation formula is defined as follows (Equation (2)):

$$VIF_i = \frac{1}{1 - {R_i}^2}(i = 1, 2, 3 \cdots) \tag{2}$$

where VIF_i refers to the variance inflation factor of each driving factor and ${R_i}^2$ refers to the unadjusted coefficient of determination for regressing the i th independent variable on the remaining independent variables [48]. A large VIF value indicates a highly collinear relationship to the other independent variables.

2.5.2. XGBoost and OP_XGBoost Regression Models

XGBoost, an advanced gradient boosting approach proposed by [49], employs classification and regression trees (CARTs) as the base classifier, relying on multiple interconnected decision trees, where the input of the subsequent decision tree is shaped by the prediction and training outcomes of the previous decision tree. Consequently, XGBoost has been widely used through data scientists, providing a parallel tree boosting that handles many ML challenges in a fast and accurate way. In this section, we briefly introduce its mathematics, for additional details; please see the original work on XGBoost model [49]. The XGBoost model can be formulated as follows (Equation (3)):

$$\hat{y}_i = \phi(\mathbf{x}_i) = \sum_{k=1}^{K} f_k(\mathbf{x}_i),\ f_k \in \mathcal{F} \tag{3}$$

where $\hat{y}_i$ denotes the predicted value, f_k corresponds to an independent tree structure with leaf weights, and $\mathcal{F}$ denotes to the set of all the possible CARTs. The objective function of XGBoost is the sum of the loss function and the regular term, respectively, to control the model accuracy and complexity [50]. The objective function in XGBoost can be formulated as follows (Equation (4)):

$$\mathcal{L}(\phi) = \sum_i l(\hat{y}_i, y_i) + \sum_k \Omega(f_k) \tag{4}$$

where

$$\Omega(f) = \gamma T + \frac{1}{2}\lambda \parallel w \parallel^2$$

where l is the convex loss function, which measures the difference between the prediction $\hat{y}_i$ and y_i target, and Ω denotes a term that penalizes the model complexity. T denotes the number of leaves in each tree and w denotes the weight associated with γ and λ, which indicate the regularization parameters.

In this study, XGBoost model is developed using the sklearn package for jupiter notebook (Python 3.9). To improve the superior performance of the model, we applied the Optuna (OP) hyper-parameter tuning technique combined with a 5-fold cross-validation [51] for dataset partitioning. The RMSE served as the objective function [52]. In general, the model construction process of this study primarily included four steps: dataset partitioning, model selection, model tuning for OP_XGBoost, and model evaluation. The optimal hyper-parameter values and descriptions for the training of the model are shown in Table 3.

Table 3. Hyper-parameter tunning.

Variables Parameter	Search Range	Description	Default	Optuna Best Values	
				Senario I	Senario II
n_estimators	[10–500]	The number of trees in the model.	100	428	425
learning_rate (eta)	[0.1–0.3]	The step size shrinkage used in each boosting round.	0.3	0.1	0.1
max_depth	[1–100]	The max depth of a tree or maximum number of splits in a tree.	6	78	8
min_child_weight	[0–30]	The minimum sum of instance weight needed in a child.	1	11	16

Table 3. *Cont.*

Variables Parameter	Search Range	Description	Default	Optuna Best Values	
				Senario I	Senario II
subsample	[0,1]	The random fraction of training data prior to growing trees to reduce overfitting.	1	0.9	1
colsample_bytree	[0.1–1]	The percentage of columns used for each tree construction.	1	0.1	0.7
lambda	[0,1]	L2 regularization parameter.	1	0.7	0.8
alpha	[0,1]	L1 regularization parameter.	0	0.7	0.7

Note: Objective = reg: squarederror, booster = gbtree, eval_metric = rmse.

2.5.3. Model Performance Evaluation

To evaluate the model performance, the datasets were randomly split into 80% training and 20% validating sets. Mean Square Error (MSE), Root Mean Squared Error (RMSE), Mean Absolute Error (MAE), and coefficient of determination (R^2) were considered four assessment metrics. All the models were resampled 500 times per grid/block unit, and the superior model was selected based on the highest R^2 and lowest MSE, RMSE, and MAE. The assessment metrics are defined as formula (Equation (5)):

$$\begin{aligned} MSE &= \frac{1}{N}\sum_{i=1}^{n}(y_i-\hat{y}_i)^2 \\ RMSE &= \sqrt{\frac{1}{N}\sum_{i=1}^{n}(y_i-\hat{y}_i)^2} \\ MAE &= \frac{1}{N}\sum_{i=1}^{n}|y_i-\hat{y}_i| \\ R^2 &= 1-\frac{\sum_i(y_i-\hat{y}_i)^2}{\sum_i(y_i-\overline{y})^2} \end{aligned} \tag{5}$$

2.5.4. SHAP Interpretation

To interpret the feature impact on the AEDR intensity, we applied SHAP (SHapley Additive exPlanations) and the partial dependence plots (PDPs). SHAP values quantify the feature importance by computing the weighted contribution of each variable across all possible feature combinations, comparing the model's prediction with and without the variable [53]. Mathematically, the SHAP values for a feature *i* are calculated as follows (Equation (6)) [54]:

$$SHAP_i = \sum_{S\subseteq N\setminus\{i\}} \frac{|S|!(|N|-|S|-1)!}{|N|!}\left[f_{S\cup\{i\}}\left(x_{S\cup\{i\}}\right)-f_S(x_S)\right] \tag{6}$$

where N denotes all the feature set, S denotes the feature subset, $|S|!$ denotes the factorial of the number of features contained in S, and $f_{S\cup\{i\}}$ and f_S denote the model trained with and without feature i, respectively. The positive, negative, or zero SHAP values indicate features increasing, decreasing, or not affecting the prediction, respectively. For instance, $SHAP_i > 0$ indicates a positive impact, and $SHAP_i < 0$ indicates a negative impact [53]. The larger the absolute value of Shapley, the stronger the contribution of the feature [55]. XGBoost and SHAP are often paired in machine learning because they together offer a comprehensive solution for prediction and interpretability. PDPs and locally weighted scatterplot smoothing (LOWESS) trend lines further visualized the complex nonlinear BE–AEDR relationships via local regression smoothing.

3. Results

3.1. AEDR Intensity Descriptive Statistics

The AEDR intensity at the grid and block scale in Tianjin Downtown were presented in Figure 3a,b. From the spatial distribution perspective, the results revealed a clear center-edge spatial structure, with a significantly higher intensity in the urban core than in the peripheral areas, particularly with high-intensity clusters in Heping, Nankai, and Hexi districts, and low-intensity clusters in Hongqiao, Hebei, and Hedong districts.

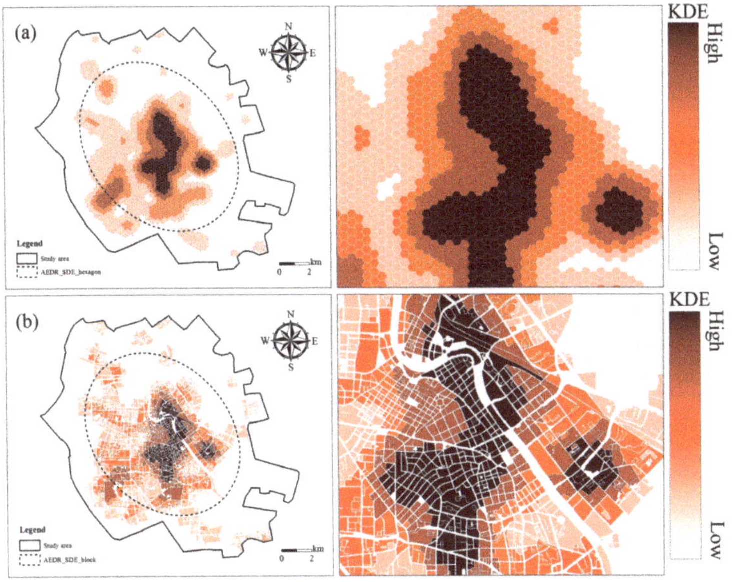

Figure 3. Intensity trend of AEDRs in Scenario I (**a**) and Scenario II (**b**).

The findings demonstrated uneven distribution of AEDRs, pinpointing the hotspot areas with high-density clusters while outlying the peripheral areas with systemic under-provision challenges.

3.2. BE Feature Screening and Correlation Analysis

The multicollinearity among 33 independent variables was assessed through VIF, excluding 10 variables with VIF > 10 values, to ensure the model's reliability. Consequently, 23 variables were retained for analysis (Figure 4a,b).

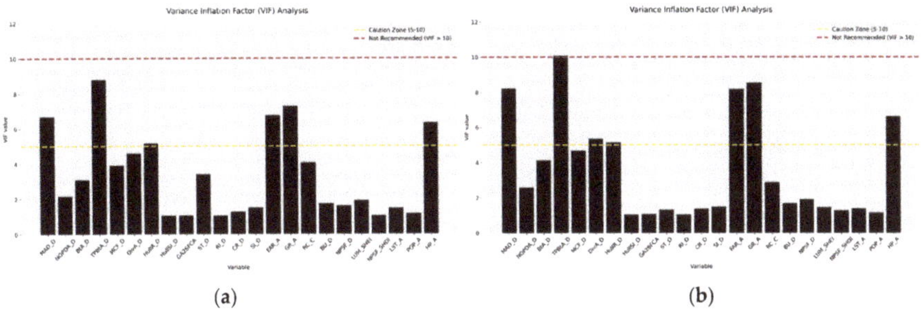

Figure 4. VIF selected features in Scenario I (**a**) and Scenario II (**b**).

Upon the Pearson correlation coefficient heatmap observation (Figure 5a,b), it is evident that there exists a significant correlation among multiple features. Strong positive correlations were observed between AEDR_D and FAR_A ($r = 0.91$ and $r = 0.92$ in SI and SII, respectively), HP_A ($r = 0.87$ and $r = 0.89$ in SI and SII, respectively), and TPBtA_D ($r = 0.85$ and $r = 0.86$ in SI and SII, respectively), suggesting AEDR concentration in high-density urban areas and transportation hubs. In contrast, several variables display notably weak correlations with AEDR_D, such as GA2SFCA ($r = -0.01$ and $r = 0.02$ in SI and SII, respectively), CR_D ($r = -0.05$ and $r = -0.06$ in SI and SII, respectively) and HullSI_D ($r = 0.00$ and $r = -0.00$ in SI and SII, respectively), reflecting potential gaps and less-served areas. Pearson correlation and VIF values of all the variables are shown in Table A2.

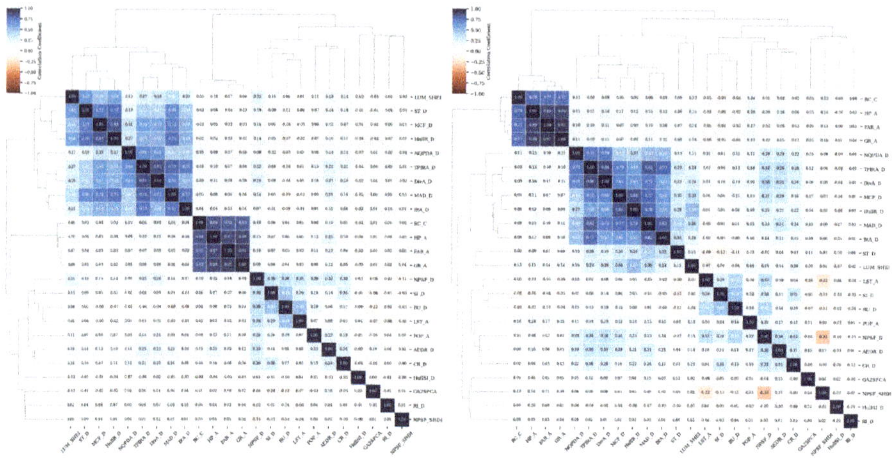

(a) (b)

Figure 5. Correlation matrix among the selected features in Scenario I (**a**) and Scenario II (**b**).

3.3. Performance Evaluation of the Prediction Models

Figure 6a,b shows the scatter plots of the models' performance predicted on the train and test sets at the grid (SI) and block scales (SII). The performance results of the 10 models (XGBoost, OP_XGBoost, LightGBM, OP_LightGBM, GBDT, OP_GBDT, AdaBoost, OP_AdaBoost, RF, OP_RF) were evaluated via MSE, RMSE, MAE, and R^2 (Tables A3 and A4).

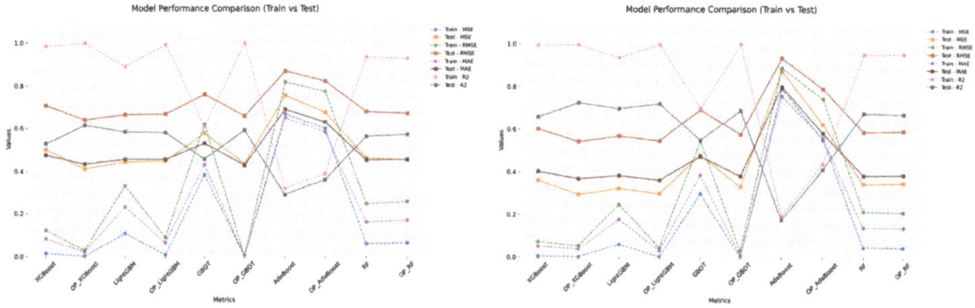

(a) (b)

Figure 6. Performance of the models in Scenario I (**a**) and Scenario II (**b**).

In SI, OP_XGBoost achieved the highest $R^2 = 0.61$ and the lowest RMSE = 0.64, while MSE = 0.41 and MAE = 0.43 outperform other models, particularly XGBoost ($R^2 = 0.53$,

RMSE = 0.71, MSE = 0.50, MAE = 0.47), LightGBM (R^2 = 0.58, RMSE = 0.67, MSE = 0.44, MAE = 0.46), OP_LightGBM (R^2 = 0.58, RMSE = 0.67, MSE = 0.45, MAE = 0.45), GBDT (R^2 = 0.46, RMSE = 0.76, MSE = 0.58, MAE = 0.53), OP_GBDT (R^2 = 0.59, RMSE = 0.66, MSE = 0.43, MAE = 0.43), AdaBoost (R^2 = 0.23, RMSE = 0.87, MSE = 0.76, MAE = 0.70), OP_AdaBoost (R^2 = 0.36, RMSE = 0.82, MSE = 0.68, MAE = 0.63), RF (R^2 = 0.56, RMSE = 0.68, MSE = 0.46, MAE = 0.45), and OP_RF (R^2 = 0.57, RMSE = 0.67, MSE = 0.45, MAE = 0.46).

In SII, the OP_XGBOOST model demonstrated even superior performance, achieving the highest R^2 = 0.72 and the lowest RMSE = 0.54, MSE = 0.30, and MAE = 0.37, which was significantly better than the XGBoost (R^2 = 0.66, RMSE = 0.60, MSE = 0.36, MAE = 0.40), LightGBM (R^2 = 0.70, RMSE = 0.57, MSE = 0.32, MAE = 0.38), OP_LightGBM (R^2 = 0.71, RMSE = 0.55, MSE = 0.30, MAE = 0.36), GBDT (R^2 = 0.55, RMSE = 0.70, MSE = 0.48, MAE = 0.47), OP_ GBDT (R^2 = 0.69, RMSE = 0.58, MSE = 0.33, MAE = 0.38), AdaBoost (R^2 = 0.18, RMSE = 0.94, MSE = 0.88, MAE = 0.80), OP_ AdaBoost (R^2 = 0.41, RMSE = 0.79, MSE = 0.63, MAE = 0.58), RF (R^2 = 0.68, RMSE = 0.59, MSE = 0.35, MAE = 0.39), and OP_ RF (R^2 = 0.67, RMSE = 0.59, MSE = 0.35, MAE = 0.39).

The notable improvements in OP_XGBoost at the block scale affirm its theoretical and practical relevance, emphasizing the adoption of OP_XGBoost at the block scale as the superior analytical approach for further spatial analysis.

3.4. Results of Modelling Interpretation

3.4.1. Feature Importance Disparities

Figures 7a–d and 8a–d showed the results of the absolute importance (AI), relative importance (RI), and rankings of independent variables in Tianjin Downtown. Feature importance (SHAP values) refers to the absolute importance (AI), inherently accounting for interactions. Both the absolute importance (AI) and relative importance (RI) were analyzed in the context of marginal and synergetic contributions. The marginal contribution denotes the isolated impact of a single feature on the model's output. The synergetic contribution denotes the hierarchical groupings of features to assess the combined impact on the model's output. The SHAP summary plot (Figures 7a and 8a) and BE-AI (Figures 7b and 8b) enabled the determination of the positive and negative contributions of feature importance. The horizontal coordinate represented the SHAP value, with the color of each sample point indicating the height of the sample value; lower sample values corresponded to higher SHAP values, indicating a negative contribution, and vice versa for positive contributions.

In terms of the marginal contribution (Figures 7c and 8c), the BE-RI displayed a continuously varying contribution trend across the two units. The top 10 variables in SI included GA2SFCA, NPSF_D, POP_A, HP_A, CR_D, TPBtA_D, NQPDA_D, SI_D, BU_D, and MAD_D, whereas other variables were negatively correlated, with AEDR intensity demonstrating lower RI effects. Consequently, the top 10 variables in SI included NPSF_D, NPSF_SHDI, GA2SFCA, CR_D, NQPDA_D, MCF_D, POP_A, TPBtA_D, MAD_D, and SI_D. The RI of the GA2SFCA showed a continuously decreasing contribution rate of 13.2% and 9.7% in the SI and SII, respectively, appearing to hold predictive importance, and ranking first in the grid model and third in the block model. Conversely, NPSF_D demonstrated a progressive increase in importance, ranking second in the grid model and first in the block model, as well as showing a continuously increasing contribution rate of 10.5% and 14.8% in the SI and SII, respectively.

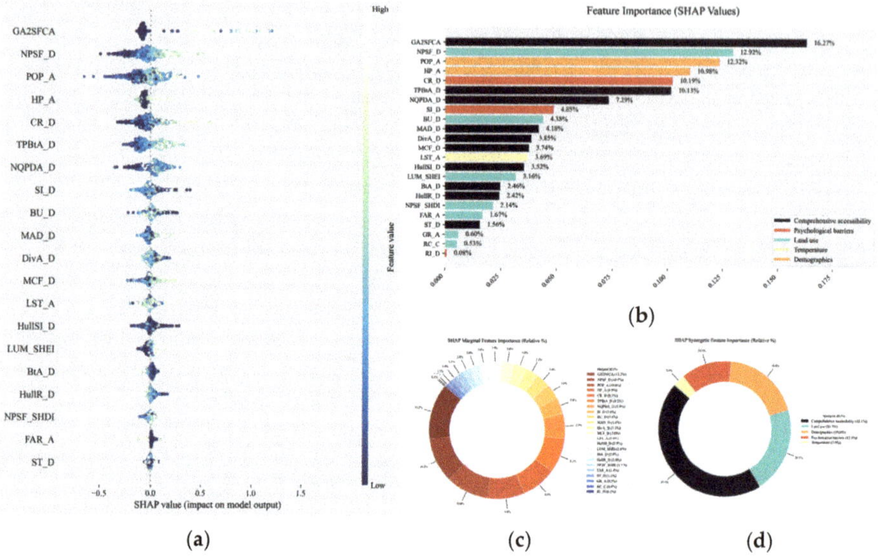

Figure 7. SHAP mean values (**a**), AI (**b**), marginal RI (**c**) and synergetic RI (**d**) in Scenario I.

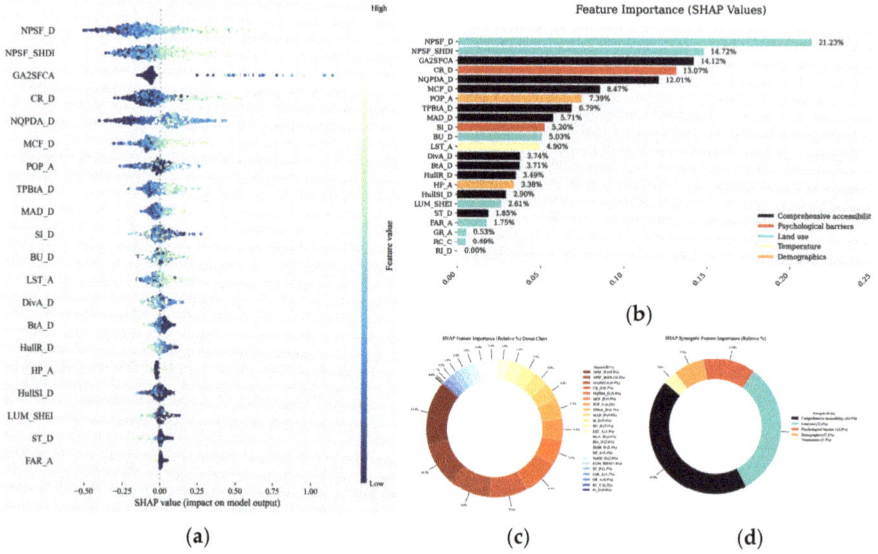

Figure 8. SHAP mean values (**a**), AI (**b**), marginal RI (**c**) and synergetic RI (**d**) in Scenario II.

In terms of the synergistic contribution (Figures 7d and 8d), the BE-RI displayed a relatively congruent contribution with a slight difference. The synergistic contribution rate of the comprehensive accessibility indicators stood at 45.1% and 43.9% in the SI and SII models, respectively. In contrast, the land-use indicators showed a higher contribution, standing at 20.7% and 32.4% in the SI and SII models, respectively, whereas the demographic indicators, with 19.0% and 7.5% in the SI and SII, showed adaptivity lower contributions. Additionally, the psychological barrier indicators demonstrated 12.3% and 12.8% and the land surface temperature indicators 3% and 3.4% in the SI and SII models, respectively. The findings revealed that comprehensive accessibility and land use play a significant role, ranking first and second in both SI and SII, underscoring the significance of the top BE features in influencing AEDR.

The findings provide two insights. First, BE features are overlooked in AEDR-related studies. In contrast, the impact of a single BE feature on AEDR varies, with some features demonstrating significant influence, while others show negative influence, highlighting the heterogeneous nature of the BE-AEDR nexus. Second, the results suggest that the influence of the BE is highly interactive with proximity to the AEDR, with the maximum influence exerted within bock pattern, which not only underscores the reason for the superior model performance but also advocates for urban designers and planners to prioritize this block pattern to maximize the effectiveness of BE-related interventions. Our findings affirm the multi-scale nature of urban environments, where certain features dominate at finer resolutions while others emerge at broader scales. This underscores the need to consider multiple spatial units to capture the full spectrum of the BE-AEDR nexus, ensuring a more robust and comprehensive urban health infrastructure planning.

3.4.2. Spatial Contribution of Independent Variables

The study calculated and analyzed the average SHAP values for each grid cell and block in Tianjin Downtown. Figures 9 and 10 illustrate the spatial distribution of SHAP values for the primary nine key BE features, highlighting the nuances of spatial patterns and reflecting spatial heterogeneity and spatial consistency trends, ultimately enhancing the underserved peripheral zones.

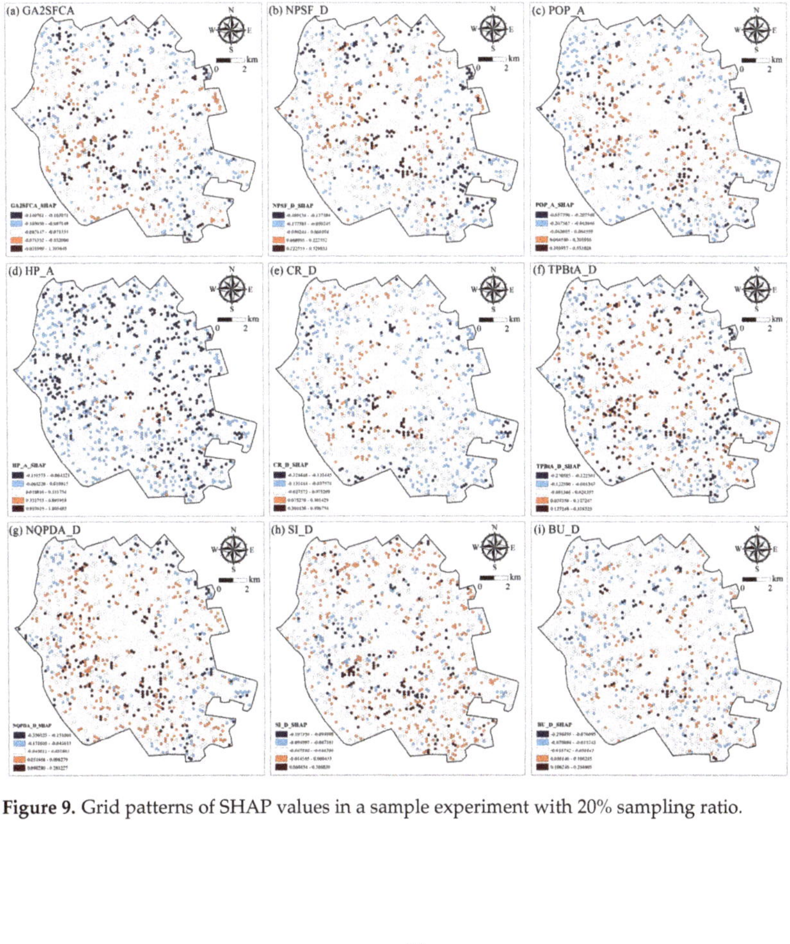

Figure 9. Grid patterns of SHAP values in a sample experiment with 20% sampling ratio.

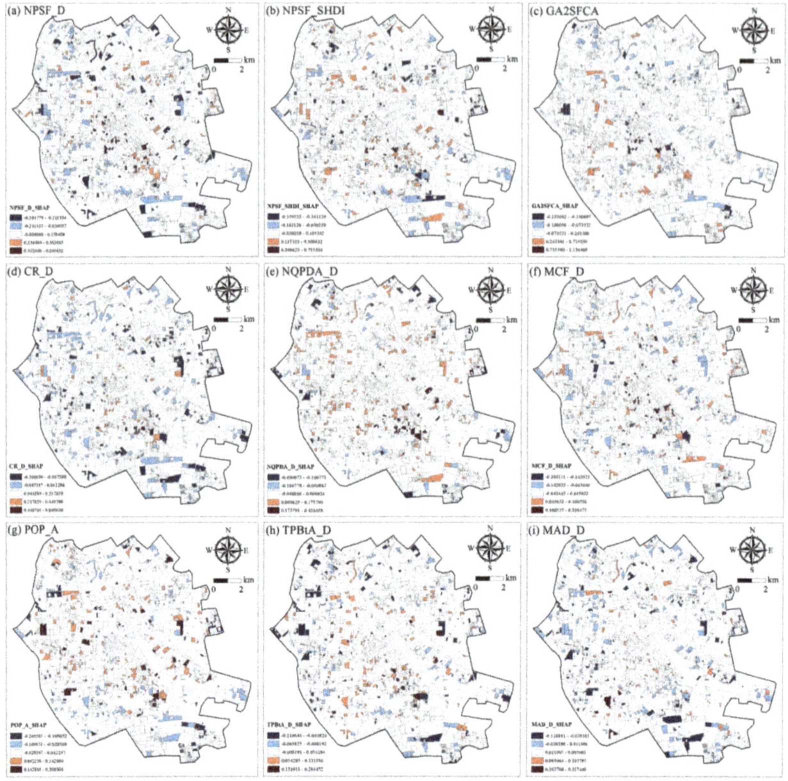

Figure 10. Block patterns of SHAP values in a sample experiment with a 20% sampling ratio.

The spatial performance of key variables revealed spatial heterogeneity and spatial consistency trends. This phenomenon highlighted the influence of spatial resolution on the interpretation of SHAP values.

At the grid scale, GA2SFCA showed strong positive contributions in the southern and eastern areas, reflecting high AED accessibility in these regions. Northern grids exhibited predominantly negative SHAP values, indicating significant gaps in AED accessibility. At the block scale, positive contributions were observed in eastern areas, suggesting finer localized accessibility. However, northern and western blocks showed more fragmented negative values. While both scales identified northern areas with limited accessibility, the block scale reveals finer spatial heterogeneity, uncovering intra-grid disparities. NPSF_D and NPSF_SHDI displayed a mixed pattern, with negative SHAP values concentrated in the urban core and western patterns, suggesting facility saturation, and positive contributions were dispersed across central, northern, and eastern patterns. Positive SHAP values emerged in southern blocks, while negative values clustered in the central areas, reinforcing the grid-level findings but with more pronounced variations across adjacent blocks. POP_A showed contrasting patterns, with positive contributions in southern and eastern grids and negative values in the north. Population influence was more spatially fragmented at the block scale, with positive values in eastern areas, while the grid scale revealed broader population trends. This phenomenon suggests that population impact on AEDR might operate at varying spatial resolutions. HP_A demonstrated a minor positive contribution across the southwest grids. The peripheral grids reflected localized negative SHAP values. The grid scale captured macro-level trends in housing price influence and smoothed the local discrepancies, reinforcing the pervasive impact of socio-economic conditions on AEDR. CR_D predominantly displayed negative contributions across the southwestern grids, implying that high crossing density hinders AED accessibility. The block scale revealed smaller patches of positive contributions in eastern and southern areas, with negative values concentrated in the north. High positive contributions of TPBtA_Ds appeared in central grids, suggesting that network connectivity enhances AED accessibility. Block scale analysis reflected similar trends, with certain blocks showing negative contributions. TPBtA_D's positive influence was consistent across both scales, highlighting network connectivity benefits. NQPDA_D showed positive SHAP values clustered in eastern, southern, and western grids, reflecting highly efficient road networks. Fragmented grids in the peripheral areas exhibited negative contributions. Similar patterns emerged at the block scale, while MAD_D and MCF_D showed fragmented contributions with emphasized micro-level accessibility challenges. SI_D demonstrated positive contributions dominating outer grids, while negative values were concentrated in the eastern areas. BU_D exhibited mixed contributions across central grids, with scattered positive values most in eastern and southern grids, highlighting potential redevelopment opportunities.

In conclusion, spatial SHAP uncovered pattern dependency, emphasizing the spatial heterogeneity and spatial consistency trends, showing how the variable contributions vary across space, while others exhibit stability. SHAP spatial maps identified underserved grids and blocks, informing targeted interventions to address AEDR development challenges.

3.4.3. Non-Linear Impact of BE Features on AEDR Intensity

To capture the inherent complexities of the feature dependence and non-linear effects of the primary nine BE features, the SHAP scatter plot and PDPs were utilized. The scatter plots indicated the degree of positive/negative features' influence on the AEDR intensity, while the fitted LOWESS curve revealed the threshold effects across grid and block patterns, as shown in Figures 11 and 12.

For comprehensive accessibility, the GA2SFCA plots showed positive effects beyond the feature values of $x \approx -0.14$ (SI) and -0.15 (SII). Further, the values plateau, indicating a relatively balanced effect on AEDR intensity. The TPBtA_D exhibited a critical threshold effect at $x \approx -0.14$ (SI) and $x \approx -0.19$ (SII), shifting from negative to positive, suggesting prioritized AEDR placement in well-connected and accessible areas. The NQPDA_D displayed an inverse U-shaped correlation with AEDR, indicating a negative–positive–negative pattern peaking around from $x \approx -0.61$ to $x \approx 2.13$ (SI), contributing negatively at both ends. While SII showed a negative–positive effect with intersection $x \approx -0.56$, characterized by stabilization thereafter. The MAD_D and MCF_D demonstrated positive impact at the threshold $x \approx 0.02$ (SII) and $x \approx 0.22$ (SII), respectively. The positive values indicated well-connected and accessible areas, while negative values indicated lower accessibility, emphasizing the significance of enhancing AEDR accessibility in underserved areas. Physiological barrier analysis revealed the CR_D's slight positive contribution, becoming more pronounced beyond $x \approx 0.25$ (SI) and $x \approx 0.19$ (SII), while SI_D exhibited a U-shaped effect, shifting from negative to positive, with the lowest threshold effect beyond $x \approx -0.85$ (SI) and the highest threshold around $x \approx 0.81$ (SI). This reflected the complex navigation dynamics, where sparsely distributed crossings and signages act as barriers, while well-planned and clustered signages improve AED response. Land-use dynamics showed the NPSF_D shifting from negative to a positive effect, with a critical threshold effect beyond $x \approx -0.08$ (SI) and $x \approx 0.01$ (SII), indicating sensitivity to NPSF density. The BU_D showed moderate positive trends below $x \approx 0.39$ (SI) then decreased gradually, indicating negative impact, possibly due to sparse building distribution, while NPSF_SHDI shifted from neutral to positive nonlinear contribution as feature values increased. Initially, the effect became evident at the x ≈ 0.09 (SII) threshold, suggesting areas with lower diversity exhibit no impact, while higher diversity exhibits positive impact, affirming the contributions of the mixed-use areas to pre-EMS service coverage. Demographic factors demonstrated HP_A's strong non-linear correlation as the housing price increased, with the threshold beyond x ≈ 1.17 (SI), characterized by better infrastructure resources. In the areas with lower housing prices, the effect was balanced and not significant, reflecting that less developed areas were underserved. POP_A showed slightly distinct trends: a negative–positive shift at x ≈ −0.12 (SI) and a V-shaped positive–negative–positive shift at x ≈ 0.18 (SII).

In general, PDPs with the threshold effect were excellent in detecting the overall non-linear BE–AEDR nexus dynamics, enhancing the model accuracy and interpretability.

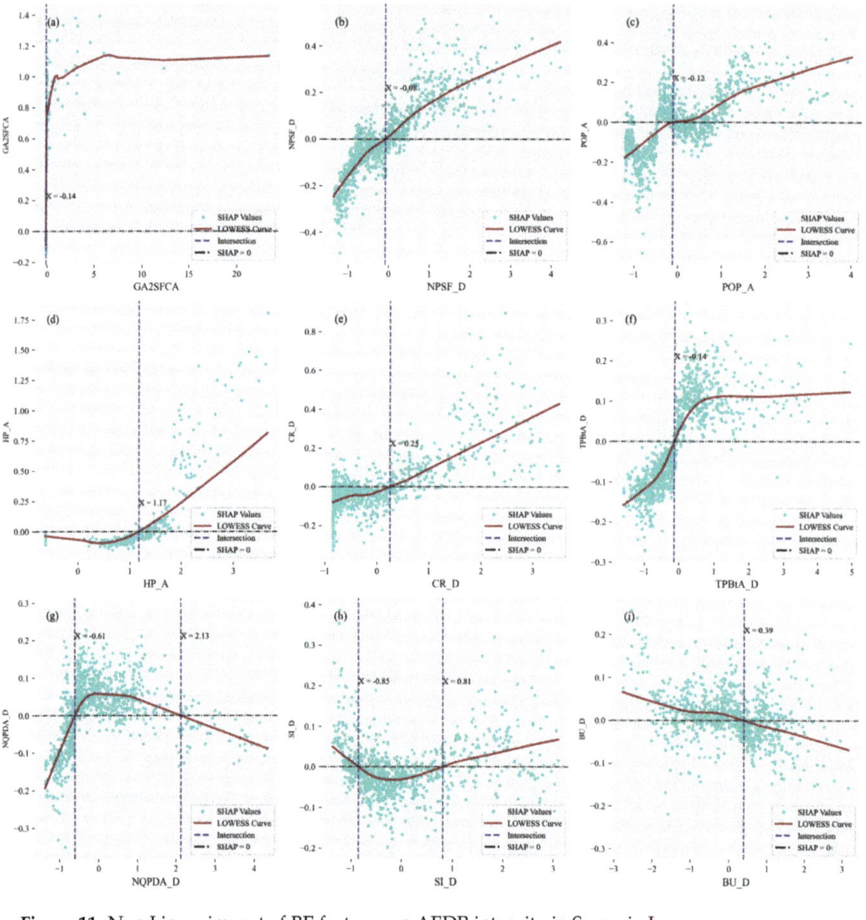

Figure 11. Non-Linear impact of BE features on AEDR intensity in Scenario I.

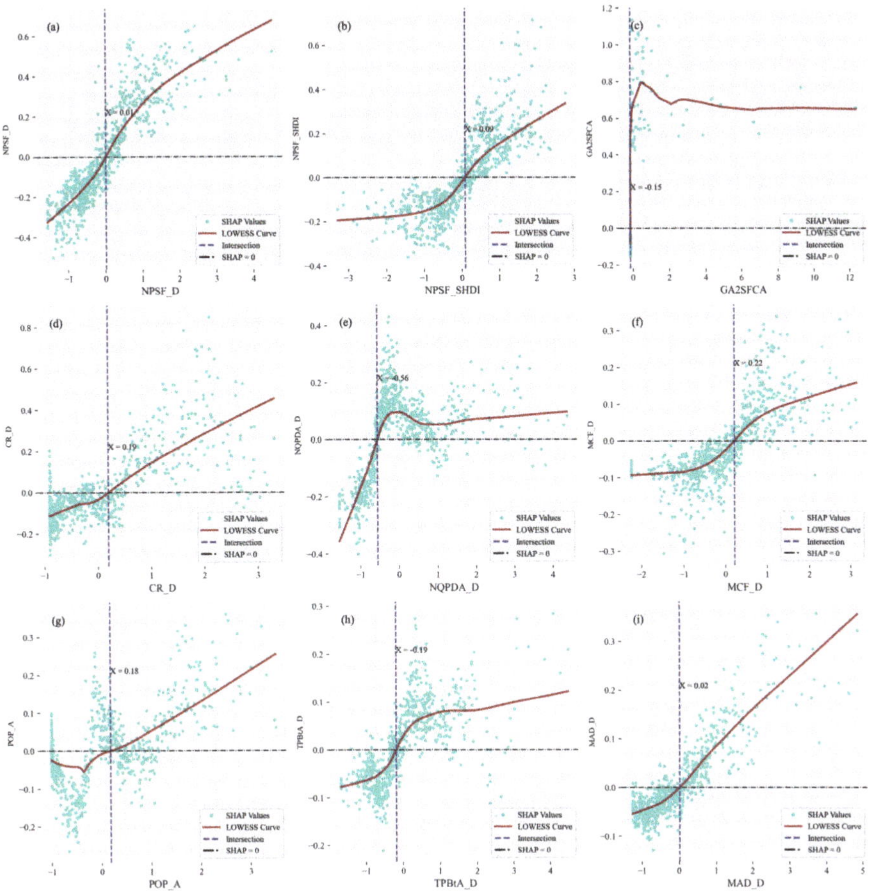

Figure 12. Non-Linear impact of BE features on AEDR intensity in Scenario II.

4. Discussion

The integration of BE considerations into AEDR planning is pivotal for enhancing pre-EMS accessibility in urban settings. This study bridges methodological and theoretical gaps by employing explainable ML models to unravel the BE–AEDR nexus, offering actionable insights for sustainable urban health planning. AEDRs have relatively dispersed geographical locations in Tianjin because they have usually been rigorously screened and jointly determined by investors, governors, and experts. Traditional AED planning studies have largely relied on linear regression or heuristic approaches, which oversimplify the intricate interactions between urban features and AEDR. This study advances the field by integrating explainable ML algorithms, notably the OP_XGBoost model optimized with SHAP. The OP_XGBoost outperformed benchmark models (e.g., XGBoost, RF, etc.) across both grid ($R^2 = 0.61$) and block ($R^2 = 0.72$) scales, demonstrating superior predictive accuracy and robustness. Unlike "black-box" models, the SHAP framework provided granular interpretability, revealing how BE features influence AEDR intensity. This methodological shift underscores the value of ML in capturing urban complexity while maintaining transparency, a critical requirement for policymakers prioritizing evidence-based decisions. Future studies could extend this approach to other cities, validating its generalizability across diverse urban morphologies. Below, we contextualize the key findings, emphasizing their academic significance and practical implications.

4.1. Bridging Accessibility and Land-Use Efficiency

The SHAP analysis highlighted pronounced disparities in feature importance across spatial resolutions. At the grid scale, comprehensive accessibility metrics like GA2SFCA dominated, contributing 13.2% to AEDR intensity, while at the block scale, nearby public service facility density (NPSF_D, 14.8%) emerged as the most influential. This divergence underscores the multi-scale nature of BE impacts: macro-scale accessibility governs broad AED placement, whereas micro-scale land-use efficiency (e.g., clustered services) becomes critical at finer resolutions. Synergistically, comprehensive accessibility and land-use indicators collectively contributed 45.1% and 43.9% to model predictions, emphasizing their centrality in AEDR planning. Eastern and southern zones exhibited strong positive contributions at the grid scale, reflecting robust AED coverage, whereas northern and western areas showed fragmented accessibility gaps, particularly at the block scale. Notably, the urban core and western zones displayed facility saturation and demonstrated unmet demand. Such insights necessitate tailored interventions, such as boosting AED deployment while targeting micro-level inefficiencies in underserved zones, like northern and western zones, to dramatically improve OHCA outcomes.

4.2. Spatial Resolution and Pattern Dependency as Game-Changers: Block-Level Granularity Redefines Urban AED Planning

The study's most striking revelation was the superior predictive performance of block-level models over grid-based ones. This aligns with urban design principles, where blocks, as functional units of pedestrian movement, better encapsulate localized BE interactions. The revealed spatial heterogeneity and consistency gaps by SHAP spatial maps advocate for multi-scale planning frameworks, where block-level granularity complements city-wide grids to address micro-level disparities.

4.3. Nonlinear Dynamics: Threshold Effects and Policy Levers

The non-linear association between the BE and AEDR could provide input for creating bystander-friendly AEDRs in high-density cities. The relationships between the built environment attributes and AEDR intensity exhibit non-linearity. The non-linear patterns offer valuable geographical insights that facilitate a deeper understanding of AEDRs within varying environmental contexts. These patterns help to clarify how different environmental factors foster specific infrastructure development in non-linear ways, ensuring resources align with the dynamic urban rhythms.

Our findings provided valuable policy implications for urban planners and policy-makers to improve future AED deployment. (1) First, since AEDR intensity was influenced by various factors, the contribution analysis prioritized the importance of the comprehensive accessibility feature for future AED placement. We note that the city center does not provide a suitable walking environment. Targeting areas with low AED accessibility, accounting for groupings of the features, can help urban planners to draw more comprehensive policies, providing diverse short-distance travel and ensuring a smooth travel system for residents' emergency requirements. (2) Second, geospatial analyses at the block scale could be beneficial for stakeholders to locate AEDs in underserved areas, reducing spatial mismatches between supply and demand. (3) Third, BE features exhibit non-linear associations with AEDR intensity, with variable-specific positive and negative thresholds. Failure to account for non-linearity may lead to underestimation of the impacts of certain variables. It is recommended that urban planners identify critical BE features to enhance AEDR usage effectively. In summary, decision-makers should consider the BE non-linear effects when formulating urban planning strategies. Understanding these effects empowers urban planners and policymakers to make more informed decisions regarding city design and planning.

5. Conclusions

AEDs are critical interventions in cardiac arrest treatment, improving OHCA survival outcomes by up to 70%. Therefore, this study established an interpretable ML-based framework and used novel datasets to uncover the complex interplay of the BE-AEDR in Tianjin Downtown.

The principal conclusions are as follows: (1) Marginally, the AEDR intensity was greatly influenced by the GA2SFCA at grid scale and NPSF_D at block scale, as well as synergistically by the comprehensive accessibility at both scales. Furthermore, the block pattern demonstrated superior performance in testing model; (2) Pattern-dependent effects existed between BE–AEDR factors, while SHAP values vary across specific patterns, emphasizing localized spatial heterogeneity and spatial consistency trends; (3) The BE-AEDR non-linear relationships were uncovered, demonstrating distinct positive and negative correlations with the threshold effects. Overall, the interpretable ML-based approach in this study demonstrated excellent predictive outcomes by setting health at the heart of the urban development approach.

Despite the robust analytical framework, this study has several limitations. First, the unavailability of OHCA incident data, as the incident spatiotemporal variations may skew AED demand predictions. Second, the analysis prioritizes pedestrian street networks, neglecting the spatiotemporal dynamics of drivers and cyclists, whose behavioral movement fluctuates, such as route preferences and speed variations. Third, the focus on the grid and block spatial units fails to address urban–rural heterogeneities in the BE–AEDR context, which could introduce variability not captured in the current model. Addressing these gaps requires multi-modal mobility data and optimized ML models, offering a more comprehensive view of urban planning and emergency preparedness, ensuring alignment with real-world needs.

Overall, this study provided scientific support for policymakers and urban planners to prioritize life-saving resource development via capturing the BE–AEDR nexus. The framework is generalizable and can be applied to settings with the same geographical features, ensuring both methodological rigor and practical applicability.

Author Contributions: Conceptualization, Sara Grigoryan; methodology, Sara Grigoryan; software, Sara Grigoryan; validation, Sara Grigoryan; formal analysis Sara Grigoryan; data curation, Sara Grigoryan; writing—original draft preparation, Sara Grigoryan; writing—review and editing, Sara Grigoryan and Nadeem Ullah; visualization, Sara Grigoryan; supervision, Yike Hu. All authors have read and agreed to the published version of the manuscript.

Funding: This research received no external funding.

Data Availability Statement: Data will be made available on request.

Conflicts of Interest: The authors declare no conflicts of interest.

Appendix A

Appendix A.1

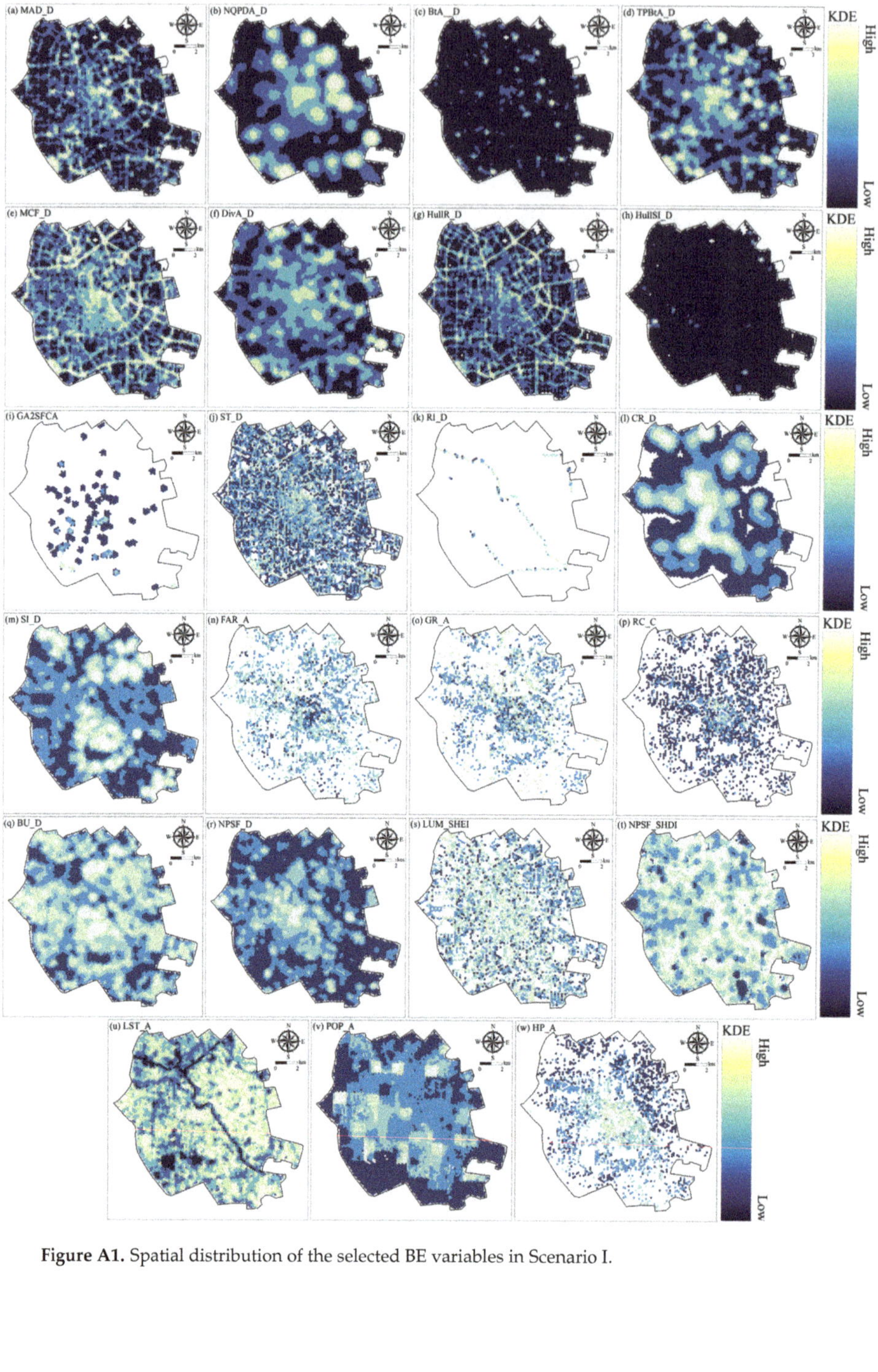

Figure A1. Spatial distribution of the selected BE variables in Scenario I.

Appendix A.2

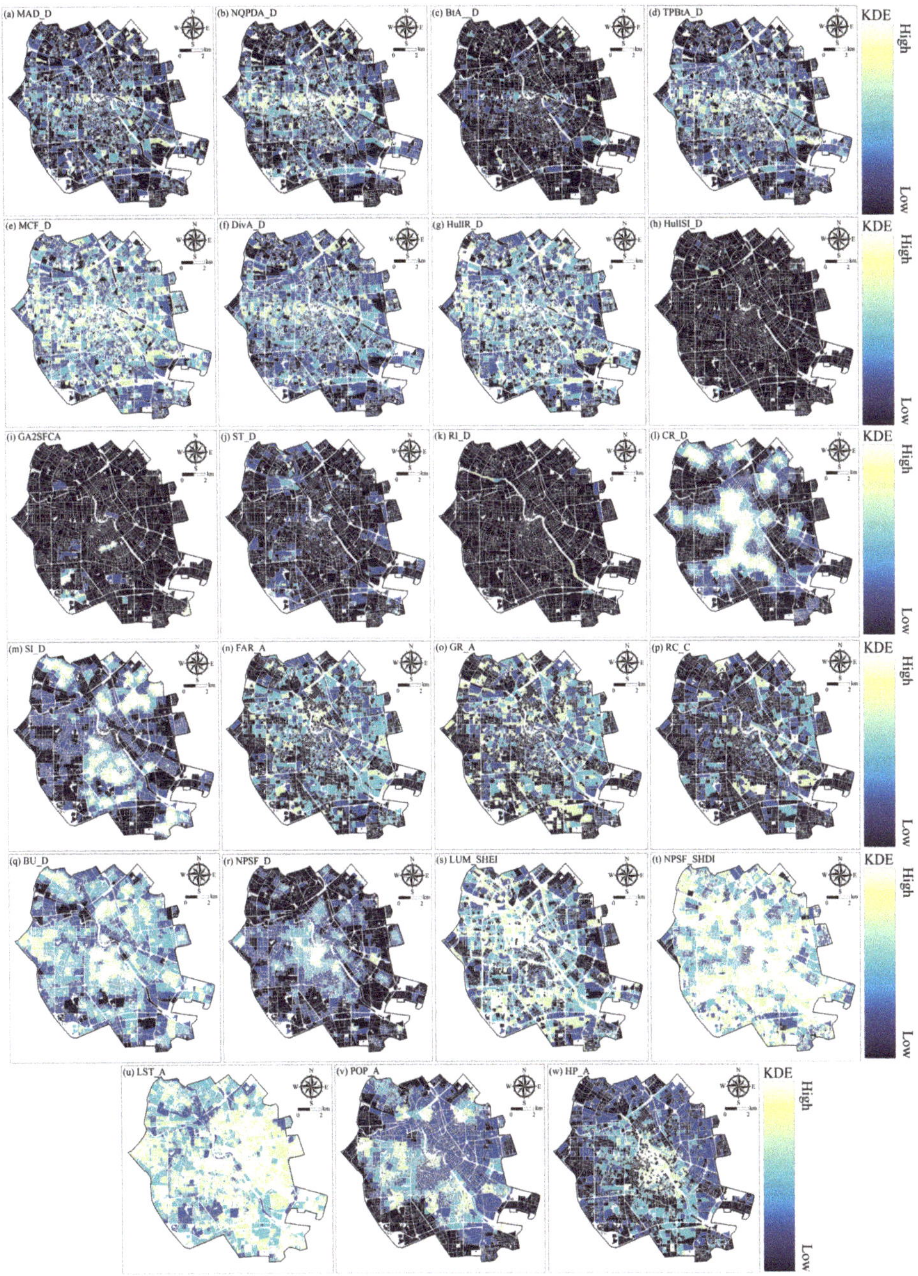

Figure A2. Spatial distribution of the selected BE variables in Scenario II.

Appendix B

Appendix B.1

Table A1. POI classification.

Level I	Level II	Number	Percentage (%)
Residential	Residences (community)	3456	3.02%
Commercial	Business and finance (company, bank, ATM, security office, etc.), commerce (convenience store, supermarket, shopping mall, store, shopping-related place, etc.), and catering (catering venue, restaurant, fast food venue, tea-coffee house, etc.)	76,551	66.81%
Industrial	Industry (factory)	142	0.12%
Transportation	Transportation facilities (railway station, subway station, bus station, taxi station, port, parking lot, etc.)	9500	8.29%
Public management and service	Administration (government institution, social organization, foreign institution, and public security), healthcare (hospital, clinic, medical service (pharmacy), EMS center, disease prevention institution), education and culture (university, college, institution, school, research institution and cultural venue, museum, exhibition hall, art gallery, library, planetarium, etc.), sport and leisure (sport stadium, golf related, recreation venue, holiday and nursing resort, cinema, park and square, tourist attraction, etc.)	24,932	21.76%

Appendix B.2

Table A2. Pearson coefficient correlation and VIF test values.

Variables	Scenario I				Scenario II			
	Pearson Coef.	*p* Value	VIF (Pre-Z-Score)	VIF (Post-Z-Score)	Pearson Coef.	*p* Value	VIF (Pre-Z-Score)	VIF (Post-Z-Score)
Lconn_D	0.31	2.20	20.74	--	0.19	1.09	1.12	--
Jnc_D	0.06	1.08	17.80	--	0.21	4.13	22.32	--
TPD_D	0.34	7.35	24.08	--	0.46	4.73	19.71	--
Ang_D	0.12	4.20	4.88	--	0.12	2.91	4.80	--
MAD_D	0.21	1.36	15.25	6.70	0.28	1.59	17.20	8.21
NQPDA_D	0.14	6.19	3.79	2.15	0.30	2.62	4.49	2.57
BtA_D	0.01	0.43	8.05	3.11	0.12	1.19	10.37	4.10
TPBtA_D	0.23	6.51	41.98	8.79	0.36	1.53	45.95	10.06
MCF_D	0.16	1.21	56.46	3.91	0.31	3.39	58.05	4.66
DivA_D	0.17	8.71	8.04	4.57	0.33	3.61	8.85	5.33
MGLA_D	0.17	1.02	70.67	--	0.32	2.88	78.26	--
HullA_D	0.10	1.98	7.46	--	0.25	2.84	5.27	--
HullP_D	0.11	1.25	70.28	--	0.27	9.81	28.83	--
HullR_D	0.06	6.91	29.06	5.16	0.21	3.34	16.61	5.12
HullB_D	0.15	8.50	4.09	--	0.27	2.42	3.77	--
HullSI_D	−0.04	0.01	1.02	1.02	−0.04	0.01	1.02	1.02
GA2SFCA	0.09	2.74	1.05	1.04	0.20	2.72	1.08	1.06

Table A2. *Cont.*

Variables	Scenario I				Scenario II			
	Pearson Coef.	p Value	VIF (Pre-Z-Score)	VIF (Post-Z-Score)	Pearson Coef.	p Value	VIF (Pre-Z-Score)	VIF (Post-Z-Score)
ST_D	0.13	1.00	6.37	3.48	0.02	0.27	1.43	1.31
RI_D	0.04	0.00	1.04	1.03	0.02	0.26	1.02	1.02
BR_D	−0.02	0.06	1.31	--	0.02	0.15	1.07	--
CR_D	0.29	1.07	1.30	1.25	0.35	1.29	1.43	1.36
SI_D	0.12	4.95	1.51	1.48	0.07	5.40	1.54	1.48
FAR_A	0.17	1.32	6.73	6.72	0.12	6.75	8.20	8.16
HP_A	0.43	1.78	6.35	6.29	0.35	8.74	6.64	6.58
GR_A	0.18	1.11	7.30	7.27	0.13	6.16	8.55	8.53
RC_C	0.39	1.45	4.06	4.04	0.18	1.70	2.88	2.87
BU_D	0.13	3.18	1.77	1.72	0.19	1.73	1.89	1.66
NPSF_D	0.33	4.31	1.73	1.59	0.36	1.94	2.09	1.90
LUM_SHEI	0.18	1.95	1.10	1.90	0.14	1.61	1.57	1.44
NPSF_SHDI	0.02	0.16	1.03	1.03	0.19	9.53	1.30	1.26
SID	0.28	1.75	25.44	--	0.40	2.29	22.26	--
LST_A	0.05	5.39	1.50	1.45	0.08	2.96	1.44	1.38
POP_A	0.13	2.25	1.18	1.15	0.10	1.34	1.15	1.14

Appendix B.3

Table A3. AEDR prediction results of each model.

Model	Scenario I							
	Training				Testing			
	MSE	RMSE	MAE	R^2	MSE	RMSE	MAE	R^2
XGBoost	0.02	0.12	0.08	0.99	0.50	0.71	0.47	0.53
OP_XGBoost	0.00	0.03	0.02	1	0.41	0.64	0.43	0.61
LightGBM	0.11	0.33	0.23	0.89	0.44	0.67	0.46	0.58
OP_LightGBM	0.01	0.09	0.07	1	0.45	0.67	0.45	0.58
GBDT	0.39	0.62	0.43	0.61	0.58	0.76	0.53	0.46
OP_GBDT	3.25	0.00	0.00	1	0.43	0.66	0.43	0.59
AdaBoost	0.67	0.82	0.65	0.32	0.76	0.87	0.70	0.23
OP_AdaBoost	0.60	0.78	0.58	0.39	0.68	0.82	0.63	0.36
RF	0.06	0.25	0.16	0.94	0.46	0.68	0.45	0.56
OP_RF	0.07	0.26	0.17	0.93	0.45	0.67	0.46	0.57

Appendix B.4

Table A4. AEDR prediction results of each model.

Model	Scenario II							
	Training				Testing			
	MSE	RMSE	MAE	R^2	MSE	RMSE	MAE	R^2
XGBoost	0.01	0.07	0.05	0.99	0.36	0.60	0.40	0.66
OP_XGBoost	0.00	0.06	0.04	1	0.30	0.54	0.37	0.72
LightGBM	0.06	0.25	0.18	0.94	0.32	0.57	0.38	0.70
OP_LightGBM	0.00	0.05	0.03	1	0.30	0.55	0.36	0.71

Table A4. *Cont.*

Model	Scenario II							
	Training				Testing			
	MSE	RMSE	MAE	R^2	MSE	RMSE	MAE	R^2
GBDT	0.30	0.55	0.39	0.70	0.48	0.70	0.47	0.55
OP_GBDT	0.00	0.03	0.01	1	0.33	0.58	0.38	0.69
AdaBoost	0.80	0.89	0.76	0.20	0.88	0.94	0.80	0.18
OP_AdaBoost	0.55	0.74	0.56	0.44	0.63	0.79	0.58	0.41
RF	0.05	0.22	0.14	0.95	0.35	0.59	0.39	0.68
OP_RF	0.05	0.21	0.14	0.95	0.35	0.59	0.39	0.67

References

1. Nichol, G.; Sayre, M.R.; Guerra, F.; Poole, J. Defibrillation for Ventricular Fibrillation: A Shocking Update. *J. Am. Coll. Cardiol.* **2017**, *70*, 1496–1509. [CrossRef] [PubMed]
2. Wong, P.P.; Low, C.T.; Cai, W.; Leung, K.T.; Lai, P.C. A Spatiotemporal Data Mining Study to Identify High-Risk Neighborhoods for Out-Of-Hospital Cardiac Arrest (OHCA) Incidents. *Sci. Rep.* **2022**, *12*, 3509. [CrossRef] [PubMed]
3. Ringh, M.; Hollenberg, J.; Palsgaard-Moeller, T.; Svensson, L.; Rosenqvist, M.; Lippert, F.K.; Wissenberg, M.; Malta Hansen, C.; Claesson, A.; Viereck, S.; et al. The Challenges and Possibilities of Public Access Defibrillation. *J. Intern. Med.* **2018**, *283*, 238–256. [CrossRef] [PubMed]
4. United Nations. *Transforming Our World: The 2030 Agenda for Sustainable Development*; United Nations: New York, NY, USA, 2015.
5. Zoghbi, W.A.; Duncan, T.; Antman, E.; Barbosa, M.; Champagne, B.; Chen, D.; Gamra, H.; Harold, J.G.; Josephson, S.; Komajda, M.; et al. Sustainable Development Goals and the Future of Cardiovascular Health: A Statement from the Global Cardiovascular Disease Taskforce. *J. Am. Heart Assoc.* **2014**, *3*, e000504. [CrossRef]
6. Fredman, D.; Haas, J.; Ban, Y.F.; Jonsson, M.; Svensson, L.; Djarv, T.; Hollenberg, J.; Nordberg, P.; Ringh, M.; Claesson, A. Use of a Geographic Information System to Identify Differences in Automated External Defibrillator Installation in Urban Areas with Similar Incidence of Public Out-Of-Hospital Cardiac Arrest: A Retrospective Registry-Based Study. *BMJ Open* **2017**, *7*, e014801. [CrossRef]
7. Brooks, S.C.; Clegg, G.R.; Bray, J.; Deakin, C.D.; Perkins, G.D.; Ringh, M.; Smith, C.M.; Link, M.S.; Merchant, R.M.; Pezo-Morales, J.; et al. Optimizing Outcomes after Out-of-Hospital Cardiac Arrest with Innovative Approaches to Public-Access Defibrillation: A Scientific Statement from the International Liaison Committee on Resuscitation. *Circulation* **2022**, *145*, e776–e801. [CrossRef]
8. Wang, Z.; Ma, L.; Liu, M.; Fan, J.; Hu, S. Summary of the 2022 Report on Cardiovascular Health and Diseases in China. *Chin. Med. J.* **2023**, *136*, 2899–2908. [CrossRef]
9. Zhang, L.; Li, B.; Zhao, X.; Zhang, Y.; Deng, Y.; Zhao, A.; Li, W.; Dong, X.; Zheng, Z.J. Public Access of Automated External Defibrillators in a Metropolitan City of China. *Resuscitation* **2019**, *140*, 120–126. [CrossRef]
10. Zhang, W.; Zhang, X.; Wu, G. The Network Governance of Urban Renewal: A Comparative Analysis of Two Cities in China. *Land Use Policy* **2021**, *106*, 105448. [CrossRef]
11. Tan, X.; Liu, X.; Shao, H. Healthy China 2030: A Vision for Health Care. *Value Health Reg. Issues* **2017**, *12*, 112–114. [CrossRef]
12. Chen, G.P.; Widener, M.J.; Zhu, M.M.; Wang, C.C. Identification of Priority Areas for Public-Access Automated External defibrillators (AEDs) in Metropolitan Areas: A Case Study in Hangzhou, China. *Appl. Geogr.* **2023**, *154*, 102922. [CrossRef]
13. Liao, S.Y.; Gao, F.; Feng, L.; Wu, J.M.; Wang, Z.X.; Chen, W.Y. Observed Equity and Driving Factors of Automated External Defibrillators: A Case Study Using WeChat Applet Data. *ISPRS Int. J. Geo-Inf.* **2023**, *12*, 444. [CrossRef]
14. Gao, F.; Lu, S.Y.; Liao, S.Y.; Chen, W.Y.; Chen, X.; Wu, J.M.; Wu, Y.J.; Li, G.Y.; Han, X. AED Inequity among Social Groups in Guangzhou. *ISPRS Int. J. Geo-Inf.* **2024**, *13*, 140. [CrossRef]
15. Folke, F.; Lippert, F.K.; Nielsen, S.L.; Gislason, G.H.; Hansen, M.L.; Schramm, T.K.; Sorensen, R.; Fosbol, E.L.; Andersen, S.S.; Rasmussen, S.; et al. Location of Cardiac Arrest in a City Center: Strategic Placement of Automated External Defibrillators in Public Locations. *Circulation* **2009**, *120*, 510–517. [CrossRef]
16. Sun, C.L.F.; Karlsson, L.; Torp-Pedersen, C.; Morrison, L.J.; Folke, F.; Chan, T.C.Y. Spatiotemporal AED Optimization is Generalizable. *Resuscitation* **2018**, *131*, 101–107. [CrossRef]
17. Dahan, B.; Jabre, P.; Karam, N.; Misslin, R.; Bories, M.C.; Tafflet, M.; Bougouin, W.; Jost, D.; Beganton, F.; Beal, G.; et al. Optimization of automated external defibrillator deployment Outdoors: An Evidence-Based Approach. *Resuscitation* **2016**, *108*, 68–74. [CrossRef] [PubMed]

18. Kwon, P.; Kim, M.J.; Lee, Y.; Yu, K.; Huh, Y. Locating Automated External Defibrillators in a Complicated Urban Environment Considering a Pedestrian-Accessible Network that Focuses on Out-of-Hospital Cardiac Arrests. *ISPRS Int. J. Geo-Inf.* **2017**, *6*, 39. [CrossRef]
19. Chrisinger, B.W.; Grossestreuer, A.V.; Laguna, M.C.; Griffis, L.M.; Branas, C.C.; Wiebe, D.J.; Merchant, R.M. Characteristics of Automated External Defibrillator Coverage in Philadelphia, PA, Based on Land Use and Estimated Risk. *Resuscitation* **2016**, *109*, 9–15. [CrossRef]
20. Lin, B.C.; Chen, C.W.; Chen, C.C.; Kuo, C.L.; Fan, I.C.; Ho, C.K.; Liu, I.C.; Chan, T.C. Spatial Decision on Allocating Automated External Defibrillators (AED) in Communities by Multi-Criterion Two-Step Floating Catchment Area (MC2SFCA). *Int. J. Health Geogr.* **2016**, *15*, 17. [CrossRef]
21. Griffis, H.M.; Band, R.A.; Ruther, M.; Harhay, M.; Asch, D.A.; Hershey, J.C.; Hill, S.; Nadkarni, L.; Kilaru, A.; Branas, C.C.; et al. Employment and Residential Characteristics in Relation to Automated External Defibrillator Locations. *Am. Heart J.* **2016**, *172*, 185–191. [CrossRef]
22. Bonnet, B.; Dessavre, D.G.; Kraus, K.; Ramirez-Marquez, J.E. Optimal Placement of Public-Access AEDs in Urban Environments. *Comput. Ind. Eng.* **2015**, *90*, 269–280. [CrossRef]
23. Kobayashi, D.; Sado, J.; Kiyohara, K.; Kitamura, T.; Kiguchi, T.; Nishiyama, C.; Okabayashi, S.; Shimamoto, T.; Matsuyama, T.; Kawamura, T.; et al. Public Location and Survival from Out-Of-Hospital Cardiac Arrest in the Public-Access Defibrillation Era in Japan. *J. Cardiol.* **2020**, *75*, 97–104. [CrossRef] [PubMed]
24. Duan, Z.; Zhao, H.; Li, Z. Non-Linear Effects of Built Environment and Socio-Demographics on Activity Space. *J. Transp. Geogr.* **2023**, *111*, 103671. [CrossRef]
25. Li, X.; Li, Y.; Jia, T.; Zhou, L.; Hijazi, I.H. The Six Dimensions of Built Environment on Urban Vitality: Fusion Evidence from Multi-Source Data. *Cities* **2022**, *121*, 103482. [CrossRef]
26. Zeng, Q.; Wu, H.; Wei, Y.; Wang, J.; Zhang, C.; Fei, N.; Dewancker, B.J. Association between Built Environment Factors and Collective Walking Behavior in Peri-Urban Area: Evidence from Chengdu. *Appl. Geogr.* **2024**, *167*, 103274. [CrossRef]
27. Liu, K.; Liao, C. Examining the Importance of Neighborhood Natural, and built Environment Factors in Predicting Older Adults' Mental Well-being: An XGBoost-SHAP approach. *Environ. Res.* **2024**, *262*, 119929. [CrossRef] [PubMed]
28. Shen, Y.; Tao, Y. Associations Between Spatial Access to Medical Facilities and Health-Seeking Behaviors: A Mixed Geographically Weighted Regression Analysis in Shanghai, China. *Appl. Geogr.* **2022**, *139*, 102644. [CrossRef]
29. Wang, Y.; Han, Y.; Luo, A.; Xu, S.; Chen, J.; Liu, W. Site Selection and Prediction of Urban Emergency Shelter based on VGAE-RF Model. *Sci. Rep.* **2024**, *14*, 14368. [CrossRef] [PubMed]
30. Chen, Y.; Zhang, X.; Grekousis, G.; Huang, Y.; Hua, F.; Pan, Z.; Liu, Y. Examining the Importance of Built and Natural Environment Factors in Predicting Self-Rated Health in Older Adults: An Extreme Gradient Boosting (XGBoost) Approach. *J. Clean. Prod.* **2023**, *413*, 137432. [CrossRef]
31. Xue, M.; Luo, Y. Dynamic Variations in Ecosystem Service Value and Sustainability of Urban System: A Case Study for Tianjin City, China. *Cities* **2015**, *46*, 85–93. [CrossRef]
32. Liu, C.; Cao, M.; Yang, T.; Ma, L.; Wu, M.; Cheng, L.; Ye, R. Inequalities in the commuting burden: Institutional Constraints and Job-Housing Relationships in Tianjin, China. *Res. Transp. Bus. Manag.* **2022**, *42*, 100545. [CrossRef]
33. Yang, H.; Jin, C.; Li, T. A Paradox of Economic Benefit and Social Equity of Green Space in Megacity: Evidence from Tianjin in China. *Sustain. Cities Soc.* **2024**, *109*, 105530. [CrossRef]
34. Li, Y.; Li, J.; Geng, J.; Liu, T.; Liu, X.; Fan, H.; Cao, C. Urban-Sub-Urban-Rural Variation in the Supply and Demand of Emergency Medical Services. *Front. Public Health* **2022**, *10*, 1064385. [CrossRef]
35. Gong, P.; Chen, B.; Li, X.; Liu, H.; Wang, J.; Bai, Y.; Chen, J.; Chen, X.; Fang, L.; Feng, S.; et al. Mapping Essential Urban Land Use Categories in China (EULUC-China): Preliminary Results for 2018. *Sci. Bull.* **2020**, *65*, 182–187. [CrossRef]
36. Song, L.; Kong, X.; Cheng, P. Supply-Demand Matching Assessment of the Public Service Facilities in 15-Minute Community Life Circle Based on Residents' Behaviors. *Cities* **2024**, *144*, 104637. [CrossRef]
37. Fan, P.Y.; Chun, K.P.; Mijic, A.; Tan, M.L.; Liu, M.S.; Yetemen, O. A Framework to Evaluate the Accessibility, Visibility, and Intelligibility of Green-Blue Spaces (GBSs) Related to Pedestrian Movement. *Urban For. Urban Green.* **2022**, *69*, 127494. [CrossRef]
38. Cooper, C.H.V. Spatial Localization of Closeness and Betweenness Measures: A Self-Contradictory but Useful form of Network Analysis. *Int. J. Geogr. Inf. Sci.* **2015**, *29*, 1293–1309. [CrossRef]
39. Hillier, B.; Iida, S. Network and Psychological Effects in Urban Movement. In *Spatial Information Theory*; Cohn, A.G., Mark, D.M., Eds.; Lecture Notes in Computer Science; Springer: Berlin/Heidelberg, Germany, 2005; Volume 3693, pp. 475–490, ISBN 978-3-540-28964-7.
40. Cooper, C.H.V.; Fone, D.L.; Chiaradia, A.J.F. Measuring the Impact of Spatial Network Layout on Community Social Cohesion: A Cross-Sectional Study. *Int. J. Health Geogr.* **2014**, *13*, 11. [CrossRef] [PubMed]
41. He, S.; Yu, S.; Wei, P.; Fang, C. A Spatial Design Network Analysis of Street Networks and the Locations of Leisure Entertainment Activities: A Case Study of Wuhan, China. *Sustain. Cities Soc.* **2019**, *44*, 880–887. [CrossRef]

42. Dai, D. Racial/Ethnic and Socioeconomic Disparities in Urban Green Space Accessibility: Where to Intervene? *Landsc. Urban. Plan.* **2011**, *102*, 234–244. [CrossRef]
43. Seong, K.; Jiao, J.; Mandalapu, A. Effects of Urban Environmental Factors on Heat-Related Emergency Medical Services (EMS) Response Time. *Appl. Geogr.* **2023**, *155*, 102956. [CrossRef]
44. Luo, Y.; Liu, Y.; Tong, Z.; Wang, N.; Rao, L. Capturing Gender-Age Thresholds Disparities in Built Environment Factors Affecting Injurious Traffic Crashes. *Travel. Behav. Soc.* **2023**, *30*, 21–37. [CrossRef]
45. Zhang, S.; Wang, L.; Shen, Y.; Zhang, Y.; Gao, Y.; Xu, T.; Zhang, Z. What Causes Emergency Medical Services (EMS) Delay? Unravel High-Risk Buildings Using Citywide Ambulance Trajectory Data. *Habitat. Int.* **2024**, *153*, 103198. [CrossRef]
46. Cheng, Q.; Sha, S. Last Defense in Climate Change: Assessing Healthcare Inequities in Response to Compound Environmental Risk in a Megacity in Northern China. *Sustain. Cities Soc.* **2024**, *115*, 105886. [CrossRef]
47. Chen, S.; Biljecki, F. Automatic Assessment of Public Open Spaces Using Street View Imagery. *Cities* **2023**, *137*, 104329. [CrossRef]
48. Zhou, Y.; Xu, K.; Feng, Z.; Wu, K. Quantification and Driving Mechanism of Cultivated Land Fragmentation under Scale Differences. *Ecol. Inform.* **2023**, *78*, 102336. [CrossRef]
49. Chen, T.; Guestrin, C. XGBoost: A Scalable Tree Boosting System. In Proceedings of the 22nd ACM SIGKDD International Conference on Knowledge Discovery and Data Mining, San Francisco, CA, USA, 13 August 2016; pp. 785–794.
50. Ma, M.; Zhao, G.; He, B.; Li, Q.; Dong, H.; Wang, S.; Wang, Z. XGBoost-Based Method for Flash Flood Risk Assessment. *J. Hydrol.* **2021**, *598*, 126382. [CrossRef]
51. Yoshida, Y.; Hayashi, Y.; Shimada, T.; Hattori, N.; Tomita, K.; Miura, R.E.; Yamao, Y.; Tateishi, S.; Iwadate, Y.; Nakada, T.A. Prehospital Stroke-Scale Machine-Learning Model Predicts the Need for Surgical Intervention. *Sci. Rep.* **2023**, *13*, 9135. [CrossRef]
52. Li, X.; Chen, J.; Chen, Z.; Lan, Y.; Ling, M.; Huang, Q.; Li, H.; Han, X.; Yi, S. Explainable Machine Learning-Based Fractional Vegetation Cover Inversion and Performance Optimization—A Case Study of an Alpine Grassland on the Qinghai-Tibet Plateau. *Ecol. Inform.* **2024**, *82*, 102768. [CrossRef]
53. He, J.; Shi, Y.; Xu, L.; Lu, Z.; Feng, M.; Tang, J.; Guo, X. Exploring the Scale Effect of Urban Thermal Environment through XGBoost Model. *Sustain. Cities Soc.* **2024**, *114*, 105763. [CrossRef]
54. Lundberg, S.; Lee, S.-I. A Unified Approach to Interpreting Model Predictions. *Adv. Neural Inf. Process. Syst.* **2017**, *30*, 1–10.
55. Zou, J.; Wang, C.; Chen, S.; Zhang, J.; Qiu, B.; Yang, H. Expanding the Associations between Built Environment Characteristics and Residential Mobility in High-Density Neighborhood Unit. *Sustain. Cities Soc.* **2024**, *116*, 105885. [CrossRef]

International Journal of
Geo-Information

MDPI

Article

Analysis of Spatial and Driving Factors of National Sanitary Resources in China Using GIS

Yujia Deng [1], Lixia Feng [2], Jeremy Cenci [3], Jiazhen Zhang [4,*] and Jun Cai [1,*]

1 College of Landscape Architecture, Sichuan Agricultural University, Chengdu 611130, China
2 School of Emergency Science, Xihua University, Chengdu 610039, China
3 Faculty of Architecture and Urban Planning, University of Mons, 7000 Mons, Belgium
4 Wales College, Lanzhou University, Lanzhou 730000, China
* Correspondence: zhangjiazhen@lzu.edu.cn (J.Z.); caijun@sicau.edu.cn (J.C.)

Abstract: Promoting health equity is key to achieving sustainable urban development. The National Sanitary Cities in China (NSCC) policy is a critical development model aimed at improving urban environments and enhancing public health. This study evaluates the selection criteria and policy impact of NSCCs, using the nearest neighbour index, geographic concentration index, imbalance index, and kernel density estimation to analyze their distribution characteristics. Additionally, it explores influencing factors using a geodetector model and spatial overlay analysis. The findings indicate a shift in NSCC selection criteria from urban sanitation to urban health, reflecting China's strategic focus on achieving health equity. The spatial distribution analysis indicates that NSCCs exhibit a clustered pattern, characterized by dual cores, dual centres, multiple scattered points, and regional extensions. NSCCs are influenced by both natural and socioeconomic factors, with economy and population, technological innovation, and informatization exerting greater influences. This study is valuable for understanding the spatial patterns of NSCCs, providing a scientific basis for promoting equitable and sustainable health resource allocation and policymaking.

Keywords: cities; China; health equity; health services; public health; national sanitary city; spatial distribution

1. Introduction

The rapid urbanization of the global population has underscored pressing urban health challenges, necessitating effective policy interventions to promote urban health development. Currently, more than half of the world's population lives in urban areas, and this proportion is expected to reach 68% by 2050 [1]. The increasing complexity of urban public health issues stems from the interplay of factors such as urban development, rising population density, environmental pollution, and climate change, all of which have profound impacts on public health [2,3]. Furthermore, urban planning and policy interventions play a crucial role in shaping residents' quality of life and overall health outcomes [4,5]. China, one of the world's most populous and urbanized nations, has faced significant public health challenges associated with its rapid urban growth [6]. Starting in 1989, the Chinese central government began to advocate for the National Sanitary Cities in China (NSCC) policy, based on the country's Patriotic Health Campaign, to improve urban sanitary conditions and enhance public health. NSCCs are nationally recognized cities that represent an exemplary level of regional health and sanitation [7]. In July 2017, the World Health Organization (WHO) presented the Chinese government with the "Award for Excellence in Social Health Governance" for the Patriotic Health Campaign's significant achievements [7].

Currently, research on the NSCC policy focuses primarily on its evaluation and impact. Related studies have revealed the importance of establishing NSCCs in improving ecological welfare performance and the multiple effects it generates [8]. Studies have focused on the core elements of urban health, such as green buildings, natural infrastructure, and community participation, exploring their roles in enhancing urban residents' quality of life [9,10]. Others have focused on healthy city planning in specific regions or countries, analyzing the socioeconomic factors influencing urban health development and policy design and implementation effectiveness [11,12]. Additionally, a few studies have taken a more macroscopic perspective, examining the relationship between healthy cities and global issues such as urban safety, ageing, and climate change [13,14]. In public health and urban planning, the effective utilization of spatial information technology (e.g., geographic information systems and remote sensing) is crucial for uncovering spatial patterns, identifying influencing factors, and promoting urban health equity and sustainable development. For example, Xie et al. used geospatial indices and ArcGIS spatial analysis to reveal the clustered distribution of leisure villages in China, highlighting the impact of natural and socioeconomic factors [15]. Similarly, Zhang et al. employed quantitative indices and the geodetector model to examine the distribution of National Forest Cities in China, linking social environmental factors to green space inequality [16]. These methods provide valuable references for analyzing the spatial patterns of NSCCs. However, existing studies on urban health often focus on singular aspects, overlooking the interplay between policies, social determinants, natural factors, and geographical disparities. This is particularly evident in the lack of research exploring how national policies can be integrated with local initiatives to tackle health inequities. Given China's vast territory and uneven distribution of cities, population, and economy, disparities in public health resources and health equity are inevitable [17,18]. Therefore, it is necessary to investigate the spatial distribution of NSCCs and the factors driving their development. Furthermore, for China, there is an urgent need to investigate how to leverage the national government's administrative mechanisms and resource advantages to create environments that meet the standards of sanitary cities and provide feasible strategies for achieving health equity. Such research is essential for clarifying the spatial dimensions of health equity, promoting health equity within the NSCC policy framework, and, on a broader scale, guiding governments at all levels to jointly create urban spaces conducive to the health of all Chinese residents, even worldwide.

This research utilized Geographic Information System software (ArcGIS 10.8), online mapping services (Google Earth), and R's GD statistical package to examine the evolution and current execution of the NSCC policy. It analyzed the spatial distribution patterns and development drivers of all cities that have appeared on the NSCC list, providing a scientific basis for developing the NSCC policy and offering new perspectives on urban health strategies. By examining national-level policies and practices, this study aimed to offer insights and solutions for the sustainable development of cities worldwide, and the research findings are expected to serve as a valuable reference for enhancing the overall resilience of cities and public health.

The paper is structured as follows: In Section 2, we present an analysis of the NSCC policy, including its origin, evolution, selection criteria, evaluation mechanisms, significance, and benefits. We describe the data sources and methodology in Section 3. In Sections 4 and 5, we provide and analyze the findings. Finally, in Sections 6 and 7, we discuss and summarize our findings and perspectives for future research.

2. Theoretical Derivation and Significance of NSCC Policy

2.1. Original NSCC Policy

In 1986, the WHO launched the "Healthy Cities" movement, which has since inspired various regions worldwide to implement healthy city construction practices tailored to their local conditions [19]. In response to this global initiative, China, through the National Patriotic Health Campaign Committee (NPHCC), began the NSCC creation campaign in 1989. The NSCC creation campaign is a government-led social health movement with extensive participation from all levels of society, based on the actual situations of Chinese cities and relying on patriotic health work with distinct Chinese characteristics. Relevant research shows that the construction of NSCCs has been a precursor to the development of healthy cities in China, and there are extensive commonalities between the two [20,21]. This suggests that the NSCC creation campaign is a positive response and localized adaptation of the global Healthy Cities movement within China's context.

2.2. Evolution Process of NSCC Policy

Since the NPHCC's initiative to establish NSCCs in 1989, the NPHCC has continuously improved the standards and evaluation management methods for NSCCs. These revisions, implemented at different stages, have been crucial in adapting to the evolving requirements of urban development and ensuring a standardized assessment and management process. The evolution of relevant policies can be divided into three distinct stages. Figure 1 illustrates the gradual shift from the creation of NSCCs to the development of a more comprehensive model of sanitary and healthy cities. From 1990 to 2020, the NPHCC cumulatively named 391 NSCCs and 71 National Sanitary Districts, accounting for more than half of China's total cities (districts).

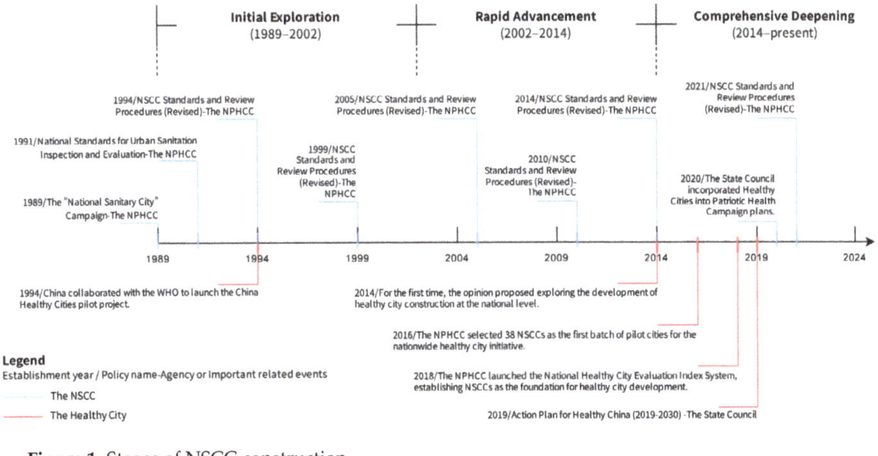

Figure 1. Stages of NSCC construction.

2.3. Evolution of Selection Criteria and Mechanisms of NSCCs

In 1989, China officially released the initial standards for creating NSCCs and established an evaluation mechanism. The aim was to ensure that improvements in sanitary conditions and the enhancement of sanitation levels progressed in tandem with Chinese urban development, marking the establishment of the NSCC policy. The revisions to the standards from 1994 to 2021 were largely consistent in content framework, with the main changes being adjustments and revisions to specific work indicators. The 2021 version of the standards includes seven aspects: patriotic health organization and management, health education and promotion, urban environmental sanitation, ecological environment, key site sanitation, food and drinking water safety, disease prevention and control, and medical services. The 2021 version of standards, revised to support the nationwide Healthy Cities initiative and integrate lessons from the COVID-19 pandemic, introduces the following changes. First, the standards strengthened the requirements for infectious disease prevention and control to actively prevent and control potential public hazards that may arise from major infectious diseases. Second, to support the implementation of the Healthy China action, the new standards added indicators for the 15 special actions of the Healthy China action. Finally, some indicators and standard content expressions were optimized, considering practical situations, economic and social development, and operability.

Regarding the evaluation mechanism, the creation of NSCCs adopts a voluntary application and level-by-level assessment. The evaluation cycle is once every three years. Successfully named cities need to pass a re-evaluation every three years to maintain their status; otherwise, they lose their designation. For example, in 2021, nine cities, including Hanzhong City in Shaanxi Province, demonstrated a decline in their work to consolidate their sanitary city status and were criticized [22]. The latest revised "NSCC Evaluation and Management Measures" simplify the evaluation procedures, reducing the original five procedures to three. The new measures replaced the previously required conditions with a scoring system and eliminated the one-vote veto. The long-term supervision mechanism has been improved, adjusting the review of NSCCs from a fixed three-year review to random inspections within three years after the designation, ensuring more dynamic and stringent supervision.

2.4. Significance and Benefits

The NSCC policy has improved urban environments and governance performance. Residents' overall score of access to an NSCC is relatively high, indicating that the policy has gained widespread recognition among the public [23]. The policy's standards and commendation mechanisms have prompted local governments to optimize their governance models and enhance overall performance. Studies have shown that the policy has increased green space, reduced industrial sulphur dioxide and wastewater emissions [24,25], and raised the proportion of urban domestic sewage treatment, waste disposal, and qualified farmers' markets [26]. The policy has also significantly improved the efficiency of environmental governance and has played a substantial role in promoting urban public services [25]. It has effectively mobilized local governments to participate actively in environmental protection, fostered learning and competition among them, and notably improved the environmental quality of cities that have successfully obtained the NSCC title. Moreover, compared to cities that have not received this title, key officials in these cities are more likely to be promoted, suggesting that the policy has had a positive impact on urban environments, public health, and officials' enthusiasm for governance, ultimately strengthening the overall performance of urban administration [20].

Relevant research indicates that establishing NSCCs effectively mitigates the impact of COVID-19, demonstrating the potential of these cities in controlling infectious diseases [27]. The creation of NSCCs has effectively promoted the development of China's health field and improved public health levels. Since the initiation of NSCC certification in 1989, relevant studies analyzing health patterns in 34 provincial-level administrative units in China from 1990 to 2017 have shown that China has made substantial progress in reducing the burden of many diseases and disabilities [28]. From 1990 to 2015, a span of 25 years, China was one of the countries with the most significant improvement in the quality and accessibility of healthcare services, among 195 countries and regions worldwide [29]. The policy has implemented a series of measures to enhance health and well-being, for instance, improving urban environmental sanitation, requiring an immunization rate exceeding

90% for age-appropriate children, promoting the standardized development of primary healthcare institutions, and implementing chronic disease prevention and control measures, among others. Since 1990, China's life expectancy has increased from 68.55 to 78.6 years (2023) [30], demonstrating the profound impact of systematic public health interventions and improved healthcare accessibility on population health.

3. Data Sources and Research Methodology

3.1. Data Sources

The NSCC list, issued by China's National Health Commission (https://en.nhc.gov.cn/), now encompasses 462 cities (excluding Hong Kong, Macao, and Taiwan). This research calibrated geographical coordinates using Google Earth and ArcGIS 10.8 to build the database, integrating data from diverse authoritative sources, such as the Chinese Academy of Sciences and national yearbooks, to analyze the influencing and driving factors. This approach allowed us to create a spatial database and visualize the effective implementation of the NSCC policy across China.

This analysis is based on the NSCC list published in December 2020. The 462 cities across 31 provinces, municipalities, and autonomous regions were included. While social organizations or institutions have released similar lists, the list issued by the central government of China is considered the most authoritative, due to the country's particular political system [31,32]. The data used in this study were sourced from the Resource and Environment Sciences and Data Platform at the Institute of Geographic Sciences and Natural Resources Research, Chinese Academy of Sciences (http://www.resdc.cn/), the China Statistical Yearbook, and the China Health Statistical Yearbook. Information on China's National Smart Cities Pilot Project was taken from the Ministry of Housing and Urban-Rural Development website (https://www.mohurd.gov.cn/), data on 3A hospitals were retrieved from the website of the National Healthcare Security Administration (https://www.nhsa.gov.cn/), and a map of China was provided by the Natural Resources Ministry's Map Technology Review Center (https://www.zrzyst.cn/). All data were accessed on 1 August 2024.

To ensure the accuracy of the evaluations for the NSCC policy, we precisely calibrated the geographical coordinates for all cities on the list. With the use of Google Earth Coordinate Picker, the central point of the city government buildings was used as the coordinate base for existing cities. For cities merged due to administrative reorganization, the newly established service management centre or government building was the central point for coordinating calibration and ensuring comprehensive and precise assessments. In total, 462 valid data points were obtained, covering all cities in the list. Subsequently, the data were imported into ArcGIS 10.8, a software tool developed by the Environmental Systems Research Institute in the USA, for data analysis and map creation. In ArcGIS 10.8, spatial coordinates were matched and projected, and data were integrated into 462 location coordinates, thus creating a spatial database for the NSCCs and visualizing their spatial distribution on a map.

3.2. Research Methodology

This study adopted well-established indices and models widely accepted in geospatial research to investigate the NSCCs. Figure 2 presents a flowchart of the research methodology. The nearest neighbour index was used to analyze the spatial distribution patterns. In contrast, the geographic concentration and imbalance indices were employed to differentiate the spatial distribution disparities. Kernel density analysis was applied to examine the spatial distribution density. The geodetector and spatial superposition models were utilized to measure the influence of natural and socioeconomic factors on the distribution.

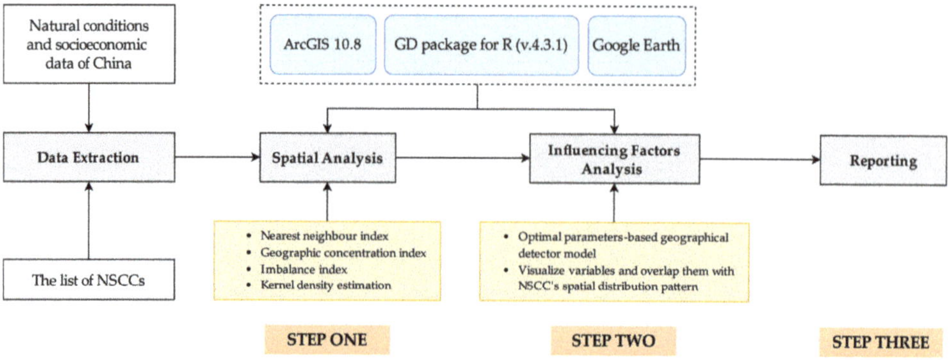

Figure 2. Research flowchart.

3.2.1. Nearest Neighbour Index

Based on the nearest neighbour index, the spatial distribution patterns of the NSCCs were evaluated [16,33]. The principle involves measuring the average distance between these cities and then comparing this measured nearest neighbour distance to the expected average nearest neighbour distance. The ratio of these distances is the nearest neighbour index, which determines the cities' spatial distribution characteristics (whether clustered, random, or dispersed). The calculation formula is as follows:

$$R = \frac{\bar{D_O}}{\bar{D_E}}; \bar{D_O} = \frac{\sum_{i=1}^{n} d_i}{n}; \bar{D_E} = \frac{0.5}{\sqrt{\frac{n}{A}}} \tag{1}$$

where R stands for the nearest neighbour index, $\bar{D_O}$ is the average of the distance between the nearest points in reality, $\bar{D_E}$ is the average between the nearest points in theory, and A is the study area. $R < 1$ indicates a clustering trend among the points: if $R = 1$, the spatial distribution of the points is random; if $R > 1$, the points tend to be dispersed.

3.2.2. Geographic Concentration Index

The geographic concentration index measures the degree of concentration in the spatial distribution of the NSCCs [34]. The G value ranges from 0 to 100, with higher G values indicating more concentrated distributions and lower G values indicating more dispersed distributions. The calculation formula is as follows:

$$G = 100 \times \sqrt{\sum_{i=1}^{n} \left(\frac{X_i}{T}\right)^2} \tag{2}$$

where G is the geographical concentration index, X_i represents the number of NSCCs in each administrative region, T is the total number of NSCCs across all regions, and n is the number of administration regions.

3.2.3. Imbalance Index

The imbalance index is used to reflect the balance of the distribution of NSCCs across different regional areas [35]. The calculation formula is as follows:

$$S = \frac{\sum_{i=1}^{n} Y_i - 50(n+1)}{100n - 50(n+1)} \tag{3}$$

where n represents the number of regions, totalling 31, and Y_i represents the cumulative percentage of NSCC in the i-th region relative to the total number. The value of S ranges from 0 to 1: $S = 0$ indicates that the NSCCs are evenly distributed across all regions; $S = 1$ means that all NSCCs are concentrated in a single region. The closer the value of S is to 1, the more uneven the distribution of NSCCs.

3.2.4. Kernel Density Estimation

The kernel density estimation method can be used to determine the clustering status of NSCCs [36]. The calculation formula is as follows:

$$f_n(x) = \frac{1}{nh}\sum_{i=1}^{n} k\left(\frac{x - X_i}{h}\right) \tag{4}$$

where fn represents the kernel density estimate, n is the number of NSCCs, k represents the kernel function, $x - Xi$ is the distance from the estimation point x to the sample Xi, and h is the search radius.

3.2.5. Optimal Parameter-Based Geographical Detector Model

The geographical detector is a statistical method widely used to explore the spatial differentiation of geographic phenomena and to identify the driving forces behind this spatial differentiation [37]. In this study, we used the "GD" package in R to implement and execute the optimal discretization method for independent variables. Using a factor detection module, we explored and identified the dominant factors influencing the distribution of NSCCs. The formula for the factor detection module is as follows:

$$q = 1 - \frac{\sum_{j=1}^{M} N_j\sigma_j^2}{N\sigma^2} \tag{5}$$

where q represents the degree to which the influencing factor explains the spatial distribution of NSCCs, with q values in the range of [0, 1]. A higher q value indicates a greater influence of the factor on the spatial distribution of NSCCs. N and σ^2 represent the study unit's total sample size and variance, respectively, and N_j and σ_j^2 denote the sample size and variance of the jth layer ($j = 1, 2, 3, \ldots, M$).

4. Results

4.1. Overview of the Study Subject

Since 1990, the NPHCC has been conducting evaluations to designate NSCCs. To date, 462 cities have been awarded the title, representing nearly 60% of all urban areas (districts) nationwide; as shown in Figure 3, the number of NSCCs generally exhibits an upward trend.

This study extracted spatial distribution data for the NSCCs and created a geographic spatial database, abstracting their distribution from a macroscopic perspective into point elements. Figure 4 illustrates the distribution of NSCCs across 31 administrative regions.

4.2. Spatial Characteristics and Structural Analysis

4.2.1. Spatial Distribution Pattern

As shown in Figure 4, the distribution of NSCCs is characterized by large clusters and small dispersions. The nearest neighbour index was used to determine the spatial distribution pattern of these point elements. With the spatial analysis tools in ArcGIS 10.8 software, the average nearest neighbour index for the NSCCs was calculated to be $R = 0.85 < 1$, and it passed the 1% significance test (p-value = 0.0000). The results reveal that the spatial distribution of NSCCs prominently features clustering within specific regional spaces.

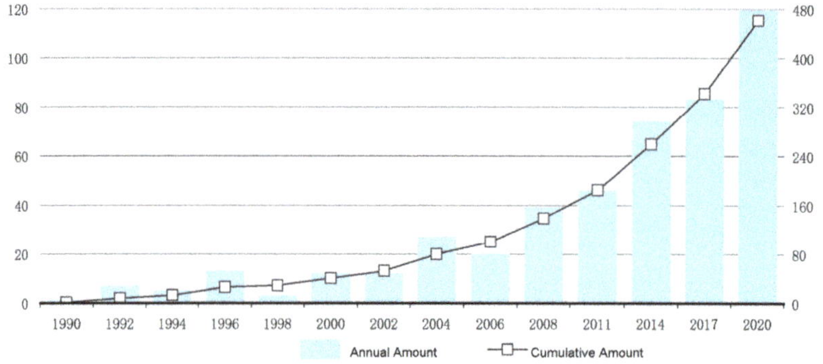

Figure 3. Number of NSCCs by period to date.

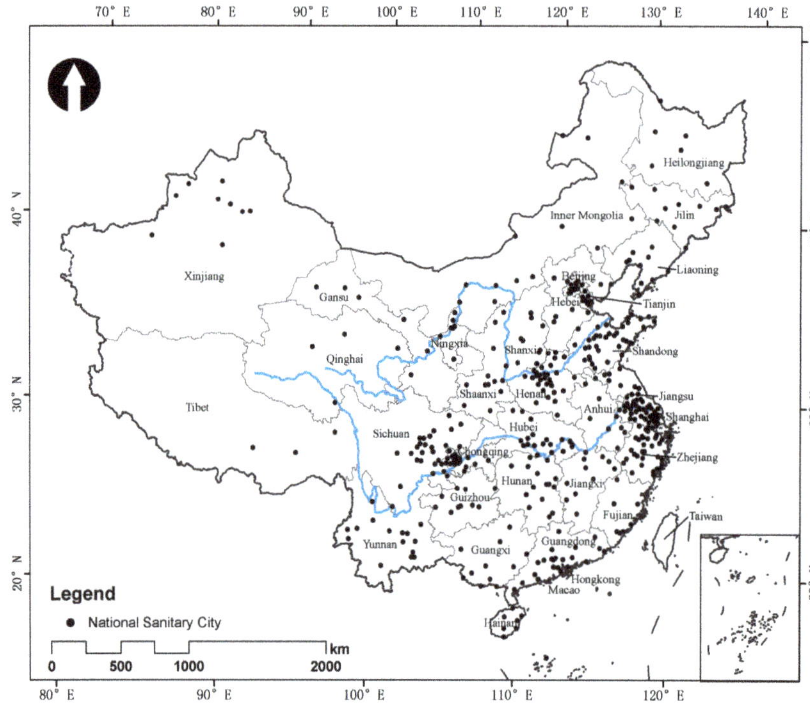

Figure 4. Spatial distribution map of NSCCs.

4.2.2. Balanced Spatial Distribution

1. Concentration analysis of spatial distribution

The concentration of the NSCC distribution was calculated using Formula (2) and the data from Table 1. The resulting geographic concentration index, G, was 21.35. If the NSCCs were evenly distributed across all administrative regions, index G' would be 17.96. Since $G > G'$, the distribution of the NSCCs is concentrated in certain administrative regions.

Table 1. Statistical distribution of NSCCs across various administrative regions.

No.	Administrative Region	NSCC Amount	Proportion/%	Cumulative Proportion/%
1	Jiangsu	41	8.87	8.87
2	Shandong	35	7.58	16.45
3	Zhejiang	34	7.36	23.81
4	Henan	31	6.71	30.52
5	Sichuan	26	5.63	36.15
6	Guangdong	22	4.76	40.91
7	Hubei	20	4.33	45.24
8	Chongqing	20	4.33	49.57
9	Shanghai	18	3.90	53.46
10	Beijing	18	3.90	57.36
11	Hunan	15	3.25	60.61
12	Yunnan	15	3.25	63.85
13	Tianjin	15	3.25	67.10
14	Shaanxi	13	2.81	69.91
15	Inner Mongolia	13	2.81	72.73
16	Jiangxi	11	2.38	75.11
17	Guizhou	11	2.38	77.49
18	Guangxi	11	2.38	79.87
19	Liaoning	10	2.16	82.03
20	Jilin	10	2.16	84.20
21	Xinjiang	9	1.95	86.15
22	Shanxi	9	1.95	88.10
23	Hainan	8	1.73	89.83
24	Hebei	7	1.52	91.34
25	Anhui	7	1.52	92.86
26	Ningxia	7	1.52	94.37
27	Fujian	7	1.52	95.89
28	Heilongjiang	6	1.30	97.19
29	Gansu	6	1.30	98.48
30	Qinghai	4	0.87	99.35
31	Tibet	3	0.65	100.00

2. Equilibrium analysis of spatial distribution

Based on the economic development levels and geographical locations, China is generally divided into three regions: eastern, central, and western [38,39]. From 2000 to 2020, the number and regional distribution of NSCCs underwent significant changes (Table 2), with the total number increasing more than 11-fold. In 2000, NSCCs were primarily concentrated in the eastern region. By 2020, the proportion in the eastern region had decreased, while the central and western regions had increased.

Table 2. Number and proportion of NSCCs in the three regions of China (2000–2020).

Region	2000		2011		2020	
	Amount	Proportion/%	Amount	Proportion/%	Amount	Proportion/%
Eastern region	33	80.48	119	64.32	215	46.54
Central region	4	9.76	32	17.30	109	23.59
Western region	4	9.76	34	18.38	138	29.87
Nationwide	41	100.00	185	100.00	462	100.00

To quantify the degree of uneven distribution, the imbalance index (Formula (3)) was applied. The resulting imbalance index for the NSCCs was $S = 0.3525$ with $0 < S < 1$, indicating an uneven distribution across the administrative regions. This demonstrates that the distribution of NSCCs across the administration regions is not uniform. The Lorenz curve, used to chart the variation in the number of NSCCs by the administration regions in Figure 5, shows an upward convex trend. Notably, the combined total of NSCCs in Jiangsu, Shandong, Zhejiang, Henan, Sichuan, Guangdong, Hubei, Chongqing, and Shanghai accounts for 53.46% of the national figure, further highlighting the uneven distribution of NSCCs.

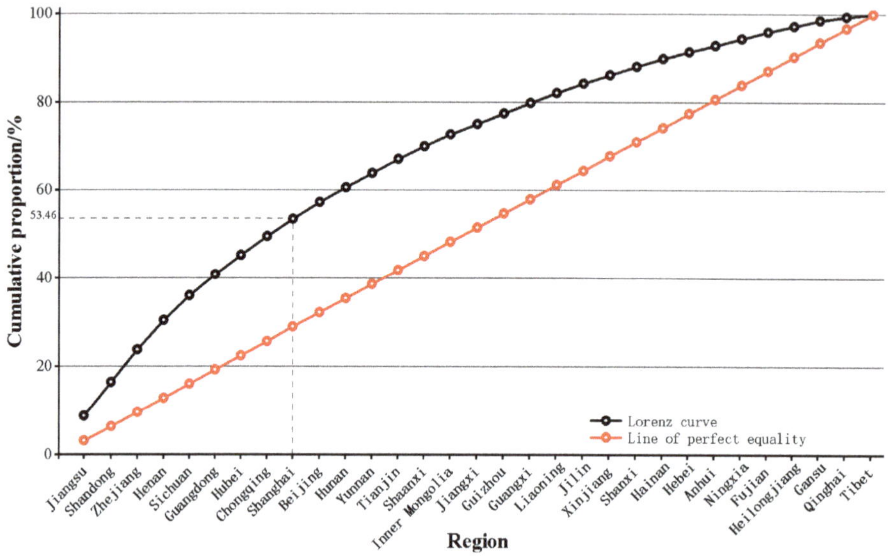

Figure 5. The Lorenz curve for the NSCC distribution by administration regions.

4.2.3. Spatial Distribution Density Characteristics

We used the kernel density tool in ArcGIS 10.8 to reveal the clustering of NSCCs. Its spatial distribution characteristics were as follows: "Dual cores, dual centres, multiple scattered points, and regional extensions", as shown in Figure 6.

Dual cores and dual centres, identified using kernel density analysis, represent different levels of spatial density: dual cores are the highest-density zones, and dual centres are secondary high-density zones. Dual cores refer to two core density areas: the Beijing–Tianjin–Hebei region (Beijing, Tianjin, and nearby Hebei), and the Yangtze River Delta region (Jiangsu, Shanghai, Anhui, and Zhejiang). Dual centres refer to two high-density central areas: one centred around Henan, comprising the provinces of Shanxi, Shaanxi, and Hubei, and the other centred around Sichuan and Chongqing, comprising the Guizhou and Hunan Provinces.

Multiple scattered points and regional expansions have formed several mid- to low-density zones. Notably, the mid- to low-density area in the southeast is a continuous high-value zone, displaying a layered distribution. In contrast, the northeast and northwest regions are primarily characterized by dispersed distributions.

Overall, the spatial distribution of NSCCs is generally higher in the east and lower in the west, denser in the south and sparser in the north, and mainly concentrated in the economically prosperous eastern regions.

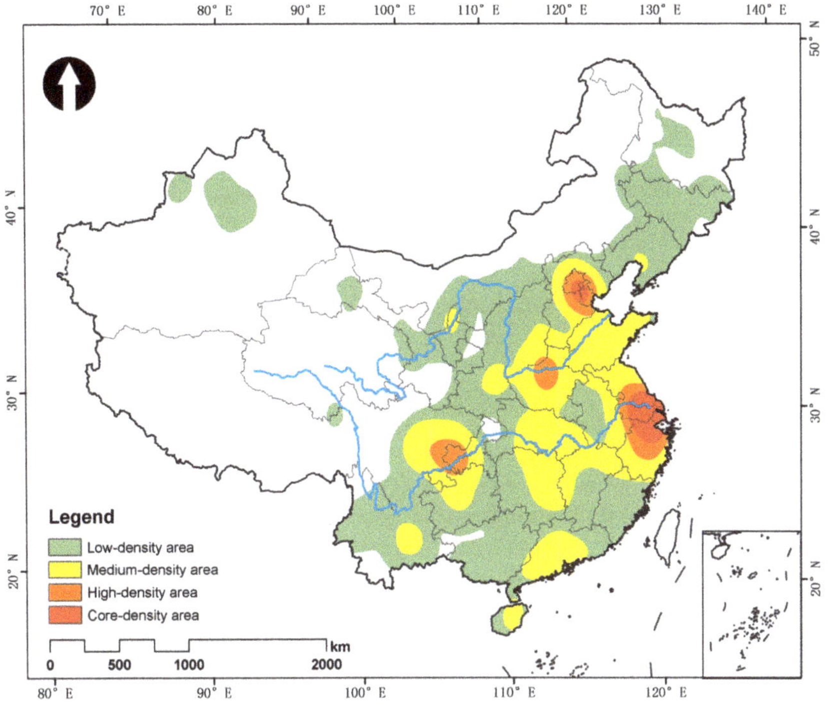

Figure 6. NSCC kernel densitometry results.

5. Driving and Influencing Factors of the Spatial Distribution of NSCCs

From the perspective of healthy cities, two main factors are crucial for understanding the spatial distribution of NSCCs: the natural environment and the socioeconomic environment [14,40], as illustrated in Figure 7.

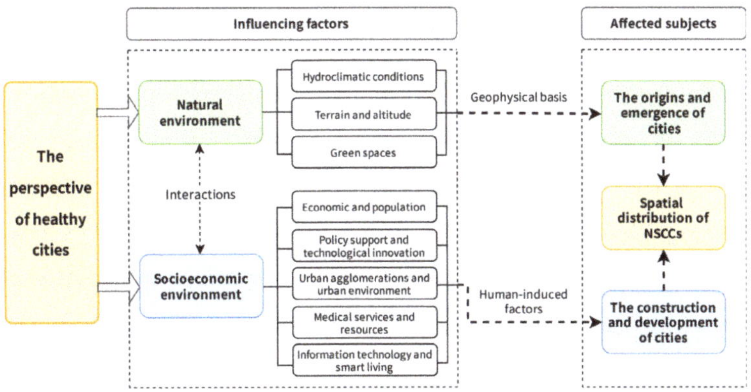

Figure 7. A framework for the analysis of factors affecting the spatial distribution of NSCCs.

5.1. Natural Environmental Factors

Cities, as densely populated settlements, exhibit intrinsic connections between their sanitary environmental and regional environmental conditions. China's diverse topography, from the 4000 m Tibetan Plateau to the varied eastern coastal landscapes [41], exerts both direct and indirect influences on human settlement patterns, economic development, and environmental protection [42,43]. Epidemiological evidence demonstrates strong associations between ambient temperature and disease incidence rates [44], while green spaces emerge as crucial determinants of urban health outcomes. These varying geographical conditions, temperature patterns, and green space distributions significantly shape the sustainable development of NSCCs.

5.1.1. Hydroclimatic Conditions

We conducted spatial overlay analysis between the NSCC distribution and China's seven climate zones [16,45]. As shown in Figure 8, nearly 87% of NSCCs are located in areas with an annual accumulated temperature over 3400 °C and annual precipitation exceeding 400 mm, indicating that environments with favourable hydrothermal conditions are conducive to establishing and developing sanitary cities. In contrast, only 2% of NSCCs are situated in the highland climate regions of the West. Recent epidemiological evidence indicates significant spatial heterogeneity in China's mortality rates under both high and low temperatures, with cold effects dominating the overall mortality burden [46]. The current pattern indicates that geographic differences in hydrothermal conditions are a major factor influencing the distribution of NSCCs, constraining the direction of their spatial spread and potential expansion areas.

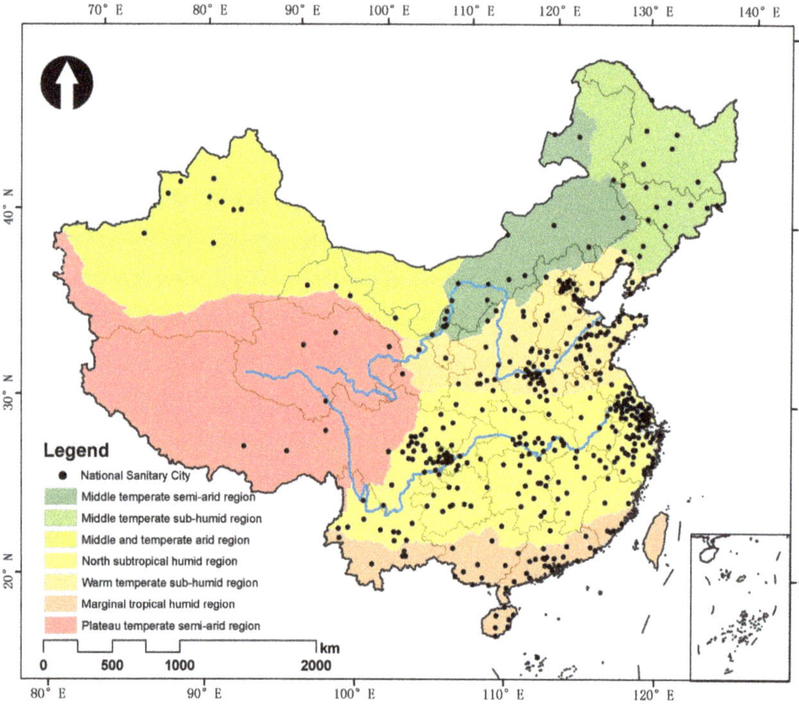

Figure 8. Spatial distribution of NSCCs overlaid with climatic factors.

5.1.2. Terrain and Altitude

Figure 9a shows that NSCCs in China are distributed across various elevations. Nearly 97% of NSCCs are located in areas below 2000 m in elevation, with the majority situated below 200 m. Only 3% of the cities are in areas where the terrain rises above 2000 m. Lower-elevation regions, which are flatter and more accessible, facilitate the aggregation and transportation of resources, making it easier to build and expand urban infrastructure and public health facilities. Additionally, these lower-altitude areas typically have denser populations, which increases the urgency and complexity of public health service needs, prompting governments and organizations to promote the development of sanitary cities more actively.

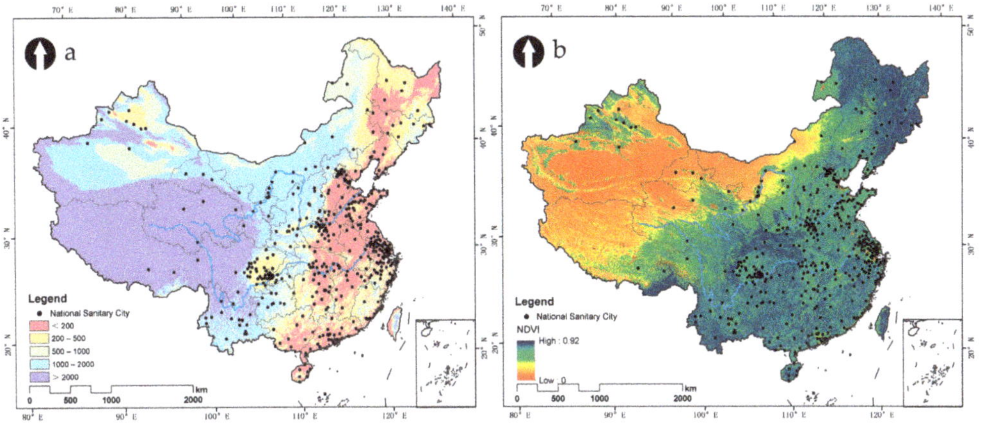

Figure 9. Spatial distribution of NSCCs overlaid with (**a**) terrain and altitude and (**b**) normalized difference vegetation index.

5.1.3. Urban Green Spaces

As shown in Figure 9b, nearly 80% of NSCCs are located in areas where the annual average NDVI (normalized difference vegetation index) ranges from 0.3 to 0.6. This indicates that most NSCCs are situated in regions with moderate vegetation cover. Such levels of vegetation cover are beneficial for improving urban environmental quality, mitigating urban heat island effects, and providing recreational green spaces for residents. In contrast, only 2.4% of NSCCs are found in areas with an annual average NDVI of 0.2 or below. Lower vegetation cover is typically associated with negative environmental factors, such as higher temperatures, poorer air quality, and limited natural habitats [47,48]. These conditions not only affect residents' daily lives but also pose challenges for these cities in meeting the environmental standards required by the NSCC policy.

5.2. Socioeconomic Factors

Based on the existing literature related to healthy cities and NSCCs [14,20,49], and referencing the standards for NSCCs, this study aggregated and examined the impact of socioeconomic factors on NSCCs from five dimensions, guided by principles of scientific rigour and data availability. Each dimension encompasses and influences multiple elements. For instance, economy and population serve as the foundation for resource allocation and health equity, shaping the capacity to implement various aspects of urban health development [50,51]. Similarly, information technology and smart living influence multiple facets of urban health—such as policy implementation, public health education, and healthcare accessibility—through digital innovation [52]. Influencing factors are shown in Table 3.

Table 3. The selection of influencing factors.

Dimensions	Factors	Units
Economic and Population	X1: Total value of secondary and tertiary industries	100 million yuan (RMB)
	X2: Urban population at year-end	persons
Policy Support and Technological Innovation	X3: Proportion of government health expenditure in total health expenditure	%
	X4: Number of patent applications	pcs
Urban Agglomerations and Urban Environment	X5: Total number of cities in provincial-level administrative regions	cities
	X6: Comprehensive utilization rate of general industrial solid waste (utilized amount/generated amount)	%
Medical Services and Resources	X7: Number of general practitioners	persons per 10,000 population
	X8: Number of beds in urban healthcare institutions	beds/1000 persons
Information Technology and Smart Living	X9: Urban broadband internet subscribers	10,000 households
	X10: Smart cities in provincial-level administrative regions	cities

5.2.1. Economic and Population

As shown in Figure 10, the output of the secondary and tertiary industries has the strongest explanatory power (0.80) for the spatial distribution of NSCCs, and this significance is statistically notable. This reflects that the level of economic development is an important foundation for the construction of NSCCs. Economically developed regions such as the Beijing–Tianjin–Hebei area and the Yangtze River Delta are two core areas in the kernel density analysis, where NSCCs are densely distributed. This indicates that higher regional economic development levels help cities meet the standards of the NSCC policy and improve the quality of their public health services and environment. Research analyzing medical geographic big data from 369 cities in China found that GDP growth is highly correlated with optimizing medical resource allocation, highlighting the key role of regional economic strength in medical resource distribution [53]. Additionally, this study found a positive correlation between economic development and a decrease in COVID-19 incidence rates, further underscoring the importance of the economy in improving public health [54]. In a sense, economic development largely determines the construction of NSCCs and the improvement of public health standards.

As indicated in Figure 10, urban population size has explanatory power (0.78) and a statistically significant impact on the spatial distribution of NSCCs. Figure 11 reveals that more than half of NSCCs are located in areas with population densities exceeding 800 people/km^2, while only 3% are found in regions with population densities below 100 people/km^2. Research shows that a 1% increase in population growth leads to a significant 1.71% increase in public health delivery system density [55]. As the population increases, the growing demand for public health services prompts establishing and expanding more public health facilities. A case study in Lanzhou, Gansu Province, found that health resources are often concentrated in densely populated areas as the urban population increases, forming a "bidirectional proximity" pattern that aligns with residents' needs [56]. This clustering effect emphasizes the role of the population as a key factor influencing the distribution of urban health resources.

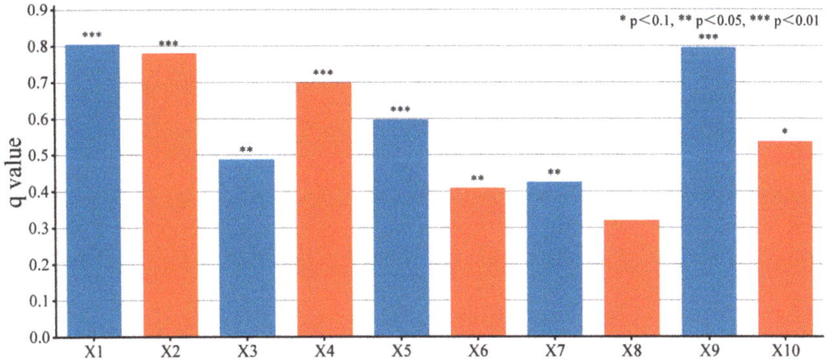

Figure 10. Single-factor analysis results from the geodetector model.

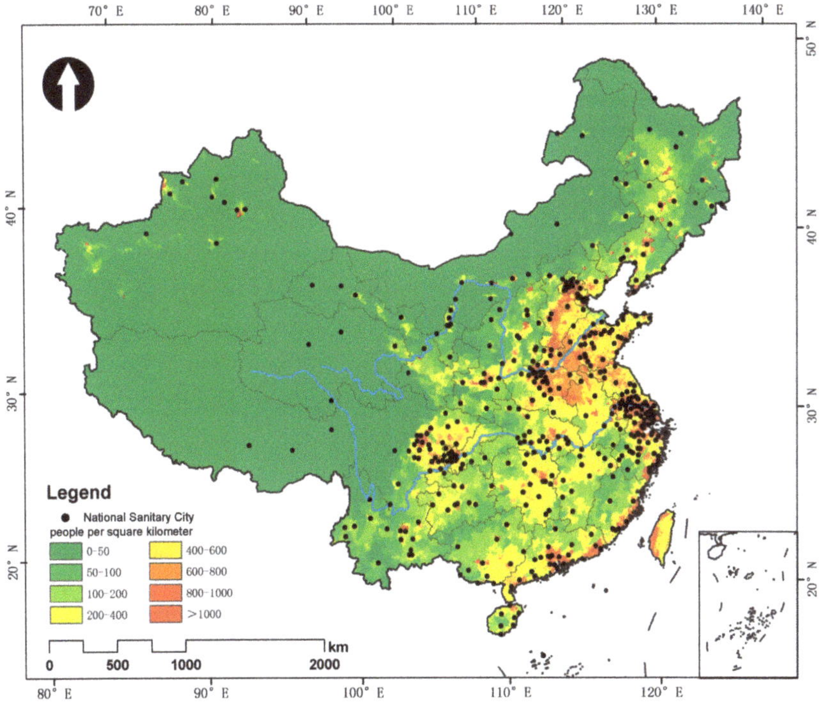

Figure 11. Spatial distribution of NSCCs overlaid with population density.

5.2.2. Policy Support and Technological Innovation

The proportion of government spending in total health expenditures reflects the orientation of policy systems and directly affects the quality, accessibility, and efficiency of public health services. Figure 10 indicates that the percentage of total health expenditure from the government has an explanatory power of 0.486 and significantly impacts the spatial distribution of NSCCs. Tan (2017) indicated that increased provincial government health expenditures positively impact public health services [57]. Additionally, Zhang and Rahman (2020) conducted a cross-national analysis of public health spending in China, and the Organization for Economic Cooperation and Development Countries further confirmed the significant role of government financial contributions in enhancing public health standards and reducing the medical burden on citizens [58].

Technological innovation is crucial for advancing public health and the development of NSCCs. Zhang et al. (2018), conducting spatial econometric analysis on 105 Chinese cities, confirmed technological innovation's positive contribution to urban green development [59]. In this context, the volume of patent applications is particularly important, as it reflects current trends and directions in technological innovation more promptly than the number of patent grants, directly demonstrating technological innovation's vitality. The spatial distribution of NSCCs is significantly influenced by the number of patent applications, as demonstrated in Figure 10, which shows an explanatory power of 0.697. This finding is further supported by the fact that nearly 50% of NSCCs are located in the eastern region of China. Hu et al. (2023) demonstrated that an increase in low-carbon patent applications in China's eastern coastal provinces indicates active technological innovation and highlights the emphasis on improving the public health environment [60]. Their study suggested that low-carbon technology innovations play a vital role in mitigating the negative impacts of climate change on public health by reducing carbon emissions and promoting environmentally friendly technologies.

5.2.3. Urban Agglomerations and Urban Environment

Given that local governments need to voluntarily apply for NSCC status, the larger the number of cities within an administrative region, the greater the potential number of NSCCs. As shown in Figure 10, the number of cities within an administrative region significantly impacts the spatial distribution of NSCCs ($q = 0.59$, $p < 0.01$). Meanwhile, spatial overlay analysis between NSCCs and Chinese urban agglomerations shows that nearly 80% of NSCCs are located within urban agglomerations, demonstrating a significant spatial alignment between the main distributions of urban agglomerations and NSCCs. Figure 12 illustrates this finding. Additionally, the "14th Five-Year Plan for the National Economic and Social Development of the People's Republic of China and the Long-Range Objectives Through the Year 2035" categorizes urban agglomeration development into three types: optimization and enhancement, development and expansion, and nurture and development [61]. As shown in Figure 12, nearly 50% of NSCCs are located within urban agglomerations prioritized for optimization and enhancement by the central government, indicating that the accumulation of NSCCs is influenced by both the uneven spatial distribution and the development of cities in China.

Additionally, as shown in Figure 10, the comprehensive utilization rate of general industrial solid waste has an explanatory power of 0.41 for the spatial distribution of NSCCs. It is statistically significant at the 0.05 level. The comprehensive utilization of industrial solid waste reduces environmental burdens and provides new resources for urban sustainable development. Jiangsu, with the highest number of NSCCs, has been promoting waste reuse since 1980. This study indicates that Jiangsu's implementation of the "Comprehensive Resource Utilization" policy has significantly benefited the environment by promoting the reuse of industrial waste [62].

5.2.4. Medical Services and Resources

The distribution of medical services, particularly general practitioners (GPs), reflects the allocation of healthcare resources across regions. As shown in Figure 10, the explanatory power of the number of GPs per 10,000 people is 0.42, which is statistically significant, indicating that medical services and resources are significant drivers affecting the spatial distribution of NSCCs. A related study analyzed the distribution patterns of GPs, highlighting their importance in ensuring equitable access to health services for populations [63]. Research covering the years 2012 to 2017 examined trends and fairness in the distribution of GPs in China. The study revealed significant nationwide growth in the number of GPs.

However, it also identified a pronounced geographical imbalance in the distribution of GPs, particularly a shortage of doctors in the western regions [64]. This disparity reflects the "more in the East, less in the West" pattern of regional medical resource allocation, which corresponds to the spatial distribution of NSCCs.

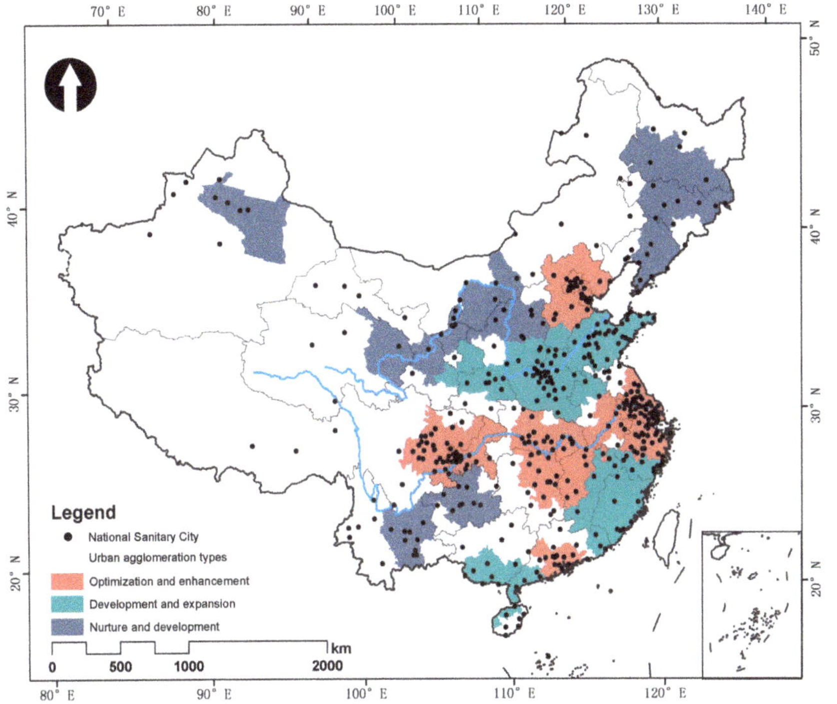

Figure 12. Spatial distribution of NSCCs overlaid with urban agglomerations.

Furthermore, under China's "Hospital Tier Management Standards", hospitals undergo an evaluation process and are classified into three levels, with each further divided into grades A, B, and C; type 3A hospitals represent the highest level of medical service in the country [65]. A spatial overlay analysis of NSCCs with 3A hospitals shows that 6.74% of administrative regions have more than 20 grade 3A hospitals and nearly a quarter of NSCCs are located within these regions, as illustrated in Figure 13. In contrast, 18.33% of administrative regions have no 3A hospitals, and only 6.72% of NSCCs are in these areas. This indicates consistency between the availability of medical services and the spatial distribution of NSCCs. The richness of medical resources, such as the number of 3A hospitals, is correlated with urban health levels. The abundance of high-quality medical resources within a region may be crucial in enhancing urban health standards.

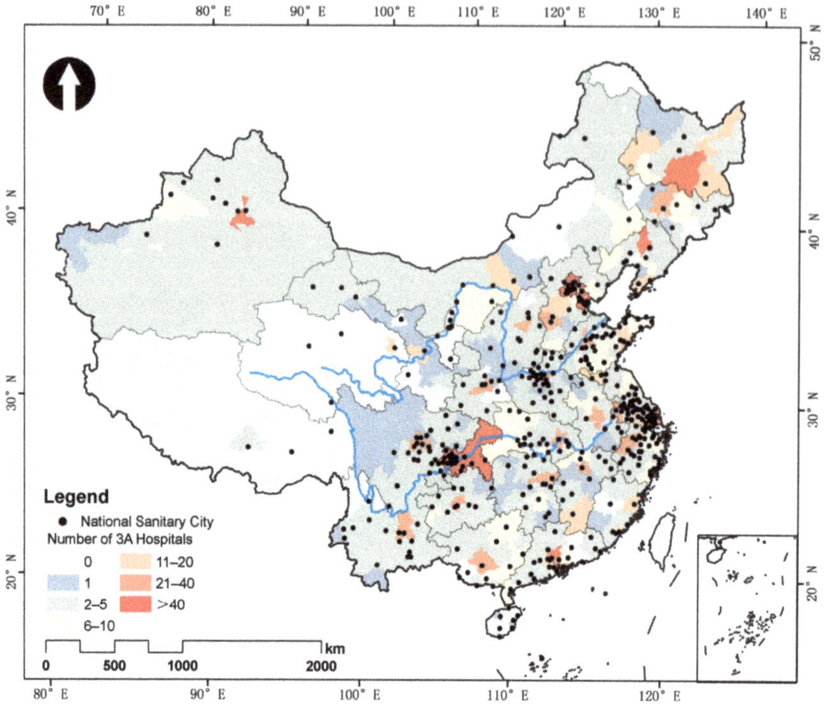

Figure 13. Spatial distribution of NSCCs overlaid with 3A hospitals.

5.2.5. Information Technology and Smart Living

The advancement of information technologies and the development of smart cities have enhanced the digitalization and intelligent management of public health services, improving the efficiency of disease prevention, health monitoring, and medical services and strengthening the emergency response capabilities of urban public health systems. Figure 10 indicates that internet broadband access has an explanatory power of 0.79 and is statistically significant, showing its significant impact on the distribution of NSCCs. Research by Kim et al. (2021) highlighted the effect of broadband internet on supporting informal caregivers by improving access to and the communication of health information, thereby easing their burden and underscoring the importance of addressing disparities in public health and bridging the digital divide [66]. Milinovich et al. (2014) demonstrated that internet searches and social media data can be utilized to monitor infectious diseases, such as influenza and dengue fever. They emphasized the potential of such data collection and analysis to optimize resource allocation and identify epidemic trends, enhancing the response capacity to public health emergencies [67].

In 2012, the State Council issued the "Interim Management Measures for National Smart City Pilot Projects", and, currently, the Ministry of Housing and Urban–Rural Development has announced 290 national-level smart city pilots. Figure 10 shows that the construction of smart cities is closely related to the distribution of NSCCs and is a significant driving factor ($q = 0.54$). Wu et al. (2022) and Wang et al. (2022) indicated that smart cities, by optimizing medical service utilization and significantly reducing haze pollution, not only effectively improve residents' health but also enhance urban environmental quality [68,69]. A systematic review by Rocha et al. (2019) further emphasizes the crucial role of smart city infrastructure in monitoring population health, environmental conditions, and promoting healthy lifestyles [70]. Additionally, the spatial overlay analysis of NSCCs and national-level smart cities, as depicted in Figure 14, shows that 93% of NSCCs are located in provincial administrative regions with more than five national smart cities and 67% in regions with more than ten smart cities. This demonstrates the consistency between the prevalence of smart health facilities and the spatial distribution of NSCCs. Since becoming an NSCC in 1995, Hangzhou's developments in the digital economy and smart city initiatives have significantly driven its progress. Innovations like the "City Brain" monitoring system, the epidemic management platform co-built with Alibaba, and the innovative "Health Code" system have shown effectiveness in controlling COVID-19 infection rates and rapid economic recovery and enhanced the efficiency and dynamic response of public health management [71].

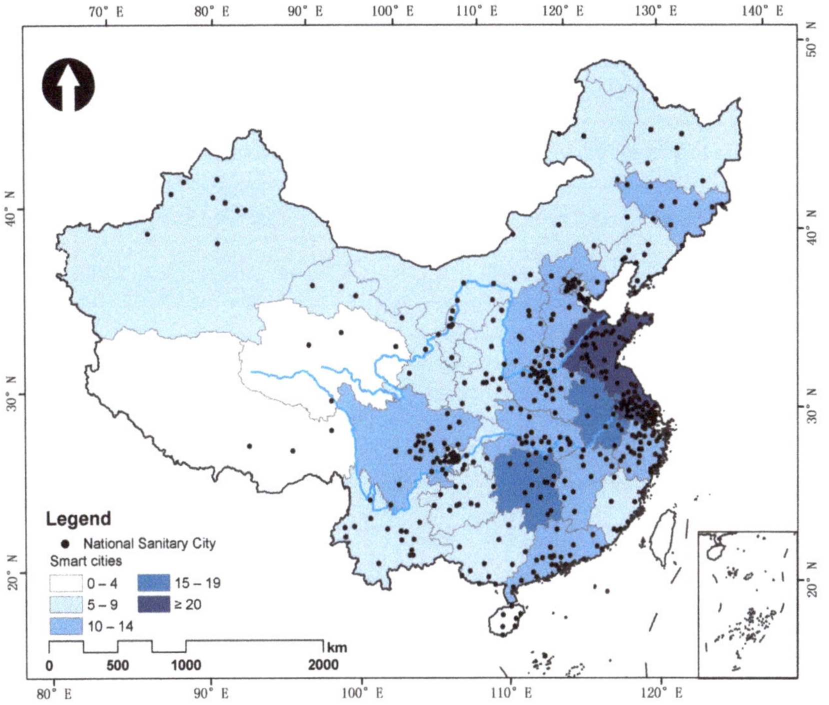

Figure 14. Spatial distribution of NSCCs overlaid with smart cities.

6. Discussion

The NSCC policy, a strategic intervention implemented by the Chinese government, was designed to improve public health and is a key development strategy for achieving health for all within China. After exploring the significance and benefits of the NSCC policy, this study utilized GIS spatial analysis methods and R analytical tools to investigate the spatial distribution of 462 NSCCs in China, as shown in Table 4, and the driving factors behind them. The main research findings are presented below.

Table 4. The spatial indices of NSCCs based on the function calculation.

No.	Function	Index
1	Nearest neighbour index	0.85
2	Geographic concentration index	21.35
3	Imbalance index	0.3525
4	Kernel density estimation	0.20–5.91

This study examined the NSCC policy, a key model of the Health Campaign in China over the past 30 years. The policy's latest criteria promote the integration of health into all policies, emphasizing the incorporation of life-cycle health management in urban planning, construction, and management, signalling a strategic shift toward health-centred development. This comprehensive approach not only strengthens urban resilience against public health challenges but also offers valuable insights for global urban health governance.

The rapid increase in the number of NSCCs highlights China's emphasis on urban health development during the urbanization process. Although the development of NSCCs trends toward regional balance, their current spatial distribution is uneven, with a greater density of NSCCs in the eastern regions compared to the central and western regions. These cities are mostly located in economically developed regions like the Yangtze River Delta and the Beijing–Tianjin–Hebei area, displaying a "two poles, two cores" distribution model. This distribution impacts not only health education and public health facilities but also disease prevention and environmental protection, directly affecting residents' health and quality of life. The geographical imbalance may lead to disparities in access to and the utilization of health resources, resulting in significant health inequalities between cities. For instance, life expectancy varies significantly across China's regions. Residents in the east, particularly in coastal areas, tend to live longer than those in the west. The Yangtze River Delta and Beijing–Tianjin–Hebei urban agglomerations have a higher life expectancy than the national average, while central and western regions generally have lower life expectancy [72]. Additionally, the results of this study demonstrate that the spatial heterogeneity in the distribution of NSCCs is influenced by multiple factors. Natural conditions such as climate and topography contribute to shaping the fundamental distribution patterns, while socioeconomic factors like economic levels, information technology, and population size amplify these imbalances. Among these factors, the disparity in economic levels is a significant factor influencing the uneven spatial distribution of NSCCs. Initially, NSCCs were highly concentrated in the eastern region, likely due to the greater degree of regional development inequality in China [73], with the eastern region being more developed than the central and western regions. However, through the implementation of targeted policies and investments, such as the "Rise of Central China" and "Great Western Development" strategies, the number of NSCCs in the central and western regions has increased significantly. Specifically, the Great Western Development policy notably enhanced the ecological foundation, service capacity, and residents' well-being in cities through systematic interventions, greatly promoting the healthy development of cities in the western region [74,75]. Although the health gap between China's eastern and western regions is narrowing [39], the average level of medical resources in western China is lower than in other regions [76,77]. This aligns with the broader pattern of socioeconomic deprivation in western China [78]. Policymakers and policy implementers should prioritize addressing regional disparities when advancing the development of healthy cities. By optimizing resource allocation strategies, strengthening infrastructure development, and enhancing healthcare service levels, they can promote more balanced urban development.

7. Conclusions

This study began with a qualitative analysis of the origin and criteria of the NSCC policy, emphasizing the importance and significance of its implementation. Subsequently, it quantitatively examined the spatial distribution characteristics and the main driving factors of NSCCs.

The NSCC policy has shifted from initially improving urban sanitation and enhancing public health to now emphasizing the co-construction and sharing of health for all. This evolution not only reflects China's continuous emphasis on strengthening public health services and health infrastructure during urbanization but also demonstrates the government's strategic adjustments in promoting health equity and resource equalization. Moreover, this policy not only improves public health and urban environments but also enhances the efficiency of urban governance and social welfare, offering effective solutions for other high-density cities facing environmental and public safety challenges.

Currently, the spatial distribution of NSCCs is uneven, primarily characterized by significant spatial clustering. Specifically, on a regional scale, it displays two core-density areas and two high-density areas, surrounded by scattered medium- and low-density areas, overall showing a laminar diffusion trend. Nationally, the NSCC distribution in the eastern regions is denser than in the west. Natural and social environmental factors are the main reasons for these policy pattern differences. Topography, climate, and other natural factors affect the spatial distribution of NSCCs to varying degrees. At the same time, socioeconomic factors, urban environments, and healthcare services are significant influencers of their distribution. Although the intent of the NSCC policy is to uniformly strengthen the public health system, the results reveal considerable regional variations. This regional disparity highlights the current policy's limitations in achieving national health equity, particularly as regions with lower socioeconomic development levels face greater challenges.

This study still has many shortcomings. Firstly, this study focused on urban-level analysis, limiting our understanding of the NSCC policy's impact on towns and villages. Future research should examine its influence on counties and towns to assess its effectiveness and mechanisms across different levels. Secondly, this study only analyzed the spatial distribution of NSCCs from a macroscopic perspective. While these methods reveal NSCC spatial patterns and their influencing factors, they emphasize associations rather than causal mechanisms. Thus, future research should include meso- and micro-level analyses, employing advanced methods (such as machine learning) and incorporating longitudinal data to examine the complex dynamics influencing NSCC policy implementation. Additionally, analyzing natural and socio-environmental factors separately may overlook their complex interactions; future research should explore integrated modelling approaches to better understand their impact on NSCCs.

This research not only emphasizes the role of geographical and socioeconomic factors in influencing policy outcomes but also reveals the urgent need for policy adjustments to address these imbalances. These findings provide critical evidence for policymakers and urban planners to improve health equity. Through recognizing the factors affecting the distribution of NSCCs, more refined and comprehensive policy interventions can be formulated based on the specific conditions of different regions. This is crucial for promoting balanced regional development, ensuring that all urban residents have equal access to health resources, and further promoting the sustainable development of urban environments.

Author Contributions: Conceptualization, Jiazhen Zhang and Jun Cai; methodology, Jiazhen Zhang; software, Yujia Deng; data curation, Yujia Deng and Lixia Feng; writing—original draft preparation, Yujia Deng; writing—review and editing, Jeremy Cenci, Jiazhen Zhang and Jun Cai; visualization, Lixia Feng; project administration, Jiazhen Zhang and Jun Cai. All authors have read and agreed to the published version of the manuscript.

Funding: This research was funded by the Sichuan Science and Technology Program, grant number 2025ZNSFSC1183.

Data Availability Statement: Not applicable.

Conflicts of Interest: The authors declare no conflict of interest.

References

1. Kundu, D.; Pandey, A.K. World Urbanisation: Trends and Patterns. In *Developing National Urban Policies: Ways Forward to Green and Smart Cities*; Kundu, D., Sietchiping, R., Kinyanjui, M., Eds.; Springer Nature: Singapore, 2020; pp. 13–49, ISBN 978-981-15-3738-7.
2. Singh, N.; Singh, S.; Mall, R.K. Chapter 17–Urban Ecology and Human Health: Implications of Urban Heat Island, Air Pollution and Climate Change Nexus. In *Urban Ecology*; Verma, P., Singh, P., Singh, R., Raghubanshi, A.S., Eds.; Elsevier: Amsterdam, The Netherlands, 2020; pp. 317–334, ISBN 978-0-12-820730-7.
3. Chaudhry, D. Climate Change and Health of the Urban Poor: The Role of Environmental Justice. *J. Clim. Change Health* **2024**, *15*, 100277. [CrossRef]
4. Mouratidis, K. Urban Planning and Quality of Life: A Review of Pathways Linking the Built Environment to Subjective Well-Being. *Cities* **2021**, *115*, 103229. [CrossRef]
5. McGreevy, M.; Harris, P.; Delaney-Crowe, T.; Fisher, M.; Sainsbury, P.; Riley, E.; Baum, F. How Well Do Australian Government Urban Planning Policies Respond to the Social Determinants of Health and Health Equity? *Land Use Policy* **2020**, *99*, 105053. [CrossRef]
6. Li, X.; Song, J.; Lin, T.; Dixon, J.; Zhang, G.; Ye, H. Urbanization and Health in China, Thinking at the National, Local and Individual Levels. *Environ. Health* **2016**, *15*, 113–123. [CrossRef] [PubMed]
7. Du, P.; Sun, B.; Pan, L.J.; Cheng, Y.B.; Li, T.T.; Wang, X.L.; Shi, L.W.; Yao, X.Y.; Shi, X.M. Achievements and Prospects on Environmental Health and Sanitary Engineering in China. *Zhonghua Yu Fang Yi Xue Za Zhi Chin. J. Prev. Med.* **2019**, *53*, 865–870. [CrossRef]
8. Li, Y.; Yang, H. The Incentive Effect of Creating a National Health City on the Ecological Welfare Performance: Based on the Evidence of Yangtze River Delta in China. *Environ. Sci. Pollut. Res.* **2023**, *30*, 83735–83759. [CrossRef]
9. Yin, S.; Chen, W.Y.; Liu, C. Urban Forests as a Strategy for Transforming towards Healthy Cities. *Urban. For. Urban. Green.* **2023**, *81*, 127871. [CrossRef]
10. Palutturi, S.; Saleh, L.M.; Rachmat, M.; Malek, J.A.; Nam, E.W. Principles and Strategies for Aisles Communities Empowerment in Creating Makassar Healthy City, Indonesia. *Gac. Sanit.* **2021**, *35*, S46–S48. [CrossRef]
11. Bafarasat, A.; Cheshmehzangi, A.; Ankowska, A. A Set of 99 Healthy City Indicators for Application in Urban Planning and Design. *Sustain. Dev.* **2023**, *31*, 1978–1989. [CrossRef]
12. Zhao, M.; Qin, W.; Zhang, S.; Qi, F.; Li, X.; Lan, X. Assessing the Construction of a Healthy City in China: A Conceptual Framework and Evaluation Index System. *Public Health* **2023**, *220*, 88–95. [CrossRef]
13. Ali, M.; Rahaman, M.; Hossain, S. Urban Green Spaces for Elderly Human Health: A Planning Model for Healthy City Living. *Land Use Policy* **2022**, *114*, 105970. [CrossRef]
14. Capolongo, S.; Rebecchi, A.; Dettori, M.; Appolloni, L.; Azara, A.; Buffoli, M.; Capasso, L.; Casuccio, A.; Conti, G.; D'Amico, A.; et al. Healthy Design and Urban Planning Strategies, Actions, and Policy to Achieve Salutogenic Cities. *Int. J. Environ. Res. Public Health* **2018**, *15*, 2698. [CrossRef]
15. Xie, Y.; Meng, X.; Cenci, J.; Zhang, J. Spatial Pattern and Formation Mechanism of Rural Tourism Resources in China: Evidence from 1470 National Leisure Villages. *ISPRS Int. J. Geo-Inf.* **2022**, *11*, 455. [CrossRef]
16. Zhang, Z.; Cenci, J.; Zhang, J. Policies for Equity in Access to Urban Green Space: A Spatial Perspective of the Chinese National Forest City Policy. *Forests* **2024**, *15*, 608. [CrossRef]
17. Tao, W.; Zeng, Z.; Dang, H.; Li, P.; Chuong, L.; Yue, D.; Wen, J.; Zhao, R.; Li, W.; Kominski, G. Towards Universal Health Coverage: Achievements and Challenges of 10 Years of Healthcare Reform in China. *BMJ Glob. Health* **2020**, *5*, e002087. [CrossRef] [PubMed]
18. Chen, J.; Lin, Z.; Li, L.; Li, J.; Wang, Y.; Pan, Y.; Yang, J.; Xu, C.; Zeng, X.; Xie, X.; et al. Ten Years of China's New Healthcare Reform: A Longitudinal Study on Changes in Health Resources. *BMC Public Health* **2021**, *21*, 2272. [CrossRef] [PubMed]
19. Fu, H.; Dai, J.; Gao, J.; Jia, Y.; Zheng, P. Healthy City Construction in China: Accomplishments and Prospects. *Chin. J. Public Health* **2019**, *35*, 1285–1288. [CrossRef]

20. Liu, S.R.; Wang, H.; Xi, T.Y. Administrative Bidding, Performance, and Political Incentives——Evidence from National Health Cities. *J. Public Manag.* **2020**, *17*, 10–20. [CrossRef]
21. Bai, Y.; Zhang, Y.; Zotova, O.; Pineo, H.; Siri, J.; Liang, L.; Luo, X.; Kwan, M.-P.; Ji, J.; Jiang, X.; et al. Healthy Cities Initiative in China: Progress, Challenges, and the Way Forward. *Lancet Reg. Health West. Pac.* **2022**, *27*, 100539. [CrossRef]
22. Announcement of the 2021 National Sanitary City and Town Reassessment Results by the National Patriotic Health Campaign Committee. Available online: http://www.nhc.gov.cn/guihuaxxs/gongwen1/202202/253a2c03dbee4cf9a952238236fda163.shtml (accessed on 7 August 2024).
23. Zheng, W.; Yao, H.; Yu, S.; Liu, J.; Hu, Y.; Wang, J. Residents' Sense of Acquisition and Influencing Factors in China's Sanitary City Initiative. *Chin. J. Epidemiol.* **2023**, *44*, 457–462. [CrossRef]
24. Wang, Y.; Pei, R.; Gu, X.; Liu, B.; Liu, L. Has the Healthy City Pilot Policy Improved Urban Health Development Performance in China? Evidence from a Quasi-Natural Experiment. *Sustain. Cities Soc.* **2023**, *88*, 104268. [CrossRef]
25. Tang, G.; Lin, M.; Xu, Y.; Li, J.; Chen, L. Impact of Rating and Praise Campaigns on Local Government Environmental Governance Efficiency: Evidence from the Campaign of Establishment of National Sanitary Cities in China. *PLoS ONE* **2021**, *16*, e0253703. [CrossRef]
26. Yue, D.; Ruan, S.; Xu, J.; Zhu, W.; Zhang, L.; Cheng, G.; Meng, Q. Impact of the China Healthy Cities Initiative on Urban Environment. *J. Urban Health* **2017**, *94*, 149–157. [CrossRef] [PubMed]
27. Gan, T.; Zhang, C.; Shen, R.; Li, B. Can the Establishment of National Sanitary Cities Better Resist the Impact of COVID-19? *Front. Public Health* **2023**, *11*, 1041355. [CrossRef]
28. Zhou, M.; Wang, H.; Zeng, X.; Yin, P.; Zhu, J.; Chen, W.; Li, X.; Wang, L.; Wang, L.; Liu, Y.; et al. Mortality, Morbidity, and Risk Factors in China and Its Provinces, 1990–2017: A Systematic Analysis for the Global Burden of Disease Study 2017. *Lancet* **2019**, *394*, 1145–1158. [CrossRef] [PubMed]
29. Barber, R.M.; Fullman, N.; Sorensen, R.J.D.; Bollyky, T.; McKee, M.; Nolte, E.; Abajobir, A.A.; Abate, K.H.; Abbafati, C.; Abbas, K.M.; et al. Healthcare Access and Quality Index Based on Mortality from Causes Amenable to Personal Health Care in 195 Countries and Territories, 1990–2015: A Novel Analysis from the Global Burden of Disease Study 2015. *Lancet* **2017**, *390*, 231–266. [CrossRef]
30. The 2023 Statistical Bulletin on the Development of China's Health Sector. Available online: https://www.gov.cn/lianbo/bumen/202408/content_6971241.htm (accessed on 4 September 2024).
31. Yang, G. What Is Historical Political Science? *Chin. Political Sci. Rev.* **2022**, *7*, 1–28. [CrossRef]
32. Feng, D.; Bao, W.; Yang, Y.; Fu, M. How Do Government Policies Promote Greening? Evidence from China. *Land Use Policy* **2021**, *104*, 105389. [CrossRef]
33. Ding, A.; Cenci, J.; Zhang, J. Links between the Pandemic and Urban Green Spaces, a Perspective on Spatial Indices of Landscape Garden Cities in China. *Sustain. Cities Soc.* **2022**, *85*, 104046. [CrossRef]
34. Dumais, G.; Ellison, G.; Glaeser, E.L. Geographic Concentration as a Dynamic Process. *Rev. Econ. Stat.* **2002**, *84*, 193–204. [CrossRef]
35. Zhang, J.; Cenci, J.; Becue, V.; Koutra, S. Research of the Industrial Heritage Category and Spatial Density Distribution in Walloon Region and Northeast China. *WIT Trans. Built Environ.* **2021**, *203*, 285. [CrossRef]
36. Wang, X.; Zhang, J.; Cenci, J.; Becue, V. Spatial Distribution Characteristics and Influencing Factors of the World Architectural Heritage. *Heritage* **2021**, *4*, 2942–2959. [CrossRef]
37. Song, Y.; Wang, J.; Ge, Y.; Xu, C. An Optimal Parameters-Based Geographical Detector Model Enhances Geographic Characteristics of Explanatory Variables for Spatial Heterogeneity Analysis: Cases with Different Types of Spatial Data. *GI Sci. Remote Sens.* **2020**, *57*, 593–610. [CrossRef]
38. Yang, Y.; Zhang, L.; Zhang, X.; Yang, M.; Zou, W. Efficiency Measurement and Spatial Spillover Effect of Provincial Health Systems in China: Based on the Two-Stage Network DEA Model. *Front. Public Health* **2022**, *10*, 952975. [CrossRef]
39. Wang, K.; Zhang, Q.; Zhang, J. Analysis on Spatial Differences and Changes of Health Level in China. *Adv. Appl. Math.* **2022**, *11*, 7524–7532. [CrossRef]
40. Ziafati Bafarasat, A.; Sharifi, A. How to Achieve a Healthy City: A Scoping Review with Ten City Examples. *J. Urban Health* **2024**, *101*, 120–140. [CrossRef]
41. Xie, S.; Yin, G.; Wei, W.; Sun, Q.; Zhang, Z. Spatial–Temporal Change in Paddy Field and Dryland in Different Topographic Gradients: A Case Study of China during 1990–2020. *Land* **2022**, *11*, 1851. [CrossRef]
42. Wang, X.-C.; Klemeš, J.J.; Dong, X.; Fan, W.; Xu, Z.; Wang, Y.; Varbanov, P.S. Air Pollution Terrain Nexus: A Review Considering Energy Generation and Consumption. *Renew. Sustain. Energy Rev.* **2019**, *105*, 71–85. [CrossRef]
43. Xi, C.; Qian, T.; Chi, Y.; Chen, J.; Wang, J. Relationship between Settlements and Topographical Factors: An Example from Sichuan Province, China. *J. Mt. Sci.* **2018**, *15*, 2043–2054. [CrossRef]
44. Chen, R.; Yin, P.; Wang, L.; Liu, C.; Niu, Y.; Wang, W.; Jiang, Y.; Liu, Y.; Liu, J.; Qi, J.; et al. Association between Ambient Temperature and Mortality Risk and Burden: Time Series Study in 272 Main Chinese Cities. *BMJ* **2018**, *363*, k4306. [CrossRef]

45. Yao, N.; Li, Y.; Lei, T.; Peng, L. Drought Evolution, Severity and Trends in Mainland China over 1961–2013. *Sci. Total Environ.* **2018**, *616–617*, 73–89. [CrossRef] [PubMed]
46. Liu, J.; Liu, T.; Burkart, K.G.; Wang, H.; He, G.; Hu, J.; Xiao, J.; Yin, P.; Wang, L.; Liang, X.; et al. Mortality Burden Attributable to High and Low Ambient Temperatures in China and Its Provinces: Results from the Global Burden of Disease Study 2019. *Lancet Reg. Health West. Pac.* **2022**, *24*, 100493. [CrossRef] [PubMed]
47. Gao, W. A Case Study of the Relationship Between Vegetation Coverage and Urban Heat Island in a Coastal City by Applying Digital Twins. *Front. Plant Sci.* **2022**, *13*, 861768.
48. Zhou, M.; Huang, Y.; Li, G. Changes in the Concentration of Air Pollutants before and after the COVID-19 Blockade Period and Their Correlation with Vegetation Coverage. *Environ. Sci. Pollut. Res.* **2021**, *28*, 23405–23419. [CrossRef] [PubMed]
49. Crane, M.; Lloyd, S.; Haines, A.; Ding, D.; Hutchinson, E.; Belesova, K.; Davies, M.; Osrin, D.; Zimmermann, N.; Capon, A.; et al. Transforming Cities for Sustainability: A Health Perspective. *Environ. Int.* **2021**, *147*, 106366. [CrossRef]
50. Johnston, B.M.; Burke, S.; Kavanagh, P.M.; O'Sullivan, C.; Thomas, S.; Parker, S. Moving beyond Formulae: A Review of International Population-Based Resource Allocation Policy and Implications for Ireland in an Era of Healthcare Reform. *HRB Open Res.* **2021**, *4*, 121. [CrossRef]
51. Marmot, M. Health Equity in England: The Marmot Review 10 Years On. *BMJ* **2020**, *368*, m693. [CrossRef]
52. Bellini, P.; Nesi, P.; Pantaleo, G. IoT-Enabled Smart Cities: A Review of Concepts, Frameworks and Key Technologies. *Appl. Sci.* **2022**, *12*, 1607. [CrossRef]
53. Wan, S.; Chen, Y.; Xiao, Y.; Zhao, Q.; Li, M.; Wu, S. Spatial Analysis and Evaluation of Medical Resource Allocation in China Based on Geographic Big Data. *BMC Health Serv. Res.* **2021**, *21*, 1084. [CrossRef]
54. You, H.; Wu, X.; Guo, X. Distribution of COVID-19 Morbidity Rate in Association with Social and Economic Factors in Wuhan, China: Implications for Urban Development. *Int. J. Environ. Res. Public Health* **2020**, *17*, 3417. [CrossRef]
55. Smith, S.A.; Mays, G.P.; Felix, H.C.; Tilford, J.M.; Curran, G.M.; Preston, M.A. Impact of Economic Constraints on Public Health Delivery Systems Structures. *Am. J. Public Health* **2015**, *105*, e48–e53. [CrossRef] [PubMed]
56. Ma, X.; Bai, Y.; Zhang, Z. Spatial Matching Analysis of Urban Health Resources and Population Distribution--A Case Study of the Central District of Lanzhou City. *Resour. Dev. Mark. Chin. J.* **2023**, *39*, 1619–1627. [CrossRef]
57. Tan, X. Explaining Provincial Government Health Expenditures in China: Evidence from Panel Data 2007–2013. *China Financ. Econ. Rev.* **2017**, *5*, 9. [CrossRef]
58. Zhang, D.; Rahman, K.M.A. Government Health Expenditure, OUT-OF-POCKET Payment and Social Inequality: A CROSS-NATIONAL Analysis of China and OECD Countries. *Int. J. Health Plan. Manag.* **2020**, *35*, 1111–1126. [CrossRef]
59. Zhang, J.; Chang, Y.; Zhang, L.; Li, D. Do Technological Innovations Promote Urban Green Development?—A Spatial Econometric Analysis of 105 Cities in China. *J. Clean. Prod.* **2018**, *182*, 395–403. [CrossRef]
60. Hu, F.; Qiu, L.; Xiang, Y.; Wei, S.; Sun, H.; Hu, H.; Weng, X.; Mao, L.; Zeng, M. Spatial Network and Driving Factors of Low-Carbon Patent Applications in China from a Public Health Perspective. *Front. Public Health* **2023**, *11*, 1121860. [CrossRef]
61. 14th Five-Year Plan for the National Economic and Social Development of the People's Republic of China and the Long-Range Objectives Through the Year 2035. Available online: http://www.gjbmj.gov.cn/n1/2021/0315/c409080-32051071.html (accessed on 15 August 2024).
62. Zhu, J.; Chertow, M.R. Greening Industrial Production through Waste Recovery: "Comprehensive Utilization of Resources" in China. *Environ. Sci. Technol.* **2016**, *50*, 2175–2182. [CrossRef] [PubMed]
63. Shu, Z.; Wang, Z.; Chen, R.; Li, M.; Lou, J.; Huang, X.; Wu, J.; Jing, L. Allocation and Development of the General Practitioner Workforce in China from 2012 to 2015: A Literature Review. *Lancet* **2017**, *390*, S91. [CrossRef]
64. Yu, Q.; Yin, W.; Huang, D.; Sun, K.; Chen, Z.; Guo, H.; Wu, D. Trend and Equity of General Practitioners' Allocation in China Based on the Data from 2012–2017. *Hum. Resour. Health* **2021**, *19*, 20. [CrossRef]
65. Liu, H.; Fang, C.; Fan, Y. Mapping the Inequalities of Medical Resource Provision in China. *Reg. Stud. Reg. Sci.* **2020**, *7*, 568–570. [CrossRef]
66. Kim, H.; Mahmood, A.; Goldsmith, J.V.; Chang, H.; Kedia, S.; Chang, C.F. Access to Broadband Internet and Its Utilization for Health Information Seeking and Health Communication among Informal Caregivers in the United States. *J. Med. Syst.* **2021**, *45*, 24. [CrossRef] [PubMed]
67. Milinovich, G.J.; Williams, G.M.; Clements, A.C.A.; Hu, W. Internet-Based Surveillance Systems for Monitoring Emerging Infectious Diseases. *Lancet Infect. Dis.* **2014**, *14*, 160–168. [CrossRef]
68. Wu, W.; Zhu, D.; Liu, W.; Wu, C.-H. Empirical Research on Smart City Construction and Public Health under Information and Communications Technology. *Socioecon. Plann. Sci.* **2022**, *80*, 100994. [CrossRef]
69. Wang, L.; Xie, Q.; Xue, F.; Li, Z. Does Smart City Construction Reduce Haze Pollution? *Int. J. Environ. Res. Public Health* **2022**, *19*, 16421. [CrossRef] [PubMed]
70. Rocha, N.P.; Dias, A.; Santinha, G.; Rodrigues, M.; Queirós, A.; Rodrigues, C. Smart Cities and Public Health: A Systematic Review. *Procedia Comput. Sci.* **2019**, *164*, 516–523. [CrossRef]

71. Zhao, W.; Zou, Y. Smart Urban Governance in Epidemic Control: Practices and Implications of Hangzhou. *Chin. Public Adm. Rev.* **2021**, *12*, 51–60. [CrossRef]
72. Zhang, Z.; Huang, Q.; Lu, Y.; Li, M.; Chen, Z.; LI, F. Analysis of Life Expectancy and the Spatial Differences of Its Influencing Factors of Chinese Residents. *J. Geo-Inf. Sci.* **2021**, *23*, 1575–1585. [CrossRef]
73. Jain-Chandra, M.S.; Khor, N.; Mano, R.; Schauer, J.; Wingender, M.P.; Zhuang, J. *Inequality in China–Trends, Drivers and Policy Remedies*; International Monetary Fund: Washington, DC, USA, 2018; ISBN 1-4843-5753-1.
74. Zhong, D.; Lu, Q.; Zhang, Y.; Li, J.; Lei, T.; Liu, C. How a Poverty Alleviation Policy Affected Comprehensive Disaster Risk Reduction Capacity: Evidence from China's Great Western Development Policy. *Int. J. Disaster Risk Reduct.* **2024**, *111*, 104656. [CrossRef]
75. Yang, F.; Yang, M.; Xue, B.; Luo, Q. The Effects of China's Western Development Strategy Implementation on Local Ecological Economic Performance. *J. Clean. Prod.* **2018**, *202*, 925–933. [CrossRef]
76. Pan, J.; Shallcross, D. Geographic Distribution of Hospital Beds throughout China: A County-Level Econometric Analysis. *Int. J. Equity Health* **2016**, *15*, 179. [CrossRef]
77. Zhang, X.; Zhao, L.; Cui, Z.; Wang, Y. Study on Equity and Efficiency of Health Resources and Services Based on Key Indicators in China. *PLoS ONE* **2015**, *10*, e0144809. [CrossRef] [PubMed]
78. Liu, Y.; Rao, K.; Wu, J.; Gakidou, E. China's Health System Performance. *Lancet* **2008**, *372*, 1914–1923. [CrossRef] [PubMed]

International Journal of
Geo-Information

MDPI

Article

Unveiling the Spatial Inequality of Accessibility to High-Quality Healthcare Resources in the Beijing–Tianjin–Hebei Urban Agglomeration of China: A Focus on the Impacts of Intercity Patient Mobility

Yandi Wang †, Lin Chen †, Binglin Liu and Zhuolin Tao *

Faculty of Geographical Science, Beijing Normal University, Beijing 100875, China;
202111051052@mail.bnu.edu.cn (Y.W.); 202111051014@mail.bnu.edu.cn (L.C.);
202011010128@mail.bnu.edu.cn (B.L.)
* Correspondence: taozhuolin@bnu.edu.cn
† These authors contributed equally to this work.

Abstract: The equality of accessibility to high-quality healthcare resources is an important issue in the development of urban agglomerations. However, comprehensive consideration of the impacts of intercity patient mobility and multilevel transportation networks is still lacking. This study develops a novel directional two-step floating catchment area method for measuring spatial accessibility to high-quality hospitals in the Beijing–Tianjin–Hebei (BTH) urban agglomeration. This method emphasizes the direction of intercity patient mobility caused by the hierarchy of high-quality healthcare resource distributions. Empirical analyses were conducted based on subdistrict-level population census data in 2020, 3-A hospital data from healthcare commissions, and door-to-door travel time data via multilevel intercity transportation networks from online maps in 2023. The analyses revealed obvious spatial inequalities in accessibility to high-quality healthcare resources in the BTH urban agglomeration, which is primarily caused by intercity inequality. Intercity patient mobility, however, can significantly mitigate the spatial inequality of healthcare accessibility within the BTH urban agglomeration. Moreover, it was determined that intracity first-mile and last-mile transfer transportation is the major barrier to intercity healthcare seeking and accessibility. This study has valuable implications for the planning and management of high-quality healthcare resources and intercity patient mobility in the BTH urban agglomeration. The developed methods are useful for measuring healthcare accessibility and inequality at the urban agglomeration scale.

Keywords: high-quality healthcare resources; accessibility; equality; urban agglomeration; intercity patient mobility

1. Introduction

Good health is at the core of basic human needs, and as such, it has gained increasing attention as socioeconomic development has continued to progress. "Good health and well-being" is highlighted as one of the 17 Sustainable Development Goals adopted by the United Nations [1]. Among the diverse determinants of health, healthcare services are of great importance and have drawn extensive attention. Access to healthcare services can be interpreted from various dimensions, e.g., accessibility, availability, accommodation, affordability, and acceptability (the five "A"s) [2]. According to the conceptual framework of Khan [3], spatial accessibility integrates the accessibility and availability dimensions, whereas aspatial accessibility refers mainly to the other three dimensions. From a spatial perspective, residents must overcome a certain distance impedance via certain transport modes to access healthcare services, the ease of which can be captured by the concept of spatial accessibility [4,5].

Spatial accessibility has been widely applied as a useful tool for evaluating the spatial configuration of healthcare and other types of services, and various methods have been developed [6–9]. Among these methods, the two-step floating catchment area (2SFCA) method has been widely applied and extended [10,11]. The inequality of spatial accessibility has been widely adopted as an operational definition and measurement of the spatial inequity of healthcare services [12,13]. Since the spatial accessibility measured using the 2SFCA method can be interpreted as potential opportunities for healthcare services per person, the inequality of spatial accessibility can directly represent the inequality of opportunities [14]. Existing studies have recognized the existence of inequality in healthcare services at various spatial scales, e.g., the city scale [15,16], the provincial scale [17,18], the national scale [19–21], the (sub-)continental scale [22,23], and even the global scale [24].

The supply of and demand for healthcare services are closely associated with the processes and patterns of urbanization. In the global context, an emerging phenomenon is that urbanized areas spread beyond the boundaries of cities, and multiple parts of urbanized areas are connected by intense socioeconomic interactions [25]. This phenomenon was first observed by Gottman [26] in the development of the concept of a metropolis. Several similar concepts have been adopted by researchers around the world, including the global city-region [27] and the megaregion [28] in the U.S. context, the polycentric urban region [29] and megacity region [25] in the European context, and the Desakota region [30] in the Asian context. In China, the concept of urban agglomeration has been proposed and widely applied in academic studies and planning practices [31]. In the National New-type Urbanization Plan issued by the central government of China [32], urban agglomerations have been endowed with the critical role of "the main form of urbanization". Owing to the intense flows of people, goods, and information between cities, transport accessibility and mobility within urban agglomerations have drawn extensive attention [33–36]. Rail, especially high-speed rail, is considered a promising and efficient solution for intercity transportation at the urban agglomeration scale [37,38].

With the emergence of urban agglomerations, the spatial accessibility of healthcare services and its inequality at the urban agglomeration scale has attracted increasing attention. Existing studies have revealed an uneven distribution of healthcare resources across cities [39,40]. Additionally, regional disparities in healthcare resources require patients to move across administrative boundaries to meet their needs, which is captured by the concept of patient mobility [41,42]. Previous studies have focused on the spatial patterns and determinants of intercity patient mobility [42–45]. A recent study demonstrated that intercity patient mobility can improve spatial accessibility to both existing and optimized high-quality healthcare resources within an urban agglomeration [46]. Furthermore, there is a tendency for core cities with more high-quality healthcare resources to offer more services to patients, which has an impact on healthcare accessibility at the urban agglomeration scale [47]. Intercity transportation (including rail) has significant impacts on the inequality of healthcare accessibility [48]. However, there is still a research gap with respect to the direction of intercity patient mobility and its impacts on the inequality of accessibility to healthcare resources at the urban agglomeration scale.

Therefore, the aim of this study is to develop a novel method for measuring spatial accessibility to healthcare services at the urban agglomeration scale. The proposed method makes marginal methodological improvements from two aspects. First, this method considers the hierarchy of high-quality healthcare services and the direction of intercity patient mobility. Second, it emphasizes the role of multilevel rail transportation networks in supporting intercity patient mobility. The Beijing–Tianjin–Hebei urban agglomeration, one of the largest urban agglomerations in China, was selected as the study area to illustrate the applicability of the proposed method.

2. Methods and Data

2.1. Study Area and Data Sources

The Beijing–Tianjin–Hebei (BTH) urban agglomeration is one of the largest and most developed urban agglomerations in China. It consists of one province (Hebei) and two provincial-level cities directly governed by the central government (Beijing and Tianjin), with a total area of 218 thousand km^2 and a population of 109.7 million. Beijing is the capital of China. Hebei Province consists of 11 prefecture-level cities, with Shijiazhuang as the provincial capital.

In China, hospitals are divided into three levels, i.e., tertiary, secondary, and primary hospitals. Each grade is further classified into three classes (A, B, and C). According to this official classification system, Grade 3 (tertiary) Class A hospitals (3-A hospitals hereafter) are widely perceived to be high-quality hospitals in China [40]. In addition, public hospitals play a vital role in the Chinese healthcare service system with respect to healthcare resources and both outpatient and inpatient services [49]. Therefore, high-quality healthcare services are represented by public 3-A hospitals. The names, addresses, and numbers of physicians and beds of 162 public 3-A hospitals were collected from the Health Commission of each city in the BTH urban agglomeration in 2023. This is an official and reliable source of hospital data in China. The spatial distribution of these 3-A hospitals is shown in Figure 1.

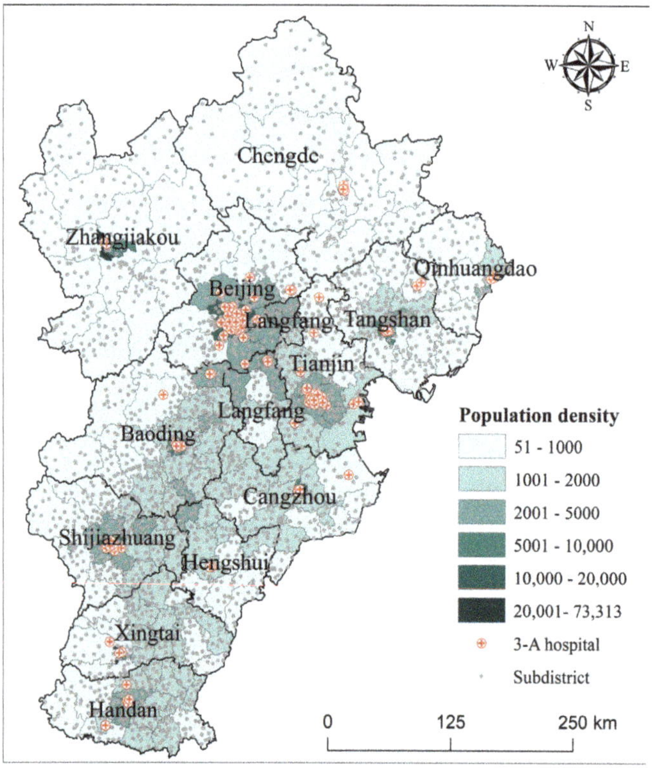

Figure 1. The distribution of subdistrict-level population density and healthcare facilities.

The town-level population data were obtained from the Seventh National Population Census of China in 2020, which is the most reliable population data source in China. These data are the latest official population census data, and town-level data are the finest census data that can be publicly accessed. There were 2987 town-level units (subdistricts hereafter) in total, including towns in rural areas and jiedaos in urban areas.

Travel time estimations rely on multisource data. The travel times between railway stations were collected from schedules on the 12306 platform (www.12306.cn (accessed on 1–15 November 2023)), the official railway ticket booking platform in China. The travel times to/from railway stations via driving or public transit were collected by leveraging the navigation application programming interface (API) of Baidu Map. This approach has been widely applied in travel time estimations owing to its comprehensive consideration of real-time traffic congestion, first-mile and last-mile walking times, transfer times, and public transit service frequencies [50].

2.2. The Directional Two-Step Floating Catchment Area Method

To improve the estimation of spatial accessibility, researchers have developed a multitude of methods, some of which include the shortest travel time method, which measures the shortest travel time from each location to the closest facility [24]; the supply-to-demand ratio method, which calculates the ratio of service supply to demand within given boundaries [19]; and the cumulative opportunities method, which sums the number of facilities within a certain travel time threshold [51]. However, these methods fail to account for the complex interactions between service supply and population demand [5,52]. The popular gravity-based methods are superior in terms of integrating accessibility and availability [53], whereas the two-step floating catchment area (2SFCA) method, which was initiated by Radke and Mu [54] and refined by Luo and Wang [10], is a popular variant of the gravity model. Owing to its understandability, the 2SFCA method has been widely applied and extended [11]. Dozens of studies have contributed methodological developments to the gravity and 2SFCA framework [53], e.g., incorporating additional distance decay functions [55,56] or variable catchment areas [57,58], considering multiple transportation modes [59,60], improving the modeling of competition effects [60–62], and incorporating actual utilization behaviors [63,64].

At the urban agglomeration scale, high-quality healthcare resources are concentrated in central cities, thus facilitating patients' travel across cities to obtain healthcare services [48]. To obtain a full picture of healthcare accessibility in an urban agglomeration, it is necessary to consider the possibility that patients might visit healthcare facilities in other cities. In other words, intercity patient mobility should be considered in the measurement of healthcare accessibility [46,48]. In existing studies, however, an unrealistic assumption was made that patients are able to select healthcare facilities located in any city within the urban agglomeration. In fact, the distribution of high-quality healthcare resources across various cities in an urban agglomeration is hierarchical, with more resources concentrated in central cities [40]. As a result, patients do not consider hospitals in all cities when seeking high-quality healthcare resources beyond the city in which they reside (or their home city). Instead, intercity patient flows should be hierarchical and directional, namely, from cities with less high-quality healthcare resources to cities with more high-quality healthcare resources [44,45,47].

According to the administrative grades of cities and quantities of high-quality healthcare resources, the cities in the BTH urban agglomeration can be classified into 4 grades (Figure 2). From highest to lowest, there is only one Grade 4 city, Beijing, where high-quality healthcare resources are the most concentrated. Existing studies have demonstrated the central role of Beijing in the country-wide intercity patient mobility network [65]. Grade

3 also includes only one city, Tianjin, which is a provincial-level city. The economic development level and quantity of 3-A hospitals are greater than those of other cities in the BTH urban agglomeration but lower than those in Beijing. Grade 2 includes two cities, Shijiazhuang and Baoding. Shijiazhuang is the current provincial capital of Hebei Province, while Baoding was the former provincial capital.

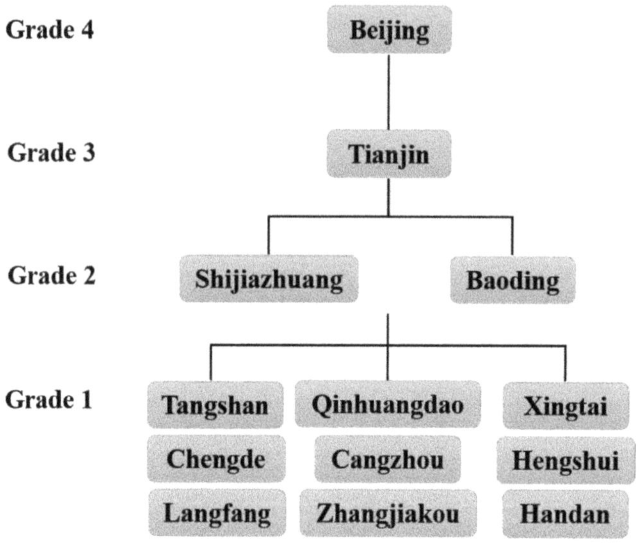

Figure 2. Hierarchy of cities in terms of the provision of high-quality healthcare resources.

In the traditional 2SFCA method, the interactions between demand and supply are restricted within the catchment area, which is usually defined as a certain travel time threshold. To account for the hierarchy and direction of patient mobility in an urban agglomeration, this study develops an extended 2SFCA method, termed the directional two-step floating catchment area (D2SFCA) method. The rationale of the D2SFCA method can be demonstrated via a two-step procedure. In the first step, the resources of each facility are allocated to all potential demand units located in the same city or in lower-grade cities. The supply–demand ratio is calculated for each facility using the following equation:

$$R_j = \frac{S_j}{\sum_{k\in\{q|C_q=C_j,\ g(C_q)<g(C_j)\}} P_k f\left(t_{kj}\right)} \quad (1)$$

where R_j is the supply–demand ratio of facility j, measured in beds per person; S_j is the supply size of facility j, represented by the number of beds; P_k is the demand size of the demand unit (subdistrict) k, represented by the age structure-adjusted population [46]; t_{kj} is the travel time from demand unit k to facility j; f is the distance decay function; C_q (C_j) denotes the city where demand unit q (facility j) is located; and function g defines the grade of the city.

In the second step, the accessibility of each unit can be calculated by summing the supply–demand ratios of all potential facilities, which can be expressed as follows:

$$A_i = \sum_{j\in\{r|C_r=C_i,\ g(C_r)>g(C_i)\}} R_j f\left(t_{ij}\right) \quad (2)$$

where A_i is the accessibility score of demand unit i; C_r denotes the city where facility r is located; and the other variables are the same as those in Equation (1). In the application of the 2SFCA method, various forms of distance decay functions have been introduced into the model, including power functions, exponential function, Kernel density functions and Gaussian functions [11]. In this study, the catchment area of each facility is determined according to the grades of the cities in the regional healthcare service system rather than according to a given threshold of travel time. Existing studies have shown that the power function outperforms other functions in modeling actual healthcare-seeking behaviors at the intercity scale in China [17]. Therefore, the distance decay function assumes a power function form in this study, which can be expressed as follows:

$$f\left(t_{ij}\right) = {t_{ij}}^{\beta} \quad (3)$$

where β is the parameter of the power function and the other variables are the same as those in Equation (1). As estimated by existing studies [17], the distance decay parameter β is approximately -1 for tertiary healthcare-seeking behaviors in Hubei Province, China, the spatial scale of which is similar to that of the BTH urban agglomeration. Therefore, β is set as -1 in this study.

2.3. Estimating Travel Time via a Multilevel Transportation Network

A challenge regarding the measurement of healthcare accessibility in urban agglomerations is the estimation of travel time. Urban agglomerations commonly feature multilevel transportation networks, including regional railways, urban metro lines, bus lines and road networks. As depicted in Figure 3, when regional railways are considered, each intercity travel to hospitals across city boundaries can be divided into three phases, i.e., home-city travel from home to railway stations, intercity travel between two railway stations, and destination-city travel from railway stations to hospitals.

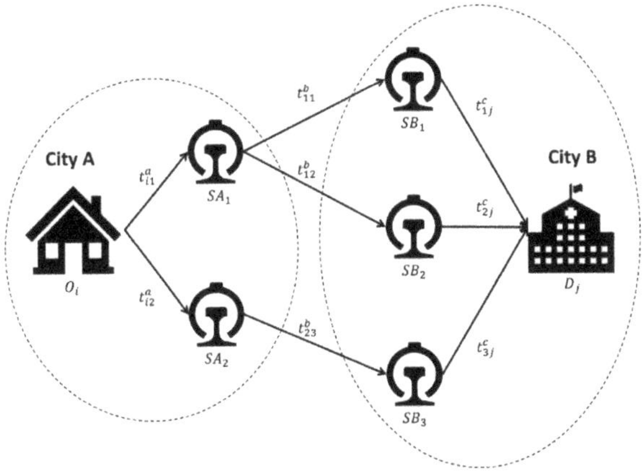

Figure 3. Illustration of intercity healthcare-seeking travel via multilevel transportation networks.

Multiple railway stations may exist in one city. When traveling between a given pair of cities, travelers may take different routes, namely, different combinations of railway stations. Generally, travel times vary across different travel routes. Therefore, it is essential to estimate the travel times of alternative routes and identify the route with the shortest travel time. As shown in Figure 3, considering two cities, A and B, patients in city A travel to city B for healthcare services. There are two railway stations (denoted by SA_k, $k = 1, 2$) in city A and three stations (denoted by SB_l, $l = 1, 2, 3$) in city B. There may be multiple railways connecting SA_k and SB_l, e.g., SA_1–SB_1, SA_1–SB_2, and SA_2–SB_3, as shown in Figure 3. In this case, for patients living at O_i in city A and visiting hospital D_j in city B, there are three alternative travel routes. The total travel times of the three routes can be estimated as follows:

$$t_{ij}^{1} = t_{i1}^{a} + t_{11}^{b} + t_{1j}^{c} \quad (4)$$

$$t_{ij}^{2} = t_{i1}^{a} + t_{12}^{b} + t_{2j}^{c} \quad (5)$$

$$t_{ij}^{3} = t_{i2}^{a} + t_{23}^{b} + t_{3j}^{c} \quad (6)$$

The shortest travel time from O_i to D_j (denoted as t_{ij}) can be identified as follows:

$$t_{ij} = min\left\{t_{ij}^{1}, t_{ij}^{2}, t_{ij}^{3}\right\} \quad (7)$$

For the intracity (both home-city and destination-city) phases of intercity travel, i.e., t_{i1}^{a} and t_{i2}^{a} for the home-city phase and t_{1j}^{c}, t_{2j}^{c} and t_{3j}^{c} for destination-city travel, patients can use various transportation modes. In this study, driving and public transit modes are considered for intracity travel to/from rail stations, which are commonly used as feeder transportation by railway travelers [66].

2.4. Decomposition of Inequality

The Gini coefficient has been widely applied to measure inequalities, including the spatial inequalities related to healthcare supply and accessibility [67,68]. Researchers further emphasize that inequalities can be decomposed into various levels. The Dagum composition method of the Gini coefficient has been widely applied to achieve such inequality decomposition [69]. In the case of spatial inequality, the whole study area is divided into a certain number of groups (or regions), and the inequalities can be decomposed into three components, namely intra-regional inequality, inter-regional inequality, and super-variable density inequality [70]. The calculation of the Dagum's Gini coefficient can be formulated as follows:

$$G = \frac{\sum_{j=1}^{k}\sum_{h=1}^{k}\sum_{i=1}^{n_j}\sum_{r=1}^{n_h}\left|y_{ji} - y_{hr}\right|}{2\mu n^2} \quad (8)$$

where y_{ij} (y_{hr}) is the accessibility score of subdistrict i (r) in region j (h); μ is the average accessibility score of all subdistricts; n is the number of subdistricts (2987 in this study); and k is the number of regions. In this study, each city is considered a region or group; therefore, there are 13 regions and n_j (n_k) denotes the number of subdistricts in region j (h). According to Dagum's decomposition method, the Gini coefficient G can be decomposed into three components:

$$G = G_w + G_{nb} + G_t \quad (9)$$

where G_w is the intracity component of the Gini coefficient, G_{nb} is the intercity component, and G_t is the super-variable density component. The formulas of the three components can be found in the original study [69], and the calculation and decomposition of Dagum's Gini coefficient were conducted in SPSSAU.

2.5. Calculation of the Proportions of Intercity and Intracity Travel Times

As previously stated, each form of intercity healthcare-seeking travel can be divided into three parts, all of which contribute to healthcare accessibility and its inequality. Based on the three phases of intercity healthcare-seeking travel, the proportions of intercity and intracity travel time can be decomposed. From the demand side, the average proportion of intracity travel time to the total travel time for each subdistrict is calculated using the following formula:

$$po_i = \frac{\sum_j \left(t_{ij}^{a} + t_{ij}^{c}\right)/t_{ij}}{m} \quad (10)$$

where po_i is the average proportion of intracity travel time from subdistrict i to all potential hospitals; j denotes hospitals; m is the number of potential hospitals that residents in subdistrict i can visit; t_{ij} is the shortest travel time from subdistrict i to hospital j; and t^a_{ij} and t^c_{ij} are the home-city and destination-city travel times, respectively, in the intracity phases.

From the supply side, the average proportion of intracity travel time to the total travel time for each hospital can be calculated as follows:

$$pd_j = \frac{\sum_i t^c_{ij}/t_{ij}}{n} \quad (11)$$

where pd_j is the average proportion of intracity travel time from all potential subdistricts to hospital j; n is the number of potential subdistricts that have access to hospital j; and the other variables are the same as those in Equation (10).

3. Results

3.1. Spatial Distribution and Equality of Healthcare Accessibility in the Intracity Scenario

The spatial distributions of healthcare accessibility at the subdistrict scale by driving or transit modes in the intracity scenario are visualized in Figure 4. The distribution of healthcare accessibility exhibits a similar pattern when considering driving or transit modes for intracity transportation. Healthcare accessibility in central urban areas is better than that in the peripheral counties. In addition, healthcare accessibility is relatively high in Beijing, Tianjin, and Shijiazhuang but low in Zhangjiakou, Langfang, and Hengshui. In the intracity scenario, such disparities in healthcare accessibility across cities are caused by the unequal distribution of high-quality healthcare resources in the BTH urban agglomeration. Within each city, healthcare accessibility decreases gradually from the city center to peripheral counties, which results from the concentration of high-quality healthcare resources in central urban areas within each city.

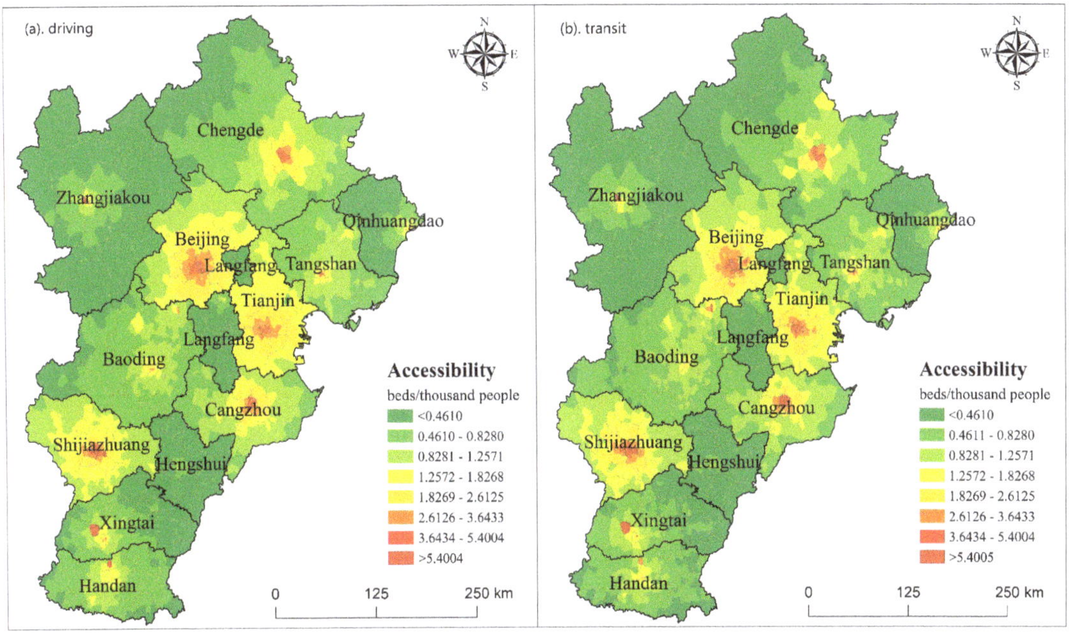

Figure 4. Healthcare accessibility by driving (**a**) or transit (**b**) in the intracity scenario.

Dagum's Gini coefficients of healthcare accessibility and three components in various scenarios are shown in Table 1. In the Intracity—Driving scenario in which intracity transportation is considered driving, the overall Gini coefficient of healthcare accessibility is 0.459, indicating obvious inequalities in the supply of healthcare resources and consequent healthcare accessibility at the subdistrict scale in the BTH urban agglomeration. By decomposing Dagum's Gini coefficient, it is found that the intracity component of the Gini coefficient is quite small (0.028, 6.1% of the overall inequality). As demonstrated above, intracity accessibility inequality is caused mainly by urban–rural disparities. In contrast, the intercity component contributes more than two-thirds (69.3%) to the overall inequality. The inequality of healthcare accessibility in the BTH urban agglomeration is caused, for the most part, by disparities between cities. In addition, the super-variable density component also contributes a certain proportion of inequality (24.6%), which means that the healthcare accessibility of some subdistricts in a city with lower average accessibility is better than that of some subdistricts in other cities with higher average accessibility. In the Intracity—Transit scenario, the overall Gini coefficient is larger than that in the Intracity—Driving scenario, indicating greater inequality in healthcare accessibility by transit mode. Similarly, the intercity component contributes approximately two-thirds (67.5%) to the overall inequality.

Table 1. Dagum's Gini coefficients of healthcare accessibility in various scenarios.

Scenario	Overall Gini Coefficient	Intracity Component	Intercity Component	Super-Variable Density Component
Intracity—Driving	0.459	0.028 (6.1%)	0.318 (69.3%)	0.113 (24.6%)
Intracity—Transit	0.466	0.029 (6.3%)	0.315 (67.5%)	0.122 (26.2%)
Intercity—Driving	0.265	0.019 (7.2%)	0.131 (49.4%)	0.116 (43.8%)
Intercity—Transit	0.297	0.020 (6.8%)	0.159 (53.7%)	0.117 (39.5%)

3.2. Spatial Distribution and Equality of Healthcare Accessibility in the Intercity Scenario

The spatial distributions of healthcare accessibility at the subdistrict scale by driving or transit mode in the intercity scenario are presented in Figure 5, which shows that healthcare accessibility is more evenly distributed in the intercity scenarios than it is in intracity scenarios (Figure 4). Similar to the intracity scenarios, healthcare accessibility also declines from central urban areas to peripheral counties, but the declining trend is weaker. However, healthcare accessibility increases in lower-grade cities, e.g., Cangzhou, Xingtai, Handan, Tangshan, and Chengde, but decreases in higher-grade cities, e.g., Beijing, Tianjin, and Shijiazhuang.

3.3. The Differences Between the Two Scenarios and the Impacts of Intercity Patient Mobility

The differences in healthcare accessibility between the intercity and intracity scenarios by driving or transit mode are presented in Figure 6. Positive values indicate that healthcare accessibility is greater in the intercity scenarios than it is in the intracity scenarios. In other words, intercity patient mobility improves healthcare accessibility in these subdistricts. Positive differences in healthcare accessibility can be observed in all Grade 1 cities, especially in the southeastern cities, i.e., Langfang, Cangzhou, Hengshui, Xingtai, and Handan. In addition, the magnitude of the positive difference in accessibility gradually decreases from the central urban areas to the peripheral counties in these cities. This finding indicates that the central areas in Grade 1 cities can benefit more in terms of healthcare accessibility due to the impacts of intercity patient mobility, whereas healthcare accessibility has decreased in Beijing, Tianjin, and Shijiazhuang. In intercity scenarios, patients living in lower-grade cities that lack high-quality healthcare resources can travel to higher-grade cities to access high-quality healthcare resources. Notably, although Baoding is also a Grade 2 city, its healthcare accessibility slightly increases in the intercity scenarios, possibly because Baoding is close to Beijing, Tianjin, and Shijiazhuang, where high-quality healthcare resources are the most concentrated. This locational advantage and the consequent benefits in healthcare accessibility can counteract some of the resources used by patients from other low-grade cities.

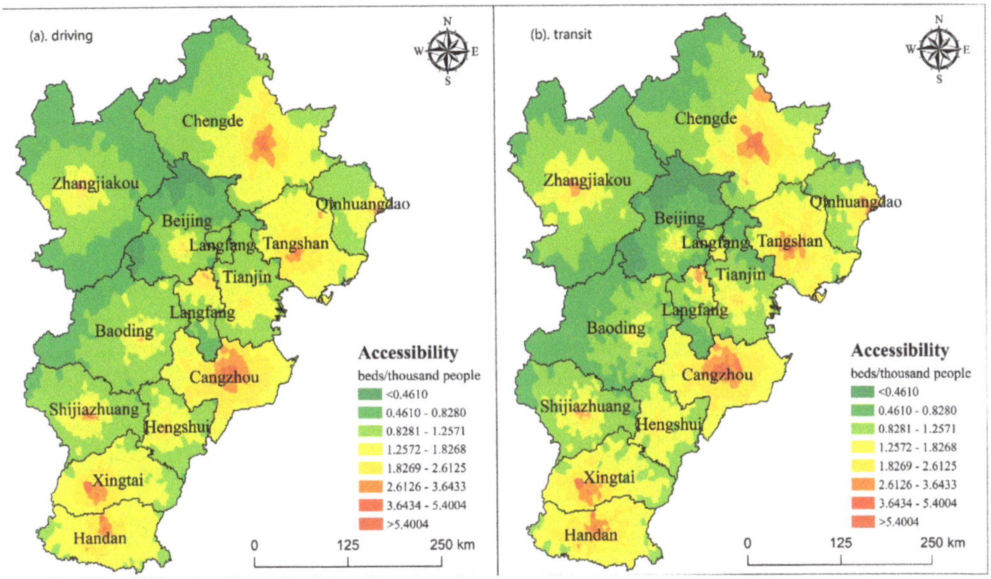

Figure 5. Healthcare accessibility by driving (**a**) or transit (**b**) in the intercity scenario.

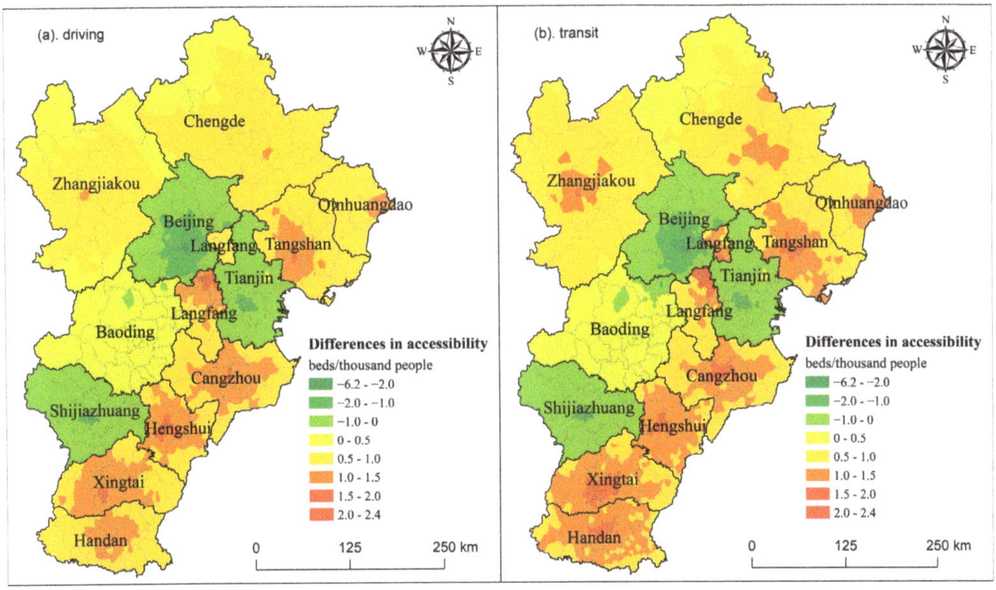

Figure 6. Differences in healthcare accessibility between the intercity and intracity scenarios by driving (**a**) or transit (**b**).

In the Intercity—Driving scenario, the overall Gini coefficient of healthcare accessibility across subdistricts in the BTH urban agglomeration is much smaller than that in the Intracity—Driving scenario (0.265 versus 0.459). Similarly, the overall Gini coefficient is also significantly lower in the Intercity—Transit scenario than in the Intracity—Transit scenario (0.297 versus 0.466; see Table 1). These differences between the intercity and intracity scenarios demonstrate that allowing intercity patient mobility can significantly mitigate the inequality of high-quality healthcare accessibility in the BTH urban agglomeration. In addition to the overall Gini coefficient, all three components decrease in the intercity scenarios compared with the intracity scenarios. However, the reduction in the intercity component is the largest among the three components, which decreases by 58.8% (from 0.318 to 0.131) or 49.5% (from 0.315 to 0.159), respectively, when driving and transit intracity transportation modes are considered.

3.4. Proportions of Intercity and Intracity Travel Times

From the demand side, the proportions of intracity travel time in the intercity scenarios by driving and transit modes are presented in Figure 7. Within each city, it is obvious that the proportion of intracity travel time increases from central urban areas to peripheral counties. At the urban agglomeration scale, the proportion is significantly greater in the areas around Beijing and gradually decreases with increasing distance from Beijing. In other words, the contribution of intercity rail transportation to healthcare accessibility is greater in areas that are further from higher-grade cities (especially Beijing).

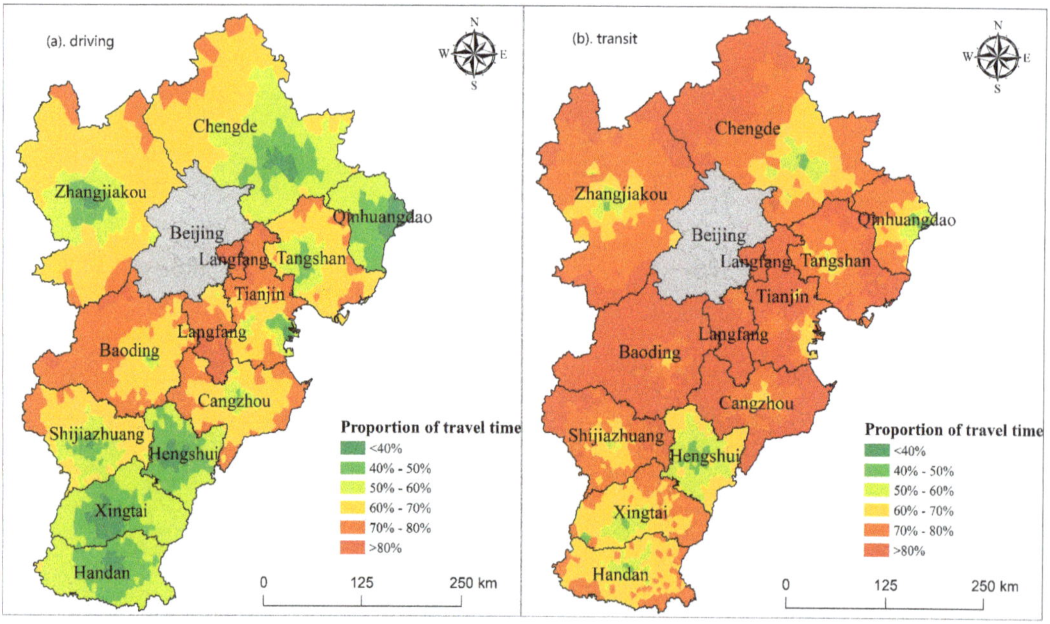

Figure 7. Proportions of intracity travel time in the intercity scenarios by driving (**a**) or transit (**b**) from the demand side.

In the Intracity—Driving scenario, the proportion of intracity travel time is more than 60% in most areas of Langfang, Baoding, Cangzhou, and Tianjin and in the peripheral counties of Zhangjiakou, Tangshan, and Shijiazhuang. In these areas, intracity travel time accounts for the majority of geographical barriers to travel for intracity, whereas intercity transportation only contributes to a limited proportion. In the Intracity—Transit scenario, the proportion of intracity travel time is more than 70% in most areas, excluding the majority of Hengshui and parts of Handan, Xingtai, Chengde, Zhangjiakou, and Qinhuangdao, which indicates obvious first-mile problems in intercity healthcare-seeking travel in these areas.

From the supply side, the proportions of destination-city travel time (i.e., travel times from rail stations to hospitals) in the intercity scenarios are presented in Figure 8, which shows that the proportion of destination-city travel time varies across hospitals within each city. In the Intercity—Driving scenario, the proportions of destination-city travel time are lower than 20% for hospitals located in central urban areas but reach 30–40% for some hospitals located far from the rail stations. In the Intercity—Transit scenario, the proportions of destination-city travel time are much greater, reaching more than 40% for many hospitals. For some peripheral hospitals, e.g., those located in northern Beijing, northern Tianjin, and northern Baoding, the proportion reaches more than 60%. These findings reveal obvious last-mile problems in intercity healthcare-seeking travel to certain 3-A hospitals. In summary, after the proportions of the intracity and intercity phases of travel time are decomposed, it is evident that although intercity rail transportation is essential for supporting intercity healthcare-seeking travels, the first-mile and last-mile problems caused by intracity transfer transportation should not be overlooked.

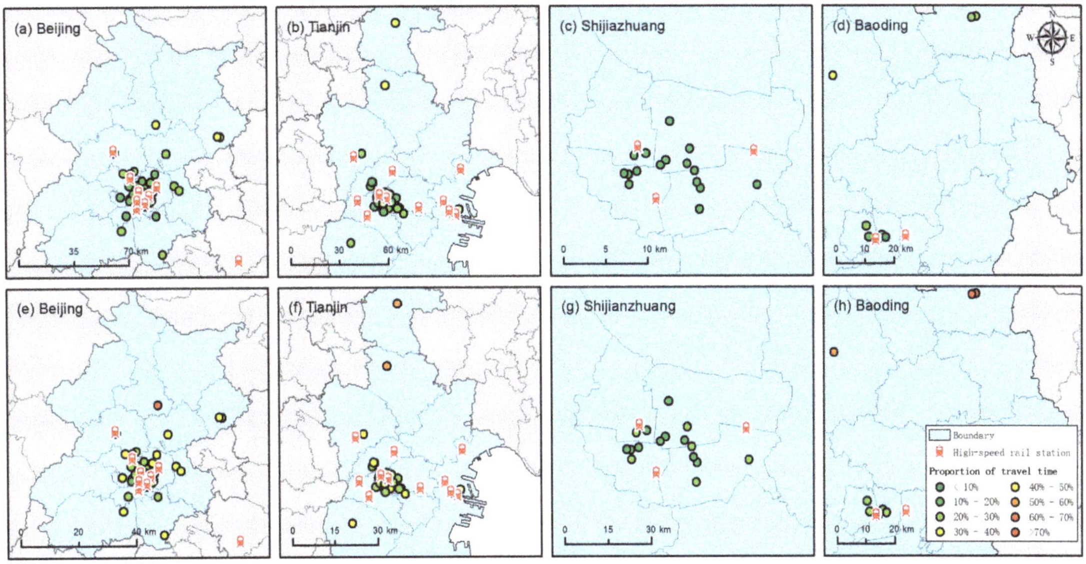

Figure 8. Proportions of destination-city travel times in intercity scenarios by driving (**a–d**) or transit (**e–h**) from the supply side.

4. Discussion

Intercity patient mobility is a common phenomenon caused by unevenly distributed high-quality healthcare resources. Given that spatial and socioeconomic integration is the fundamental feature of urban agglomerations, mitigating the inequality of spatial accessibility to high-quality healthcare resources at the urban agglomeration scale has become a focus. However, a full picture of the spatial inequality of healthcare accessibility at the urban agglomeration scale is still lacking because the hierarchy of high-quality healthcare resource distribution and the impacts of intercity rail transportation are being ignored. This study contributes to this field by developing a novel method for measuring healthcare accessibility at the urban agglomeration scale that incorporates the hierarchy of high-quality healthcare services, the direction of intercity patient mobility and the role of multilevel rail transportation networks.

The results revealed obvious spatial inequalities in the spatial accessibility of high-quality healthcare resources (3-A hospitals) in the BTH urban agglomeration. In intracity scenarios, it is assumed that patients would select hospitals within the city in which they reside. Therefore, the estimated healthcare accessibility in the intracity scenarios reflects the supply level of high-quality healthcare resources relative to demand. Although healthcare accessibility is relatively high in higher-grade cities (especially Beijing, Tianjin, and Shijiazhuang), it exhibits obvious urban–rural disparities within each city. These findings confirm the need to consider the hierarchy of high-quality healthcare resources and the direction of intercity patient mobility in the measurement of healthcare accessibility on the urban agglomeration scale, which is also consistent with existing studies [46,47]. Dagum's Gini coefficient was then applied to decompose the intracity and intercity components of the inequality of healthcare accessibility. The intercity component, i.e., the inequality of healthcare accessibility between cities, accounts for the majority of accessibility inequality, thus suggesting that to mitigate the spatial inequalities of healthcare accessibility at the urban agglomeration scale, the key is to narrow the gaps in high-quality healthcare resources among cities.

The healthcare accessibility and the accompanying inequalities in intracity and intercity scenarios are further compared. The differences between these scenarios reflect the impacts of intercity patient mobility on the inequalities in healthcare accessibility. The inequality of healthcare accessibility is obviously lower in the intercity scenarios than in the intracity scenarios. In addition, although both the intracity and intercity inequality components decrease, the intercity component decreases more. This finding indicates that given the uneven distribution of high-quality healthcare resources in the BTH urban agglomeration, intercity patient mobility, i.e., the flow of patients across city boundaries, significantly mitigates the inequalities, especially the intercity inequality, of healthcare accessibility.

Notably, our findings are consistent with those of existing studies in the Changsha–Zhuzhou–Xiangtan urban agglomeration [47] and the Shenzhen–Dongguan–Huizhou agglomeration [46]. However, as only the driving mode is considered in these studies, the crucial role of rail transportation in intercity travel is overlooked. In addition to considering the direction of intercity patient mobility, this study also improves the measurement of urban agglomeration-scale healthcare accessibility by incorporating multilevel intercity transportation networks, i.e., multiple rail stations within a city, multiple rail lines connecting a pair of cities, and first- and last-mile transfer transportation to/from rail stations via driving or transit. This improved method more accurately estimates intercity patients' travel time to hospitals.

Furthermore, we separated intercity healthcare-seeking travels into intracity (including home-city and destination-city) and intercity phases. The proportions of intracity travel time to total travel time were calculated from both the demand and supply sides. From the demand side, the proportion of intracity travel time shows obvious disparities across subdistricts and is significantly greater in the areas around Beijing. When patients use the transit mode in the intracity phase, the proportion of intracity travel time is quite high, reaching more than 70% in most areas. This finding indicates that intracity transportation, i.e., first-mile and last-mile transfer transportation, is the major barrier to intercity healthcare accessibility. On the supply side, our analyses demonstrate that hospitals distant from rail stations are more likely to suffer from the last-mile intracity transportation dilemma.

This study sheds light on the methodological development of spatial accessibility measurement in urban agglomerations or other functional areas where intercity connections play a vital role. First, it is necessary to account for intercity interactions between demand and supply as well as the structure or hierarchy of such interactions. By contrast, traditional analyses limited to a single city might lead to biased results. Second, door-to-door travel time estimation is essential for accurate measurement of spatial accessibility at a cross-city scale.

These findings can also provide valuable practical implications for policymaking and planning of healthcare resources. First, the configuration of high-quality healthcare resources within an urban agglomeration should emphasize intercity coordination. On the one hand, higher-grade cities not only provide high-quality healthcare services to local patients but also service patients from lower-grade cities. Therefore, more high-quality healthcare services should be allocated to the central cities of an urban agglomeration. On the other hand, policy countermeasures should be put forward to facilitate intercity patient mobility, e.g., improving intercity healthcare accessibility, promoting cross-city settlement of medical insurance, and making it more convenient to schedule appointments. Second, it is suggested to strengthen intracity transportation connections between rail stations and high-grade hospitals in the central cities.

We acknowledge that there are limitations to this study. First, only travel time costs between stations and from/to stations are considered in measuring healthcare accessibility, whereas other costs, e.g., waiting and transfer time costs within stations and economic costs, are not taken into account. Second, although our focus is on spatial accessibility to healthcare resources, future studies should focus on socioeconomic barriers to intercity patient mobility and accessibility. Third, while the hierarchy of high-quality healthcare resources and the direction of intercity patient mobility are important assumptions in this study, they are not substantiated based on actual intercity healthcare-seeking behaviors. Greater effort is needed to re-examine our findings by considering patients' actual behaviors and using the data to support the findings. Fourth, all 3-A hospitals were included in this study. However, these hospitals have different specializations or functions and varied compositions of departments. Therefore, the influences by intercity patient mobility might vary across hospitals. Future studies could better distinguish between the different types of hospitals and consider the heterogeneity in patients' preferences. Fifth, it is assumed that intercity travels are based on railway mode, while the possibility that some patients might travel by driving across cities was overlooked in this study.

5. Conclusions

While spatial inequalities regarding the accessibility to high-quality healthcare resources on the urban agglomeration scale are an important issue, they face challenges due to intense socioeconomic interactions and patient mobility between cities. This study developed a novel directional 2SFCA method for revealing the spatial inequalities of accessibility to 3-A hospitals in the BTH urban agglomeration, with a focus on the impacts of intercity patient mobility. To address the methodological challenges posed by the characteristics of urban agglomerations, our method emphasizes the direction of intercity patient mobility caused by the hierarchy of high-quality healthcare resource distribution. To reveal the impacts of intercity patient mobility, multilevel intercity rail transportation connecting various cities and intracity transfer transportation by driving or transit are considered when estimating door-to-door travel times.

The results revealed obvious spatial inequalities in the accessibility of high-quality healthcare resources in the BTH urban agglomeration. Intercity inequalities, i.e., disparities between cities, account for more than two-thirds of the overall accessibility inequalities. Although intercity patient mobility can significantly mitigate the spatial inequalities of healthcare accessibility within the BTH urban agglomeration, intracity first-mile and last-mile transfer transportation is the major barrier to intercity healthcare accessibility. Hence, this study has valuable implications for the planning and management of high-quality healthcare resources and intercity patient mobility in the BTH urban agglomeration. The developed methods are useful for measuring healthcare accessibility and inequalities at the urban agglomeration scale.

Author Contributions: Conceptualization, Zhuolin Tao; methodology, Yandi Wang, Lin Chen, Binglin Liu and Zhuolin Tao; software, Yandi Wang, Lin Chen and Binglin Liu; validation, Yandi Wang, Lin Chen, Binglin Liu and Zhuolin Tao; formal analysis, Yandi Wang, Lin Chen, Binglin Liu and Zhuolin Tao; investigation, Zhuolin Tao; resources, Zhuolin Tao; data curation, Yandi Wang, Lin Chen and Binglin Liu; writing—original draft preparation, Yandi Wang, Lin Chen and Zhuolin Tao; writing—review and editing, Yandi Wang, Lin Chen and Zhuolin Tao; visualization, Yandi Wang, Lin Chen and Binglin Liu; project administration, Zhuolin Tao; funding acquisition, Zhuolin Tao. All authors have read and agreed to the published version of the manuscript.

Funding: This research was funded by the National Natural Science Foundation of China, grant numbers 42471262 and 42101189.

Data Availability Statement: All data used in this study are free to access.

Acknowledgments: The authors would like to thank the editor and anonymous reviewers for their suggestions.

Conflicts of Interest: The authors declare no conflicts of interest.

References

1. The United Nations (UN). *Sustainable Development Goals 3*; The United Nations (UN): New York, NY, USA, 2015.
2. Penchansky, R.; Thomas, J.W. The concept of access: Definition and relationship to consumer satisfaction. *Med. Care* **1981**, *19*, 127–140. [CrossRef] [PubMed]
3. Khan, A.A. An integrated approach to measuring potential spatial access to health care services. *Socio Econ. Plan. Sci.* **1992**, *26*, 275–287. [CrossRef] [PubMed]
4. Guagliardo, M.F. Spatial accessibility of primary care: Concepts, methods and challenges. *Int. J. Health Geogr.* **2004**, *3*, 3. [CrossRef] [PubMed]
5. McGrail, M.R. Spatial accessibility of primary health care utilising the two step floating catchment area method: An assessment of recent improvements. *Int. J. Health Geogr.* **2012**, *11*, 50. [CrossRef]
6. Park, Y.; Guldmann, J. Understanding disparities in community green accessibility under alternative green measures: A metropolitan-wide analysis of Columbus, Ohio, and Atlanta, Georgia. *Landsc. Urban Plan.* **2020**, *200*, 103806. [CrossRef]
7. Sharma, G.; Patil, G.R. Spatial and social inequities for educational services accessibility—A case study for schools in Greater Mumbai. *Cities* **2022**, *122*, 103543. [CrossRef]
8. Sharma, G.; Patil, G.R. Urban spatial structure and equity for urban services through the lens of accessibility. *Transp. Policy* **2024**, *146*, 72–90. [CrossRef]
9. Xiong, Q.; Liu, Y.; Xing, L.; Wang, L.; Ding, Y.; Liu, Y. Measuring spatio-temporal disparity of location-based accessibility to emergency medical services. *Health Place* **2022**, *74*, 102766. [CrossRef]
10. Luo, W.; Wang, F. Measures of spatial accessibility to health care in a GIS environment: Synthesis and a case study in the Chicago region. *Environ. Plan. B Plan. Des.* **2003**, *30*, 865–884. [CrossRef]
11. Wang, F. Measurement, optimization and impact of healthcare accessibility: A methodological review. *Ann. Assoc. Am. Geogr.* **2012**, *102*, 1104–1112. [CrossRef]
12. Oliver, A.; Mossialos, E. Equity of access to health care: Outlining the foundations for action. *J. Epidemiol. Community Health* **2004**, *58*, 655–658. [CrossRef] [PubMed]
13. Whitehead, J.; Pearson, A.L.; Lawrenson, R.; Atatoa-Carr, P. How can the spatial equity of health services be defined and measured? A systematic review of spatial equity definitions and methods. *J. Health Serv. Res. Policy* **2019**, *24*, 270–278. [CrossRef] [PubMed]
14. Wang, F.; Tang, Q. Planning toward equal accessibility to services: A quadratic programming approach. *Environ. Plan. B Plan. Des.* **2013**, *40*, 195–212. [CrossRef]
15. Du, X.; Liu, M.; Luo, S. Exploring Equity in a Hierarchical Medical Treatment System: A Focus on Determinants of Spatial Accessibility. *ISPRS Int. J. Geo Inf.* **2023**, *12*, 318. [CrossRef]
16. Vallée, J.; Shareck, M.; Le Roux, G.; Kestens, Y.; Frohlich, K.L. Is accessibility in the eye of the beholder? Social inequalities in spatial accessibility to health-related resources in Montréal, Canada. *Soc. Sci. Med.* **2020**, *245*, 112702. [CrossRef]

17. Tao, Z.; Cheng, Y.; Du, S.; Feng, L.; Wang, S. Accessibility to delivery care in Hubei Province, China. *Soc. Sci. Med.* **2020**, *260*, 113186. [CrossRef]
18. Ghorbanzadeh, M.; Kim, K.; Erman Ozguven, E.; Horner, M.W. Spatial accessibility assessment of COVID-19 patients to healthcare facilities: A case study of Florida. *Travel Behav. Soc.* **2021**, *24*, 95–101. [CrossRef]
19. Yan, X.; He, S.; Webster, C.; Yu, M. Divergent distributions of physicians and healthcare beds in China Changing patterns, driving forces, and policy implications. *Appl. Geogr.* **2022**, *138*, 102626. [CrossRef]
20. Jia, P.; Wang, Y.; Yang, M.; Wang, L.; Yang, X.; Shi, X.; Yang, L.; Wen, J.; Liu, Y.; Yang, M.; et al. Inequalities of spatial primary healthcare accessibility in China. *Soc. Sci. Med.* **2022**, *314*, 115458. [CrossRef]
21. Ye, P.; Ye, Z.; Xia, J.; Zhong, L.; Zhang, M.; Lv, L.; Tu, W.; Yue, Y.; Li, Q. National-scale 1-km maps of hospital travel time and hospital accessibility in China. *Sci. Data* **2024**, *11*, 1130. [CrossRef]
22. Falchetta, G.; Hammad, A.T.; Shayegh, S. Planning universal accessibility to public health care in sub-Saharan Africa. *Proc. Natl. Acad. Sci. USA* **2020**, *117*, 31760–31769. [CrossRef] [PubMed]
23. Juran, S.; Broer, P.N.; Klug, S.J.; Snow, R.C.; Okiro, E.A.; Ouma, P.O.; Snow, R.W.; Tatem, A.J.; Meara, J.G.; Alegana, V.A. Geospatial mapping of access to timely essential surgery in sub-Saharan Africa. *BMJ Glob. Health* **2018**, *3*, e000875. [CrossRef] [PubMed]
24. Weiss, D.J.; Nelson, A.; Vargas-Ruiz, C.A.; Gligorić, K.; Bavadekar, S.; Gabrilovich, E.; Bertozzi-Villa, A.; Rozier, J.; Gibson, H.S.; Shekel, T.; et al. Global maps of travel time to healthcare facilities. *Nat. Med.* **2020**, *26*, 1835–1838. [CrossRef] [PubMed]
25. Hall, P.; Pain, K. *The Polycentric Metropolis: Learning from Megacity Regions in Europe*; Earthscan: London, UK, 2006.
26. Gottmann, J. Megalopolis or the Urbanization of the Northeastern Seaboard. *Econ. Geogr.* **1957**, *33*, 189–200. [CrossRef]
27. Scott, A.J. *Global City-Regions: Trends, Theory, Policy*; Oxford University Press: New York, NY, USA, 2001.
28. Florida, R.; Gulden, T.; Mellander, C. The rise of the mega-region. *Camb. J. Reg. Econ. Soc.* **2008**, *1*, 459–476. [CrossRef]
29. Kloosterman, R.; Musterd, S. The Polycentric Urban Region: Towards a Research Agenda. *Urban Stud.* **2001**, *38*, 623–633. [CrossRef]
30. McGee, T.G. The Emergence of Desakota Regions in Asia: Expanding a Hypothesis. In *The Extended Metropolis: Settlement Transition Is Asia*; Ginsburg, N., Koppel, B., McGee, T.G., Eds.; University of Hawaii Press: Honolulu, HI, USA, 1991.
31. Fang, C.; Yu, D. Urban agglomeration: An evolving concept of an emerging phenomenon. *Landsc. Urban Plan.* **2017**, *162*, 126–136. [CrossRef]
32. The State Council of China. *The National New-Type Urbanization Plan*; The State Council of China: Beijing, China, 2014.
33. Dash Nelson, G.; Rae, A. An Economic Geography of the United States: From Commutes to Megaregions. *PLoS ONE* **2016**, *11*, e0166083. [CrossRef]
34. Huang, H.; Xia, T.; Tian, Q.; Liu, T.; Wang, C.; Li, D. Transportation issues in developing China's urban agglomerations. *Transp. Policy* **2020**, *85*, A1–A22. [CrossRef]
35. Marull, J.; Font, C.; Boix, R. Modelling urban networks at mega-regional scale: Are increasingly complex urban systems sustainable? *Land Use Policy* **2015**, *43*, 15–27. [CrossRef]
36. Zhang, W.; Fang, C.; Zhou, L.; Zhu, J. Measuring megaregional structure in the Pearl River Delta by mobile phone signaling data: A complex network approach. *Cities* **2020**, *104*, 102809. [CrossRef]
37. Lin, X.; Yang, J.; MacLachlan, I. High-speed rail as a solution to metropolitan passenger mobility: The case of Shenzhen-Dongguan-Huizhou metropolitan area. *J. Transp. Land Use* **2018**, *11*, 1257–1270. [CrossRef]
38. Ross, C. Transport and megaregions: High-speed rail in the United States. *Town Plan. Rev.* **2011**, *82*, 341–356. [CrossRef]
39. Harrington, D.W.; Rosenberg, M.W.; Wilson, K. Comparing health status and access to health care in Canada's largest metropolitan areas. *Urban Geogr.* **2014**, *35*, 1156–1170. [CrossRef]
40. Yu, M.; He, S.; Wu, D.; Zhu, H.; Webster, C. Examining the Multi-Scalar Unevenness of High-Quality Healthcare Resources Distribution in China. *Int. J. Environ. Res. Public Health* **2019**, *16*, 2813. [CrossRef]
41. Brekke, K.R.; Levaggi, R.; Siciliani, L.; Straume, O.R. Patient mobility and health care quality when regions and patients differ in income. *J. Health Econ.* **2016**, *50*, 372–387. [CrossRef]
42. Koylu, C.; Delil, S.; Guo, D.; Celik, R.N. Analysis of big patient mobility data for identifying medical regions, spatio-temporal characteristics and care demands of patients on the move. *Int. J. Health Geogr.* **2018**, *17*, 32. [CrossRef]
43. Beraldo, S.; Collaro, M.; Marino, I. Patient migration as a response to the regulation of subnational healthcare budgets. *Reg. Stud.* **2023**, *57*, 2207–2219. [CrossRef]
44. Ding, J.; Yang, C.; Wang, Y.; Li, P.; Wang, F.; Kang, Y.; Wang, H.; Liang, Z.; Zhang, J.; Han, P.; et al. Influential factors of intercity patient mobility and its network structure in China. *Cities* **2023**, *132*, 103975. [CrossRef]
45. Wang, X.; Nie, X. The uneven distribution of medical resources for severe diseases in China: An analysis of the disparity in inter-city patient mobility. *Appl. Geogr.* **2024**, *165*, 103226. [CrossRef]
46. Zhong, Q.; Wu, J.; Tao, Z. Intercity patient mobility can improve healthcare accessibility and equality in metropolitan areas: A case study of Shenzhen metropolitan area, China. *Appl. Geogr.* **2024**, *171*, 103383. [CrossRef]

47. Li, C.; Wang, J. A hierarchical two-step floating catchment area analysis for high-tier hospital accessibility in an urban agglomeration region. *J. Transp. Geogr.* **2022**, *102*, 103369. [CrossRef]
48. Zhang, H.; Zhou, B.-B.; Liu, S.; Hu, G.; Meng, X.; Liu, X.; Shi, H.; Gao, Y.; Hou, H.; Li, X. Enhancing intercity transportation will improve the equitable distribution of high-quality health care in China. *Appl. Geogr.* **2023**, *152*, 102892. [CrossRef]
49. Yip, W.; Fu, H.; Chen, A.T.; Zhai, T.; Jian, W.; Xu, R.; Pan, J.; Hu, M.; Zhou, Z.; Chen, Q.; et al. 10 years of health-care reform in China: Progress and gaps in Universal Health Coverage. *Lancet* **2019**, *394*, 1192–1204. [CrossRef]
50. Tao, Z.; Yao, Z.; Kong, H.; Duan, F.; Li, G. Spatial accessibility to healthcare services in Shenzhen, China: Improving the multi-modal two-step floating catchment area method by estimating travel time via online map APIs. *BMC Health Serv. Res.* **2018**, *18*, 345. [CrossRef]
51. Chen, K.; Zhao, P.; Qin, K.; Kwan, M.; Wang, N. Towards healthcare access equality: Understanding spatial accessibility to healthcare services for wheelchair users. *Comput. Environ. Urban Syst.* **2024**, *108*, 102069. [CrossRef]
52. Yang, D.; Goerge, R.; Mullner, R. Comparing GIS-based methods of measuring spatial accessibility to health services. *J. Med. Syst.* **2006**, *30*, 23–32. [CrossRef]
53. Stacherl, B.; Sauzet, O. Gravity models for potential spatial healthcare access measurement: A systematic methodological review. *Int. J. Health Geogr.* **2023**, *22*, 34. [CrossRef]
54. Radke, J.; Mu, L. Spatial decomposition, modeling and mapping service regions to predict access to social programs. *Geogr. Inf. Sci.* **2000**, *2*, 105–112. [CrossRef]
55. Dai, D. Black residential segregation, disparities in spatial access to health care facilities, and late-stage breast cancer diagnosis in metropolitan Detroit. *Health Place* **2010**, *16*, 1038–1052. [CrossRef]
56. Luo, W.; Qi, Y. An enhanced two-step floating catchment area (E2SFCA) method for measuring spatial accessibility to primary care physicians. *Health Place* **2009**, *15*, 1100–1107. [CrossRef] [PubMed]
57. McGrail, M.R.; Humphreys, J.S. Measuring spatial accessibility to primary health care services: Utilising dynamic catchment sizes. *Appl. Geogr.* **2014**, *54*, 182–188. [CrossRef]
58. Langford, M.; Higgs, G.; Fry, R. Multi-modal two-step floating catchment area analysis of primary health care accessibility. *Health Place* **2016**, *38*, 70–81. [CrossRef]
59. Mao, L.; Nekorchuk, D. Measuring spatial accessibility to healthcare for populations with multiple transportation modes. *Health Place* **2013**, *24*, 115–122. [CrossRef] [PubMed]
60. Delamater, P.L. Spatial accessibility in suboptimally configured health care systems: A modified two-step floating catchment area (M2SFCA) metric. *Health Place* **2013**, *24*, 30–43. [CrossRef]
61. Luo, J. Integrating the Huff Model and Floating Catchment Area Methods to Analyze Spatial Access to Healthcare Services. *Trans. GIS* **2014**, *18*, 436–448. [CrossRef]
62. Shao, Y.; Luo, W. Supply-demand adjusted two-steps floating catchment area (SDA-2SFCA) model for measuring spatial access to health care. *Soc. Sci. Med.* **2022**, *296*, 114727. [CrossRef]
63. Wang, J.; Du, F.; Huang, J.; Liu, Y. Access to hospitals: Potential vs. observed. *Cities* **2020**, *100*, 102671. [CrossRef]
64. Wei, Z.; Bai, J.; Feng, R. Evaluating the spatial accessibility of medical resources taking into account the residents' choice behavior of outpatient and inpatient medical treatment. *Socio Econ. Plan. Sci.* **2022**, *83*, 101336. [CrossRef]
65. Wei, W.; Xiang, B. Spatial pattern of cross-city medical network and supply-demand relationship of medical facilities in China: Based on cross-city medical internet data. *Geogr. Res.* **2024**, *43*, 701–717.
66. Jia, W.; Huang, Z.; Bao, J.; Shen, W. Spatiotemporal differences in the accessibility of scenic spots based on door-to-door travel by high-speed rail: A case study of Shanghai-Nanjing intercity travel. *Tour. Trib.* **2023**, *38*, 148–159.
67. Dai, G.; Li, R.; Ma, S. Research on the equity of health resource allocation in TCM hospitals in China based on the Gini coefficient and agglomeration degree: 2009–2018. *Int. J. Equity Health* **2022**, *21*, 145. [CrossRef] [PubMed]
68. Skaftun, E.K.; Verguet, S.; Norheim, O.F.; Johansson, K.A. Geographic health inequalities in Norway: A Gini analysis of cross-county differences in mortality from 1980 to 2014. *Int. J. Equity Health* **2018**, *17*, 64. [CrossRef] [PubMed]
69. Dagum, C. A New Approach to the Decomposition of the Gini Income Inequality Ratio. *Empir. Econ.* **1997**, *22*, 515–531. [CrossRef]
70. Peng, R.; Huang, J.; Deng, X. Spatiotemporal evolution and influencing factors of the allocation of social care resources for the older adults in China. *Int. J. Equity Health* **2023**, *22*, 222. [CrossRef]

International Journal of
Geo-Information

MDPI

Article

Leveraging a Cooler, Healthier, and Decarbonized School Commute: City-Scale Estimation and Implications for Nanjing, China

Lifei Wang [1], Ziqun Lin [1], Zhen Xu [1,*] and Lingyun Han [2]

1 College of Landscape Architecture, Nanjing Forestry University, Nanjing 210037, China; wanglifei@njfu.edu.cn (L.W.); linziqun@njfu.edu.cn (Z.L.)
2 School of Geography, Jiangsu Second Normal University, Nanjing 210013, China; hanlingyun@jssnu.edu.cn
* Correspondence: xuzhen@njfu.edu.cn

Abstract: An important aspect of a well-designed urban form is supporting active school travel by adolescents, as it has positive effects on physical activity, healthy lifestyles, and reducing vehicle-related carbon emissions. To achieve this, it is necessary to provide sufficient shading and fewer detours on home–school routes, especially in an era of frequent heatwaves. Analyzing the school travel environment at the city scale is essential for identifying practical solutions and informing comprehensive urban policy-making. This study proposes a framework for investigating, assessing, and intervening in home–school routes in Nanjing, China, emphasizing a dual assessment of commuting routes based on the pedestrian detour ratio and shading ratio. This work reveals that approximately 34% of middle school households in Nanjing face challenges in walking to and from school, with only 24.18% of walking routes offering fewer detours and sufficient shade. We advocate reengineering urban forms by reducing barriers to facilitate shortcuts, thereby providing school-age students with better access to cooler and healthier environments, aiming to promote walking and reduce car dependence. The findings may encourage more families to engage in active commuting and serve as a lever to drive school decarbonization and combat climate warming. Our work, with transferability to other cities, can assist urban designers in piloting urban (re)form incrementally and pragmatically to promote sustainable urban agendas.

Keywords: active school travel; walkability; urban form; shaded sidewalks; landscape analytics; urban design

1. Introduction

Over the past few years, the substantial carbon emissions from human activities, notably from car traffic, have exacerbated urban warming [1]. This has led to frequent extreme weather events, such as heatwaves, which severely threaten the physical health of residents, particularly vulnerable groups like children. Due to the severe negative impacts on the environment, economy, and society, there is a growing public consensus that heavy reliance on internal combustion engines for urban transportation is unsustainable [2]. The pressing call for a shift to sustainable urban mobility is reflected in arguments for reassigning city street space in favor of active transport and achieving a vision of "streets for people", moving away from the notion of "streets for traffic" [3]. This vision is increasingly embraced and expanded by planners and decision-makers who are attempting to transform the street network and urban form to promote walkability. A conducive walking environment on city streets lays the groundwork for essential urban functions like social interaction, leisure, and play [4]. This is vividly exemplified by the daily school commutes of adolescents [5].

For school-aged children (typically between the ages of 11 and 17), commuting to and from school is a fundamental part of their daily life [6]. Active school travel (AST) is recognized as a vital source of increased physical activity outside school, exposure to nature, street experiences, independent mobility, spatial cognition, and social interactions for adolescents [5,7]. Advocacy for AST has become a prominent public policy initiative in many cities worldwide, some of which have been successfully converted into infrastructure projects like Safe Routes to School and Walking School Bus [8]. At the same time, educational institutions are also considered pioneers and major stakeholders in addressing climate change and reducing energy consumption [9,10]. Cultivating sustainable travel habits at a young age could foster lifelong practice and inspire future generations to adopt sustainable travel behavior [11].

An important goal in urban planning and management is to support AST by adolescents, as it has positive effects on physical activity, healthy lifestyles, and reducing vehicle-related carbon emissions [5]. However, long routes and numerous detours on the way to school may reduce the desire to walk and increase students' exposure to heat [12,13]. Specifically, students sometimes choose longer routes to avoid the sun. Once the route exceeds walking distance, or there is simply no shady alternative, they have to drive to school, creating more congestion and carbon emissions. This is how poor street design can cause disorder, pollution, and other urban problems.

In China, walking is a common choice due to parking difficulties, poor cycling conditions, and the "attending nearby schools" policy. Although the Chinese government aims to assign children to nearby schools to avoid long commutes, a Beijing study found that over 80% of students have a school commute exceeding 5 km, indicating that the "attending nearby schools" policy does not guarantee shorter school commutes [14]. China's urban morphology is indeed characterized by large, walled institutions and residential compounds, which may create challenges such as spatial fragmentation, reduced mobility, and potential barriers for vulnerable groups like children [15]. The characteristic of gated communities often hinders walking, requiring pedestrians to take longer detours to reach their destinations. This will increase the risk of excessive heat exposure.

Some scholars have noticed this and have attempted to propose solutions through urban morphology, school catchment planning, and urban management practices [16,17]. Solid research has demonstrated that positive commuting behavior is greatly influenced by home–school distance and street connectivity [18,19]. Shortcuts in road networks have been shown to effectively encourage positive commuting behaviors by diverting students away from traffic noise and pollution [18]. Seeking support from urban greening, such as street trees and roadside green spaces, may be also potential solutions.

Yet, the detours and urban morphological factors in traditional research have not been combined with related nature-based solutions in recent studies, especially in regions with unique residential forms like China. Cultural norms and policies uniquely shape walking behaviors in China, particularly for children commuting to school, presenting both challenges and opportunities for urban planners to focus on the intersection of urban morphology, pedestrian mobility, and urban greening. Significant gaps persist in understanding the commuting environments of students in China, and studies on how urban (re)form knowledge can drive urban policies and planning for mainstreaming remain limited.

To address these gaps, this study uses Nanjing as a case study to extensively examine the shading and detour factors along school routes for middle school students in the central urban area. The goal is to expand the understanding of children's commuting environments in regions with unique urban forms like China. We hypothesize that students will choose the best route recommended by Baidu Maps (the leading online mapping service in China, which relies on the travel patterns of the majority to suggest routes) and assess the extent of exposure to direct sunlight and detours along these routes. We aim to explore potential shortcuts and interventions to improve these issues, promoting AST, reducing car dependency, and lowering carbon emissions. The final results will provide a set of processes for investigation, evaluation, and intervention, with the potential for application in other regions. This work also contributes to the existing literature on Chinese urban management and child geography.

This study's outline is as follows. Section 2 provides a more detailed description of AST, heat exposure along commuting routes, and school decarbonization initiatives. Section 3 presents the case study city, methods, and datasets. Section 4 assesses shading and detour factors along school routes, along with potential carbon emissions. Section 5 discusses measures for optimizing urban morphology and concludes with a practical set of processes for addressing these issues. Sections 6 and 7 summarize this study.

2. Literature Review

2.1. Active School Travel

Active school travel (AST) was first proposed in the early 2000s. This concept refers to school-aged children or adolescents, aged 7–14, commuting to school using active transportation modes such as walking, biking, or other non-motorized vehicles [5]. Many studies have found that urban form helps predict travel mode to and from school [20]. Route distance has been interpreted as the strongest predictor of AST. The distance thresholds that determine AST vary depending on the mode of transportation. Research indicates that a home distance of 1.5 km from school is identified as the threshold for Canadian students to shift from driving to alternative modes such as walking or biking [21]. In another study, it was found that most pedestrians reside within 1.5 miles of their destination, while cyclists typically live within 2.5 miles [22]. Further evidence in Beijing reveals that nearly half (47.5%) of students live within 2 km of their school, with walking being their primary mode of travel. For distances between 2 and 6 km, cycling becomes the main mode [23]. The distance threshold is profoundly influenced by the diverse urban forms and spatial configurations. Owing to the substantial heterogeneity among Chinese cities and the scarcity of existing research, it is challenging to establish a definitive threshold for this study. Consequently, a threshold of 1600 m, which has generally been accepted in the academic literature, is employed as a benchmark to explore walking routes [24,25].

Additionally, in the field of urban morphology, numerous scholars have employed space syntax theory and geographic information system (GIS) technologies to examine the physical structure of walkable street networks, thereby evaluating pedestrian movement patterns [26–28]. The connectivity and integration of street networks are impressive factors in predicting urban mobility [27]. Research has also revealed that connecting cul-de-sacs and improving pedestrian pathways can significantly alleviate traffic congestion [25]. The pedestrian detour ratio (PDR) is another excellent predictor of AST. This metric reflects the permeability of the urban road network. A PDR less than 1.3 indicates a neighborhood grid street pattern with relatively small blocks, while a value greater than 1.6 suggests irregular streets and cul-de-sacs [29].

In mainland China, relevant research is not yet mature. A report from Guangzhou, China, indicates a positive correlation between green space, the number of vehicles, and the likelihood of AST [30]. It also mentions the potential impact of China's unique urban forms, while other studies in Nanjing, Nanchang, and other areas have more specifically raised concerns that gated community forms hinder AST [31,32]. Another study of children's transportation in Shanghai shows that improving connectivity is a low-cost measure that significantly promotes children's safety in getting to school [33].

The existing literature in China primarily relies on self-reported data from students to explore their travel characteristics. The limited studies available have merely observed the impacts of gated communities without delving deeper into the issue or providing corresponding planning recommendations. Therefore, this work is essential. Based on online map data, this study examines the main travel routes of students and specifically investigates the detours caused by gated communities, aiming to propose relevant interventions.

2.2. Heat Exposure for Commuters

Devising natural and design-based solutions to combat urban heat waves has become an important urban planning issue. Urban tree canopy is a key nature-based solution for cooling cities. Many solid studies have proven the substantial cooling effects of tree cover and building shade [34]. Research indicates that the temperature difference between shaded and unshaded areas can be as much as 20 °C [34]. When selecting their paths, urban pedestrians frequently consider shade as a top priority [12].

More specific measures have gained attention for providing shade on routes. For example, strategically selecting and planting street trees near schools or using smartphone apps for adaptive route planning can provide students with cooler and more comfortable commuting environments [13,35]. In cities such as Melbourne, Sydney, and Barcelona, projects like 'WayfinderHeat' have developed and evaluated adaptive route planning using a smartphone app to provide precise shade distributions at the street level [36,37]. Other research and measures include developing a Cool Walkshed Index (CWI) to assess shaded areas and exploring suitable options for cooling infrastructure [38,39].

A study in Poland highlights the necessity of balancing walking distance and exposure to greenery for children's health, even if it means taking longer routes [17]. Although studies have attempted to promote thermal safety through designs such as road orientation, street tree canopy, and catchment modeling [40,41], these efforts typically focus on local and micro-scale designs. Comprehensive urban-level studies to assess shaded routes for school commutes in China still remain unclear.

2.3. School-Based Decarbonization

Active transport plays a significant role in the efforts towards school decarbonization. Evidence has shown a strong potential for replacing short car trips with more sustainable modes in students' commuting patterns between home and university [42], and transitioning from cars to walking or public transport can significantly reduce carbon dioxide emissions [11]. A report from Beijing indicates that students' AST can effectively promote low-carbon practices [43].

Scholars are increasingly interested in carbon accounting for schools. A European Union initiative, Euronet 50/50, is dedicated to supporting the transition to a low-carbon economy in schools. The program aims to help school communities raise awareness and promote changes in attitudes to enable responsible decisions, including selecting more sustainable transport alternatives (walking, cycling, or public transport) [44]. As a global leader in climate action, China has set the goal of achieving carbon neutrality by 2060. The 14th Five-Year Plan highlights the importance of reducing carbon emissions from urban transportation. Promoting non-motorized transportation in schools (including primary, secondary, and higher education) effectively contributes to rapid urban decarbonization.

The modeling of emissions is generally regarded as a challenging task, due to the great variety of vehicle types, road conditions, and ways of driving. In view of the difficulty of collecting detailed travel data and the lack of a comprehensive methodology for the estimation of carbon emissions from travel, some studies use GIS to calculate travel distance for estimating the carbon footprints [45,46]. Another study utilizes IPCC carbon emission inventory data to estimate carbon emissions according to travel distance [47]. In addition, a separate study applies origin–destination (OD) analysis to quantify CO_2 emissions for each route [48].

Although there are many studies on the carbon footprint and lifecycle decarbonization of schools, their reference value for China is limited by various cultural and policy factors. Further exploration is required to evaluate the impact of AST on carbon emissions in Chinese schools. In this study, considering the priority of quickly drawing attention to the relationship between school commuting behavior and urban carbon emissions, GIS technology and travel distance are used to estimate carbon emissions, thereby bypassing data barriers and complex calculation formulas.

3. Methodology

3.1. Study Area

In this study, we selected the central urban area of Nanjing as the research area, covering approximately 330.25 km^2 and a population of about 3.66 million. Nanjing (31°14′ to 32°37′N, 118°22′ to 119°14′E) is the capital city of Jiangsu Province, China, and plays a key role in the Yangtze River Delta region, one of China's most developed in terms of education and economics. Similar to most major cities in China, Nanjing has undergone extensive urbanization and motorization. By 2024, the number of privately owned cars in Nanjing reached 2.49 million, and it continues to grow by over 100,000 vehicles annually. Residents are increasingly relying on cars for commuting, resulting in substantial carbon emissions.

The 2023 China Climate Report reveals that the national average temperature hit an all-time high. The country experienced the second highest number of high-temperature days and the fourth highest number of extreme heat events in history [49]. Prolonged heatwaves make walking-based commuting increasingly unsustainable. Even for relatively short home–school distances, parents often opt to drive their children to avoid excessive sun exposure. This behavior exacerbates urban congestion, air pollution, and noise.

We studied our hypotheses and framework in Nanjing, China, aiming to serve as a pioneer and provide a demonstrative model. The study area covers Xuanwu, Gulou, Qinhuai, Jianye, and parts of Qixia and Yuhuatai, and the dataset includes 61 public middle schools and 3238 residential communities. The spatial distributions of these schools are shown in Figure 1.

3.2. Data Analysis Metrics

The data analysis metrics used in the study are as follows (Table 1 and Figure 2).

(1) School Catchment: Based on the Chinese educational policy of "attending nearby schools", each public middle school corresponds to a school catchment and the locations and basic information of residential communities within each catchment have been recorded. The delineation of school catchments was based on policy documents released by the educational bureaus of various administrative districts in Nanjing in 2024. Residential community information was gathered by scraping Nanjing real estate information in 2024 from the "Beike Zhaofang" website. The data were collected in February 2024. We obtained the population data by cross-referencing the residential community's information with the data from the Seventh National Census. All school catchments in this study are visualized using GIS, as shown in Figure 1.

(2) School Commute Route: We acquired the routes from the school to the residential communities based on Baidu Map's path planning service to simulate the school commute route. Baidu Maps is the largest and most widely used online map service in China. The road network selected in this study is based on the most frequently chosen pedestrian routes in the Baidu Maps route planning service. Relevant indicators are all based on these routes. A total of 3238 routes were generated, each starting from the main gate location of the school and ending at the geometric center of each residential community. Every route includes information such as crow-fly distance, route distance, number of turns, and number of road crossings. Furthermore, according to the literature review, we evaluated the potential for active school commuting behavior based on the route distance in three scenarios. Scenario A represents segments within 1000 m, where active commuting behavior is highly likely to occur. Scenario B represents segments between 1000 m and 1600 m, where such behavior may occur. Scenario C represents segments over 1600 m, where such behavior is less likely to occur.

(3) Pedestrian Detour Ratio (PDR): Gated communities may create more detours for school commuting routes (Figure 2d). We used the pedestrian detour ratio (PDR) to measure the directness of school commute walking routes. The PDR is commonly used to quantify the minimum additional walking distance beyond the crow-fly distance that is required for a commuter to reach a destination. The formula is shown as follows:

$$PDR_{ij} = \frac{S_{ij}}{C_{ij}} \tag{1}$$

where PDR_{ij} is the pedestrian detour ratio between origin i and destination j, S_{ij} is the distance of the shortest walking path between i and j, and C_{ij} is the crow-fly distance from i to j.

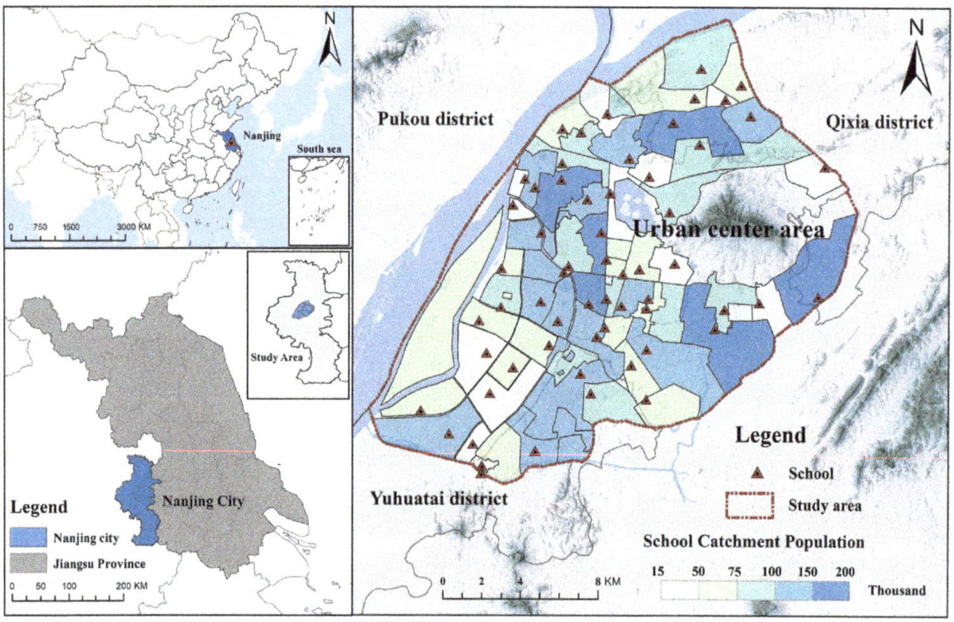

Figure 1. Spatial distributions of the schools in the study area of Nanjing.

Table 1. Relevant data analysis metrics and description.

School Catchment	The catchments are defined according to the "attending nearby schools" policy, including some residential communities.
School Commute Route	Data from Baidu Maps' path planning service simulated the school commute routes and were divided into three scenarios regarding AST based on distances of 1000 and 1600 m.
Pedestrian Detour Ratio (PDR)	It is used to measure the directness of school commute walking routes.
Pedestrian Shade Ratio (PSR)	It is used to assess the shading and cooling effects along commute routes.
Carbon Emissions	These data estimate the CO_2 emissions generated by car commuting to school.

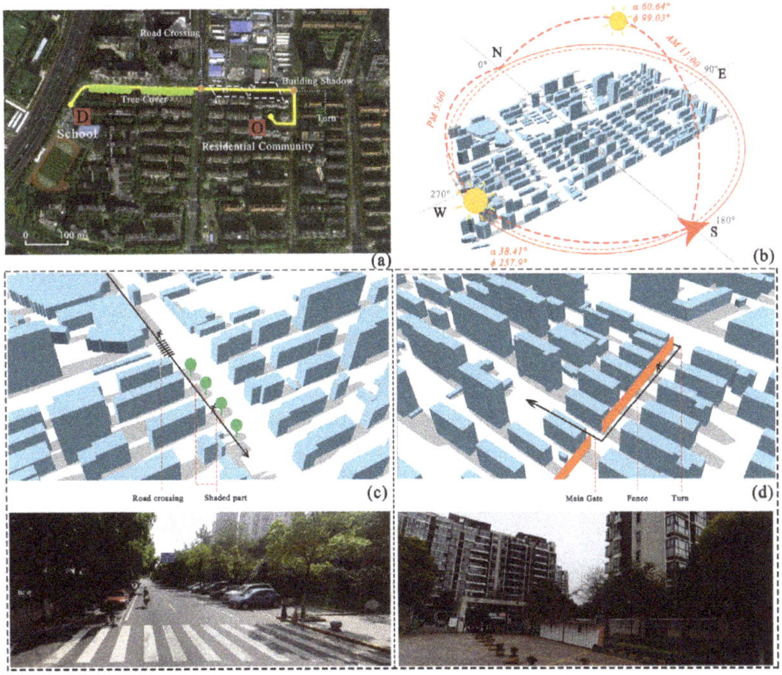

Figure 2. (**a**) Schematic of school–home walking route. (**b**) Schematic of sun and shadow. (**c**,**d**) Local route modeling and photographs of walking routes.

(4) Pedestrian Shade Ratio (PSR): According to the literature review, many solid studies have already demonstrated that building shadows and tree cover can effectively reduce street temperatures. In this study, the pedestrian shade ratio is used to assess the shading and cooling effects along commute routes. The formula is shown as follows:

$$PSR_{ij} = \frac{D_{ij}}{S_{ij}} \tag{2}$$

where PSR_{ij} is the pedestrian shade ratio between origin i and destination j, D_{ij} represents the physical length in the shade (affected by tree cover and building shadows) between i and j, and S_{ij} is the school commute route from school i to resident j. Tree cover data were sourced from the 2 m spatial resolution Urban Tree Cover Product [50]. Building shadows derived from the 2024 Baidu Maps Nanjing building data were processed to simulate their shadows under sunlight using ArcGIS.

According to field surveys, the midday dismissal time for middle school students in Nanjing is between 11:00 a.m. and 12:00 p.m., the afternoon school start time is between 1:30 p.m. and 2:00 p.m., and the afternoon dismissal time is between 5:00 p.m. and 6:00 p.m. To account for as many schools as possible, the selected time points should be as early as possible within the given time intervals. At the same time, the minimum level of shading provided by tree canopies should be chosen to ensure the worst-case scenario. Taking 24 June 2024 in Nanjing, China, as an example, the solar altitudes at 11:00 a.m., 1:30 p.m., and 5:00 p.m. are 60.64°, 51.37°, and 38.41°, respectively, while the solar azimuths are 99.03°, 165.23°, and 257.9°. Among these times, the shadow under the tree canopy is smallest at 11:00 a.m. Additionally, we conducted a sensitivity analysis at the three time points and found that the impact on the research results was minimal. Therefore, we chose the shading at 11:00 a.m. to represent the commuting times of students in Nanjing for the analysis.

(5) Carbon Emissions: For home–school distances that are less likely to promote active school commuting behaviors, we assume that the mode of transportation for commuting in these residential communities is by car. However, the precise methods for calculating vehicle carbon emissions are not yet clear. Therefore, based on the IPCC carbon emission inventory data and relevant studies [47,51], we used the following formula to estimate the carbon emissions generated by commuting.

$$CT_{rij} = \sum_{1}^{n} D_{ij} * Q_j * T_j * F * 2 \quad (3)$$

$$CT_{si} = \sum_{1}^{m} CT_{rij} \quad (4)$$

In the formula, CT_{rij} represents the weekly carbon emissions (kg) generated by commuting from school i to residential community j. n is the number of households in the residential community, D_{ij} is the home–school commute distance (km) between i and j, Q_j is the number of trips per day, and T_j is the number of school days per week. F is the carbon emission factor of the vehicle ($kgCO_2/km$). The factor of 2 represents a round trip. On the other hand, CT_{si} represents the total weekly carbon emissions (kg) for school catchment si, and m is the number of residential communities in school catchments.

4. Result

A total of 3238 commuting routes for 61 schools in the study area have been reviewed. Based on relevant research [25], we set the walking distance threshold for school commuting at 1600 m, assuming that households living beyond this distance would opt for car commuting. Therefore, in the two scenarios mentioned in Section 2.3, households in scenarios A and B walk, while households in scenario C drive. There are 1188 residential communities (36.69%) within 1000 m, 1273 (39.31%) between 1000 and 1600 m, and 1108 (34.22%) beyond 1600 m. The spatial distributions of these residential communities are shown in Figure 3.

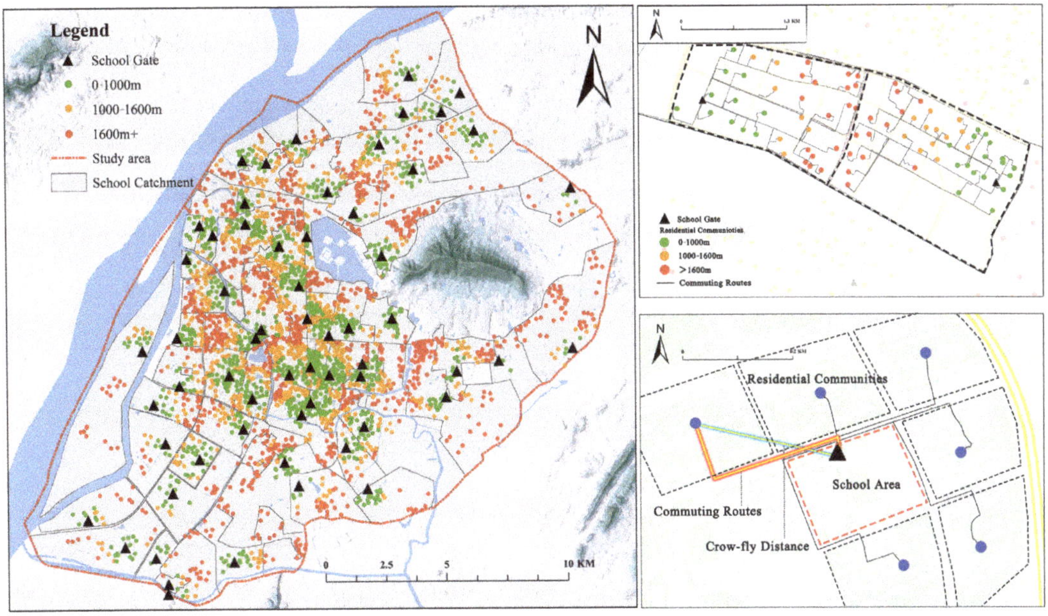

Figure 3. Spatial distribution of residential communities by different routes distance.

An overall number of 2130 commuting routes within 1600 m has been obtained. The metrics for these routes are shown in Table 2. In the central urban area of Nanjing, the average crow-fly distance from residential communities to schools is 651 m (Figure 4c), with a maximum distance of 1468 m and a minimum distance of 34 m. Of these routes, 1843 residential communities have a crow-fly distance of less than 1000 m, accounting for 86.53%.

Table 2. Metrics of walking routes.

	Min	Max	Mean	Median	SD
Crow-fly distance	34 m	1468 m	651 m	644 m	298 m
Route distance	81 m	1598 m	929 m	939 m	368 m
PDR	1.02	5.97	1.52	1.41	0.45
PSR	0	0.98	0.30	0.28	0.19
Turn	0	16.00	5.11	5.00	2.48
Road crossing	0	6.00	1.34	1.00	1.01
Population ratio	11.00%	100.00%	64.95%	65.00%	22.56%

The average distance of school commute routes within the study area is 929 m (Figures 4c and 5). There are 314 residential communities (14.74%) within 500 m and 1188 communities (55.77%) within 1000 m. Assuming an average walking speed of 1.2 m per second for adolescents, more than half of the adolescents in the central urban area of Nanjing can walk to school within 15 min. Of the 61 schools, 44 have average route distances within 1000 m (Figure 6a).

Assuming an average of one school-aged child per household, 57.62% of adolescents have commuting routes within 1000 m based on the number of households in each residential community. At the school catchment level, an average of 64.95% of households have commuting distances within 1600 m (Figure 6b). The lowest percentage is in the Jinling Affiliated Middle School in Jianye District, where only 11.00% of adolescents have commuting distances within 1600 m. In contrast, all households in the catchment of Nanjing No. 9 Middle School, Huadian Middle School, and Liren Middle School fall within this distance range. Only 16 schools have less than 50% of households within the range, mostly located in Xuanwu and Yuhua Districts, including the southeast and northwest areas of Zijin Mountain, while districts with higher percentages are mainly located in the central old city area.

The average PDR for all commuting routes is 1.52, with a median of 1.41, a maximum of 5.97, and a minimum of 1.02 (Figure 4a). Of these routes, 1489 (69.91%) have a PDR more than 1.3, 513 (24.08%) more than 1.6, and 304 (14.27%) more than 1.8. At the school catchment level, only one of the 61 catchments has an average PDR below 1.3, while 19 catchments have an average PDR over 1.6 (Figure 6c). For residential communities with commuting distances more than 1000 m, 619 communities (29.06%) have a PDR more than 1.3, and 159 (7.46%) more than 1.6. Longer route distances and higher PDRs indicate lower urban permeability between residential communities and schools.

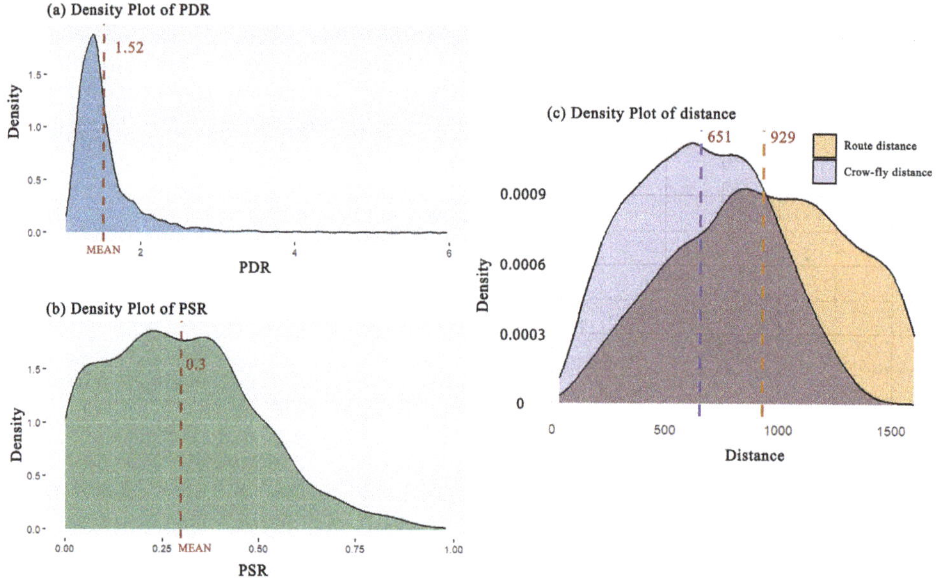

Figure 4. Density plot of PDR (a), PSR (b), and distance (c).

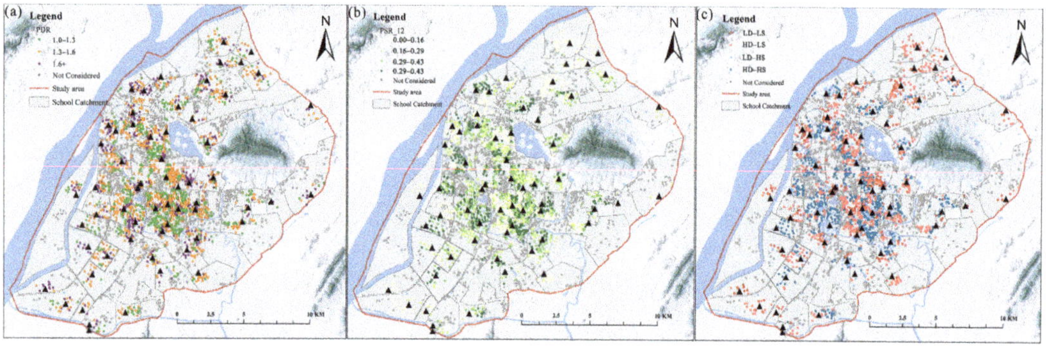

Figure 5. PDR values (a) and PSR values (b) for various residential communities, and the evaluation of high and low values (c).

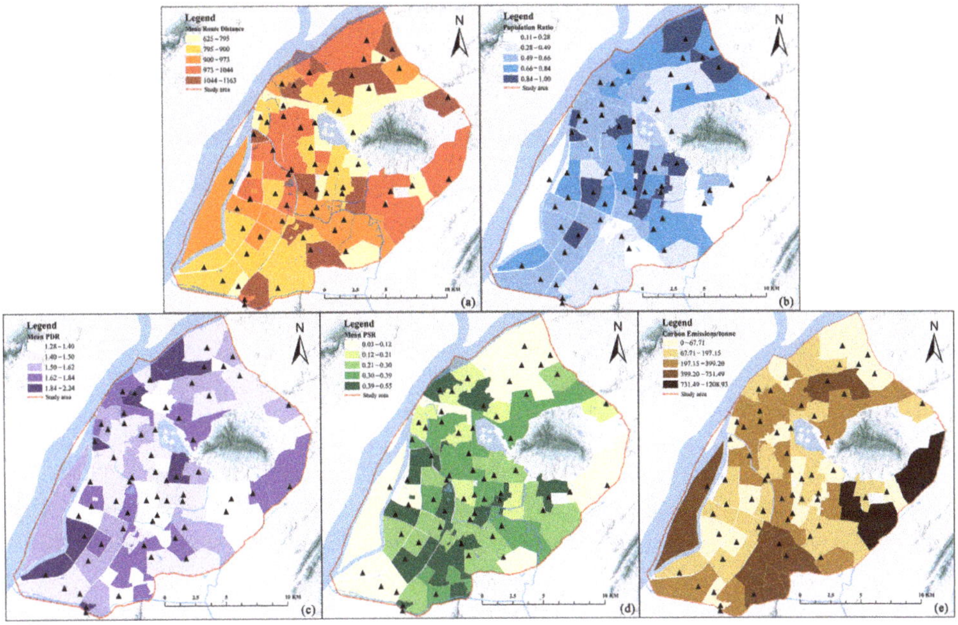

Figure 6. (**a**) Average walking distance per school district, (**b**) proportion of students walking to school per school district, (**c**) average PDR of walking routes per school district, (**d**) average PSR of walking routes per school district, (**e**) average estimated commuting carbon emissions per school district.

The average PSR for all commuting routes is 0.30, with a median of 0.28, a maximum of 0.98, and a minimum of 0 (Figure 4b). Of these routes, 757 (35.54%) have a PSR below 0.2, and 320 (15.02%) have a PSR above 0.5. At the school catchment level, 34 out of 61 catchments have an average PSR below 0.3. It is evident that low PSR values are mostly located at the edges of the central urban area (Figure 6d). A higher PSR indicates that there are more shaded areas and less heat exposure along the commuting routes for adolescents.

Based on the relevant literature reviewed in Section 2, we assessed the shading and detours on commuting routes in different residential communities using two levels: PDR and PSR, with corresponding thresholds of 1.6 and 0.3, respectively (Figure 5a,b). According to the results, residential communities were categorized into four types: low-quality detour and low-quality shading (LD-LS), high-quality setour and low-quality shading (HD-LS), low detour and high shading (LD-HS), and high detour and high shading (HD-HS) (Figure 5c). It was found that 32.52% of the residential communities in the study area had low-quality shading, and 16.06% had low-quality detours. Among them, 273 residential communities (8.43%) fell into the LD-LS category, while 24.18% fell into the HD-HS category. The quadrant chart in Figure 7 clearly illustrates the average conditions of each school district (Figure 7). From the map, we are able to quickly identify the school districts that have issues. In Figure 5, the red areas represent low-quality shading. The peripheral areas, due to insufficient urban development and lack of greenery, exhibit generally poor quality in both detours and shading, particularly in several northern residential communities. Notably, there are also some deficiencies in the central area, such as low-quality shading at Five Junior High School and Wen Shu Secondary School, and low-quality detours at Jianye Junior High School and Meiyuan Secondary School. While there may not be a large value for shorter route detours, the overly dense problematic situation may be that there is a barrier of some sort, which still has refinement needs and implications.

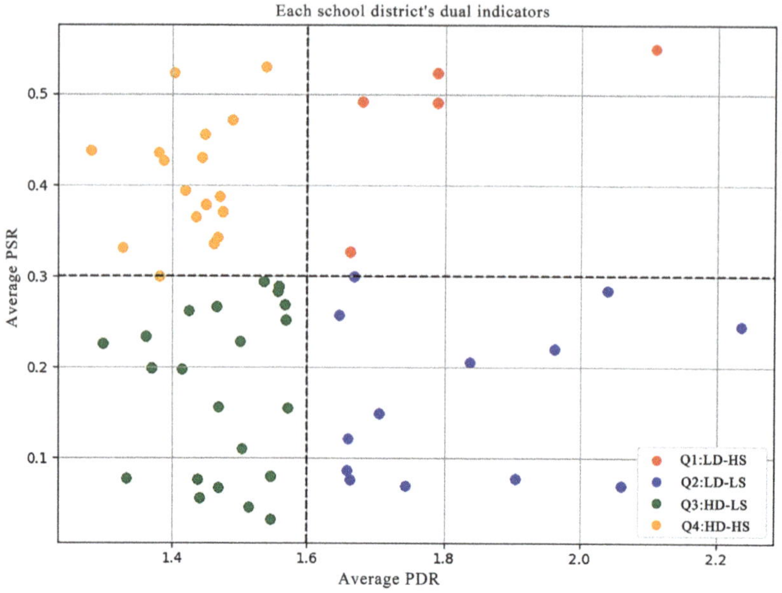

Figure 7. Each school district's dual indicators.

Commuting routes with distances exceeding 1600 m yielded 1108 home–school paths, with an average distance of 2003 m. It is estimated that the average weekly carbon emissions from commuting to school for households in Nanjing's central urban area amount to 11 tons. The proportion of residential communities relying on motorized commutes is 34.22%. Two notable high emission values are observed in these school catchments, both located in the southeastern part of the study area, specifically Xingzhi Secondary School and Maqun No. 1 Middle School. These two areas are characterized by their proximity to the edges of the central urban area and their coverage of relatively large regions. Some communities within the Xingzhi Secondary School Catchment are primarily inhabited by rural resettlers. Compared to the well-integrated school communities in the central area, these areas bear higher costs to support students' commutes. These findings underscore potential social disparities and spatial inequalities: communities on the outskirts face not only challenges related to their identity and the threat of falling back into poverty but also varying degrees of access to educational opportunities.

5. Discussion

As heatwaves become more common, school students are increasingly vulnerable. If no action is taken, this could result in greater reliance on motorized school travel for students from car-owning households, while posing a higher health risk for students who must walk or bike. The purpose of identifying these issues is not merely to improve macro-level statistics but to provide precise, efficient, and waste-free solutions. Typically, urban core areas have more developed infrastructure (including urban canopies) and denser populations than peripheral areas. In edge areas, public consensus is relatively easier to achieve on measures such as increasing tree coverage, narrowing streets, or optimizing the locations of future schools. However, in high-density core areas, such measures often face significant challenges and controversies. In these regions, small-scale, low-cost interventions may prove particularly effective.

5.1. Reduce the Fence in Gated Community

Reducing barriers to create shortcuts is an effective strategy. In many cities, large, gated communities or institutional campuses occupy vast areas, hindering pedestrian movement. For example, the route from No. 130 Bancang Street to No. 13 Suojin School could be significantly shortened for young pedestrians by partially or entirely removing certain fences (Figure 8a). This adjustment would expand the street network and enhance urban connectivity. Similar to Chevalier's suggestion for road intersections in Shanghai, this proposal also highlights the potential positive impacts of minimal interventions. However, a more specific analysis is still needed for different regions [33].

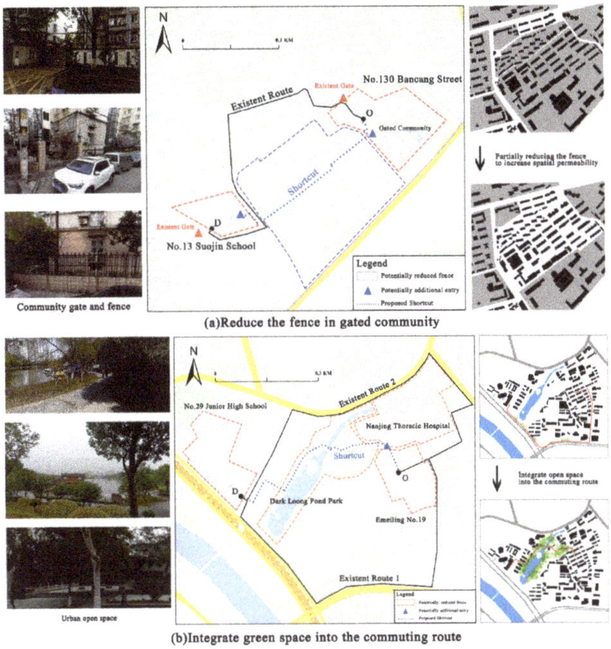

Figure 8. (**a**) Reduce the fence in gated community. (**b**) Integrate green space into the commuting route.

Furthermore, allowing schools to have multiple entry points may also shorten travel distances for students. Utilizing GIS technology to analyze the spatial distribution of students' residential locations and traffic flow data enables school administrators to optimize campus entrance and exit layouts, thereby enhancing connectivity between the campus and pedestrian traffic. This approach offers multiple advantages: it reduces walking distances, particularly in areas with a high density of residential units, improves commuting efficiency, and alleviates traffic congestion during peak hours.

Sharing the internal routes for transient through-access may also be a solution. This approach allows for better land utilization in high-density urban areas by temporarily designating land as school travel corridors and enhances campus safety by minimizing students' exposure to external roadways.

Such temporary use is expected to serve as a catalyst for urban transformation and change, allowing communities to participate in the physical process of urban development and providing participants with different spatial experiences [52]. This approach of temporary use reveals the value of testing, similar to many common strategies in active transportation and other urban design practices [53]. Once successful, it can be further developed and made permanent; even if the results are not satisfactory, it can be easily removed without incurring significant costs.

5.2. Integrate Green Space into the Commuting Route

Langenheim et al. and other researchers have focused on minimizing the solar radiation impact on students by analyzing tree canopy structure, height, and species choice [13]. But this may not be applicable for post-construction evaluation and retrofitting. Alternatively, utilizing existing green spaces presents another viable solution. Green or shaded areas between schools and homes have the potential to serve as pedestrian walkways (Figure 8b). Although incorporating green spaces into school routes may increase the actual physical distance, it could result in a lower perceived distance. Reducing detours can be a trade-off for seeking shade [54,55]. Reports indicate that maximizing exposure to greenery requires selecting routes that are 9.5% longer than the shortest available routes [17]. However, the findings of this study reveal an alternative perspective: the increased distance associated with seeking greenery may be attributed to the prevalence of excessive walls.

In neighborhoods with low permeability and high detour rates, enhancing the openness of parks could integrate urban greening into the commuting environment. This approach may simultaneously reduce walking distances and increase exposure to greenery. Notably, some megacities in China, such as Beijing and Shanghai, have already pioneered initiatives to open up park boundaries and under-canopy spaces, providing residents with more activity spaces. Moreover, green space corridors can help students avoid noise, vehicle emissions, and the risks of traffic accidents. This nation-based solution unlocks the potential of existing resources and is sufficiently flexible to address economic and social challenges.

5.3. School-Based Decarbonization

Universities may potentially be candidates for carbon credits within existing trading frameworks, owing to their reduction in energy use and greenhouse gas release. Specifically, the proposal here considers including school catchment carbon emissions in trading and evaluation programs. Additional greenhouse gas emissions from each school could be converted into energy credits or taxes, allowing participation in the carbon market. Carbon emissions also could be used as a metric to drive effective school catchment planning and foster active commuting practices. A modest change to the current incentive system would achieve the intended effect. Even small and simple decarbonization initiatives at the school and individual family level are crucial for combating global warming, given China's vast population. A comprehensive application of this practice across all schools would aid in advancing national sustainability.

Scholars in various fields such as transportation, urban planning, and others have already called for active commuting, more efficient urban design, and multiple pathways for decarbonization strategies. In line with the principle of "only measurable is manageable," quantifying carbon emissions has become a prerequisite for formulating decarbonization strategies [56,57]. One popular approach is through the development and deployment of a comprehensive travel survey across all university affiliates to measure commute mode split and frequency [58,59].

Decarbonizing schools has been recognized as a decarbonization action with tremendous potential and responsibility, but the complex scenarios of local policies constrain its progress. Currently, most studies involve complex indicators and require costly social surveys, which hinder public understanding and the rapid advancement of decarbonization efforts. This study employs a simple, straightforward quantification method based on commuting routes to facilitate action among various stakeholders, filling the research gap on school decarbonization in China.

5.4. Framework and Other Intervention

Given the predictable patterns of students' commuting times and directions, it becomes feasible to pinpoint critical locations and prioritize routes for through-travel and shortcuts. This enables the development of detailed measures for evaluating specific routes and communities. This study outlines a framework for identifying, evaluating, and intervening at an urban scale, aiming to promote cooler, healthier, and decarbonized school commutes (Figure 9). It begins by delineating school catchments based on current conditions and using online map services to obtain school–home routes. Various indicators are then employed to quantify the characteristics of these routes, with a comprehensive analysis and evaluation of problematic areas. This study proceeds to examine these areas in detail and implements targeted, small-scale planning, design, and intervention measures for remediation and improvement. This framework can also be beneficially adopted by universities, local authorities, and other public institutions alike.

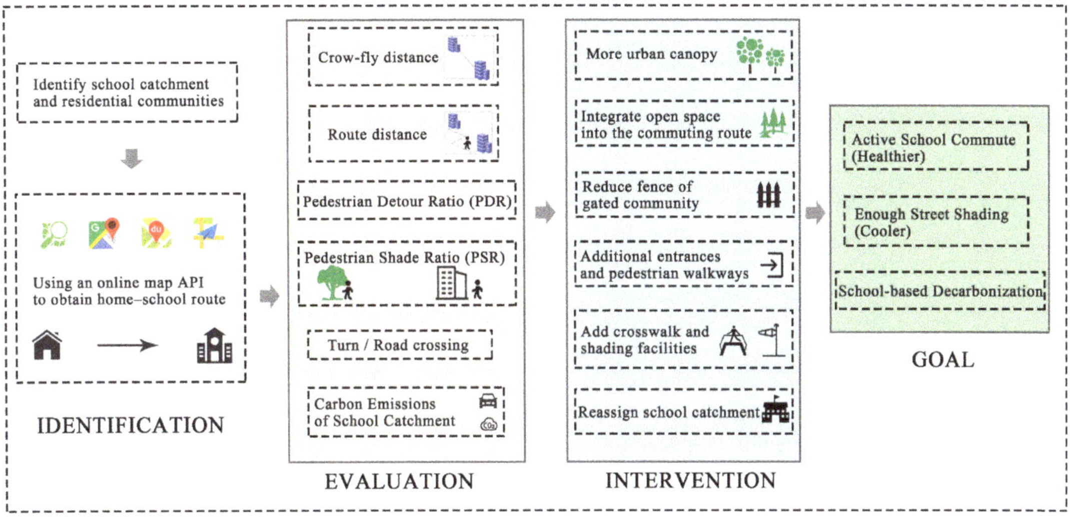

Figure 9. A framework for identifying, evaluating, and intervening at the urban scale.

School catchments are often delineated by service radius, which is the Euclidean (crow-fly) distance between the school and home, a practice that is consistent with regulations in many countries [24,60]. As outlined in the National Code for the Design of Schools (GB 50099-2011), the standard service radius for junior high schools in China is 1000 m. However, the study findings show that many students actually travel considerably farther than the crow-fly distance between their homes and the school, due to factors such as cul-de-sacs, property walls, and topographic features, which all contribute to more sinuous routes. This aligns with observed realities and the consensus of many researchers [18,61,62]. Our results further highlighted the cost associated with sinuous routes and emphasized the need for school catchment planning to prioritize route distance over crow-fly distance. At the same time, PDR, street network connectivity, and relevant theories and indicators of spatial syntax are also suitable methods for assessing students' travel patterns.

In the aftermath of epidemics, there is a shift towards more controlled and protected living environments, driven by the enduring effects of epidemic management strategies on societal behaviors and living arrangements. These effects include, but are not limited to, remnants of enclosed management and ongoing awareness of isolated communities. Gated compounds in China represent both a legacy and a prevailing norm, necessitating long-term consideration and resolution by policymakers and urban planners [63]. Demolishing the walls of residential communities may not be an overly radical measure, at least it may not have been before the pandemic. In 2016, the Chinese government even introduced a policy that called for the complete removal of walls to alleviate urban congestion and utilize idle resources within communities [64]. Due to complex factors such as conflicting interests, social norms, and security concerns, compounded by the onset of the pandemic, this planning initiative was ultimately abandoned. Things have changed now. Currently, China is promoting the opening of boundary-free parks and school sports resources. Changes in urban form are also possible. A suitable approach to address potential limitations is to gradually and systematically open up. Residents sauntering in communities may offer "street eye and neighborhood surveillance" [65]. Additionally, the widespread presence of surveillance cameras in Chinese cities also contributes to a sense of security for families.

6. Limitations

This study has several limitations. It specifically examines the central area of Nanjing, a megacity in China. Access to socioeconomic and school travel data about Chinese households is limited, making it challenging for researchers to obtain accurate information. The threshold for walking distance to school depends on various factors, including topography, street networks, building layouts, and social norms. Research on this issue in Chinese cities is still insufficient, and the exact distance threshold remains unclear.

Additionally, issues related to travel modes influenced by household income disparities cannot be adequately addressed. Future research could integrate social surveys to obtain more precise and targeted information, and incorporate additional dimensions of influencing factors, such as street-level air quality, noise, household income, travel habits, etc. Based on the available data, more refined studies on socio-economic stratification and age group segmentation could be conducted to gain a deeper understanding of the commuting characteristics of Chinese middle school students.

Meanwhile, the Chinese government has not yet released carbon emission coefficients for various types of motor vehicles or data on household transportation, and there is no standardized method for estimating carbon emissions. The calculation method used in this study is based on the existing literature, which employs GIS analysis and travel distance estimates, and remains relatively rough. Nevertheless, this study can serve as a method to bypass data barriers, facilitating quick communication with planners and enhancing public understanding, while also providing a foundation for further calculations.

7. Conclusions

This study uses Nanjing, China, as a case study to examine the potential of community forms and existing urban greening to provide shade and reduce detours at the urban scale. The research demonstrates how gated urban forms detour school commuting routes and identifies which home-to-school routes are severely exposed to heat. Given that school commute times and directions are predictable, we propose a practical and universal framework to assess and identify vulnerable areas and implement targeted interventions.

We found that approximately 34% of middle school families in Nanjing face challenges with walking to school, while only 37% can conveniently access schools on foot. The average PDR for all commuting routes is 1.52, with 70% exceeding 1.3. The PSR is 0.3, with 36% of values falling below 0.2. This indicates that 36% of families experience significant heat exposure on home–school routes. We advocate for the dual assessment of commuting routes using both the PDR and PSR. In Nanjing, only 24.18% of routes are guaranteed to have minimal detours and adequate shade.

The research findings are expected to swiftly and directly identify the challenges (long walking distances and limited shaded areas) faced by middle school students in Nanjing in terms of walking to school. By precisely pinpointing these existing issues, low-cost interventions can be implemented to address them in a targeted manner. This paper offers several recommendations for urban management and planning design, including reducing the walls of certain gated communities, adding school entrances and exits based on residential locations, opening internal pathways of public institutions, temporarily utilizing idle spaces, and integrating existing urban greenery into commuting routes. These interventions aim to enhance pedestrian permeability and optimize urban form through micro-scale transformations and the integration of existing resources. Such changes would not only provide school-age students with better access to cooler and healthier environments but also encourage more families to adopt active commuting habits, thereby serving as a lever to promote school decarbonization and mitigate climate warming. We emphasize that, although these interventions are designed for specific cases, they can also address broader issues encountered in multiple areas.

This research provides an integrated analysis of urban form and management, school commuting, and school decarbonization. The findings fill a gap in related research within Chinese cities and can be applied to other cities to reveal how salutary shortcuts can be exploited from adverse urban forms, leading to cooler, healthier, and more sustainable urban travel environments.

Author Contributions: Conceptualization, Lifei Wang and Lingyun Han; methodology, Lifei Wang and Zhen Xu; software, Lifei Wang and Ziqun Lin; validation, Lifei Wang, Zhen Xu and Ziqun Lin; formal analysis, Lifei Wang; investigation, Lifei Wang; resources, Zhen Xu and Lingyun Han; data curation, Lifei Wang; writing—original draft preparation, Lifei Wang; writing—review and editing, Lifei Wang and Zhen Xu; visualization, Lifei Wang and Ziqun Lin; supervision, Zhen Xu and Lingyun Han; project administration, Zhen Xu; funding acquisition, Zhen Xu. All authors have read and agreed to the published version of the manuscript.

Funding: This work was supported by National Natural Science Foundation of China [No. 52078254], Humanities and Social Sciences Foundation of the Ministry of Education of China [18YJCZH043], and Priority Academic Program Development of Jiangsu Higher Education Institutions.

Data Availability Statement: The original contributions presented in the study are included in the article material, further inquiries can be directed to the corresponding author.

Conflicts of Interest: The authors declare no conflict of interest.

References

1. Newman, P. Cool planning: How urban planning can mainstream responses to climate change. *Cities* **2020**, *103*, 102651. [CrossRef]
2. Loo, B.P. Walking towards a happy city. *J. Transp. Geogr.* **2021**, *93*, 103078. [CrossRef]
3. Bertolini, L. The next 30 years: Planning cities beyond mobility? *Eur. Plan. Stud.* **2023**, *31*, 2354–2367. [CrossRef]
4. Bertolini, L. From "streets for traffic" to "streets for people": Can street experiments transform urban mobility? *Transp. Rev.* **2020**, *40*, 734–753. [CrossRef]
5. Lam, H.Y.; Jayasinghe, S.; Ahuja, K.D.; Hills, A.P. Active school commuting in school children: A narrative review of current evidence and future research implications. *Int. J. Environ. Res. Public Health* **2023**, *20*, 6929. [CrossRef]
6. McDonald, N.C. Children's mode choice for the school trip: The role of distance and school location in walking to school. *Transportation* **2008**, *35*, 23–35. [CrossRef]
7. Khan, A.; Mandic, S.; Uddin, R. Association of active school commuting with physical activity and sedentary behaviour among adolescents: A global perspective from 80 countries. *J. Sci. Med. Sport* **2021**, *24*, 567–572. [CrossRef]
8. McDonald, N.C.; Steiner, R.L.; Lee, C.; Rhoulac Smith, T.; Zhu, X.; Yang, Y. Impact of the safe routes to school program on walking and bicycling. *J. Am. Plan. Assoc.* **2014**, *80*, 153–167. [CrossRef]

9. Aghamolaei, R.; Fallahpour, M. Strategies towards reducing carbon emission in university campuses: A comprehensive review of both global and local scales. *J. Build. Eng.* **2023**, *76*, 107183. [CrossRef]
10. Barron, A.R.; Parker, B.J.; Sayre, S.S.; Weber, S.S.; Weisbord, D.J. Carbon pricing approaches for climate decisions in US higher education: Proxy carbon prices for deep decarbonization. *Elem. Sci. Anth.* **2020**, *8*, 42. [CrossRef]
11. Pantelaki, E.; Caspani, A.C.; Maggi, E. Impact of home-school commuting mode choice on carbon footprint and sustainable transport policy scenarios. *Case Stud. Transp. Policy* **2024**, *15*, 101110. [CrossRef]
12. Azegami, Y.; Imanishi, M.; Fujiwara, K.; Kusaka, H. Effects of solar radiation in the streets on pedestrian route choice in a city during the summer season. *Build. Environ.* **2023**, *235*, 110250. [CrossRef]
13. Langenheim, N.; White, M.; Tapper, N.; Livesley, S.J.; Ramirez-Lovering, D. Right tree, right place, right time: A visual-functional design approach to select and place trees for optimal shade benefit to commuting pedestrians. *Sustain. Cities Soc.* **2020**, *52*, 101816. [CrossRef]
14. Liao, C.; Dai, T. Is "Attending Nearby School" Near? An analysis of travel-to-school distances of primary students in Beijing using Smart card data. *Sustainability* **2022**, *14*, 4344. [CrossRef]
15. Liu, A.; Kelobonye, K.; Zhou, Z.; Xu, Q.; Xu, Z.; Han, L. School commuting mode shift: A scenario analysis for active school commuting using GIS and online map API. *ISPRS Int. J. Geo-Inf.* **2020**, *9*, 520. [CrossRef]
16. Basu, R.; Colaninno, N.; Alhassan, A.; Sevtsuk, A. Hot and bothered: Exploring the effect of heat on pedestrian route choice behavior and accessibility. *Cities* **2024**, *155*, 105435. [CrossRef]
17. Khanian, M.; Łaszkiewicz, E.; Kronenberg, J.; Sikorska, D. Urban heterogeneity of the trade-offs between exposure to greenery and walking distance in children's home–school routes. *Appl. Geogr.* **2024**, *173*, 103437. [CrossRef]
18. Clark, A.F.; Bent, E.A.; Gilliland, J. Shortening the trip to school: Examining how children's active school travel is influenced by shortcuts. *Environ. Plan. B Plan. Des.* **2016**, *43*, 499–514. [CrossRef]
19. Smith, M.; Hawley, G.; Mackay, L.; Hosking, J.; Mackie, H.; Ikeda, E.; Egli, V.; Ellaway, A.; Witten, K. Impact of changing road infrastructure on children's active travel: A multi-methods study from Auckland, New Zealand. *J. Transp. Health* **2020**, *18*, 100868. [CrossRef]
20. Lidbe, A.; Li, X.; Adanu, E.K.; Nambisan, S.; Jones, S. Exploratory analysis of recent trends in school travel mode choices in the US. *Transp. Res. Interdiscip. Perspect.* **2020**, *6*, 100146. [CrossRef]
21. Mammen, G.; Stone, M.R.; Buliung, R.; Faulkner, G. School travel planning in Canada: Identifying child, family, and school-level characteristics associated with travel mode shift from driving to active school travel. *J. Transp. Health* **2014**, *1*, 288–294. [CrossRef]
22. Nelson, N.M.; Foley, E.; O'gorman, D.J.; Moyna, N.M.; Woods, C.B. Active commuting to school: How far is too far? *Int. J. Behav. Nutr. Phys. Act.* **2008**, *5*, 1. [CrossRef]
23. Zhang, R.; Yao, E.; Liu, Z. School travel mode choice in Beijing, China. *J. Transp. Geogr.* **2017**, *62*, 98–110. [CrossRef]
24. Ikeda, E.; Stewart, T.; Garrett, N.; Egli, V.; Mandic, S.; Hosking, J.; Witten, K.; Hawley, G.; Tautolo, E.S.; Rodda, J.; et al. Built environment associates of active school travel in New Zealand children and youth: A systematic meta-analysis using individual participant data. *J. Transp. Health* **2018**, *9*, 117–131. [CrossRef]
25. Kontou, E.; McDonald, N.C.; Brookshire, K.; Pullen-Seufert, N.C.; LaJeunesse, S. US active school travel in 2017: Prevalence and correlates. *Prev. Med. Rep.* **2020**, *17*, 101024. [CrossRef]
26. Hossain, S.T.; Al-Ramadan, B.; Bilal, M.; Altuwaijri, H.A. Enhancing Accessibility in Public Spaces: A Computational Study of Hatirjheel Lakefront Using Space Syntax. *ISPRS Int. J. Geo-Inf.* **2025**, *14*, 29. [CrossRef]
27. Şahin Körmeçli, P. Analysis of walkable street networks by using the space syntax and GIS techniques: A case study of Çankırı City. *ISPRS Int. J. Geo-Inf.* **2023**, *12*, 216. [CrossRef]
28. Hacar, Ö.Ö.; Gülgen, F.; Bilgi, S. Evaluation of the space syntax measures affecting pedestrian density through ordinal logistic regression analysis. *ISPRS Int. J. Geo-Inf.* **2020**, *9*, 589. [CrossRef]
29. Scoppa, M.; Bawazir, K.; Alawadi, K. Walking the superblocks: Street layout efficiency and the sikkak system in Abu Dhabi. *Sustain. Cities Soc.* **2018**, *38*, 359–369. [CrossRef]
30. Wang, X.; Liu, Y.; Yao, Y.; Zhou, S.; Zhu, Q.; Liu, M.; Helbich, M. Adolescents' environmental perceptions mediate associations between streetscape environments and active school travel. *Transp. Res. Part D Transp. Environ.* **2023**, *114*, 103549. [CrossRef]
31. Sun, G.; Wallace, D.; Webster, C. Unravelling the impact of street network structure and gated community layout in development-oriented transit design. *Land Use Policy* **2020**, *90*, 104328. [CrossRef]
32. Han, L.; Xu, Z.; Sabel, C. Exploring the potential of urban (re) form: Modifying gated communities to shorten school travel distance in Nanjing, China. *Environ. Plan. B Urban Anal. City Sci.* **2021**, *48*, 2536–2553. [CrossRef]
33. Chevalier, A.; Charlemagne, M. When connectivity makes safer routes to school: Conclusions from aggregate data on child transportation in Shanghai. *Transp. Res. Interdiscip. Perspect.* **2020**, *8*, 100267. [CrossRef]
34. Morakinyo, T.E.; Balogun, A.A.; Adegun, O.B. Comparing the effect of trees on thermal conditions of two typical urban buildings. *Urban Clim.* **2013**, *3*, 76–93. [CrossRef]

35. Deilami, K.; Rudner, J.; Butt, A.; MacLeod, T.; Williams, G.; Romeijn, H.; Amati, M. Allowing users to benefit from tree shading: Using a smartphone app to allow adaptive route planning during extreme heat. *Forests* **2020**, *11*, 998. [CrossRef]
36. Igoe, D.P.; Downs, N.J.; Parisi, A.V.; Amar, A. Evaluation of shade profiles while walking in urban environments: A case study from inner suburban Sydney, Australia. *Build. Environ.* **2020**, *177*, 106873. [CrossRef]
37. Neset, T.S.; Navarra, C.; Graça, M.; Opach, T.; Wilk, J.; Wallin, P.; Andersson, L.; Cruz, S.S.; Monteiro, A.; Rød, J.K. Navigating urban heat–Assessing the potential of a pedestrian routing tool. *Urban Clim.* **2022**, *46*, 101333. [CrossRef]
38. Xiong, K.; He, B.J. Planning for heat-resilient educational precincts: Framework formulation, cooling infrastructure selection and walkable routes determination. *Sustain. Cities Soc.* **2024**, *101*, 105183. [CrossRef]
39. AlKheder, S. The relation between walkability in hot arid regions and the built environment: The case of Kuwait in the Arabian Gulf. *J. Urban. Int. Res. Placemaking Urban Sustain.* **2023**, 1–25. [CrossRef]
40. Meng, Y.; Wang, J.; Xi, C.; Han, L.; Feng, Z.; Cao, S.J. Investigation of heat stress on urban roadways for commuting children and mitigation strategies from the perspective of urban design. *Urban Clim.* **2023**, *49*, 101564. [CrossRef]
41. White, M.; Kimm, G.; Langenheim, N. Pedestrian access modelling with tree shade–won't someone think of the children. *Procedia Eng.* **2017**, *198*, 139–151. [CrossRef]
42. Ribeiro, P.J.; Fonseca, F. Students' home-university commuting patterns: A shift towards more sustainable modes of transport. *Case Stud. Transp. Policy* **2022**, *10*, 954–964. [CrossRef]
43. Wu, D.; Ma, L.; Yan, X. Exploring zonal heterogeneities of primary school students' commute-mode choices through a geographically weighted regression model. *J. Geogr. Sci.* **2024**, *34*, 804–833. [CrossRef]
44. Pietrapertosa, F.; Tancredi, M.; Salvia, M.; Proto, M.; Pepe, A.; Giordano, M.; Afflitto, N.; Sarricchio, G.; Di Leo, S.; Cosmi, C. An educational awareness program to reduce energy consumption in schools. *J. Clean. Prod.* **2021**, *278*, 123949. [CrossRef]
45. Kuonen, S. Estimating greenhouse gas emissions from travel–a GIS-based study. *Geogr. Helv.* **2015**, *70*, 185–192. [CrossRef]
46. Zhang, J.; Ai, Q.; Ye, Y.; Deng, S. A hybrid estimation of carbon footprints for urban commuting transportation via path reconstruction. *Environ. Plan. B Urban Anal. City Sci.* **2024**, *51*, 456–478. [CrossRef]
47. Rong, P.; Zhang, L.; Qin, Y.; Xie, Z.; Li, Y. Spatial differentiation of daily travel carbon emissions in small-and medium-sized cities: An empirical study in Kaifeng, China. *J. Clean. Prod.* **2018**, *197*, 1365–1373. [CrossRef]
48. Määttä-Juntunen, H.; Antikainen, H.; Kotavaara, O.; Rusanen, J. Using GIS tools to estimate CO2 emissions related to the accessibility of large retail stores in the Oulu region, Finland. *J. Transp. Geogr.* **2011**, *19*, 346–354. [CrossRef]
49. Zhang, S.; Zhang, C.; Cai, W.; Bai, Y.; Callaghan, M.; Chang, N.; Chen, B.; Chen, H.; Cheng, L.; Dai, H.; et al. The 2023 China report of the Lancet Countdown on health and climate change: Taking stock for a thriving future. *Lancet Public Health* **2023**, *8*, e978–e995. [CrossRef]
50. He, D.; Shi, Q.; Liu, X.; Zhong, Y.; Zhang, L. Generating 2m fine-scale urban tree cover product over 34 metropolises in China based on deep context-aware sub-pixel mapping network. *Int. J. Appl. Earth Obs. Geoinf.* **2022**, *106*, 102667. [CrossRef]
51. Shen, Y.S.; Lin, Y.C.; Cheah, W.; Lin, J.; Xu, L.; Li, Y. Influences and pathways of urban form and lifestyle on carbon emission reduction. *Urban Clim.* **2022**, *46*, 101325. [CrossRef]
52. Madanipour, A. Temporary use of space: Urban processes between flexibility, opportunity and precarity. *Urban Stud.* **2018**, *55*, 1093–1110. [CrossRef]
53. Dong, J.; Guo, R.; Guo, F.; Cai, J. Potential evaluation and implementation strategy for pocket park construction in high-density urban areas: A case study in dalian, China. *Front. Archit. Res.* **2024**, *13*, 319–334. [CrossRef]
54. Wolf, H.; Vierø, A.R.; Szell, M. CoolWalks: Assessing the Potential of Shaded Routing for Active Mobility in Urban Street Networks. *arXiv* **2024**, arXiv:2405.01225. [CrossRef]
55. Cirrincione, L.; Di Dio, S.; La Gennusa, M.; Peri, G.; Rizzo, G.; Scaccianoce, G. Changing commuters' mobility behaviors of university campuses: Environmental and energy comparisons. In *E3S Web of Conferences*; EDP Sciences: Les Ulis, France, 2021; Volume 312, p. 12003.
56. Clabeaux, R.; Carbajales-Dale, M.; Ladner, D.; Walker, T. Assessing the carbon footprint of a university campus using a life cycle assessment approach. *J. Clean. Prod.* **2020**, *273*, 122600. [CrossRef]
57. Valls-Val, K.; Bovea, M.D. Carbon footprint in Higher Education Institutions: A literature review and prospects for future research. *Clean Technol. Environ. Policy* **2021**, *23*, 2523–2542. [CrossRef] [PubMed]
58. Yanez Vargas, J.; Klein-Banai, C. Guide to estimating multi-modal commuting greenhouse gas emissions. *Sustain. J. Rec.* **2020**, *13*, 119–126. [CrossRef]
59. Crotti, D.; Grechi, D.; Maggi, E. Reducing the carbon footprint in college mobility: The car commuters' perspective in an Italian case study. *Environ. Impact Assess. Rev.* **2022**, *92*, 106702. [CrossRef]
60. Giles-Corti, B.; Wood, G.; Pikora, T.; Learnihan, V.; Bulsara, M.; Van Niel, K.; Timperio, A.; McCormack, G.; Villanueva, K. School site and the potential to walk to school: The impact of street connectivity and traffic exposure in school neighborhoods. *Health Place* **2011**, *17*, 545–550. [CrossRef]

61. Buliung, R.N.; Larsen, K.; Faulkner, G.E.; Stone, M.R. The "path" not taken: Exploring structural differences in mapped-versus shortest-network-path school travel routes. *Am. J. Public Health* **2013**, *103*, 1589–1596. [CrossRef]
62. Banerjee, T.; Uhm, J.; Bahl, D. Walking to school: The experience of children in inner city Los Angeles and implications for policy. *J. Plan. Educ. Res.* **2014**, *34*, 123–140. [CrossRef]
63. Zou, J.; Wang, C.; Chen, S.; Zhang, J.; Qiu, B.; Yang, H. Expanding the associations between built environment characteristics and residential mobility in high-density neighborhood unit. *Sustain. Cities Soc.* **2024**, *116*, 105885. [CrossRef]
64. Yang, S.; Tan, W.; Yan, L. Evaluating accessibility benefits of opening gated communities for pedestrians and cyclists in China: A case study of Shanghai. *Sustainability* **2021**, *13*, 598. [CrossRef]
65. Jacobs, J. *The Death and Life of Great American Cities*; Random House: Manhattan, NY, USA, 1961.

International Journal of
Geo-Information

MDPI

Article

Spatial Prediction of High-Risk Areas for Asthma in Metropolitan Areas: A Machine Learning Approach Applied to Tehran, Iran

Alireza Mohammadi [1,*], Elahe Pishgar [2] and Juan Aguilera [3]

1 Department of Geography and Urban-Rural Planning, Faculty of Social Sciences, University of Mohaghegh Ardabili, Ardabil 5619911367, Iran
2 Department of Geography, Faculty of Geography, University of Tehran, Tehran 1417853933, Iran; epishagar2018@gmail.com
3 Center for Community Health Impact, UTHealth Houston School of Public Health, El Paso, TX 79902, USA
* Correspondence: a.mohammadi@uma.ac.ir

Abstract: Asthma prevalence in large urban areas of developing countries is a significant public health concern, with increased rates driven by various socioeconomic and environmental factors. This study aims to predict asthma risk in Tehran, a major urban center in Iran. Data from 1473 asthma patients, alongside demographic, socioeconomic, air quality, environmental, weather, and healthcare access variables, were analyzed using geographic information systems (GIS) and remote sensing techniques. Three ensemble machine learning algorithms—Random Forest (RF), Gradient Boosting Machine (GBM), and Extreme Gradient Boosting (XGBoost)—were applied to model and predict asthma risk. A Negative Binomial Regression Model (NBRM) identified seven key predictors: population density, unemployment rate, particulate matter ($PM_{2.5}$ and PM_{10}), nitrogen dioxide (NO_2), sulfur dioxide (SO_2), neighborhood deprivation index, and road intersection density. Among the algorithms, GBM outperformed the others, with a training RMSE of 0.56 and a test RMSE of 1.07, demonstrating strong generalization. Additionally, GBM achieved the highest R-squared values (0.95 for training and 0.76 for testing) and lower MAE values (0.43 for training and 0.88 for testing). Effective pattern recognition was confirmed by EV values of 0.95 for training and 0.75 for testing, along with a Moran's I value of 0.17, indicating minimal spatial autocorrelation.

Keywords: large cities; spatial analysis; sociodemographic; built environment; ambient air pollution; urban heat islands; healthcare facilities; Sentinel-5; google earth engine; Landsat 8

1. Introduction

Asthma, a primary non-communicable disease, affects both children and adults, with the highest prevalence among children. It causes inflammation and narrowing of the airways, leading to symptoms like coughing, wheezing, breathlessness, and chest tightness [1]. Approximately 300 million people have asthma all over the world, with 250,000 deaths attributed to the disease annually, most of which are preventable [2]. As of a 2023 study, asthma prevalence varied across continents: Asia (3.44%), Africa (3.67%), South America (4.90%), Europe (5.69%), North America (8.29%), and Oceania (8.33%); among global asthma cases, 26.70% were severe, 30.99% were eosinophilic, 48.95% included allergic rhinitis, and 7.0% to 25.40% included nasal polyps [3]. Asthma is often underdiagnosed and undertreated, particularly in low- and middle-income countries [1]. Various studies have reported the prevalence of asthma in Iran in recent years at around 8.9% (95% confidence interval (CI): 8.5–9.3) [4,5].

Furthermore, demographic and socioeconomic factors like population density, aging, illiteracy, and unemployment are linked to higher rates of asthma prevalence and mortality in large urban areas [6]. High population density increases exposure to air pollution and asthma [7,8]. Aging populations may experience worsened asthma symptoms due to age-related changes [9,10]. Low literacy levels can hinder effective asthma management, leading to more severe outcomes [11]. Unemployment, often tied to lower socioeconomic status, limits access to healthcare and may increase exposure to asthma environmental triggers [12,13].

Previous studies have also shown that exposure to ambient air pollutants, including particulate matter ($PM_{2.5}$ and PM_{10}), nitrogen dioxide (NO_2), ozone (O_3), and sulfur dioxide (SO_2), is a significant risk factor for asthma prevalence [14–17] Particulate matter, consisting of tiny particles suspended in the air, can penetrate deep into the respiratory system, triggering airway inflammation and exacerbating asthma symptoms [18]. NO_2, primarily emitted from vehicles and industrial sources, has been associated with increased asthma incidence and severity, likely due to its irritant effects on the airways [19,20]. Increased levels of O_3, a highly reactive gas formed by the interaction of sunlight with pollutants like NO_2, were linked to asthma attacks and decreased lung function among individuals residing in urban centers [21]. SO_2, primarily emitted from industrial processes and power plants, can irritate the airways and exacerbate respiratory conditions such as asthma [20].

Large urban areas in developing countries also pose significant built environmental risks for asthma onset or fatality. A study has indicated that the prevalence, severity, and morbidity of asthma have significantly increased among residents in low-income urban areas [21]. Poor-quality urban environments, characterized by socioeconomic disadvantage, inadequate access to healthcare, and poor housing conditions, contribute to the exacerbation of asthma symptoms in deprived areas [22–25]. Road intersection density, often associated with high traffic volume and vehicular emissions, is another significant determinant of asthma prevalence [25,26]. The proximity of residential areas to busy roads increases exposure to traffic-related air pollutants, such as particulate matter and nitrogen oxides, which can aggravate asthma symptoms and respiratory inflammation [27].

According to previous studies [28,29], the Normalized Difference Vegetation Index (NDVI), a green space and vegetation density measure, has been inversely associated with asthma prevalence. Higher levels of greenery in neighborhoods are linked to improved air quality, reduced pollution exposure, and enhanced respiratory health outcomes [28,29]. Exposure to industrial emissions, including SO_2 and volatile organic compounds, is a known risk factor for asthma prevalence [30]. Additionally, proximity to fuel stations in urban areas, characterized by emissions from gasoline and diesel vehicles, is associated with increased asthma prevalence due to heightened exposure to benzene, a known respiratory irritant [31]. Urban heat islands (UHIs), where cities are hotter than surrounding areas due to human activities, worsen with climate change, leading to higher asthma prevalence and severity. Increased temperatures amplify air pollutants like ozone (O_3) and particulate matter ($PM_{2.5}$), which trigger asthma symptoms [32,33].

Climate change also prolongs heat waves and the pollen season, further aggravating asthma [34]. Urban areas experience high temperatures due to extreme climate conditions, worsening asthma by intensifying pollutants like ozone and particulate matter. Longer heat waves and extended pollen seasons also aggravate asthma [34]. Some studies confirmed that limited access to healthcare facilities in large cities of developing countries exacerbates asthma by delaying diagnosis, reducing treatment adherence, and hindering symptom management [35,36].

In Tehran, the capital city of Iran, it was estimated that the average asthma prevalence was 13.4% [37], exceeding the country's overall average asthma prevalence of 8.9%. Certain studies indicated that asthma among adults in Tehran was 11.73% [5]. In children, the highest reported prevalence was 32% in Tehran, while in adolescents, it was 37% [38]. Previous research on asthma in Tehran has frequently explored the correlation between asthma and patient lifestyle [39], the link between asthma and food allergies or environmental pollutants [40], and the economic implications [41] associated with asthma. Some studies have also examined asthma's spatial dimensions and spatial modeling within Tehran city using ensemble machine learning algorithms [42–44].

Spatial epidemiology is the application of theory and methods from epidemiology, geography, and statistics to describe spatial distributions of health outcomes and to analyze associations with possible causes to inform intervention and improve health [45]. Utilizing geographic information systems (GIS) for spatial analysis of asthma is essential for comprehending its prevalence in urban areas and informing prevention and management strategies [42,46,47]. Various geostatistical modeling techniques, including spatial regression [48], Bayesian [49], and machine learning algorithms (MLAs), integrate geographical and environmental data to identify patterns and correlations with asthma incidence [42].

Geographically Weighted Regression (GWR), Multiscale Geographically Weighted Regression (MGWR), Spatial Lag Model (SLM), Spatial Error Model (SEM), Bayesian Spatial Models, and Spatial Autoregressive Models (SAR) are primarily statistical or econometric models that incorporate spatial dependencies and structures [50]. These methods are valued for their interpretability and ability to model spatial relationships and dependencies explicitly [51]. However, they are not typically classified as machine learning algorithms (MLAs). Among the various machine learning algorithms, Random Forest (RF), Gradient Boosting Machine (GBM), and Extreme Gradient Boosting (XGBoost) are ensemble algorithms that have been specifically adapted for spatial count data. These algorithms capture complex, non-linear relationships, making them practical for regression and prediction tasks. While GBM improves accuracy by iteratively optimizing residual errors, RF minimizes overfitting by averaging multiple decision trees. Large spatial datasets benefit greatly from XGBoost's scalability and regularization. To balance bias, variance, and overfitting, grid search and cross-validation were used to optimize the hyperparameters for all algorithms, including the number of trees, learning rate, and regularization terms. These algorithms were selected because of their versatility and resilience in identifying significant predictors and interactions in spatial epidemiological settings [42,52].

Machine learning (ML), which offers improved disease prediction, risk assessment, and individualized treatment skills, has emerged as a key instrument in medical research in recent years. The ability of machine learning algorithms like Random Forest (RF), Gradient Boosting Machine (GBM), and XGBoost to capture intricate, non-linear correlations between risk factors is demonstrated by successful applications in domains including diabetes, cardiovascular illnesses, and cancer [53–55], as well as in the prediction of infectious diseases such as COVID-19 [56]. In the context of asthma, machine learning (ML) is an emerging method that enhances conventional statistical techniques by offering more precise forecasts and insights into the incidence of asthma. Although there are currently few studies on machine learning in asthma risk prediction [42–44], newer studies show how ML is increasingly used to advance knowledge and direct focused public health initiatives. By using cutting-edge machine learning techniques to forecast asthma risk in Tehran, this work adds to this trend while tackling the city's problems with extreme air pollution, urban heat island effects, and healthcare inequities. The study intends to further the integration of machine learning in asthma epidemiology by improving spatial risk prediction and informing public health initiatives using these methods.

This study fills essential gaps in the body of knowledge regarding the prevalence of asthma in Tehran. Although the prevalence of asthma in the city has been studied in previous years, machine-learning-based regression techniques for predicting spatial risk have not been widely applied. Furthermore, sociodemographic, built-environmental, and environmental factors—like air pollution, urban heat islands, and healthcare accessibility—have not all been thoroughly incorporated into a single spatial framework in previous studies. This study uses the Binomial Negative Regression Model (BNRM), geographic information systems (GIS), and sophisticated ensemble machine learning techniques, such as Random Forest (RF), Gradient Boosting Machine (GBM), and Extreme Gradient Boosting (XGBoost), to close these gaps. These resources pinpoint high-risk areas and offer helpful information for focused public health initiatives. The study uses extensive spatial regression models and a larger dataset to improve prediction accuracy and policy relevance. Tehran is a critical case study because of its extreme air pollution, notable urban heat island effects, and inequalities in access to healthcare. Asthma risks are increased by the city's congested urban environment and industrial pollution, underscoring the necessity of efficient spatial modeling. This study contributes to a more thorough understanding of asthma prevalence by concentrating on Tehran and provides a solid framework for predicting spatial risk in highly polluted urban environments. It focuses on combining socioenvironmental factors to identify high-risk locations, which will help direct focused public health programs in the city.

2. Materials and Methods

2.1. Study Setting

Tehran, Iran's capital, covers 730 square kilometers with a population density of about 11,000 per square kilometer. It has over 8 million residents within the city and more than 15 million in the metropolitan area [57]. The city, divided into 22 districts and 350 neighborhoods, provides a unique environment for studying asthma prevalence and risk factors. The city experiences a semi-arid climate marked by hot summers and cold winters, resulting in diverse seasonal air quality challenges [58,59]. Tehran's urban heat island effects are significant, with temperature variations of up to 7 °C between urban and rural areas, influenced by dense construction and limited green spaces [60]. Approximately 7.5% of Tehran's population is 65 years or older, the illiteracy rate is 7%, and the unemployment rate was reported to be about 7% [61].

Tehran is one of the world's most polluted cities. It faces significant air pollution challenges, with elevated levels of particulate matter ($PM_{2.5}$ and PM_{10}) exceeding safe thresholds, reaching 30–50 $\mu g/m^3$ for $PM_{2.5}$ and 70–100 $\mu g/m^3$ for PM_{10} during peak pollution seasons [62]. Additionally, NO_2 levels persistently average 50–60 $\mu g/m^3$, surpassing the WHO limit of 40 $\mu g/m^3$. Ozone (O_3) concentrations can spike to 150 $\mu g/m^3$ in summer due to photochemical reactions from vehicular and industrial emissions, while SO_2 levels are generally lower, averaging 20–30 $\mu g/m^3$ with occasional industrial spikes [63,64].

According to calculations based on OSM data using a geographic information system, Tehran's urban infrastructure showcases a high road intersection density, notably exceeding 400 intersections per square kilometer in central districts. Furthermore, according to the calculation based on Landsat 8 images, the city's average Normalized Difference Vegetation Index (NDVI) was 0.3, indicating moderate vegetation cover, with higher values observed in the greener northern areas. The city has 6.5 m^2 of green area for every person [65]. Proximity to industrial zones, particularly in the outskirts, exposes residents to significant industrial emissions [66]. There are about 120 public and private hospitals in Tehran, and about 60 hospitals provide services to asthma patients [61]. However, the spatial distribution of these hospitals is uneven, and local access to them varies. Figure 1 illustrates the location of the study area, the distribution of hospitals that have admitted patients with asthma, and the spatial distribution of asthma cases from 2020 to 2023.

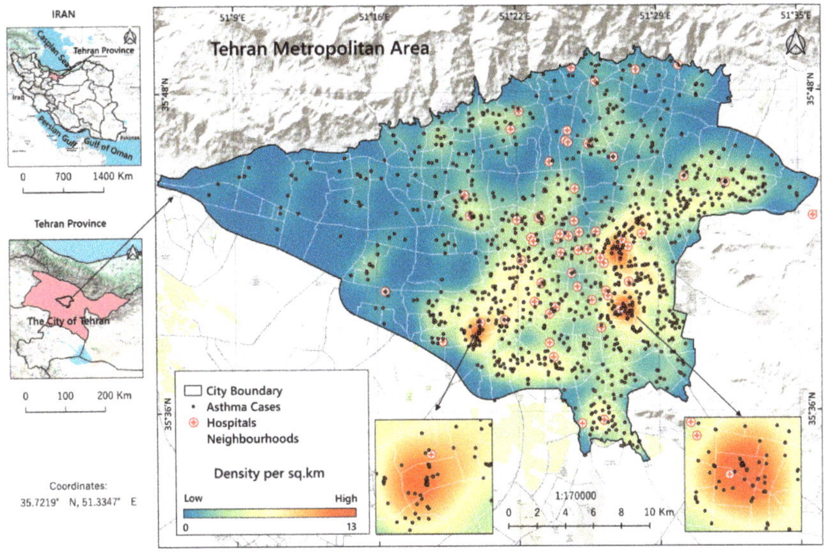

Figure 1. Spatial distribution map of asthma cases and their density in the study area.

2.2. Data Source and Its Processing

We employed a comprehensive dataset containing spatial and non-spatial data, consisting of 1 dependent variable and 15 independent variables selected based on existing literature. This dataset can be categorized into four primary groups: (1) census datasets, (2) remote sensing data acquired from Landsat 8 and Sentinel-5 satellite products, (3) GIS datasets, and (4) open-source datasets, which incorporate spatial data obtained from OpenStreetMap. The asthma data (response variable) consisted of information on 2179 patients, collected in Excel format from 70 hospitals affiliated with the Ministry of Health and Medical Education (MHME), spanning the period from 6 July 2020, to 2 August 2023, with an assigned ethics code number.

After incomplete or outlier cases were eliminated, 1473 patients made up the final sample for analysis. To protect patient privacy, the data were geocoded using the UTM coordinate system, which represents locations as neighborhood-level point features. This method allowed for spatial analysis while maintaining patient confidentiality. This secondary data analysis was approved as ethical and per the Ministry of Health and Medical Education's guidelines. The confirmed asthma diagnoses in the area during the designated study period are represented by the asthma cases included in this analysis. The study's reproducibility was ensured by adhering to a protocol that described the data integration and spatial analysis methodology. Although the data offer insightful information about the distribution of asthma, this study does not purport to provide a thorough epidemiological evaluation of all asthma cases in the study area.

Figure 2 shows the research methodology flowchart.

Patient information included age, sex, date of admission, date of discharge, hospitalization outcome (discharged, complete recovery, partial recovery, and death), and patient address. We used the patient addresses from the original dataset to create the point data for the dependent variable. These addresses were geocoded to determine each case's exact geographic coordinates (latitude and longitude). Following this, the data were aggregated into 350 neighborhoods within Tehran city and compiled as asthma cases (N = 1473) (dependent variable) in a shapefile. The indicators considered are provided in Table 1, based on existing literature and data availability for the city. Population data and data on elderly individuals (aged 65 and older) were extracted from the 2016 census data [67]. The proportion of illiterate people (%) among individuals aged 6 and above and the proportion of unemployed people (%) among individuals in the labor force aged 15 to 64 were calculated for the 350 neighborhoods using census data. Additionally, information on the neighborhood deprivation index (percentage of deteriorated buildings in each neighborhood) was obtained from Tehran Municipality, indicating areas with deprived buildings.

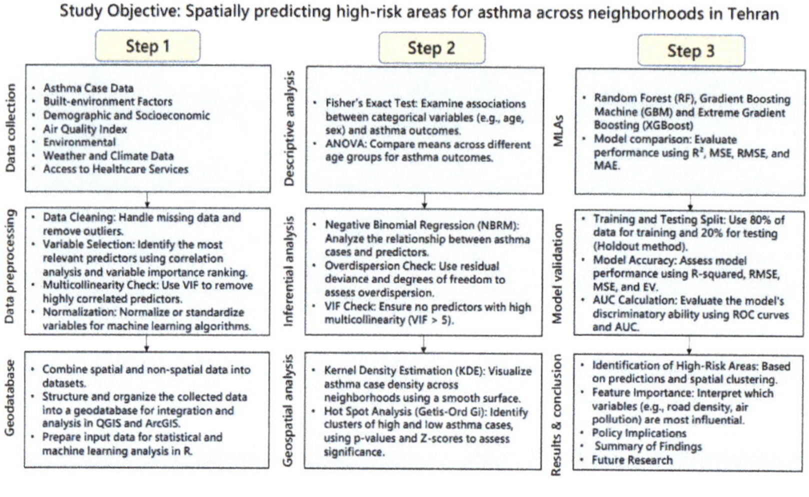

Figure 2. Research methodology flowchart.

Table 1. Indicators identified from the literature review to examine the relationship between asthma prevalence and neighborhood characteristics in Tehran (2020–2024).

Aspects	Indicator	Spatial Database and Data Type	Source
Demographic and Socioeconomic	V1: Population density (per sq.km)	Census, ESRI shapefile	[67]
	V2: Proportion of elderly (%)	Census, ESRI shapefile	[67]
	V3: Proportion of illiterate people (%)	Census, ESRI shapefile	[67]
	V4: Proportion of unemployed people (%)	Census, ESRI shapefile	[67]
Air Quality Index	V5: Particulate matter (AAI include $PM_{2.5}$ and PM_{10})	Sentinel-5, Raster	Google Earth Engine
	V6: Nitrogen dioxide (NO_2)	Sentinel-5, Raster	Google Earth Engine
	V7: Ozone (O_3)	Sentinel-5, Raster	Google Earth Engine
	V8: Sulfur dioxide (SO_2)	Sentinel-5, Raster	Google Earth Engine
Environmental	V9: Neighborhood deprivation index (%)	Land use map, ESRI shapefile	Tehran municipality, OpenStreetMap
	V10: Road intersection density (per square kilometers)	OSM, ESRI shapefile, and Raster	OpenStreetMap
	V11: Normalized Difference Vegetation Index (NDVI)	Landsat 8, Raster	Google Earth Engine
	V12: Exposure to industrial emissions	Land use map, OSM, ESRI shapefile	OpenStreetMap
	V13: Proximity to fuel stations	Land use map, OSM, ESRI shapefile	Tehran Municipality, OpenStreetMap
Weather and Climate	V14: Urban heat islands (UHIs)	Landsat 8, Raster	Google Earth Engine
Access and Utilization of Healthcare Services	V15: Access to healthcare facilities	Land use map, OSM, ESRI shapefile	Tehran municipality, OpenStreetMap

Data on the most common air pollutants, including offline high-resolution imagery of the UV Aerosol Index (UVAI), also known as the Absorbing Aerosol Index (AAI), and levels of nitrogen dioxide (NO_2), ozone (O_3), and sulfur dioxide (SO_2), were extracted using the Sentinel-5 Precursor, a satellite launched on 13 October 2017 by the European Space Agency to monitor air pollution. We employed the Google Earth Engine (GEE) cloud-based geospatial analysis platform to extract all city-level pollutant concentrations with a uniform cell size of 10 m. To calculate road intersection density (per square kilometer), we extracted all intersections from the road network using OpenStreetMap (OSM) data with QGIS software (version 3.36.3). The Normalized Difference Vegetation Index (NDVI) is a quantitative index of greenness ranging from 0 to 1, where 0 represents minimal or no greenness, and 1 represents maximum greenness [68]. The Normalized Difference Vegetation Index (NDVI) formula is typically represented as:

$$\mathrm{NDVI} = \frac{(\mathrm{NIR} - \mathrm{Red})}{(\mathrm{NIR} + \mathrm{Red})} \quad (1)$$

NIR denotes near-infrared reflectance, while Red signifies red reflectance. NDVI is a pivotal metric within remote sensing analytical products employed for vegetation assessment [69]. NDVI was determined using Landsat 8 imagery. For Landsat 8, the NDVI calculation is expressed as (Band 5 − Band 4)/(Band 5 + Band 4) [70].

Data regarding the locations of industrial sites (V12), fuel stations (V13), and healthcare facilities (V15) were extracted from the city's land use vector map, obtained from the Tehran City Municipality. To calculate V12, we computed the spatial density of industrial units per square kilometer. For variable V13, we used the Euclidean distance method to calculate the distance (in meters) between the neighborhood center and fuel stations. The proximity of these locations to the 350 neighborhoods' centroids was assessed using Euclidean distance tools in ArcGIS Pro. To calculate V15, we computed the spatial density of health centers (such as hospitals) per square kilometer. These data were subsequently cross-referenced with OpenStreetMap datasets.

Urban heat islands (UHIs) are characterized by elevated temperatures in urban areas compared to their rural surroundings, primarily due to human activities. Land surface temperature (LST) is a key metric for identifying UHIs, with urban areas typically exhibiting higher LSTs due to heat-absorbing surfaces and reduced vegetation cover [71]. The UHIs were quantified using the USGS Landsat 8 Level 2, Collection 2, Tier 1 product via Google Earth Engine (GEE). A commonly used formula for LST calculation from satellite imagery is derived from Planck's law, which relates the radiance detected by the sensor to the surface temperature. The formula is expressed as follows [68,72]:

$$\mathrm{LST} = \frac{K_2}{\ln\left(\frac{K_1}{T_B} + 1\right)} - 273.15 \quad (2)$$

where LST represents the land surface temperature in degrees Celsius, and K_1 and K_2 denote calibration constants specific to the sensor utilized. T_B signifies the brightness temperature recorded by the sensor. This formula stems from the fundamental principles of Planck's law and the Stefan–Boltzmann law, elucidating the correlation between the emitted radiance from a surface and its temperature [68,72].

Particulate matter (AAI, including $PM_{2.5}$ and PM_{10}) (V5), nitrogen dioxide (NO_2) (V6), ozone (O_3) (V7), sulfur dioxide (SO_2) (V8), and the Normalized Difference Vegetation Index (NDVI) (V11) and urban heat islands (UHIs) (V14) from Landsat 8 were among the environmental and air quality variables that we extracted using Google Earth Engine. Mean values were compiled for every spatial unit after raster data had been pre-processed to match neighborhood polygons spatially. We used the remote sensing variables' annual average values for compatibility with the 2020–2023 aggregated asthma data. Additionally, using the Sentinel-5 data's temporal coverage and spatial consistency, the spatial–temporal relationships between these variables and asthma prevalence were examined.

After preparing the spatial layers for each predictive variable, all selected spatial data indicators were transformed to the UTM Projection, WGS-84 Datum, Zone 39 N, with a uniform cell size of 30 m resolution to prevent any spatial output errors. The values of each variable (averaging where necessary) were then extracted for each neighborhood and stored in a geodatabase using ArcGIS Pro, maintaining the same coordinate system.

Figure 3 illustrates the spatial distribution of predictor value ranges across the study area, collected at the neighborhood level, which serves as the spatial analysis unit.

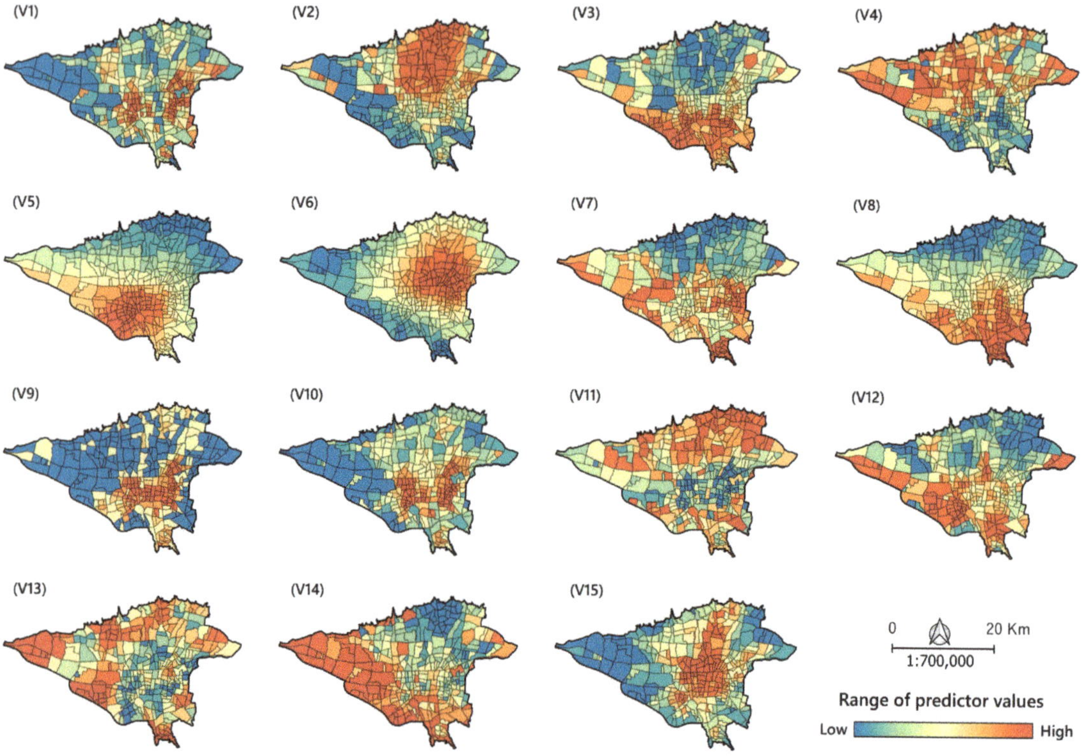

Figure 3. Spatial distribution maps of initial predictors in the study area.

2.3. Analytical Methods

2.3.1. Statistical Methods Used for Descriptive Analysis

We employed Fisher's exact test, an extension of the Chi-squared analysis [73], to evaluate the association between age, sex, and disease outcome to determine their independence under the null hypothesis. Additionally, analysis of variance (ANOVA) serves as a valuable statistical method for assessing disparities among the means of three or more groups, akin to an extension of the t-test for comparing multiple independent samples [74]. In this study, ANOVA was employed to assess the differences in mean ages across distinct age groups—categorized as "children" (age < 12), "adolescents" (age between 12 and 17), "adults" (age between 18 and 59), and "elderly" (age 60 and above)—concerning various disease outcome categories.

2.3.2. Statistical Methods Used for Inferential Analysis

Negative Binomial Regression Model (NBRM)

There are various methods to detect localized influential predictors in regression analysis, such as Explanatory Regression (ER), Ordinary Least Squares (OLS), and Generalized Linear Models (GLMs) [75]. GLMs are particularly noted for their effectiveness in pinpointing the most significant predictors in count data, especially when overdispersion is present. We assessed overdispersion by comparing the residual deviance to the degrees of freedom.

While machine learning algorithms are better than simple regressors in fitting data with multicollinearity, multicollinearity can affect model interpretability and feature importance across different machine learning algorithms [76]. Therefore, first, we ran a multicollinearity test to find predictors with high variance inflation factor (VIF) issues in R-Studio using the "car" package [77]. We removed highly correlated predictors according to previous studies (VIF > 5) [42]. We removed only one variable (V14) with the highest correlation (VIF = 5.2).

In the next step, Negative Binomial Regression (NBRM) was employed using the "MASS" package in R-Studio [78] to examine the relationship between asthma cases and predictors in this study. This method is ideal for counting data with overdispersion, a common issue in ecological and health studies [79]. NBRM extends Poisson regression to accommodate this variability, providing a better fit and more reliable estimates of coefficients and inference. In the generalized linear model framework, NBRM (Equation (3)) models the total count of events (Y) within a defined space–time interval, parameterized from a Poisson–gamma mixture as described by Hilbe [80], or equivalently, as the count of failures before achieving the $(1/\alpha)$th success. The NBRM model can be written as [81]:

$$\Pr(y_i|x_i) = \frac{\Gamma(y_i + \alpha^{-1})}{y_i!\Gamma(\alpha^{-1})}\left(\frac{\alpha^{-1}}{\alpha^{-1}+\mu_i}\right)^{\alpha-1}\left(\frac{\mu_i}{\alpha^{-1}+\mu_i}\right)^{y_i} \quad (3)$$

The formula represents the probability mass function of Negative Binomial Regression (NBRM), where $\Pr(y_i|x_i)$ denotes the probability of observing y_i events given predictor variables x_i. The function incorporates parameters α and μ_i, which describe the dispersion and mean, respectively. This equation is crucial for modeling count data with overdispersion, accommodating scenarios where the variance exceeds the mean, as commonly encountered in ecological and health studies [81].

2.3.3. Geospatial and Spatial Statistics Methods for Spatial Analysis

Kernel Density Estimation (KDE)

A well-known quartic type of kernel density estimation (KDE) method [82] was applied to create a heat map with a 30-square-meters cell size resolution, mapping asthma cases within the study area. This method assesses asthma case density per square kilometer using a smooth, continuous surface fitted over observed data points. It employs a quartic (biweight) kernel to enhance spatial visualization and capture patterns effectively, enabling detailed mapping and nuanced modeling of event distribution [83]. The optimal bandwidth size was determined using the mean random distance (RD mean) method [84]. A bandwidth of 1000 m, based on RD mean calculations, was selected for its effectiveness in producing a smooth density map.

The Hot Spot Analysis (Getis-Ord Gi*)

The Getis-Ord Gi* statistic, known as hot spot analysis (HAS), is a cluster mapping technique employed in health-related analysis to examine event density in specific locations [85]. Hot spots are areas with concentrated incidents vital for disease prevention [86].

The Gi* statistic identifies local spatial autocorrelation through Z score and p-value, indicating clusters of high or low values [86]. Significant Z scores arise when a feature's local sum and neighbors differ significantly from the overall sum, suggesting non-random clustering [87]. Using point feature patterns, the Gi* statistic has been widely used to pinpoint hot and cold spots [88]. This study utilized the Getis-Ord Gi* statistic to detect hot and cold spots of asthma occurrences based on sample data at the neighborhood level, applying the "K nearest neighbors" (KNN) method for spatial relationship conceptualization [86]. In spatial analysis, K nearest neighbors (KNN) identify the K closest polygons to a target based on metrics like Euclidean distance, which are ideal for detecting clusters or patterns involving neighboring polygons. This method is flexible, allowing us to adjust K for tailored proximity analysis and understand spatial relationships among features [85,86].

Our analysis used the false discovery rate (FDR), a statistical technique to manage false positives among significant outcomes during multiple-hypothesis testing. By lowering critical p-values, FDR addresses the heightened likelihood of false positives due to multiple comparisons, thereby enhancing accuracy in identifying genuinely significant findings in extensive datasets or spatial analyses [85,86].

The KDE creates a smooth surface to visualize event density, highlighting areas of high concentration without assessing statistical significance. At the same time, HAS (Getis-Ord Gi*) uses Z-scores and p-values to identify statistically significant clusters of high and low values, providing an analytical approach to detect local spatial autocorrelation [86].

2.3.4. Methods for Spatial Predictions Using MLAs

Among various types of machine learning algorithms, Random Forest (RF), Gradient Boosting Machine (GBM), and XGBoost algorithms were chosen for regression and prediction analysis. These MLAs are well-suited for spatial regression analysis due to their ability to manage complex relationships, large datasets, and noise. They enhance predictive accuracy, reveal key factors, and offer robust, generalizable insights into asthma prevalence [43,44,89].

Random Forest (RF)

Random Forest Regression (RF) is an ensemble-supervised machine learning algorithm developed by Leo Breiman and Adele Cutler, which creates models and generates predictions using an adaptation of the Random Forest algorithm [90]. The RF algorithm was designed and formulated for regression and prediction tasks. It constructs multiple decision trees using the bagging technique with bootstrapped samples, which involves generating random samples from the input data and training decision trees on these samples [91]. Developed by Ho in 1995 [92] and extended by Breiman in 2001 [93], RF is valued for its ease of implementation, speed, and high performance. For regression, it predicts by averaging the outputs of individual trees, reducing overfitting through majority voting. The algorithm ensures uncorrelated decision trees by selecting random feature subsets for training, which reduces model variance and enhances prediction accuracy, making it a robust choice for regression and prediction tasks. If implemented accordingly, RF can be adapted for count data, primarily through Poisson regression trees [91]. The RF algorithm constructs a model using a bagging technique, where multiple decision trees are created in parallel with random subsets of the training data. Each tree votes on an outcome, and the RF algorithm aggregates these votes for prediction. This ensemble method addresses overfitting issues of individual trees, resulting in a robust and intuitive model that requires fewer parameters [90].

Gradient Boosting Machine (GBM)

GBM is a robust machine learning algorithm used for regression tasks. It builds an ensemble of decision trees sequentially, where each new tree corrects the errors made by the previous ones by fitting them to the residuals. This technique uses weak learners (simple decision trees) and employs the mean squared error loss to improve the model progressively. Key features of GBM include the learning rate, which controls the contribution of each tree, and regularization techniques that prevent overfitting by limiting tree depth and applying penalties [94]. The algorithm also incorporates early stopping, monitoring performance on a validation set to halt training when improvement ceases while providing extensive hyperparameter tuning options for precise control over model complexity. Known for its high accuracy and ability to handle large datasets [95], GBM is highly effective in various practical applications. It offers superior performance in data-driven tasks and competitive machine learning challenges [96].

Extreme Gradient Boosting (XGBoost)

The XGBoost is an advanced implementation of GBM, recognized for its efficiency, flexibility, and optimization. It excels in handling sparse data, leveraging parallel processing, and utilizing weighted quantile sketching to enhance accuracy and scalability on large datasets. XGBoost supports custom loss functions, integrates built-in cross-validation, and is extensively used in competitive environments and industry applications for classification, regression, and ranking, owing to its strong performance and rich feature set [97].

MLA Implementation Procedure

Packages "randomForest" [93], "gbm", and "xgboost" [97] were used in the R-Studio software (Version 2024.12.0+467), respectively, to run the algorithms. Similar settings were applied when running the algorithms to perform the same analyses and compare the model outputs. We uploaded the input database, including the six most significant predictors and our response variable (asthma cases), to the algorithms in R-Studio as a comma-separated file (*.csv). Next, we split the data into training and test sets to evaluate the model's performance. We set 100 as the number of trees for each algorithm. To validate MLAs, 80% of the data is typically allocated for training, while the remaining 20% is reserved for testing using the holdout method. The holdout method is a technique in machine learning in which the dataset is split into separate training and testing sets to evaluate model performance [98].

MLAs Accuracy Assessment

The most commonly used validation metrics for count data in MLAs, including R-squared (R^2), root mean squared error (RMSE), mean squared error (MSE), mean absolute error (MAE), and explained variance (EV) or variance explained (VE), were applied to measure model performance and select the best model for analysis and interpretation [99]. R-squared (R^2) in machine learning measures how well a regression model fits the data, with values ranging from 0 to 1 indicating poor to perfect fit, respectively [99]:

$$R^2 = 1 - \frac{\sum_{i=1}^{n} (predicted_i - actual_i)^2}{\sum_{i=1}^{n} (actual_i - mean(actual))^2} \quad (4)$$

MSE is a metric used in regression analysis to measure the average squared differences between predicted and actual values. It provides a way to quantify the overall quality of a model's predictions, where lower MSE values indicate better performance [99]:

$$MSE = \frac{1}{n}\sum_{i=1}^{n}(predicted_i - actual_i)^2 \quad (5)$$

where the number of observations is represented by n.

RMSE in regression quantifies average prediction errors by taking the square root of the average squared differences between predicted and actual values, indicating prediction accuracy. Lower RMSE values signify better alignment between predicted and actual outcomes, indicating superior model performance in minimizing prediction errors [100]:

$$RMSE = \sqrt{\frac{1}{n}\sum_{i=1}^{n}(predicted_i - actual_i)^2} \quad (6)$$

MAE is a metric that measures the average absolute differences between predicted and actual values. It provides a straightforward way to quantify the magnitude of errors in a model's predictions, where lower MAE values indicate better predictive accuracy [99]:

$$MAE = \frac{1}{n}\sum_{i=1}^{n}|predicted_i - actual_i| \quad (7)$$

In statistics, explained variation (EV) measures the proportion to which a mathematical model accounts for a given dataset's variation (dispersion). EV measures how well predictors (in regression) account for variability in the response variable or total dataset. Higher EV values indicate greater explanatory power, which is crucial for assessing model effectiveness or dimensionality reduction success [101]. We applied all suitable metrics to measure MLA's performance using the "caret" package designed for MLAs [102].

After applying the MLAs, the Global Moran's Index (GMI) was employed to assess spatial autocorrelation in model residuals, offering insights into potential spatial dependencies. This index is instrumental in identifying whether the residuals demonstrate significant spatial clustering or dispersion across the study area, which aids in selecting the most suitable model. The GMI is defined as follows [86,90]:

$$I = \frac{n\left(\sum_{i=1}^{n}\sum_{j=1}^{n} w_{ij}(x_i - \overline{x})(x_j - \overline{x})\right)}{\left(\sum_{i=1}^{n}\sum_{j=1}^{n} w_{ij}\right)\left(\sum_{i=1}^{n}(x_i - \overline{x})^2\right)} \quad (8)$$

where n represents the total number of spatial units (in this case, the number of neighborhoods in the Tehran metropolitan area); x_i denotes the standardized death rate of overall cancers per 100,000 people in the neighborhood; I is the mean death rate across all counties; and w_{ij} represents the spatial weight between neighborhood i and j. Moran's Index (I) ranges from −1 to +1, with values further from zero indicating stronger (positive or negative) spatial autocorrelation [103]. To compute the GMI, training and test data residuals were assigned as value fields for each study unit. This was followed by applying the GMI using GeoDa software (Version 1.22.0.4) [104].

3. Results

3.1. Non-Spatial Descriptive Findings

According to the sample data's temporal trend of asthma prevalence, 1473 cases occurred over four years. Just two cases, or 0.14% of the total, were reported in 2020. This rose sharply to 823 cases (55.86%) in 2022 after increasing significantly to 46 cases (3.12%) in 2021. In 2023, there was a decrease, though, with 602 cases (40.88%). Data analysis revealed that the average age of the patients was 53 years. Among all cases, 47.5% (n = 699) were female, and 52.5% (n = 774) were male. Among all cases (N = 1473), 2.02%

(n = 28) were adolescents, 38.6% (n = 569) were adults, 12.61% (n = 186) were children, and 46.77% (n = 690) were elderly. Examining the relationship between age groups and asthma using Fisher's exact test showed a significant (p-value < 0.00) relationship between age groups and asthma. However, the results indicated that the relationship was not significant (p-value > 0.05) between gender and asthma prevalence, showing no substantial difference in the disease prevalence between genders. The average length of hospital stay of the patients was five days. The time distribution of the data shows that nearly 60% of the patients were admitted from February to July. Upon analysis, it was found that within the studied samples, 41.61% (n = 614) had achieved complete recovery, 11.12% (n = 163) had passed away, 11.83% (n = 172) were discharged, and 35.54% (n = 524) had partially recovered. The results of the ANOVA test indicated that the age group variable has a highly significant effect on the outcome of death ($p < 2 \times 10^{-16}$). Among the total deaths due to asthma (614 cases), 53% (n = 85) were men. Notably, the highest proportion of mortality was observed among the elderly age group (8.81%), followed by adults (2.24%).

3.2. *Spatial Analysis Findings*

3.2.1. KDE Method Results

In a study of 350 neighborhoods, the KDE map revealed significant variability in asthma cases. The mean KDE value is 3.4, with a standard deviation of 2.38 and a range of 11.73. The maximum and minimum KDE values are 11.77 and 0.04, respectively. Notably, 161 neighborhoods (approximately 46%) have KDE values exceeding 3.4 cases per square kilometer, indicating higher asthma burdens in these areas (see Figure 1).

3.2.2. Hot Spot Analysis Results

The "hot spot" analysis identified 87 hot spots (24.9%, with p-value < 0.05 and Gi* statistic > 1) and 88 cold spots (25.1%, with p-value < 0.05 and Gi* statistic > −1). Hot spots have significantly higher asthma cases, while cold spots have significantly lower concentrations. The spatial distribution of these spots reveals that areas with hot spots and high asthma burden are in the west and east of the city center, indicating localized clusters of high asthma incidence (see Figure 4).

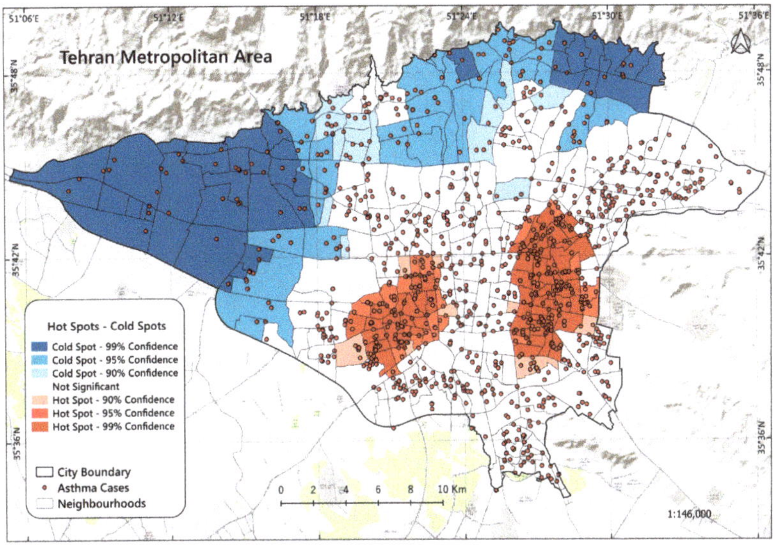

Figure 4. The spatial distribution of asthma case hot spots and cold spots within the study area.

3.3. Results from Negative Binomial Regression Model (NBRM)

In our analysis of the factors affecting the distribution of asthma cases in Tehran, we employed a Negative Binomial Regression Model (NBRM) to account for overdispersion in the count data. The predictors included variables V1 through V15, with the response variable being the count of asthma cases. We calculated each predictor's variance inflation factor (VIF) to address multicollinearity. A VIF value exceeding 5 indicates potential multicollinearity issues. Predictors with VIF values greater than 5, such as V14, were removed iteratively. The final set of predictors included in our NBRM were free of significant multicollinearity. We assessed overdispersion by comparing the residual deviance to the degrees of freedom. The ratio of deviance to degrees of freedom was 0.632, indicating no significant overdispersion in the model. We employed a stepwise selection method to refine the model further. The final model, selected based on the lowest Akaike information criterion (AIC), is summarized in Table 2.

Table 2. Initial summary of negative binomial regression model coefficients.

Predictor	Estimate	Std. Error	z Value	Pr (>|z|)
V1	1.9×10^{-5}	4.9×10^{-6}	3.8×10^{0}	1.5×10^{-4} ***
V2	-3.2×10^{-2}	1.9×10^{-2}	-1.6×10^{0}	1.0×10^{-1}
V3	8.8×10^{-3}	1.1×10^{-2}	7.7×10^{-1}	4.4×10^{-1}
V4	-3.2×10^{-2}	4.1×10^{-2}	-7.7×10^{-1}	4.4×10^{-1}
V5	1.4×10^{0}	6.2×10^{-1}	2.2×10^{0}	2.6×10^{-2} *
V6	2.3×10^{3}	5.9×10^{2}	3.9×10^{0}	1.1×10^{-4} ***
V7	-1.4×10^{2}	2.2×10^{2}	-6.3×10^{-1}	5.3×10^{-1}
V8	5.2×10^{3}	1.6×10^{3}	3.3×10^{0}	1.1×10^{-3} **
V9	-5.6×10^{-3}	2.2×10^{-3}	-2.6×10^{0}	1.0×10^{-2} *
V10	5.9×10^{-4}	1.5×10^{-4}	4.0×10^{0}	7.6×10^{-5} ***
V11	9.5×10^{-1}	1.1×10^{0}	8.7×10^{-1}	3.8×10^{-1}
V12	3.4×10^{-3}	4.6×10^{-3}	7.4×10^{-1}	4.6×10^{-1}
V13	-2.1×10^{-5}	3.6×10^{-5}	-5.7×10^{-1}	5.7×10^{-1}
V14	-2.7×10^{-2}	4.1×10^{-2}	-6.6×10^{-1}	5.1×10^{-1}
V15	6.7×10^{-3}	2.3×10^{-2}	2.9×10^{-1}	7.7×10^{-1}

Significance codes: 0—'***', 0.001—'**', 0.01—'*', 0.05—'.', 0.1—' ', 1, AIC = 1219.

The lack of significant overdispersion and multicollinearity issues validated the model's robustness. The stepwise selection process further optimized the model, ensuring the inclusion of only the six most relevant predictors. The final model emphasizes several key factors that significantly impact the distribution of asthma cases in Tehran. Variables V1 (population density), V4 (proportion of unemployed people (%)), V5 (particulate matter including $PM_{2.5}$ and PM_{10}), V6 (nitrogen dioxide (NO_2)), V8 (sulfur dioxide (SO_2)), V9 (neighborhood deprivation index (%)), and V10 (road intersection density) consistently emerged as significant across model iterations, highlighting their influence as the most critical predictors in our next analysis and MLA predictions (Table 3).

Table 3. Stepwise selected model summary.

Predictor	Estimate	Std. Error	z Value	Pr (>|z|)
V1	1.97×10^{-5}	3.07×10^{-6}	6.433758	1.24×10^{-10} ***
V4	−0.07422	0.034637	−2.14278	0.032131 *
V5	1.404977	0.470555	2.985788	0.002828 **
V6	1865.001	413.0592	4.515094	6.33×10^{-6} ***
V8	4250.563	1240.331	3.426957	0.00061 ***
V9	−0.00491	0.002075	−2.36894	0.017839 *
V10	0.000556	0.000138	4.041288	5.32×10^{-5} ***

Significance codes: 0—'***', 0.001—'**', 0.01—'*', 0.05—'.', 0.1—' ', 1, AIC = 1210.

3.4. Results and Performance of MLAs

The evaluation of various machine learning algorithms (MLAs) for predicting the response variable "asthma cases" across different neighborhoods offers insights into the performance of Random Forest (RF), Gradient Boosting Machine (GBM), and XGBoost. The evaluation metrics, including RMSE (root mean squared error), R-squared, MAE (mean absolute error), explained variance (EV), and Moran's I, help assess each model's fit to the training data and its ability to generalize to unseen test data, as well as the spatial randomness of residuals. These metrics are universally applicable and highly relevant for RF, GBM, and XGBoost regression models. In this study, we used 20% of the spatial data for testing. The MLA diagnostics are summarized in Table 4.

Table 4. Summary of MLA diagnostics.

MLAs	RMSE		R-Squared		MAE		EV		Moran's I
	(Train)	(Test)	(Train)	(Test)	(Train)	(Test)	(Train)	(Test)	(Train)
RF	0.56	1.08	0.96	0.75	0.40	0.84	1	0.74	0.29
GBM	0.56	1.07	0.95	0.76	0.43	0.88	0.95	0.75	0.17
XGBoost	0.22	1.21	0.99	0.69	0.16	0.91	0.99	0.68	0.12

The Random Forest algorithm demonstrates moderate performance, with a training RMSE of 0.56 and a test RMSE of 1.08, indicating a good fit on the training data but reduced performance on the test data. The R-squared values are 0.96 for the training set and 0.75 for the test set, suggesting that the algorithm explains a significant portion of the variance in the response variable, though less effectively on the test data. The MAE values are 0.40 for training and 0.84 for testing, highlighting higher prediction errors on unseen data. The explained variance (EV) values of 1.00 for training and 0.74 for testing further indicate that the algorithm performs well on the training data but may not generalize as effectively. The Moran's I value of 0.29 indicates moderate spatial autocorrelation in the residuals.

The Gradient Boosting algorithm performs slightly better, with a training RMSE of 0.56 and a test RMSE of 1.07, suggesting strong generalization compared to the Random Forest algorithm. The R-squared values are 0.95 for training and 0.76 for testing, reflecting good explanatory power for the variance in the data. The MAE values of 0.43 for training and 0.88 for testing indicate slightly lower prediction errors than the Random Forest algorithm. Additionally, the EV values of 0.95 for training and 0.75 for testing suggest effective pattern capture without substantial overfitting. The Moran's I value of 0.17 suggests lower spatial autocorrelation in the residuals compared to the Random Forest.

The XGBoost algorithm achieves the lowest training RMSE of 0.22 and the highest training R-squared of 0.99, indicating an almost perfect fit on the training data. However, the test RMSE of 1.21 and test R-squared of 0.69 suggest a notable decline in performance on the test data, implying potential overfitting. The MAE values are 0.16 for training and 0.91 for testing, showing minimal errors on the training set but higher errors on the test set. The EV values of 0.99 for training and 0.68 for testing further confirm that XGBoost may be overfitting to the training data. Additionally, Moran's I value of 0.12 indicates the lowest level of spatial autocorrelation in the residuals among the three algorithms, suggesting that XGBoost may handle spatial dependencies more effectively.

Among the Random Forest (RF), Gradient Boosting Machine (GBM), and XGBoost algorithms evaluated, GBM emerged as the best performer. It achieved the lowest test RMSE (1.07), high R-squared values (0.95 for training and 0.76 for testing), and strong explained variance (EV) values (0.95 for training and 0.75 for testing), indicating a superior balance between training and test performance. The algorithm also exhibited minimal spatial autocorrelation in residuals, with a Moran's I value of 0.17, making it the most robust and suitable for predicting asthma cases in this dataset.

The XGBoost algorithm, while showing the lowest training RMSE (0.22) and highest training R-squared (0.99), demonstrated a significant decline in performance on the test data (test RMSE of 1.21 and test R-squared of 0.69), suggesting potential overfitting. Its Moran's I value of 0.12 indicates the lowest spatial autocorrelation in residuals, which is a positive aspect. Still, the overall model performance on test data was not as strong as GBM. The Random Forest algorithm had a test RMSE of 1.08, with R-squared values of 0.96 for training and 0.75 for testing, showing fair performance. However, it had a higher level of spatial autocorrelation in residuals (Moran's I value of 0.29) compared to GBM and XGBoost.

In sum, the GBM algorithm is the most suitable for this regression task. It offers a well-balanced and robust performance across various metrics, including minimal spatial autocorrelation, making it the best choice among this dataset's three algorithms for predicting asthma cases.

The variable importance diagnostics from the Gradient Boosting Machine (GBM) algorithm using R-Studio indicate that V1 (6.49%), V5 (4.53%), V9 (6.86%), and V10 (36.53%) are the most influential predictors for asthma occurrence, with V10 being the most significant. In contrast, V4 (1.2%), V6 (2.25%), and V8 (2.28%) contribute minimally to the model's predictive power. Mapping the most essential variables provides a detailed view of asthma occurrence by highlighting spatial patterns and trends. Figure 5 displays the spatial distribution of the values of the most important predictors in the study area at a high-resolution scale (100-cell size) based on the Gradient Boosting algorithm, our best-fitting model.

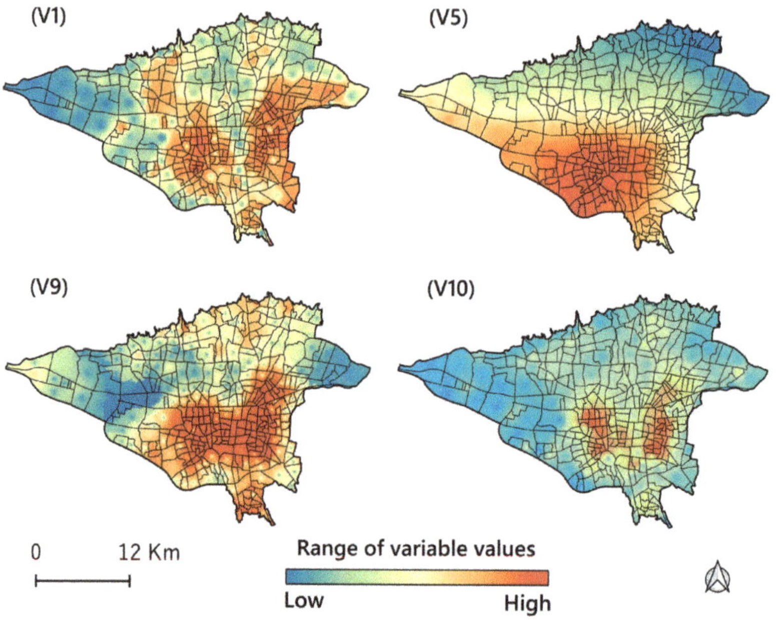

Figure 5. The Gradient Boosting algorithm determined spatial distribution maps of the most significant predictor values in the study area. Legend: V1: population density; V5: particulate matter including $PM_{2.5}$ and PM_{10}; V9: neighborhood deprivation index (%), which shows the most deprived areas; V10: road intersection density per square kilometers.

3.5. Visualizing Risk Prediction of Disease

The primary outcome of our study is a risk map developed using key predictors to assess the probability of asthma in the study area (Figure 6). Utilizing our best-fitting Gradient Boosting Machine (GBM) algorithm, validated with appropriate metrics, we generated a risk prediction map to evaluate the likelihood of asthma occurrence. To assess the model's accuracy, we employed a bivariate choropleth map in ArcGIS Pro version 3.2 [105]. This map compares the actual vs. predicted risk of asthma occurrence across various urban neighborhoods as determined by the GBM algorithm. The map demonstrates a strong agreement (R^2 = 0.92) between the model's predicted values and the observed asthma incident count per neighborhood. In a scatter plot, the R^2 value, or the coefficient of determination, measures how well the independent variable(s) explain the variance in the dependent variable. R^2 ranges from 0 to 1, where a value closer to 1 indicates that the data points fit the regression line well, meaning a strong relationship between the variables. Red line represents the identity line, indicating perfect prediction where observed values exactly match predicted values. Conversely, an R^2 closer to 0 suggests a weak relationship, with the data points more widely scattered around the red line.

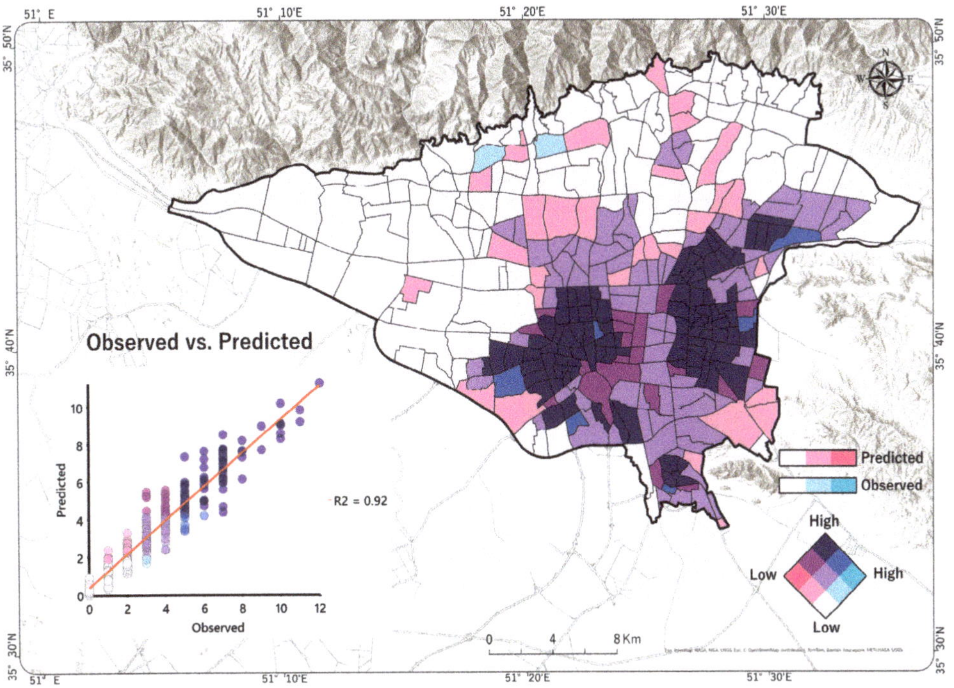

Figure 6. Spatial distribution map of locations with varying asthma occurrence risk probability levels within the study area.

Created in QGIS (QGIS Development Team, 2024), the map is designed for a straightforward interpretation, with high-risk neighborhoods highlighted. Based on the GBM model's results (Figure 6), around 164 neighborhoods (46.85%), home to an estimated 4,400,000 people (52% of the city's total population), are identified as high-risk areas, with predicted values exceeding the mean of approximately 3.42. The map indicates that the southwest and southeast regions near the city center have the highest risk of asthma occurrence. These insights can guide public health interventions and resource allocation, ensuring that high-risk areas receive the necessary attention to mitigate asthma risks.

4. Discussion

This study revealed significant age-related differences in asthma prevalence and outcomes, with a notable relationship between age groups and asthma incidence. Our findings showed that elderly patients with asthma are at a higher risk for morbidity and mortality from their asthma than younger patients, as corroborated by previous studies [106–108]. Asthma morbidity and mortality are higher in the elderly due to underdiagnosis, comorbidities, and physiological changes like reduced lung elasticity and muscle strength. Immunosenescence, characterized by diminished immune responses and increased systemic inflammation that occurs with age, exacerbates asthma and infection risks [107,108]. Underutilization and reduced effectiveness of inhaled corticosteroids, coupled with airway remodeling, further elevate asthma risks. Additionally, age-related changes in lung structure, such as decreased chest wall compliance and increased airway obstruction, contribute to the severity of asthma in older adults [107,108].

In contrast, according to our findings, gender did not significantly correlate with asthma prevalence. Asthma prevalence is similar across genders due to balancing factors: boys have higher rates in childhood, while women have higher rates in adulthood due to hormonal influences and symptom reporting [109,110]. These opposing trends result in comparable overall prevalence. Genetic and environmental factors contributing to asthma risk also do not show strong gender bias, further equalizing prevalence rates between males and females [109,110].

Seasonal trends were observed, with most hospital admissions occurring from February to July, highlighting potential environmental or lifestyle factors influencing asthma exacerbations. According to previous studies [111–114], respiratory infections such as colds and flu are more common during these months, triggering asthma exacerbations [111]. Additionally, springtime increases pollen levels from trees, grasses, and flowers, leading to heightened allergic reactions in asthmatics. Changes in weather, including sudden temperature fluctuations and humidity [112,113] and increasing air pollutants [114], can also aggravate asthma symptoms. These combined factors contribute to the higher rate of asthma hospital admissions during this period.

Applying KDE analysis to 350 neighborhoods revealed significant spatial variability in asthma cases, with nearly half experiencing elevated asthma rates. The "hot spot" analysis further identified clusters of high and low asthma incidence, with notable concentrations of hot spots in the west and east of the city center. These results suggest localized factors affecting asthma prevalence and underscore the need to uncover underlying causes and guide targeted public health interventions. Asthma occurrences vary across large urban areas due to various environmental and socioeconomic factors and air pollutants, with some of these factors explored in this study. Higher asthma occurrences in specific neighborhoods are linked to elevated levels of air pollutants resulting from drought, traffic, and industrial activities [26]. Poor urban design, characterized by limited green spaces, combined with socioeconomic disparities, further impacts asthma occurrences, as lower-income areas face higher exposure to pollutants and have reduced access to healthcare [28,29]. Additionally, local climate and weather patterns can exacerbate asthma symptoms, leading to significant spatial differences in asthma occurrences within urban settings [112–114].

Using a validated and robust NBRM that exhibited no issues with overdispersion or multicollinearity, we identified population density (V1), proportion of unemployed people (V4), particulate matter (including $PM_{2.5}$ and PM_{10}) (V5), nitrogen dioxide (NO_2) (V6), sulfur dioxide (SO_2) (V8), neighborhood deprivation (V9), and road intersection density (V10) as the most significant predictors of asthma distribution (Table 3). These results underscore the critical influence of environmental characteristics (including built environment characteristics), air pollutants, and socioeconomic conditions on asthma prevalence. We will discuss these influential factors in detail in the following sections, as they were identified as the most significant predictors by our robust machine learning algorithm analysis results.

Among the MLAs evaluated for predicting asthma cases, the GBM emerged as the top performer. It achieved the lowest prediction errors, highest R-squared values, and superior explained variance, indicating a strong balance between training and test performance. Additionally, the GBM algorithm demonstrated minimal spatial autocorrelation in residuals, making it the most robust and suitable algorithm for this dataset. The GBM findings highlighted road intersection density (V10), neighborhood deprivation index (V9), population density (V1), and particulate matter (V5) as the most influential predictors of asthma occurrence, with road intersection density being the most significant. In contrast, sulfur dioxide (V8), nitrogen dioxide (V6), and the proportion of unemployed people (V4) contributed minimally to the model's predictive power. This underscores the reliability and effectiveness of the GBM algorithm, making it a valuable tool for similar predictive tasks in the future.

According to the GBM algorithm, road intersection density (V10) predicts asthma cases significantly. Increased traffic congestion at intersections leads to higher emissions of pollutants such as particulate matter and nitrogen dioxide, exacerbating respiratory conditions and reducing air quality, contributing to the development and worsening of asthma symptoms [26]. Urban neighborhood deprivation (V9) is linked to asthma due to various interconnected factors, such as limited access to healthcare, higher pollution levels, poor housing conditions, increased stress, and greater exposure to environmental hazards. These conditions contribute to higher rates of respiratory problems, including asthma, in deprived and impoverished areas [21–23]. Population density (V1) is also associated with asthma due to higher pollution levels, increased exposure to allergens, and more frequent respiratory infections in densely populated areas. These factors collectively contribute to a higher prevalence of asthma [7,8]. Particulate matter ($PM_{2.5}$ and PM_{10}) (V5) is significantly associated with asthma. Fine particles ($PM_{2.5}$) can penetrate the lungs, causing inflammation and aggravating cardiovascular and respiratory conditions [14]. Increased levels of $PM_{2.5}$ are linked to a 2–3% rise in asthma symptoms among children. Similarly, elevated PM_{10} concentrations are correlated with more frequent emergency room visits and hospital admissions for asthma, underscoring the substantial impact of particulate matter on asthma prevalence and severity [14,15,32–34].

The primary outcome of this study was the creation of a risk map using the Gradient Boosting Machine (GBM) algorithm to evaluate asthma occurrence across different neighborhoods. This map compared predicted asthma risks with observed cases and identified several high-risk areas, notably in the southwest and southeast zones near the city center. Compared to findings from previous studies [42–44], our use of various machine learning algorithms (MLAs) and a broader set of predictors enabled us to predict areas with the highest disease risk with greater reliability and accuracy. This approach confirmed earlier results and provided more nuanced insights into the spatial distribution of asthma risk, enhancing the robustness and precision of our predictive modeling.

4.1. Strengths, Limitations, and Future Directions

This study utilized GIS, remote sensing (RS), and ensemble machine learning algorithms, specifically GBM, to predict asthma-prone areas in urban settings. Identifying key predictors such as population density, particulate matter ($PM_{2.5}$ and PM_{10}), neighborhood deprivation index, and road intersection density yields a detailed risk map of Tehran's high-risk areas. These findings offer critical insights for targeted public health interventions, assisting community planners and administrators in managing asthma and optimizing resource allocation. However, several limitations must be acknowledged. The study may not fully account for age-related complexities, gender differences, or all the environmental and lifestyle factors that influence asthma. Spatial variability suggests that localized factors influence prevalence, but the study may not account for all contributing variables. Reliance on specific data sources, such as satellite imagery and census data, may result in biases in spatial resolution, temporal variability, and data coverage. For example, remote sensing data may have limitations in accurately capturing fine-scale variations in urban environments, whereas census data may not fully reflect population dynamics or specific subpopulations. Furthermore, excluding factors such as urban heat islands and socioeconomic disparities risks overlooking essential determinants. These data-related biases may limit the results' generalizability, so caution is advised when applying these findings to other settings with different environmental or social characteristics.

Future research should incorporate more comprehensive data and additional variables to enhance predictive accuracy. Moreover, while machine learning algorithms are robust and predictive, they are computationally intensive and prone to overfitting, require extensive tuning, and can face obstacles of interpretability, outliers, and imbalanced data.

4.2. Policy Implications

The study's conclusions have ramifications for public health initiatives and urban development strategies meant to reduce the prevalence of asthma. The reported regional variations in Tehran's asthma prevalence highlight the need for a focused and localized strategy. Strict air quality monitoring, emission control in busy locations, and the encouragement of cleaner modes of transportation, especially in impoverished and highly populated neighborhoods, are all essential components of successful programs. Green space and buffer zone integration must be prioritized in urban development to lower pollution exposure and enhance air quality.

Addressing inequities in asthma outcomes requires improved access to healthcare services in high-risk communities and more public health surveillance. Additionally, the study highlights the need to address age-related vulnerabilities, particularly the increased risks older populations face due to comorbidities and decreased lung function. Tailored healthcare interventions, such as early diagnosis and better management strategies, are crucial to meeting their needs. Public awareness campaigns and infrastructure investments aimed at reducing traffic congestion can help minimize environmental triggers of asthma. Furthermore, addressing socioeconomic disparities through improved housing, education, and economic development initiatives can play a key role in mitigating the burden of asthma.

Important insights into the function of essential predictors such as particulate matter, neighborhood deprivation, and traffic intersection density were obtained by applying machine learning models, especially GBM. These results highlight the need for evidence-based decisions to efficiently distribute resources and create interventions focusing on high-risk locations. Metropolitan planners and legislators may promote healthier and more resilient areas by enacting egalitarian, data-driven, and locally relevant policies.

5. Conclusions

In this study, we integrated GIS, remote sensing (RS), and ensemble machine learning algorithms to predict asthma-prone areas in urban environments. Our results indicate that ensemble machine learning algorithms effectively identify asthma risk areas, with the Gradient Boosting Machine (GBM) algorithm demonstrating superior accuracy compared to other algorithms. Key predictors in our model were population density, particulate matter ($PM_{2.5}$ and PM_{10}), neighborhood deprivation index, and road intersection density.

The resulting asthma risk map highlighted higher-risk areas in the southern and western parts of Tehran near the city center, where increased population density and transportation contribute significantly to air pollution levels. Such risk maps provide valuable tools for community planners and administrators to manage and mitigate asthma in these regions. Additionally, our findings offer essential insights for guiding public health interventions and optimizing resource allocation to address asthma risks in the most affected neighborhoods.

Supplementary Materials: The following supporting information can be downloaded at: https://www.mdpi.com/article/10.3390/ijgi14030105/s1, Table S1: Data.

Author Contributions: Conceptualization, Alireza Mohammadi; methodology, Alireza Mohammadi; software, Alireza Mohammadi; validation, Alireza Mohammadi; formal analysis, Alireza Mohammadi; investigation, Elahe Pishgar; resources, Elahe Pishgar; data curation, Alireza Mohammadi; writing—original draft preparation, Alireza Mohammadi; writing—review and editing, Juan Aguilera; visualization, Alireza Mohammadi; supervision, Alireza Mohammadi; project administration, Alireza Mohammadi; funding acquisition, Alireza Mohammadi. All authors have read and agreed to the published version of the manuscript.

Funding: This research was funded by the University of Mohaghegh Ardabili, Iran, under grant number 14341. The funder provided financial support for the study, and the grant number has been verified for accuracy.

Data Availability Statement: The original contributions presented in this study are included in the Supplementary Material. Further inquiries can be directed to the corresponding author.

Acknowledgments: The authors thank the Masih Daneshvari Hospital (Tehran) for making the data accessible. The authors express gratitude to the University of Mohaghegh Ardabili (Iran), for extending the opportunity to conduct this research. Moreover, the authors wish to convey their profound gratitude to the editor-in-chief for their supportive comments and suggestions.

Conflicts of Interest: The authors declare no conflicts of interest.

References

1. World Health Organization. Asthma. Available online: https://www.who.int/news-room/fact-sheets/detail/asthma (accessed on 9 September 2024).
2. Merhej, T.; Zein, J.G. Epidemiology of Asthma: Prevalence and Burden of Disease. *Adv. Exp. Med. Biol.* **2023**, *1426*, 3–23. [CrossRef] [PubMed]
3. Rabe, A.P.J.; Loke, W.J.; Gurjar, K.; Brackley, A.; Lucero-Prisno, D.E. Global Burden of Asthma, and Its Impact on Specific Subgroups: Nasal Polyps, Allergic Rhinitis, Severe Asthma, Eosinophilic Asthma. *J. Asthma Allergy* **2023**, *16*, 1097–1113. [CrossRef] [PubMed]
4. Seyedrezazadeh, E.; Gilani, N.; Ansarin, K.; Yousefi, M.; Sharifi, A.; Rouhi, A.H.J.; Aftabi, Y.; Najmi, M.; Dastan, I.; Moghaddam, M.P. Economic Burden of Asthma in Northwest Iran. *Iran. J. Med. Sci.* **2023**, *48*, 156–166. [CrossRef] [PubMed]
5. Fazlollahi, M.R.; Najmi, M.; Fallahnezhad, M.; Sabetkish, N.; Kazemnejad, A.; Bidad, K.; Shokouhi Shoormasti, R.; Mahloujirad, M.; Pourpak, Z.; Moin, M. The Prevalence of Asthma in Iranian Adults: The First National Survey and the Most Recent Updates. *Clin. Respir. J.* **2018**, *12*, 1872–1881. [CrossRef] [PubMed]
6. Holmes, L.; Enwere, M.; Williams, J.; Ogundele, B.; Chavan, P.; Piccoli, T.; Chinaka, C.; Comeaux, C.; Pelaez, L.; Okundaye, O.; et al. Black–White Risk Differentials in COVID-19 (SARS-CoV2) Transmission, Mortality and Case Fatality in the United States: Translational Epidemiologic Perspective and Challenges. *Int. J. Environ. Res. Public Health* **2020**, *17*, 4322. [CrossRef] [PubMed]
7. Shin, S.; Bai, L.; Burnett, R.T.; Kwong, J.C.; Hystad, P.; van Donkelaar, A.; Lavigne, E.; Weichenthal, S.; Copes, R.; Martin, R.V.; et al. Air Pollution as a Risk Factor for Incident Chronic Obstructive Pulmonary Disease and Asthma: A 15-Year Population-Based Cohort Study. *Am. J. Respir. Crit. Care Med.* **2021**, *203*, 1138–1148. [CrossRef] [PubMed]
8. Aslam, R.; Sharif, F.; Baqar, M.; Nizami, A.S.; Ashraf, U. Role of Ambient Air Pollution in Asthma Spread among Various Population Groups of Lahore City: A Case Study. *Environ. Sci. Pollut. Res.* **2023**, *30*, 8682–8697. [CrossRef] [PubMed]
9. Nanda, A.; Baptist, A.P.; Divekar, R.; Parikh, N.; Seggev, J.S.; Yusin, J.S.; Nyenhuis, S.M. Asthma in the Older Adult. *J. Asthma* **2020**, *57*, 241–252. [CrossRef] [PubMed]

10. Khosa, J.K.; Louie, S.; Moreno, P.L.; Abramov, D.; Rogstad, D.K.; Alismail, A.; Matus, M.J.; Tan, L.D. Asthma Care in the Elderly: Practical Guidance and Challenges for Clinical Management-A Framework of 5 "Ps.". *J. Asthma Allergy* **2023**, *16*, 33–43. [CrossRef]
11. Zaeh, S.E.; Ramsey, R.; Bender, B.; Hommel, K.; Mosnaim, G.; Rand, C. The Impact of Adherence and Health Literacy on Difficult-to-Control Asthma. *J. Allergy Clin. Immunol. Pract.* **2022**, *10*, 386–394. [CrossRef]
12. Jabre, N.A.; Keet, C.A.; McCormack, M.; Peng, R.; Balcer-Whaley, S.; Matsui, E.C. Material Hardship and Indoor Allergen Exposure among Low-Income, Urban, Minority Children with Persistent Asthma. *J. Community Health* **2020**, *45*, 1017–1026. [CrossRef] [PubMed]
13. Perez, M.F.; Coutinho, M.T. An Overview of Health Disparities in Asthma. *Yale J. Biol. Med.* **2021**, *94*, 497–507.
14. Qin, P.; Luo, X.; Zeng, Y.; Zhang, Y.; Li, Y.; Wu, Y.; Han, M.; Qie, R.; Wu, X.; Liu, D.; et al. Long-Term Association of Ambient Air Pollution and Hypertension in Adults and in Children: A Systematic Review and Meta-Analysis. *Sci. Total Environ.* **2021**, *796*, 148620. [CrossRef] [PubMed]
15. Singh, G.K.; Rai, S.; Jadon, N. Major Ambient Air Pollutants and Toxicity Exposure on Human Health and Their Respiratory System: A Review. *J. Environ. Manag. Tour.* **2021**, *12*, 1774–1788. [CrossRef]
16. Ayres-Sampaio, D.; Teodoro, A.C.; Sillero, N.; Santos, C.; Fonseca, J.; Freitas, A. An Investigation of the Environmental Determinants of Asthma Hospitalizations: An Applied Spatial Approach. *Appl. Geogr.* **2014**, *47*, 10–19. [CrossRef]
17. Alvarez-Mendoza, C.I.; Teodoro, A.; Freitas, A.; Fonseca, J. Spatial Estimation of Chronic Respiratory Diseases Based on Machine Learning Procedures—An Approach Using Remote Sensing Data and Environmental Variables in Quito, Ecuador. *Appl. Geogr.* **2020**, *123*, 102273. [CrossRef]
18. Sonwani, S.; Madaan, S.; Arora, J.; Suryanarayan, S.; Rangra, D.; Mongia, N.; Vats, T.; Saxena, P. Inhalation Exposure to Atmospheric Nanoparticles and Its Associated Impacts on Human Health: A Review. *Front. Sustain. Cities* **2021**, *3*, 690444. [CrossRef]
19. Naclerio, R.; Ansotegui, I.J.; Bousquet, J.; Canonica, G.W.; D'Amato, G.; Rosario, N.; Pawankar, R.; Peden, D.; Bergmann, K.C.; Bielory, L.; et al. International Expert Consensus on the Management of Allergic Rhinitis (AR) Aggravated by Air Pollutants: Impact of Air Pollution on Patients with AR: Current Knowledge and Future Strategies. *World Allergy Organ. J.* **2020**, *13*, 100106. [CrossRef]
20. Manisalidis, I.; Stavropoulou, E.; Stavropoulos, A.; Bezirtzoglou, E. Environmental and Health Impacts of Air Pollution: A Review. *Front. Public Health* **2020**, *8*, 14. [CrossRef]
21. Altman, M.C.; Kattan, M.; O'Connor, G.T.; Murphy, R.C.; Whalen, E.; LeBeau, P.; Calatroni, A.; Gill, M.A.; Gruchalla, R.S.; Liu, A.H.; et al. Associations between Outdoor Air Pollutants and Non-Viral Asthma Exacerbations and Airway Inflammatory Responses in Children and Adolescents Living in Urban Areas in the USA: A Retrospective Secondary Analysis. *Lancet Planet. Health* **2023**, *7*, e33–e44. [CrossRef]
22. Keet, C.A.; McCormack, M.C.; Pollack, C.E.; Peng, R.D.; McGowan, E.; Matsui, E.C. Neighborhood Poverty, Urban Residence, Race/Ethnicity, and Asthma: Rethinking the Inner-City Asthma Epidemic. *J. Allergy Clin. Immunol.* **2015**, *135*, 655–662. [CrossRef] [PubMed]
23. Sullivan, P.W.; Ghushchyan, V.; Kavati, A.; Navaratnam, P.; Friedman, H.S.; Ortiz, B. Health Disparities Among Children with Asthma in the United States by Place of Residence. *J. Allergy Clin. Immunol. Pract.* **2019**, *7*, 148–155. [CrossRef]
24. Roy, S.; Majumder, S.; Bose, A.; Chowdhury, I.R. The Rich-Poor Divide: Unravelling the Spatial Complexities and Determinants of Wealth Inequality in India. *Appl. Geogr.* **2024**, *166*, 103267. [CrossRef]
25. Stewart, I.T.; Clow, G.L.; Graham, A.E.; Bacon, C.M. Disparate Air Quality Impacts from Roadway Emissions on Schools in Santa Clara County (CA). *Appl. Geogr.* **2020**, *125*, 102354. [CrossRef]
26. Khreis, H. Traffic, Air Pollution, and Health. In *Advances in Transportation and Health*; Elsevier: Amsterdam, The Netherlands, 2020; pp. 59–104.
27. Gasana, J.; Dillikar, D.; Mendy, A.; Forno, E.; Ramos Vieira, E. Motor Vehicle Air Pollution and Asthma in Children: A Meta-Analysis. *Environ. Res.* **2012**, *117*, 36–45. [CrossRef] [PubMed]
28. Yu, H.; Zhou, Y.; Wang, R.; Qian, Z.; Knibbs, L.D.; Jalaludin, B.; Schootman, M.; McMillin, S.E.; Howard, S.W.; Lin, L.Z.; et al. Associations between Trees and Grass Presence with Childhood Asthma Prevalence Using Deep Learning Image Segmentation and a Novel Green View Index. *Environ. Pollut.* **2021**, *286*, 117582. [CrossRef] [PubMed]
29. Zeng, X.W.; Lowe, A.J.; Lodge, C.J.; Heinrich, J.; Roponen, M.; Jalava, P.; Guo, Y.; Hu, L.W.; Yang, B.Y.; Dharmage, S.C.; et al. Greenness Surrounding Schools Is Associated with Lower Risk of Asthma in Schoolchildren. *Environ. Int.* **2020**, *143*, 105967. [CrossRef] [PubMed]
30. Buteau, S.; Shekarrizfard, M.; Hatzopolou, M.; Gamache, P.; Liu, L.; Smargiassi, A. Air Pollution from Industries and Asthma Onset in Childhood: A Population-Based Birth Cohort Study Using Dispersion Modeling. *Environ. Res.* **2020**, *185*, 109180. [CrossRef]

31. Ly, B.-T.; Kajii, Y.; Nguyen, T.-Y.L.; Shoji, K.; Van, D.-A.; Do, T.-N.N.; Nghiem, T.-D.; Sakamoto, Y. Characteristics of Roadside Volatile Organic Compounds in an Urban Area Dominated by Gasoline Vehicles, a Case Study in Hanoi. *Chemosphere* **2020**, *254*, 126749. [CrossRef]
32. Arunab, K.S.; Mathew, A. Quantifying Urban Heat Island and Pollutant Nexus: A Novel Geospatial Approach. *Sustain. Cities Soc.* **2024**, *101*, 105117. [CrossRef]
33. Aghamohammadi, N.; Ramakreshnan, L.; Supramanian, R.K.; Lim, Y.C. Climate Change Adaptation and Public Health Strategies in Malaysia. In *Climate Change and Human Health Scenarios: International Case Studies*; Springer: Berlin/Heidelberg, Germany, 2023; pp. 99–113.
34. D'Amato, G.; Chong-Neto, H.J.; Monge Ortega, O.P.; Vitale, C.; Ansotegui, I.; Rosario, N.; Haahtela, T.; Galan, C.; Pawankar, R.; Murrieta-Aguttes, M.; et al. The Effects of Climate Change on Respiratory Allergy and Asthma Induced by Pollen and Mold Allergens. *Allergy Eur. J. Allergy Clin. Immunol.* **2020**, *75*, 2219–2228. [CrossRef] [PubMed]
35. Simich, C.S.; Jones, M.P. Chapter Asthma. In *Urban Emergency Medicine*; Cambridge University Press & Assessment: Cambridge, UK, 2023; p. 98.
36. Yasaratne, D.; Idrose, N.S.; Dharmage, S.C. Asthma in Developing Countries in the Asia-Pacific Region (APR). *Respirology* **2023**, *28*, 992–1004. [CrossRef] [PubMed]
37. Sabeti, Z.; Ansarin, K.; Seyedrezazadeh, E.; Asghari Jafarabadi, M.; Zafari, V.; Dastgiri, S.; Shakerkhatibi, M.; Gholampour, A.; Ghanbari Ghozikali, M.; Ghasemzadeh, R.; et al. A Comparison of Asthma Prevalence in Adolescents Living in Urban and Semi-Urban Areas in Northwestern Iran. *Hum. Ecol. Risk Assess.* **2021**, *27*, 2051–2068. [CrossRef]
38. Rahimian, N.; Aghajanpour, M.; Jouybari, L.; Ataee, P.; Fathollahpour, A.; Lamuch-Deli, N.; Kooti, W.; Kalmarzi, R.N. The Prevalence of Asthma among Iranian Children and Adolescent: A Systematic Review and Meta-Analysis. *Oxid. Med. Cell. Longev.* **2021**, *2021*, 6671870. [CrossRef] [PubMed]
39. Shariat, M.; Rostamian, E.; Moayeri, H.; Shariat, M.; Sharifi, L. A Review on the Relation between Obesity and Vitamin D with Pediatric Asthma, and a Report of a Pilot Study in Tehran, Iran: Review Article. *Tehran Univ. Med. J.* **2020**, *78*, 274–283.
40. Masoud, F.; Kashi, G. Air Pollution on Mortality from Asthma in Tehran during the Years 1391 to 1394. *Iran. J. Allergy Asthma Immunol.* **2018**, *17*, 181–182.
41. Sharifi, L.; Pourpak, Z.; Fazlollahi, M.R.; Bokaie, S.; Moezzi, H.R.; Kazemnejad, A.; Moin, M. Asthma Economic Costs in Adult Asthmatic Patients in Tehran, Iran. *Iran. J. Public Health* **2015**, *44*, 1212–1218.
42. Razavi-termeh, S.V.; Sadeghi-niaraki, A.; Choi, S.M. Spatial Modeling of Asthma-prone Areas Using Remote Sensing and Ensemble Machine Learning Algorithms. *Remote Sens.* **2021**, *13*, 3222. [CrossRef]
43. Razavi-Termeh, S.V.; Sadeghi-Niaraki, A.; Choi, S.M. Spatio-Temporal Modelling of Asthma-Prone Areas Using a Machine Learning Optimized with Metaheuristic Algorithms. *Geocarto Int.* **2022**, *37*, 9917–9942. [CrossRef]
44. Razavi-Termeh, S.V.; Sadeghi-Niaraki, A.; Choi, S.M. Asthma-Prone Areas Modeling Using a Machine Learning Model. *Sci. Rep.* **2021**, *11*, 1912. [CrossRef] [PubMed]
45. Morrison, C.N.; Mair, C.F.; Bates, L.; Duncan, D.T.; Branas, C.C.; Bushover, B.R.; Mehranbod, C.A.; Gobaud, A.N.; Uong, S.; Forrest, S.; et al. Defining Spatial Epidemiology: A Systematic Review and Re-Orientation. *Epidemiology* **2024**, *35*, 542–555. [CrossRef] [PubMed]
46. Kappas, M. GIS and Remote Sensing for Public Health. In *Geospatial Data Science in Healthcare for Society 5.0*; Springer: Berlin/Heidelberg, Germany, 2022; pp. 79–97.
47. Cushing, A.M.; Khan, M.A.; Kysh, L.; Brakefield, W.S.; Ammar, N.; Liberman, D.B.; Wilson, J.; Shaban-Nejad, A.; Espinoza, J. Geospatial Data in Pediatric Asthma in the United States: A Scoping Review Protocol. *JBI Evid. Synth.* **2022**, *20*, 2790–2798. [CrossRef] [PubMed]
48. Studies, P. Spatial Analysis and Determinants of Asthma Health and Health Services Use Outcomes in Ontario. Master's Thesis, University of Ottawa, Ottawa, ON, Canada, 2016.
49. Spyroglou, I.I.; Spöck, G.; Chatzimichail, E.A.; Rigas, A.G.; Paraskakis, E.N. A Bayesian Logistic Regression Approach in Asthma Persistence Prediction. *Epidemiol. Biostat. Public Health* **2018**, *15*, e12777-1–e12777-14. [CrossRef]
50. Roy, S.; Chowdhury, I.R. Intoxication in the City: Investigating Spatial Patterns and Determinants of Drugs and Alcohol-Related Illegal Activities in India's Geostrategic Corridor. *Appl. Geogr.* **2024**, *171*, 103386. [CrossRef]
51. Grekousis, G. *Spatial Analysis Methods and Practice: Describe-Explore-Explain Through GIS*; Cambridge University Press: Cambridge, UK, 2020; ISBN 9781108614528.
52. Amaral, J.L.M.; Sancho, A.G.; Faria, A.C.D.; Lopes, A.J.; Melo, P.L. Differential Diagnosis of Asthma and Restrictive Respiratory Diseases by Combining Forced Oscillation Measurements, Machine Learning and Neuro-Fuzzy Classifiers. *Med. Biol. Eng. Comput.* **2020**, *58*, 2455–2473. [CrossRef]
53. Placido, D.; Yuan, B.; Hjaltelin, J.X.; Zheng, C.; Haue, A.D.; Chmura, P.J.; Yuan, C.; Kim, J.; Umeton, R.; Antell, G.; et al. A Deep Learning Algorithm to Predict Risk of Pancreatic Cancer from Disease Trajectories. *Nat. Med.* **2023**, *29*, 1113–1122. [CrossRef] [PubMed]

54. Zhang, L.; Wang, Y.; Niu, M.; Wang, C.; Wang, Z. Machine Learning for Characterizing Risk of Type 2 Diabetes Mellitus in a Rural Chinese Population: The Henan Rural Cohort Study. *Sci. Rep.* **2020**, *10*, 4406. [CrossRef]
55. Oikonomou, E.K.; Khera, R. Machine Learning in Precision Diabetes Care and Cardiovascular Risk Prediction. *Cardiovasc. Diabetol.* **2023**, *22*, 259. [CrossRef]
56. Razavi-Termeh, S.V.; Sadeghi-Niaraki, A.; Farhangi, F.; Choi, S.-M. COVID-19 Risk Mapping with Considering Socio-Economic Criteria Using Machine Learning Algorithms. *Int. J. Environ. Res. Public Health* **2021**, *18*, 9657. [CrossRef]
57. World Population Review. *Sharjah Population 2024*; World Population Review: Walnut, CA, USA, 2024.
58. Maghrebi, M.; Danandeh Mehr, A.; Karrabi, S.M.; Sadegh, M.; Partani, S.; Ghiasi, B.; Nourani, V. Spatiotemporal Variations of Air Pollution during the COVID-19 Pandemic across Tehran, Iran: Commonalities with and Differences from Global Trends. *Sustainability* **2022**, *14*, 16313. [CrossRef]
59. Dehghan, A.; Khanjani, N.; Bahrampour, A.; Goudarzi, G.; Yunesian, M. The Relation between Air Pollution and Respiratory Deaths in Tehran, Iran- Using Generalized Additive Models. *BMC Pulm. Med.* **2018**, *18*, 49. [CrossRef] [PubMed]
60. Kiavarz, M.; Hosseinbeigi, S.B.; Mijani, N.; Shahsavary, M.S.; Firozjaei, M.K. Predicting Spatial and Temporal Changes in Surface Urban Heat Islands Using Multi-Temporal Satellite Imagery: A Case Study of Tehran Metropolis. *Urban Clim.* **2022**, *45*, 101258. [CrossRef]
61. Management and Planning Organization of Tehran Province. *Results of the 2015 Census of Tehran Province and City*; MPO: Tehran, Iran, 2016.
62. Mohammadi, A.; Pishgar, E.; Fatima, M.; Lotfata, A.; Fanni, Z.; Bergquist, R.; Kiani, B. The COVID-19 Mortality Rate Is Associated with Illiteracy, Age, and Air Pollution in Urban Neighborhoods: A Spatiotemporal Cross-Sectional Analysis. *Trop. Med. Infect. Dis.* **2023**, *8*, 85. [CrossRef]
63. Khoshakhlagh, A.H.; Mohammadzadeh, M.; Morais, S. Air Quality in Tehran, Iran: Spatio-Temporal Characteristics, Human Health Effects, Economic Costs and Recommendations for Good Practice. *Atmos. Environ. X* **2023**, *19*, 100222. [CrossRef]
64. Banirazi Motlagh, S.H.; Pons-Valladares, O.; Hosseini, S.M.A. City-Scale Model to Assess Rooftops Performance on Air Pollution Mitigation; Validation for Tehran. *Build. Environ.* **2023**, *244*, 110746. [CrossRef]
65. Ramyar, R.; Saeedi, S.; Bryant, M.; Davatgar, A.; Mortaz Hedjri, G. Ecosystem Services Mapping for Green Infrastructure Planning–The Case of Tehran. *Sci. Total Environ.* **2020**, *703*, 135466. [CrossRef] [PubMed]
66. Gheshlaghpoor, S.; Abedi, S.S.; Moghbel, M. The Relationship between Spatial Patterns of Urban Land Uses and Air Pollutants in the Tehran Metropolis, Iran. *Landsc. Ecol.* **2023**, *38*, 553–565. [CrossRef]
67. Statistical Centre of Iran (SCI). *Tehran City Housing and Income Census Data and Reports 2016*; Statistical Centre of Iran: Tehran, Iran, 2022.
68. Roy, S.; Bose, A.; Majumder, S.; Roy Chowdhury, I.; Abdo, H.G.; Almohamad, H.; Abdullah Al Dughairi, A. Evaluating Urban Environment Quality (UEQ) for Class-I Indian City: An Integrated RS-GIS Based Exploratory Spatial Analysis. *Geocarto Int.* **2022**, *38*, 2153932. [CrossRef]
69. Huang, S.; Tang, L.; Hupy, J.P.; Wang, Y.; Shao, G. A Commentary Review on the Use of Normalized Difference Vegetation Index (NDVI) in the Era of Popular Remote Sensing. *J. For. Res.* **2021**, *32*, 1–6. [CrossRef]
70. U.S. Geological Survey. USGS Landsat Normalized Difference Vegetation Index | U.S. Geological Survey. Available online: https://www.usgs.gov/landsat-missions/landsat-normalized-difference-vegetation-index (accessed on 20 June 2024).
71. Santamouris, M.; Cartalis, C.; Synnefa, A.; Kolokotsa, D. On the Impact of Urban Heat Island and Global Warming on the Power Demand and Electricity Consumption of Buildings—A Review. *Energy Build.* **2015**, *98*, 119–124. [CrossRef]
72. Kumari, B.; Tayyab, M.; Shahfahad; Salman; Mallick, J.; Khan, M.F.; Rahman, A. Satellite-Driven Land Surface Temperature (LST) Using Landsat 5, 7 (TM/ETM+ SLC) and Landsat 8 (OLI/TIRS) Data and Its Association with Built-Up and Green Cover Over Urban Delhi, India. *Remote Sens. Earth Syst. Sci.* **2018**, *1*, 63–78. [CrossRef]
73. Ufondu, A.N.; Shukla, U.C.; Stambaugh, C.; Huber, K.E.; Stambaugh, N. Categorical Variable Analyses: Chi-Square, Fisher's Exact, Mantel–Haenszel. In *Translational Radiation Oncology*; Eltorai, A.E.M., Bakal, J.A., Kim, D.W., Wazer, D.E., Eds.; Academic Press: Cambridge, MA, USA, 2023; pp. 165–170, ISBN 9780323884235.
74. Jones, G.P.; Stambaugh, C.; Stambaugh, N.; Huber, K.E. Analysis of Variance. In *Translational Radiation Oncology*; Eltorai, A.E.M., Bakal, J.A., Kim, D.W., Wazer, D.E., Eds.; Academic Press: Cambridge, MA, USA, 2023; pp. 171–177, ISBN 9780323884235.
75. ESRI. How Exploratory Regression Works. Available online: https://pro.arcgis.com/en (accessed on 26 October 2022).
76. Chan, J.Y.; Leow, S.M.; Bea, K.T.; Cheng, W.K.; Phoong, S.W.; Hong, Z.-W.; Lin, J.-M.; Chen, Y.-L. A Correlation-Embedded Attention Module to Mitigate Multicollinearity: An Algorithmic Trading Application. *Mathematics* **2022**, *10*, 1231. [CrossRef]
77. Fox, J.; Weisberg, S. *An R Companion to Applied Regression*, 3rd ed.; Sage: Thousand Oaks, CA, USA, 2011.
78. Venables, W.N.; Ripley, B.D. *Modern Applied Statistics with S*, 4th ed.; Springer: New York, NY, USA, 2002; ISBN 0-387-95457-0.
79. Stevens, R.S.; Dean, M.D.; Miller, J.S.; Dougald, L.E. Monitoring Crash Impacts of Exceptions to Entrance Spacing Standards: Lessons Learned from Virginia. *Case Stud. Transp. Policy* **2020**, *8*, 648–657. [CrossRef]
80. Hilbe, J.M. *Negative Binomial Regression*; Cambridge University Press: Cambridge, UK, 2007; ISBN 9780511811852.

81. Cappai, S.; Rolesu, S.; Coccollone, A.; Laddomada, A.; Loi, F. Evaluation of Biological and Socio-Economic Factors Related to Persistence of African Swine Fever in Sardinia. *Prev. Vet. Med.* **2018**, *152*, 1–11. [CrossRef]
82. Silverman, B.W. *Density Estimation: For Statistics and Data Analysis*; Routledge: London, UK, 2018; ISBN 9781351456173.
83. Carlos, H.A.; Shi, X.; Sargent, J.; Tanski, S.; Berke, E.M. Density Estimation and Adaptive Bandwidths: A Primer for Public Health Practitioners. *Int. J. Health Geogr.* **2010**, *9*, 39. [CrossRef] [PubMed]
84. Chun, Y.; Griffith, D.A. *Spatial Statistics and Geostatistics: Theory and Applications for Geographic Information Science and Technology*; Sage Publishing: Thousand Oaks, CA, USA, 2012.
85. ESRI. ArcGIS Pro Help. Available online: https://pro.arcgis.com/en/pro-app/latest/help/main/welcome-to-the-arcgis-pro-app-help.htm (accessed on 10 June 2024).
86. Mitchel, A. Volume 2: Spartial Measurements and Statistics. In *The ESRI Guide to GIS Analysis*; ESRI Press: Bucharest, Romania, 2005; Volume 2.
87. Bornmann, L.; de Moya Angeon, F. Hot and Cold Spots in the US Research: A Spatial Analysis of Bibliometric Data on the Institutional Level. *J. Inf. Sci.* **2019**, *45*, 84–91. [CrossRef]
88. Ord, J.K. Art Getis and local spatial statistics. *J. Geogr. Syst.* **2024**, *26*, 191–200. [CrossRef]
89. Farahani, M.; Razavi-Termeh, S.V.; Sadeghi-Niaraki, A. A Spatially Based Machine Learning Algorithm for Potential Mapping of the Hearing Senses in an Urban Environment. *Sustain. Cities Soc.* **2022**, *80*, 103675. [CrossRef]
90. Environmental Systems Research Institute (ESRI). ArcGIS Professional GIS Help. Available online: https://pro.arcgis.com/en/pro-app/latest/help (accessed on 4 August 2024).
91. Mienye, I.D.; Sun, Y. A Survey of Ensemble Learning: Concepts, Algorithms, Applications, and Prospects. *IEEE Access* **2022**, *10*, 99129–99149. [CrossRef]
92. Ho, T.K. Random Decision Forests. In Proceedings of the International Conference on Document Analysis and Recognition, ICDAR, Montreal, QC, Canada, 14–16 August 1995; IEEE: New York, NY, USA, 1995; Volume 1, pp. 278–282.
93. Breiman, L. Random Forests. *Mach. Learn.* **2001**, *45*, 5–32. [CrossRef]
94. Friedman, J.H. Greedy Function Approximation: A Gradient Boosting Machine. *Ann. Stat.* **2001**, *29*, 1189–1232. [CrossRef]
95. Miller, A.; Panneerselvam, J.; Liu, L. A Review of Regression and Classification Techniques for Analysis of Common and Rare Variants and Gene-Environmental Factors. *Neurocomputing* **2022**, *489*, 466–485. [CrossRef]
96. Natekin, A.; Knoll, A. Gradient Boosting Machines, a Tutorial. *Front. Neurorobot.* **2013**, *7*, 21. [CrossRef] [PubMed]
97. Chen, T.; Guestrin, C. XGBoost: A Scalable Tree Boosting System. In Proceedings of the ACM SIGKDD International Conference on Knowledge Discovery and Data Mining, San Francisco, CA, USA, 13–17 August 2016; pp. 785–794.
98. Raschka, S. Model Evaluation, Model Selection, and Algorithm Selection in Machine Learning. *arXiv* **2018**, arXiv:arXiv1811.12808.
99. Dagli, B.Y. Application of a Statistical Regression Technique for Dynamic Analysis of Submarine Pipelines. *J. Mar. Sci. Eng.* **2024**, *12*, 955. [CrossRef]
100. Eastman, J.R. *TerrSet Geospatial Monitoring and Modeling System*; Clark University: Worcester, MA, USA, 2016; pp. 345–389. Available online: https://www.clarku.edu/centers/geospatial-analytics/terrset/ (accessed on 12 June 2024).
101. Barbur, V.A.; Montgomery, D.C.; Peck, E.A. *Introduction to Linear Regression Analysis*; John Wiley & Sons: Hoboken, NJ, USA, 1994; Volume 43, ISBN 1119578752.
102. Kuhn, M. Building Predictive Models in R Using the Caret Package. *J. Stat. Softw.* **2008**, *28*, 1–26. [CrossRef]
103. Vilinová, K. Spatial Autocorrelation of Breast and Prostate Cancer in Slovakia. *Int. J. Environ. Res. Public Health* **2020**, *17*, 4440. [CrossRef] [PubMed]
104. Anselin, L. GeoDa [software]. Version 1.22.0.4. 2023. Available online: https://geodacenter.github.io/ (accessed on 10 June 2024).
105. ESRI ArcGIS Pro. *ArcGIS PRO Modul. 4—Data Anal*; University of Toronto: Toronto, ON, Canada, 2022; p. 3.
106. Pishgar, E.; Fanni, Z.; Tavakkolinia, J.; Mohammadi, A.; Kiani, B.; Bergquist, R. Mortality Rates Due to Respiratory Tract Diseases in Tehran, Iran during 2008-2018: A Spatiotemporal, Cross-Sectional Study. *BMC Public Health* **2020**, *20*, 1414. [CrossRef] [PubMed]
107. D'Amato, G.; Vitale, C.; Molino, A.; Stanziola, A.; Sanduzzi, A.; Vatrella, A.; Mormile, M.; Lanza, M.; Calabrese, G.; Antonicelli, L. Asthma-Related Deaths. *Multidiscip. Respir. Med.* **2016**, *11*, 37. [CrossRef] [PubMed]
108. Dunn, R.M.; Busse, P.J.; Wechsler, M.E. Asthma in the Elderly and Late-Onset Adult Asthma. *Allergy Eur. J. Allergy Clin. Immunol.* **2018**, *73*, 284–294. [CrossRef] [PubMed]
109. Fuhlbrigge, A.L.; Jackson, B.; Wright, R.J. Gender and Asthma. *Immunol. Allergy Clin. N. Am.* **2002**, *22*, 753–789. [CrossRef]
110. Oraka, E.; Kim, H.J.E.; King, M.E.; Callahan, D.B. Asthma Prevalence among US Elderly by Age Groups: Age Still Matters. *J. Asthma* **2012**, *49*, 593–599. [CrossRef] [PubMed]
111. Chan, K.-P.F.; Kwok, W.-C.; Ma, T.-F.; Hui, C.-H.; Tam, T.C.-C.; Wang, J.K.-L.; Ho, J.C.-M.; Lam, D.C.-L.; Sau-Man Ip, M.; Ho, P.-L. Territory-Wide Study on Hospital Admissions for Asthma Exacerbations in the COVID-19 Pandemic. *Ann. Am. Thorac. Soc.* **2021**, *18*, 1624–1633. [CrossRef] [PubMed]
112. Bagheri, O.; Moeltner, K.; Yang, W. Respiratory Illness, Hospital Visits, and Health Costs: Is It Air Pollution or Pollen? *Environ. Res.* **2020**, *187*, 109572. [CrossRef]

113. Chen, Y.; Kong, D.; Fu, J.; Zhang, Y.; Zhao, Y.; Liu, Y.; Chang, Z.; Liu, Y.; Liu, X.; Xu, K.; et al. Associations between Ambient Temperature and Adult Asthma Hospitalizations in Beijing, China: A Time-Stratified Case-Crossover Study. *Respir. Res.* **2022**, *23*, 38. [CrossRef] [PubMed]
114. Ko, F.W.S.; Lau, L.H.S.; Ng, S.S.; Yip, T.C.F.; Wong, G.L.H.; Chan, K.P.; Chan, T.O.; Hui, D.S.C. Respiratory Admissions before and during the COVID-19 Pandemic with Mediation Analysis of Air Pollutants, Mask-Wearing and Influenza Rates. *Respirology* **2023**, *28*, 47–55. [CrossRef]

International Journal of
Geo-Information

MDPI

Article

A 3D Model-Based Framework for Real-Time Emergency Evacuation Using GIS and IoT Devices

Noopur Tyagi [1], Jaiteg Singh [1,*], Saravjeet Singh [1] and Sukhjit Singh Sehra [2]

[1] Chitkara University Institute of Engineering and Technology, Chitkara University, Rajpura 140401, Punjab, India; noopur.tyagi@chitkara.edu.in (N.T.); saravjeet.singh@chitkara.edu.in (S.S.)
[2] Department of Physics & Computer Science, Wilfrid Laurier University, Waterloo, ON N2L 3C5, Canada; ssehra@wlu.ca
* Correspondence: jaiteg.singh@chitkara.edu.in

Abstract: Advancements in 3D modelling technology have facilitated more immersive and efficient solutions in spatial planning and user-centred design. In healthcare systems, 3D modelling is beneficial in various applications, such as emergency evacuation, pathfinding, and localization. These models support the fast and efficient planning of evacuation routes, ensuring the safety of patients, staff, and visitors, and guiding them in cases of emergency. To improve urban modelling and planning, 3D representation and analysis are used. Considering the advantages of 3D modelling, this study proposes a framework for 3D indoor navigation and employs a multiphase methodology to enhance spatial planning and user experience. Our approach combines state-of-the art GIS technology with a 3D hybrid model. The proposed framework incorporates federated learning (FL) along with edge computing and Internet of Things (IoT) devices to achieve accurate floor-level localization and navigation. In the first phase of the methodology, Quantum Geographic Information System (QGIS) software was used to create a 3D model of the building's architectural details, which are required for efficient indoor navigation during emergency evacuations in healthcare systems. In the second phase, the 3D model and an FL-based recurrent neural network (RNN) technique were utilized to achieve real-time indoor positioning. This method resulted in highly precise outcomes, attaining an accuracy rate over 99% at distances of no less than 10 metres. Continuous monitoring and effective pathfinding ensure that users can navigate safely and effectively during emergencies. IoT devices were connected with the building's navigation software in Phase 3. As per the performed analysis, it was observed that the proposed framework provided 98.7% routing accuracy between different locations during emergency situations. By improving safety, building accessibility, and energy efficiency, this research addresses the health and environmental impacts of modern technologies.

Keywords: smart infrastructure; emergency evacuation; machine learning; edge computing; GIS; 3D model; indoor positioning; safety and security

1. Introduction

Evacuation planning in emergency situations is crucial to any healthcare facility. In an event of unforeseen crises, the safe evacuation of patients, staff, and visitors is of prime importance to minimize the risk to human lives. Safe evacuation is a crucial process and involves the identification and promulgation of optimal evacuation routes in real time considering the unique challenges and complexities of healthcare environments [1–3]. A healthcare facility accommodates susceptible populations, including patients, with different levels of mobility or who are dependent on special equipment, which may further complicate route planning within a healthcare setting. In this regard, besides patients' lives, sophisticated infrastructure, medical equipment, and hazardous chemicals also mandate careful route planning to ensure safe evacuation in cases of emergencies [4,5]. Due to hospital complexity, standard evacuation strategies often fail to evacuate quickly and effectively. Modern Information and Communications Technology (ICT) systems provide real-time tracking, best route recommendations, and improved emergency decision-making to improve evacuation preparation. Furthermore, emergency situations are dynamic and require flexible, adaptable, and scalable evacuation plans that can be put into place very fast based on changeable circumstances [6,7]. The potential of using 3D modelling, GIS, and emerging technologies in enhancing wayfinding in healthcare facilities during emergency situations has not been fully considered [8]. Despite this potential of 3D modelling and so many advanced technologies in creating ICT-based evacuation methods, the former still has a foundational role. Table 1 provides a summary of ICT-based evacuation methods. Table 1 enumerates ICT-based evacuation planning systems, detailing their inputs, advantages, and disadvantages.

Table 1. Summary of existing ICT-based evacuation methods.

Methods	Description	Key Inputs and Variables	Advantages	Disadvantages	Reference
Universal Design of ICT for Emergency Management	The focus of the study is on creating tools that are accessible through various ICTs in emergency situations, thereby including people with disabilities.	Assessments of user needs, standards for accessibility, methods for communication.	Encourages inclusiveness in emergency management, hence ensuring safety of diverse groups as a whole.	Implementation may require high amounts of resources and requires extensive training for users and responders.	[9]
Intelligent Evacuation Route Planning	This approach focused on developing optimal evacuation channels through algorithms based on maximum flow theories at times of crisis.	Configuration of structure, number of evacuees, conditions of route.	Efficient route planning saves more time in evacuation and is flexible to various conditions.	May require complex calculations and data entry; effectiveness depends on accurate data acquisition	[10]
Integration of sensor network and BIM	For real-time collection and monitoring, BIM is combined with sensors	IoT connectivity, BIM data, sensor information (temperature, humidity, occupancy, etc.)	Improves data accuracy through enhanced monitoring of building conditions	High implementation cost, complexity in integration	[11,12]
Building Information Model	An intelligent evacuation system using BIM	Environmental sensor data (temperature, smoke, humidity, etc.), historical incident data, simulation parameters, communication protocols, user location data	Real-time guidance	Requires accurate BIM and costly to implement	[13]

Current ICT-based solutions have many benefits, but they often lack spatial depth and real-time adaptation for complex healthcare contexts. Three-dimensional modelling improves spatial visualization, route planning, and real-time guidance, especially in healthcare settings where mobility-challenged patients need additional help. Three-dimensional modelling is the process of creating a digital representation of a physical object in three dimensions. The 3D model helps to provide realistic modelling of cities and buildings. In healthcare facility evacuation planning, which entails developing a virtual image of the entire institution, including all the rooms, hallways, and exits, the 3D modelling approach provides user-centric and better spatial solutions [14]. The 3D models provides a deeper understanding of the structure of a building compared to a 2D approach [15]. Three-dimensional modelling provides better visualization in various ways within healthcare settings. For example, if a patient needs to locate medical facilities, specialist rooms, or a specific ward within a hospital, then an application with 3D modelling of the building can make this easy. A detailed and realistic perspective makes it easier for patients to navigate the hospital more efficiently to improve their overall experience and reduce the time spent in searching for places/locations [4,15]. For the easy navigation in indoor environments, a 3D model comprises the following basic elements:

1. Building: A building is one of the main elements of an indoor area and represents the complete or part of the indoor area. This can be termed the BGroup and includes different elements.
2. Floor: Different levels in a building represent the floors. This can be termed the FGroup and is represented by a set of elements that range from 1 to n, depending upon the maximum accessible floors within the building.
3. Locations: The collection of ordered pairs of values for different locations. Each location is represented by a value on the x-axis and y-axis (x, y). The values (x0, y0) represent the lower bounds, and (x0 + length) and (y0 + width) represent the upper limits.

Augmented reality, virtual reality, and digital twins boost our ability to simulate, visualize, and interact with the hospital environment during emergencies by using the advantages of 3D modelling. These technologies improve emergency planning models' immersion and accuracy. Technologies like augmented reality, virtual reality, and digital twins are merged together to replicate an actual building [16–18]. Three-dimensional modelling can be put into place to improve visualization by using blueprints, building information models, and data gathered for indoor structure plans. Three-dimensional modelling can further help in improving spatial awareness of medical facilities, optimizing resource allocation, and enhancing navigation in hospitals in the healthcare domain. A number of applications are supported through 3D modelling for navigation, evacuation routing, emergency planning, disaster response, and localization [19,20]. Simulation allows the user to interact with a virtual environment as they interact with a real environment. The accuracy of the 3D model can be increased by integrating qualitative data and information from other sources, such as technologies and existing databases [21]. Three-dimensional modelling also attracts researchers and experts from various fields who use a simulation approach to gather information and enhance applications. Capturing, manipulating, transporting, projecting, and sharing the visualization is an important process [22,23]. Informative data would be beneficial for construction analysis, emergency applications, and urban area planning. For sustainable urban development, it is necessary to incorporate sustainability concepts into urban modelling. In order to provide intelligent routing and optimum navigation services, 3D modelling uses edge computing devices (Raspberry Pi, edge servers, and LiDAR sensors) and Internet of Things (IoT) devices (such as Bluetooth beacons, edge gateways, and IMUs) [24]. To determine the location of an object, wireless localization is commonly used within a building. By using Wi-Fi signals and Bluetooth low-energy (BLE) signals, precise positioning can be accomplished. GIS software (3.24.1 version of QGIS, ArcGIS Pro 3.0), positioning sensors (LiDAR), IoT devices, and Universal Asynchronous Receivers/Transmitters (UARTs) are a few examples of tools that can be used for effective indoor mapping and positioning as well as for situational awareness during emergencies. Integrating indoor positioning technologies with GIS enables the real-time tracking of patients, staff, and healthcare facilities.

To make the process easier, python tools and plugins such as QGIS2threejs can be used [25]. In an indoor environment, it is challenging to provide the precise location of an object, but the use of Received Signal Intensity Indicator (RSSI) in wireless systems helps to check the communication and signal strength to find the exact location [26]. RSSI with machine learning improves the accuracy of localization. In an indoor environment, FL serves as a useful alternative for secure connection during localization and routing in data-sensitive devices. ML is a computational approach that enables computers to acquire information from data without explicit programming [18]. To predict the spatial coordinates of the user, ML utilizes the RSSI data. FL helps to train the model using multiple devices while ensuring that their data are private and not compromising the central server. In indoor localization, FL allows devices to train a model collaboratively using RSSI data from different locations. Integrating RSSI-based ML with FL ensures the privacy of sensitive data while optimizing navigation and resource allocation. The collective training improves the indoor navigation accuracy and related applications. An integrated indoor navigation system that comprises FL, edge computing, and IoT devices to create indoor navigation systems is shown in Figure 1. This integration significantly improves the traffic flow, asset tracking, and localization in indoor environments by including Wi-Fi, RFID, and IoT sensors.

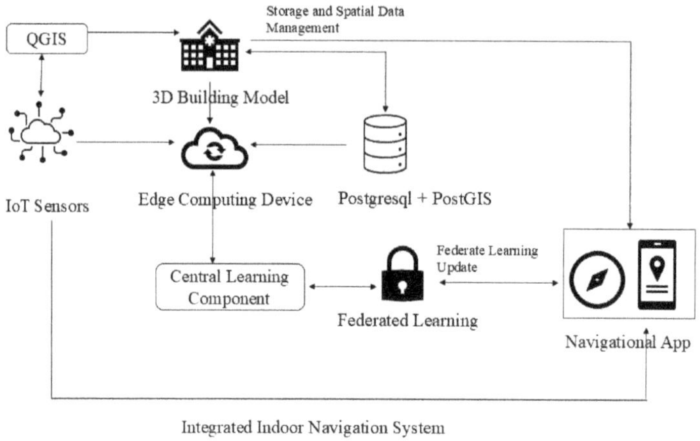

Figure 1. Integrating FL, edge computing, and IoT devices to create indoor navigation systems.

Considering the limitations of indoor environments, this study presents a novel framework for emergency evacuation in indoor environments by using the data of IoT devices and a 3D model for navigational activities. In this study, the basic requirement of navigation, i.e., indoor localization, is achieved by using FL and ML on edge devices. The highlights of the proposed framework can be summarized as follows:

1. The development of an innovative indoor navigation system for healthcare facilities that prioritizes safety and efficiency, especially during emergencies by leveraging GIS technology to convert traditional 2D maps into interactive 3D models.
2. The provision of a more comprehensible and informational spatial representation of the structure. Additionally, we suggest utilizing machine learning and FL to precisely identify the user's location within the building based on RSSI signals.
3. An indoor application that may provide real-time routing and navigation in emergency situations by utilizing existing infrastructure and 3D model.

A key factor motivating this research relates to determining the best way of executing emergency evacuations in complex healthcare environments, in which a combination of vulnerable patients and medical equipment poses specific challenges. Conventional frameworks for evacuations lack the flexibility and precision that are required in specialized environments, such as the inclusion of real-time data and the evolution of patient-specific strategies for evacuation. This work fills the existing gaps by proposing a novel framework that incorporates FL, IoT-based real-time data collection, and dynamic indoor navigation with the aim of creating more secure and efficient evacuation operations in healthcare buildings. The paper will be structured as follows: Section 2 will examine previous studies on the subject matter. Section 3 will explain the methodology used to create a 3D model and its uses for emergency evacuation. In Section 4, the investigation results will be presented, along with a comprehensive analysis of the collected data. Finally, Section 5 will summarize the findings and provide valuable perspectives for future research.

2. Research Work

Indoor navigation is becoming essential in healthcare environments, as prompt access to places can greatly influence patient outcomes. This section examines numerous studies that utilize modern technologies for efficient indoor navigation, emphasizing the distinct issues presented by healthcare facilities. Indoor navigation within healthcare facilities should enhance the patient and visitor experience by reducing the stress of finding locations. A building information model (BIM) can be changed into a 3D ontology-based indoor navigation model to support emergency evacuation [27]. To obtain effective door-to-door navigation, these models require consideration of building geometry, semantics, and real-time dynamic changes in the environment [28]. For the first responder, there is a need for rapid model generation for decision support and situational awareness [1]. Different technologies, like Wi-Fi, LiDAR, and Bluetooth, have been used for building modelling, localization, and navigation inside healthcare buildings. To analyze and visualize the energy performance of buildings more efficiently and accurately, a framework was proposed [29]. Additionally, mobile augmented reality applications have been developed to simulate building evacuations, allowing users to visualize 3d models of buildings and their routes on smartphones [30]. Few researchers have presented the potential benefits of using BIM for building simulation, modelling, enhanced communication and collaboration, and building performance optimization [31–33]. In addition to this, research has been conducted to demonstrate how GIS may increase the precision of building simulations, especially when integrated with BIM, and support sustainable building, urban design, and operation [34–36]. To create a 3D model, an automated technique for the 3D modelling of a topological indoor navigation network was presented [37]. For visual indoor localization, sophisticated tools like LiDAR and cameras were used. But this apparatus does not support the semantic comprehension that is needed for effective 3D modelling [37]. Several studies have discussed how versatile QGIS is when it comes to building 3D representations of outdoor environments for various applications. These studies used game engines and other relevant tools. Similarly to outdoor modelling, a smartphone-based application was presented [38]. This application used deep learning for autonomous map maintenance and a grid-based pathfinding method. Additionally, edge computing has been widely used due to its low latency, bandwidth reduction, reliability, and real-time processing. Edge caching, edge training, edge inference, and edge offloading are the four main components of edge intelligence, centred on improving data processing speed, quality, and privacy close to the data source through AI-driven systems. This shows that the impact of ML and DL is affected by emphasizing the spread of IoT devices. Edge intelligence, or edge AI, takes a close look at concepts including cloud, edge, and fog computing, as well as existing methods and use cases. To improve data processing speed, and privacy near data sources, this can be achieved through edge caching, edge training, edge inference, and edge offloading in AI-driven systems [39]. This highlights how important ML, particularly DL, is in emphasizing the increase in IoT devices. Edge intelligence and edge AI closely examine ideas like cloud, edge, and fog computing as well as use cases and existing methods. Edge AI is the intersection of edge computing and artificial intelligence. Model accuracy, energy consumption, and latency are evaluated for deploying DL methods at the network edge [40]. To make a real-time prediction, ML algorithms such as KNN, SVM, and neural networks are used in positioning systems. Data mining in the IoT can enhance 3D localization [41]. Table 2 lists some recent works in the field of indoor navigation, localization, and tracking.

Comparing indoor positioning and navigation technology shows real-time localization and accuracy improvements. Emergency evacuation scenarios require a rapid response and precision, yet these solutions vary. For instance, Wi-Fi RSSI fingerprints have great accuracy but may have latency in dynamic situations where movement and obstruction updates are critical [47]. FL aggregates real-time data from distributed sources without compromising privacy, making it ideal for emergency situations where IoT sensor or mobile device data must be quickly processed and acted upon. Densely fused variational autoencoders paired with reinforcement learning also have good accuracy and responsiveness and develop optimal paths over time. This feature helps emergency algorithms adapt to new risks. However, simpler Kalman filter-based QR code localization can navigate indoors but cannot adjust to the live data inputs needed for evacuation. In analyzing these methodologies, frameworks with IoT integration and FL capabilities, like those described in this paper, show potential for emergency responses. They provide real-time adaptability, high localization accuracy, and data privacy for unanticipated and crucial emergency evacuations in complicated healthcare settings. These features push evacuation systems toward more resilient, dynamically satisfying patient-specific and situational needs.

Table 2. An overview of research work in the field of indoor localization and navigation.

Ref	Purpose	Dataset	Tool/Technologies	Results
[42]	Indoor Localization	WIFI Data	RSSI fingerprint + SVM, KNN + Principle Component Analysis (PCA)	Maximum accuracy of 90%
[43]	Position Estimation	Accelerometer and gyroscope reading	Artificial Neural Network (ANN) and Kalman filter	Predicted location with RMSE of 2.38
[44]	Indoor Localization	Unlabeled crowd-sourced RSS fingerprint data	FL + stacked autoencoder	Maximum accuracy of around 99%
[45]	Indoor Tracking and Navigation	Dataset using Monte Carlo method	Message-based time difference in arrivals (TDOA) equations	Highest localization errors in 2D and 3D of 7.5 cm and 11.2 cm, respectively.
[46]	Indoor Localization and Navigation	Wi-Fi RSSI data	Densely fused variational autoencoder + deep reinforced learning using Markov decision process	95.99% mean accuracy
[38]	Indoor Localization and Navigation	QR Code	Extended Kalman filter	-

Three-dimensional modelling is essential for creating accurate spatial representations that can enhance navigation and the sense of visualization while evacuating buildings in emergency situations. These models greatly help responders in navigating difficult places and in directing people to safety by providing a better understanding of evacuation routes and the locations of risks [1]. For instance, 3D models of buildings have been very instrumental in easing evacuation within buildings by providing needed views that enhance the accuracy and efficiency of evacuation. Additionally, training and simulation exercises resort to 3D models, since it is possible to have responders and building dwellers familiarize themselves with various evacuation situations [44]. This realistic representation, although resource-intensive and requiring technical expertise to use efficiently, can be tested with various scenarios, and it can reveal bottlenecks on evacuation routes.

This technology has also been found to be a facilitator of IoT in the collection and transmission of real-time data during evacuations due to emergencies. IoT devices monitor the building parameters—including occupancy levels and potential fires, among other parameters—and thus, the availability of such information increases the chances of better decision-making during an emergency [48]. In addition, further integration of BIM and IoT could increase occupant safety by increasing the updating of building information. For example, smart exit signs and IoT-based public address systems should be able to automatically offer real-time customized evacuation instructions. With these systems come the benefits of safety and situational awareness, but there are downsides, too, which include dependency on technology that is susceptible to cyberattacks, system failures, and concerns about issues of confidentiality and privacy [48].

This study focuses on the importance of cutting-edge technologies like 3D modelling, GIS, and machine learning for emergency evacuation and indoor navigation, particularly in complex structures like hospitals [49]. Healthcare facilities have particular challenges, such as safely evacuating patients with different degrees of mobility and adjusting to the dynamic nature of emergency circumstances [50]. For quick and effective responses, an intelligent evacuation system can be created by combining real-time sensor data with BIM, edge computing, and IoT devices [51]. Based on the literature studied, 3D modelling can offer a more accurate and user-focused spatial depiction of healthcare facilities. For efficient route planning in an emergency situation, the combination of GIS and 3D modelling presents a promising solution [52]. To increase the localization accuracy, FL and ML can be important considerations to enable effective evacuation in a delicate healthcare environment while maintaining data privacy [53]. There is still a gap in the literature regarding the use of 3D modelling and developing technologies for thorough evacuation planning in healthcare facilities, despite the improvements in ICT-based evacuation methods [54,55]. In order to address this gap, this study proposes a novel framework that leverages 3D modelling, GIS, and ML/FL to create effective, real-time indoor navigation for healthcare settings. The proposed framework aims to maximize evacuation routes and improve patient safety.

An integrated indoor navigation system, as shown in Figure 1, provides a significant benefit for healthcare environments. This system optimizes patient flow, asset tracking, and staff efficiency by integrating data from sources, including Wi-Fi, RFID, and IoT sensors, with advanced computing and spatial data management. This system's ability to provide real-time location information and navigation can enhance patient satisfaction by reducing wait times and improving overall efficiency.

3. Methodology

This research study is based on three interrelated stages of indoor navigation, as shown in Figure 2. With significant implications for emergency rescue operations, health, and environmental sustainability, each phase is strategically designed to contribute to the development of an accurate and dependable three-dimensional indoor navigation system tailored for emergency scenarios. Detailed descriptions of these phases are provided in the following subsections.

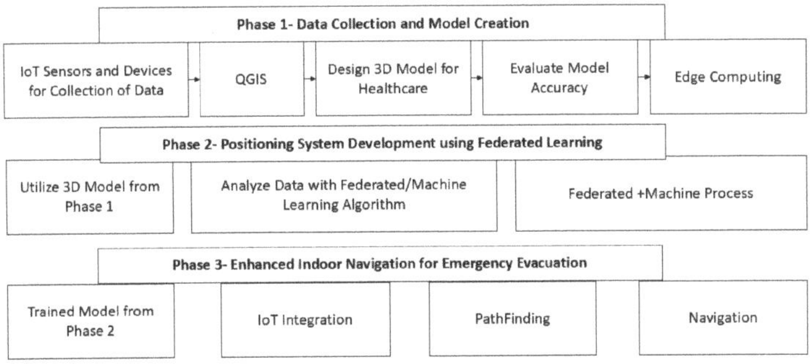

Figure 2. Three-dimensional indoor navigation system from Phase 1 to Phase 3.

3.1. Technologies

In this study, an RNN and FL approach is used for determining the users' location in the healthcare system. RNN is used to handle and classify the sequential data. An RNN is a type of neural network that can memorize the previous input because of the feed-forward feature. FL is used to train the RNN and enable us to conduct data analysis while maintaining the integrity of the stored data. The FL-inspired framework is elaborated upon in Figure 3. FL involves three main components: a server, a communication architecture, and an individual client acting as a consumer. To protect privacy, especially when it comes to indoor positioning in 3D spaces, FL uses a decentralized data storage strategy [56–58]. This approach protects the user's private information and data of critical locations.

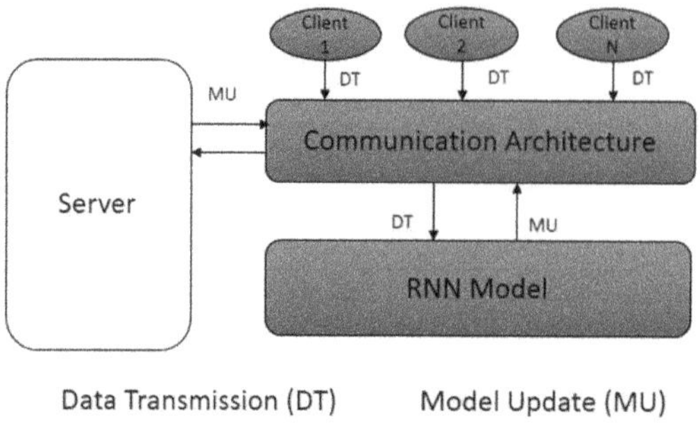

Figure 3. Federated learning framework.

The integration of FL and RNNs for indoor positioning can significantly enhance emergency responses and rescue operations in the following ways:

Emergency Medical Responses: In cases of mass causalities, administration can use FL to train models on local patient data without disclosing sensitive information. This allows for the real-time tracking of patients and resource allocation [59].

Disaster Response Coordination: Several agencies can use FL to exchange information about affected populations without compromising personal privacy. This collaboration can strengthen situational awareness and improve response strategies [60].

Search and Rescue Operations: The proposed method can facilitate data sharing in different teams (police, fire department, medical teams) during search and rescue operations while protecting the privacy of individuals' information [61].

The fundamental principle of FL is collaborative model training, which is different from the conventional approach of centralizing datasets. Each customer's data are stored locally on their personal device (e.g., smartphone, IoT) and utilized for personalized training [62]. This means that the raw data will never leave the device. The customized training enhances the global positioning model without transmitting the raw data to the central server or other clients. Fingerprint localization is used to precisely and accurately determine the location of the device. In fingerprint localization, higher accuracy can be achieved by reducing entropy loss. The main objective of FL is to improve the accuracy of the 3D indoor location model by reducing the average loss across several training clients, as denoted by Equation (1).

$$\mathrm{minL(w)} = (1/\mathrm{v}) * \sum(\mathrm{i} = 1 \text{ to } \mathrm{p})\mathrm{li(w)} \tag{1}$$

In Equation (1), li(w) represents the loss function which is used to determine the weight values that are lost throughout the client-side training process. The variable "w" indicates the weight values associated with the 3D positioning model. The function L(w) represents minimal values, which can be calculated by dividing the total number of function values (v) by the sum of the individual function values li(w). FL is a state-of-the-art technique that calculates optimal weight values to reduce loss across clients using a cutting-edge method.

3.2. Development of 3D Model

QGIS 3D building model development comprises three steps. The first step involves importing architectural data from CAD files and geographical sources, such as floor plans and building height dimensions, to create the basic model. Next, accurate indoor navigation is achieved by measuring rooms, floors, and building heights using various devices. In this study, LiDAR data were used to assess room heights and structural elements and compare them to 2D floor plans to build a realistic 3D model. The zones included high ceilings, stairwells, and split-level rooms. Each zone's LiDAR height data were modelled independently to accurately depict 3D structural height variations, as shown in Figure 4. This division required lobby and hallway representation. This ensured that the navigation model incorporated emergency evacuation and reliable indoor navigation [63].

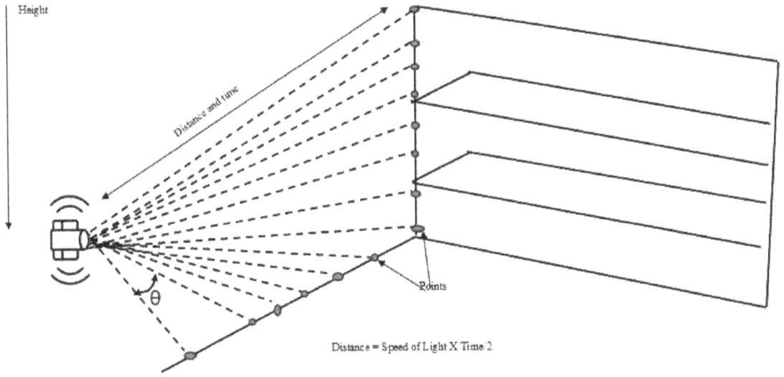

Figure 4. LiDAR data collection.

Further, the QGIS2threejs plugin was used to convert the 2D blueprint into a developed 3D model containing all levels and interior spaces. This 3D model was also verified using BIM to check the accuracies. After creating the 3D model, a few essential steps were performed to ensure the proper preprocessing of data with regard to the required RSSI data in the indoor location. There were 470 Wi-Fi access points placed inside the building in such a way that statistics about RSSI could be generated. The other 390 active access points were taken down to zero, since those that were weak or even signal-less were removed from the list. The data were normalized to ensure the H-RNN and FL model provided input in a consistent manner.

This study employed QGIS (Version 3.24.1) software along with BIM to develop a 3D model of the building. This process involved data collection and processing QGIS data and rendering it through BIM for footprint marking and visualization. Figure 5 depicts the conceptual process of creating the 3D model in QGIS, whereby raw data from maps, blueprints, and locations were processed with the QGIS2threejs plugin for three-dimensional visualization. The DB Manager plugin was used to store spatial data in the PostgreSQL database. LiDAR sensors (TFmini) delivered exact height readings for structural components, facilitating correct modelling for emergency situations. Points of Interest, including access points, emergency equipment, and safe zones, were incorporated to facilitate rescue operations. Figure 6 illustrates the three-dimensional model with evacuation pathways and emergency exits.

In the second phase, to accurately determine the position of users inside a building, FL can be applied for 3D indoor positioning during an emergency. The next sub section provides more details about the second phase.

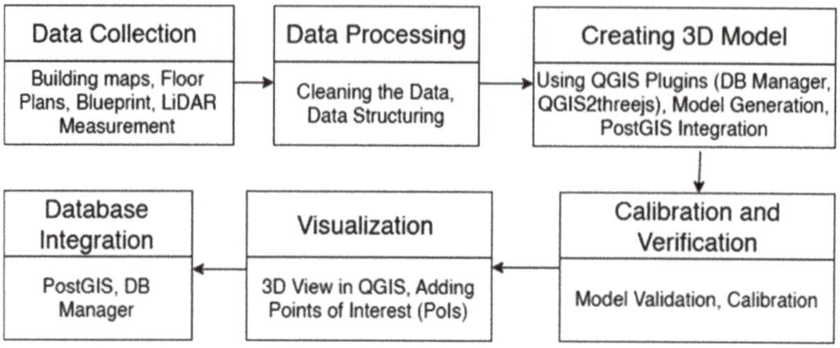

Figure 5. The conceptual flow of creating the 3D model in QGIS.

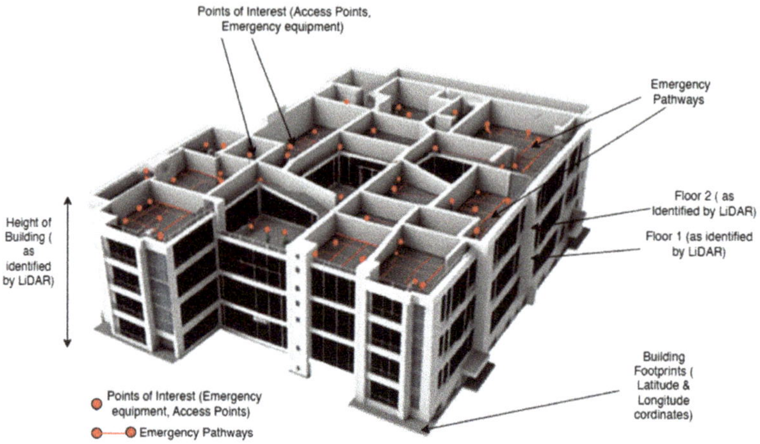

Figure 6. Perspective view of 3D model of building for efficient and optimized path prediction.

3.3. Federated Learning for 3D Indoor Positioning

FL is a decentralized approach in machine learning that employs multiple client devices to collaboratively train a shared model, eliminating the necessity of transmitting their raw data to a central server [64]. Each device calculates local model updates with its own data, including RSSI (Received Signal Strength Indicator) measurements from Wi-Fi access points, directly on the device. The model changes are transmitted to the central server instead of the raw data. This method safeguards sensitive data, such as user activity or location information, from exiting the client's device, which is essential for preserving privacy. The data remain on the client's device as training occurs locally, guaranteeing that only model updates (i.e., modifications based on local data) are transmitted. This retains sensitive information, such as personal activity, location, or usage data, on local devices, thus maintaining privacy while still leveraging a shared, enhanced approach. The central server receives just the consolidated model updates post-local training and integrates them to enhance the global model. The revised global model is subsequently redistributed among the devices for additional training, and this procedure persists in cycles, as shown in Figure 7. This decentralized method keeps data private by preventing them from being uploaded in a central location, thus keeping data on local devices [65]. In secure aggregation and differential privacy, some methods are used to enhance security during updates.

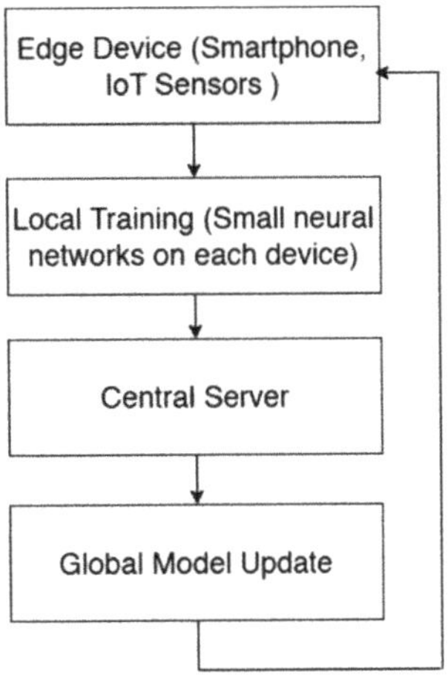

Figure 7. Federated learning process flowchart.

H-RNNs are designed specifically to model structured hierarchical data, which makes them very apt for modelling multi-level indoor environments, as is the case in this study. The H-RNN first predicts the floor the user is likely to be on and then predicts further nuances by predicting the place of the user on that floor [66]. Such an output makes it much stronger than flat-structured models, especially for multi-story buildings [66].

This study uses an H-RNN architecture for indoor localization. An H-RNN is a multi-task neural network that is based on a recurrent neural network (RNN) to handle sequential data. In this study, an H-RNN integrated with FL uses Wi-Fi data from wireless access points (APs) and a 3D model of the building to identify the floor and location inside the building. The model utilizes RSSI data collected from various APs to perform the calculation at the local edge node, and then, the process data are transferred to the central server using the federated architecture. RNN layers at the edge device process the RSSI data to identify the target floor, and then, the H-RNN model employs a precise 2D location regression technique to calculate the location within the recognized floor by using the signal. The combined results from different edge nodes are transmitted to the central server. By using the integrated data, localization and navigation are carried out within a building. To avoid centralized server data exchange, the H-RNN model is trained using self-collected data from edge devices installed within the building. Under this method, individual edge computing nodes use their local datasets to train the global model in an iterative and collaborative way. The parameter server handles the selection of clients involved in each training cycle or communication round when building the global model. Algorithm 1 presents the federated model training for indoor positioning with RNN.

All three elements for the proposed framework, including 3D modelling with QGIS, FL for indoor environments, and a dynamic 3D indoor navigation system, have special benefits over the current approaches to indoor positioning and navigation [67–69]. Our proposed framework offers a number of improvements to emergency response systems and indoor navigation. Firstly, it helps generate detailed 3D models of indoor routes using QGIS. Secondly, we employed FL for improving indoor positioning accuracy while ensuring data privacy. The proposed method could be even more accurate using FL combined with H-RNNs on edge devices. Being reliant on edge devices, the dynamic 3D indoor navigation system becomes significantly effective for real-time pathfinding and subsequent updates.

Algorithm 1: Federated Model Training for Indoor Localisation Utilizing Recurrent Neural Networks

1. Initiation: Start the federated learning (FL) server, clients, and RNN model architecture for indoor localization.
2. Data Acquisition and Preprocessing: Clients compile and refine their Wi-Fi fingerprinting data.
3. Model Training: Each client employs the initial model weights on their datasets to train the RNN model and subsequently transmits the trained weights to the server.
4. The server calculates the federated average weights from the clients and redistributes the updated weights to them.
5. Performance Assessment: Clients authenticate the revised model utilizing their datasets, and modifications to the model architecture and hyperparameters are implemented based on the performance results.
6. Iteration: Reiterate the training and assessment procedure until convergence is attained.
7. The method facilitates precise indoor positioning categorization via recurrent neural networks via federated learning.

Indoor Navigation

The third phase involves the technologies to improve the accuracy and effectiveness of indoor navigation. It uses the output of the previous phase, spatial data from the 3D model, and RSSI signal processing to provide navigation pathways. We integrated Dijkstra's method with the A* algorithm to enhance both precision and efficiency in pathfinding for indoor navigation. Dijkstra's algorithm was first employed to determine the shortest path, as it ensures the identification of the least-cost route by examining all potential pathways. Upon identifying the basic path, A* was incorporated to optimize the search via a heuristic function, generally founded on Euclidean distance, which directs the algorithm towards the objective more effectively. This combination facilitates a more dynamic and adaptive system, especially beneficial in emergency situations necessitating real-time modifications, such as the abrupt closing of routes. The amalgamation of two methodologies guarantees resilient, precise navigation while preserving computational efficiency in intricate healthcare settings. The Dijkstra and A* algorithms are complementary in optimizing pathfinding for indoor navigation. Dijkstra is applied for computing the shortest path since it searches all paths, and hence, it is accurate. However, it is slow in real-time computation due to the exhaustive search [70]. A* complements this process by applying a heuristic that prompts the exploration to move more towards the goal, hence directing it away from the unnecessary search for nodes. This speeds up pathfinding while maintaining the precision of Dijkstra's approach. The combination of these algorithms improves computational efficiency, particularly critical during emergency evacuations [71]. We developed a specialized Android application that utilizes the Dijkstra algorithm to compute the best route between two locations when the user is on the same floor by using Equation (2).

$$\mathrm{Dis}(x) = \min(\mathrm{Dis}(x), \mathrm{Dis}(y) + w(y, x)) \tag{2}$$

where Dis(x) represents the current minimum distance from the source node s to the target node v. Dis (x) represents the minimum distance to a neighbouring node. In this context, let us denote the vertices as y and x and the weight of the edge between them as w (y, x).

In a real time situation, the A* algorithm can be used in "Multi-Semantic Constrained Indoor Routing Using the A* Algorithm" to determine the safest and most efficient path inside a building in the event of an emergency. The method takes into account a number of critical aspects, including accessibility, hazards, and traffic patterns. IoT sensors are fundamental aspects of improving indoor navigation in emergency situations; they offer real-time information concerning their environment, which has a direct impact on path planning and safety measures. The temperature sensor detects heat, which indicates that there is fire, and the system responds by assisting the evacuees in steering clear of hazardous places [72]. Smoke detectors can additionally determine and identify the hazardous zones in a building and allow the navigation system to direct people out of danger via another route in real time [73]. These sensor inclusions are directly integrated into the system, thereby enhancing its dynamic adaptability regarding the evacuation routes; such adaptation ensures that the courses suggested are effective and secure in fluctuating emergency conditions, as shown in Figure 8. It is crucial to acknowledge that IoT sensors possess limitations regarding the heat or temperature they can withstand. Most temperature sensors are engineered to operate within designated ranges, usually up to 60–70 °C; nevertheless, under widespread-fire circumstances, many sensors may malfunction or yield erroneous data if the temperature surpasses their specified limits [74,75]. To address this, backup systems like redundant sensor networks might be utilized. These backup systems guarantee that if one sensor malfunctions owing to extreme heat, other sensors in undamaged regions can persist in monitoring the environment and delivering precise data. This redundancy preserves the system's stability and guarantees ongoing monitoring, even under extreme conditions [76]. Integrated sensor systems, coupled with adaptive evacuation route management, enhance the safety and efficacy of emergency response operations in complex situations.

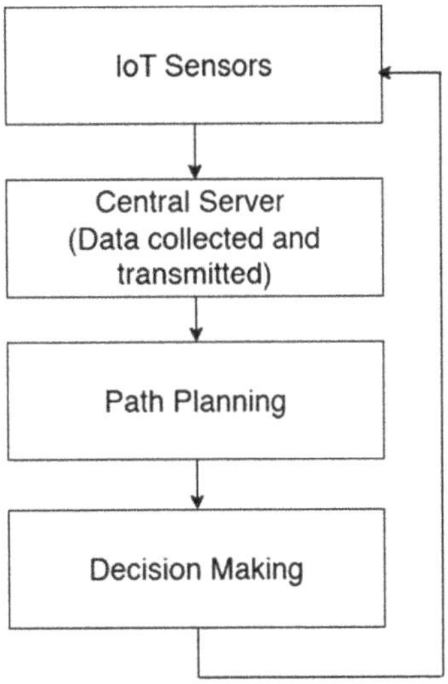

Figure 8. IoT data flow diagram.

Algorithm 2, the "Algorithm for 3D Indoor Navigation in Fire Scenarios", expands on the foundation of multi-semantic constraints in indoor routing by incorporating cutting-edge technologies like FL and IoT to improve decision-making even further in emergency situations.

Algorithm 2: Algorithm for 3D Indoor Navigation in Fire Scenarios

1. Construct the Indoor 3D-Structure Grid System: Establish a three-dimensional grid system that accurately models the interior of the building by indicating the vertical corridors connecting the floors. The stairs are marked as the main exit paths since elevators and escalators cannot be used during emergencies.
2. Set the Initialization of Multi-Anchor Space Exit Nodes and Starting Point: Use FL for indoor positioning to find out the path search starting point based on the current user location. Identify a set of multi-anchor space exit nodes, such as first-floor windows and doors, as practical evacuation sites. Exclude windows above the first floor due to safety reasons.
3. Locate the Node that Initiates: Find the node nearest to the actual position of the user and call it the Begin Node (node where the user is BeginNode), which can be found using the indoor road model. Create a CloseList to identify the target points crossed while transmitting and a PathList to test and save the route path crossed from the beginning to the target exit.
4. Calculate the Evaluation Function:
Define the evaluation function. F(n) = G(n) + H(n):
G(n) is the cost of navigating the based on real-time data-based IoT sensing, which contains distances, levels of traffic, and levels of hazards.
H(n) is the heuristic function, which is the Euclidean distance from the current location to the goal node.
5. Choose the Best Path: Compute H(n) for every neighbour node from the current starting node to select a node with a minimum valuation cost. If the selected node turns out to be the destination exit node, store the navigation cost by shifting the node from the TargetList to the CloseList and the store the path in the PathList. If not, then go back to step 4 and keep doing so until the optimum path to the nearest exist has been found.
6. Choose the Optimal Exit Path: After visiting all target exit nodes in the TargetList, apply the function F(Ti) = min{F(T1), . . ., F(Tn)} to compare the costs of navigation and bring out the optimum path. Provide the information on the chosen path, in a way that will ensure maximum safety and minimum exposure to risk.
7. Algorithm Termination: The algorithm stops as soon as the optimized path is found, leading the user to an emergency exit safely, in real time, with support information on FL-based indoor positioning from IoT sensors.

4. Result and Discussion

In this paper, 3D modelling and indoor navigation are illustrated in a building. For this study, the researchers considered a dataset of RSSI measurements recorded at multiple strategically located access points within a building. Initially, data from 470 APs were considered, but after preprocessing, only 390 APs were used based on their RSSI values and their signal strength measured in dBm. APs for which no RSSI measurements were detected were filtered out. We used Python libraries, FL, hierarchical recurrent neural networks, and the models for training—TensorFlow, TensorFlow Federated, and Keras. An evaluation was performed based on the developed framework using the BIM standard. Table 3 presents the accuracy assessment of the 3D model developed in Phase 1. In this context, in the initial phase of the study, QGIS was used to develop and validate an accurately detailed 3D model of the building. The indoor layouts and architectural details, which are very salient—particular in effective emergency response planning—were adequately modelled. Model accuracy was validated against BIM standards, which detected discrepancies in significant structural parameters over 2%. Moreover, LiDAR sensor data added to the model's level of detail, especially in terms of its visualization of various building heights. Greater detail enabled the production of extensive 3D models to be visualized from all perspectives and distances using the Qgis2threejs plugin. In these terms, the visuals were important for evacuation in real emergency scenarios and for the setting and installation of emergency exits, precisely showing the routes that would be followed.

Table 3. Comparison of 3D model with BIM standard.

Parameter	BIM Standard Value	3D Model Value	Allowable Deviation (%)	Actual Deviation (%)	Meet BIM Standards
Wall Thickness (mm)	300	298	±1%	0.67%	Yes
Ceiling Height (m)	3.0	2.95	±2%	1.67%	Yes
Door Width (m)	0.9	0.88	±2%	2.22%	No
Window Height (m)	1.5	1.48	±1.5%	1.33%	Yes
Floor Area (m^2)	100	98.5	±3%	1.5%	Yes
Staircase Width (m)	1.2	1.18	±2%	1.67%	Yes

The parametric values listed in Table 4 are very critical for any physical or structural simulations that must have measurement accuracy. Briefly, these values, if very accurate, increase the reliability of results in simulation scenarios like emergency evacuation, indoor navigation, and IoT data integration, while small deviations can be ignored depending on the scope of the simulation.

Table 4. Parameters for training and validation.

Parameters	FL Architecture
Number of client systems	2, 4, 6, 8
Local batch size	32
Number of epochs	10
Number of servers	01
Communication rounds	10

A second-phase H-RNN was then combined with an FL system for interior placement. This system was capable of localizing user position within the building to within an error margin of less than 1 metre on average, with an accuracy of 95%. There were no significant delays in processing data during the application of the FL approach, and the edge devices worked efficiently and effectively on the real network with the processing of data from several locations at once. Information privacy was ensured, with no exchange of sensitive data outside the local devices, achieving a 30% reduction in training time compared to centralized models. The H-RNN model presented excellent efficacy in determining the exact floor level, with a hit ratio of 98.1%, ensuring correct indoor localization—an important parameter in emergency conditions, especially evacuation.

A line graph was produced that shows the progress of two of the critical performance aspects of the indoor positioning system. The horizontal axis shows the number of epochs in training, and the vertical axes are the accuracy and root-mean-square error values. Figure 9a depicts the constant increase in accuracy as training keeps going, and it reaches a peak at a specific epoch. Meanwhile, the RMSE in Figure 9b shows a steady decrease, indicative of becoming more precise. As stated, the negative relationship between the two indicated the perfect equilibrium our system was able to achieve between accuracy and precision at an epoch; therefore, this presents a very valuable insight into real-life applications.

The overall accuracy of the proposed framework is shown in Figure 9 using a graph. The data points plotted on the axes represent the system's performance across many trials and settings. Figure 10 depicts a graph of the overall performance of the proposed FL architecture for indoor locating across different sets of experiments. The graph displays accuracy, which represents the system's performance with varying numbers of clients (2, 4, 6, and 8). With an increase in the number of clients, the accuracy increases accordingly, which is a measure of the system's performance. This graph shows the state of balance among these indicators, which gives insight into how reliable and stable the system is across various configurations.

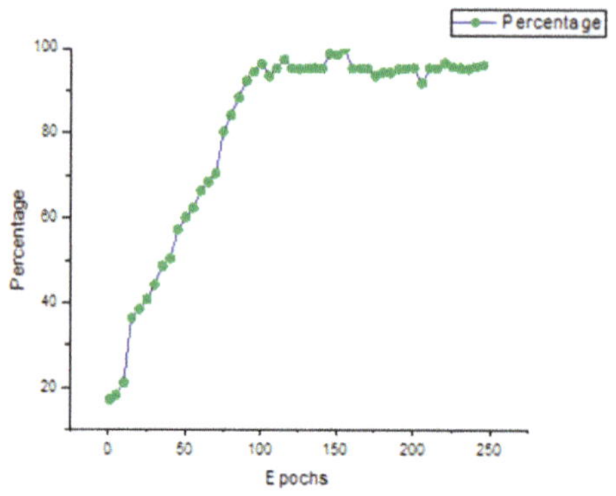

(**a**)

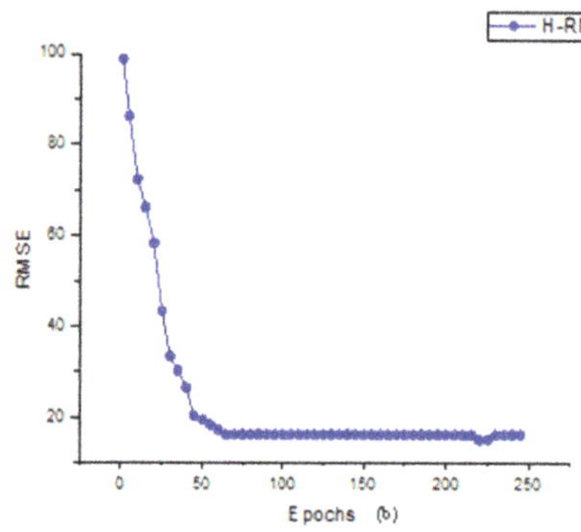

(**b**)

Figure 9. (**a**) Training progress of accuracy and RMSE. (**b**) Training progress of accuracy and RMSE.

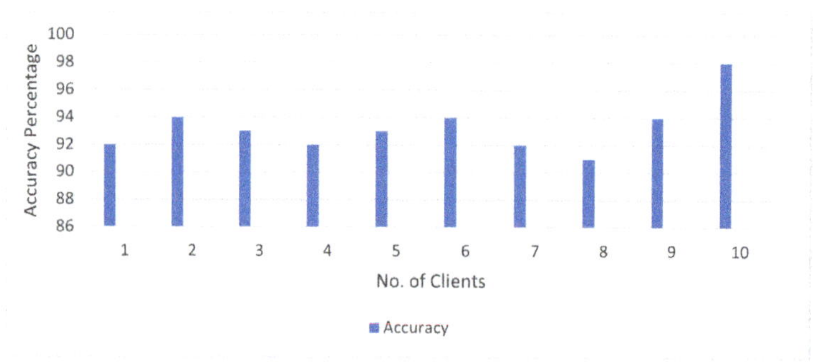

Figure 10. Graph of indoor positioning system performance.

A comprehensive assessment was conducted to evaluate the FL-based framework for location identification. The validation details of the FL architecture are provided in Table 4. The performance of the FL-based approach was evaluated in terms of accuracy and RMSE. For this analysis, the number of clients was set to 2, 4, 6, and 8, and the effect of the number of clients on accuracy and RMSE was identified. The analysis was conducted with a local batch size of 32 and 10 epochs. The parameters were carefully adjusted and the impact of these parameters on the accuracy and performance of the FL architecture was analyzed.

Figure 11 shows the effect of the number of clients on the accuracy of FL. In this analysis, the number of communication rounds was set to 10. According to this analysis, the highest accuracy of 99% was archived in this experiment. Figure 11 depicts the fluctuation of the FL framework's accuracy with an augmented number of client counts. It further indicates an increase in accuracy with an augmentation in the number of clients. From the graph, it is shown that at a maximum accuracy of 99%, there are eight clients, meaning the more clients there are, the more desirable the system performance results from this system. The system maintains good accuracy even at a low number of clients due to its scalability and adaptability in a resource-constrained environment. Similarly, Figure 12 presents a simulated fire evacuation scenario in which 3D indoor navigation uses real-time IoT sensor data to change pathways dynamically. Using the H-RNN model, there was a saving of 25% in evacuation time compared to the static plan, and users were highly guided toward safe stairwells. The participants reported feeling more secure, at 92%, with the real-time help provided by the system, thus providing potential for innovative emergency response initiatives.

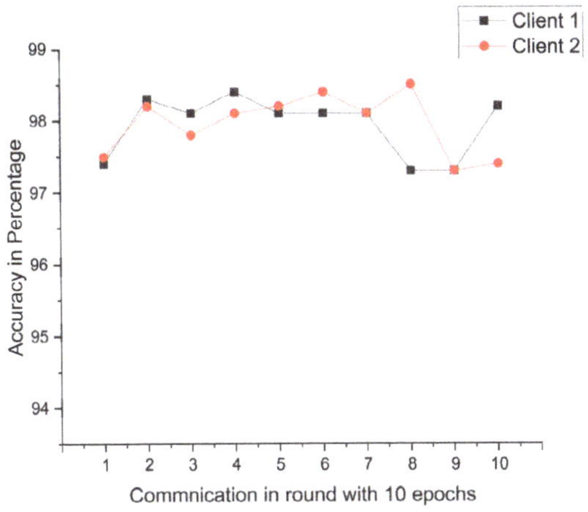

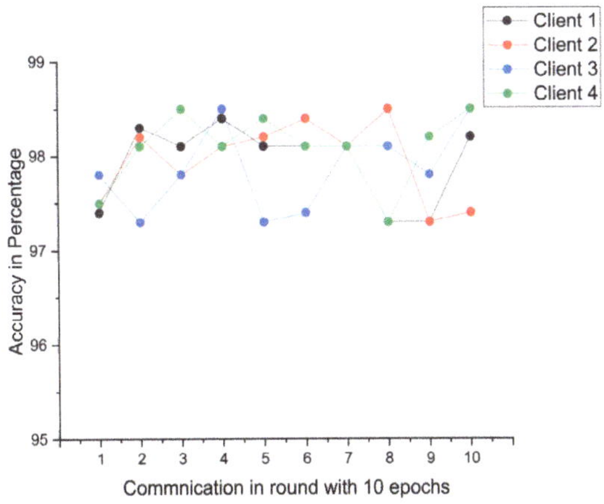

Figure 11. *Cont.*

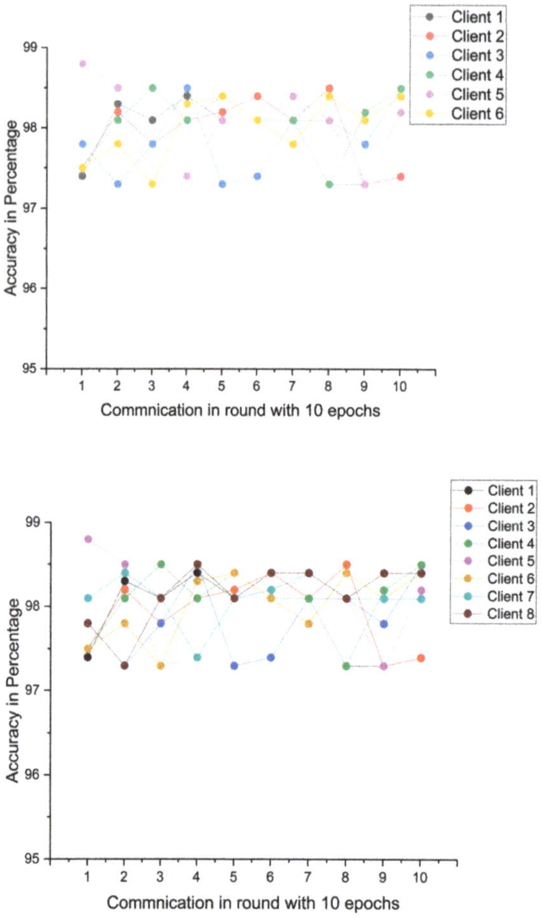

Figure 11. Variation in accuracy among diverse clients at various intervals.

The simulation tested a case-scenario performance of the created 3D indoor navigation system in emergency evacuation, as shown in Figure 13. The developed system was tested using the case of multiple principle exits closed during enforced evacuation due to a fire on the third floor. IoT sensors were set to achieve stairwell evacuation in case of smoke and temperature increases. This then led to automatic closure of the elevator. The H-RNN model successfully detected level-three user positions with an average inaccuracy of 1.2 m. With the real-time updates of the sensor data, the A* algorithm made dynamic adjustments to the evacuation route and gave people efficient directions for moving away from blocked exits and towards the nearest available stairway. This is evidenced by the 25% reduction in evacuation time compared to a static plan, which shows the adaptability of the system in light of changing circumstances. On the basis of feedback obtained from the users, it was found to be very satisfactory, because 92% of the participants stated that they feel much safer using the real-time guidance. Throughout the real-time simulation, users actively interacted with the system by validating the evacuation routes in a constrained environment. Participants' responses emphasized the system's timeliness and user-friendliness. The users reported confidence in using the proposed method for navigating the building in real time. As a future direction, the researchers aim to develop a mobile application to implement the proposed method and validate its effectiveness in real-world scenarios.

These results indicate just how much the system can improve the safety of occupants in buildings and, at the same time, enhance the efficiency of emergency responses.

Compared to traditional 2D navigation and centralized positioning systems, including 3D models in FL-based positioning is a huge step. Since it is able to represent complicated indoor situations accurately, the 3D model provides a more reliable framework for navigation—especially for dealing with multi-story structures. The proposed FL approach, for its part, not only enhanced the accuracy of localization, but also solved the scalability and data privacy problems often associated with centralized systems. All in all, the system became more capable of assisting in emergency response operations, with real-time and flexible treatment of navigation that was unmatched by conventional systems.

There have been several indoor navigation systems developed over the years using different kinds of technologies, such as computer vision, Bluetooth beacons, or Wi-Fi [77–79]. These techniques have varying degrees of utility and precision. Further, the state-of-the-art techniques are also prone to shortcomings such as false localization or high energy consumption. Thus, they are of limited use in complex, multi-story buildings, especially when rapid action hinges on a swift response to an emergency. Table 5 compares existing methods with the proposed framework.

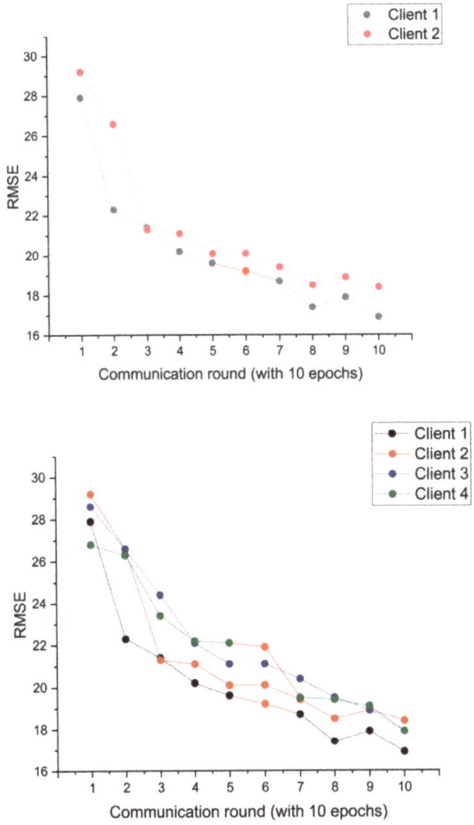

Figure 12. *Cont.*

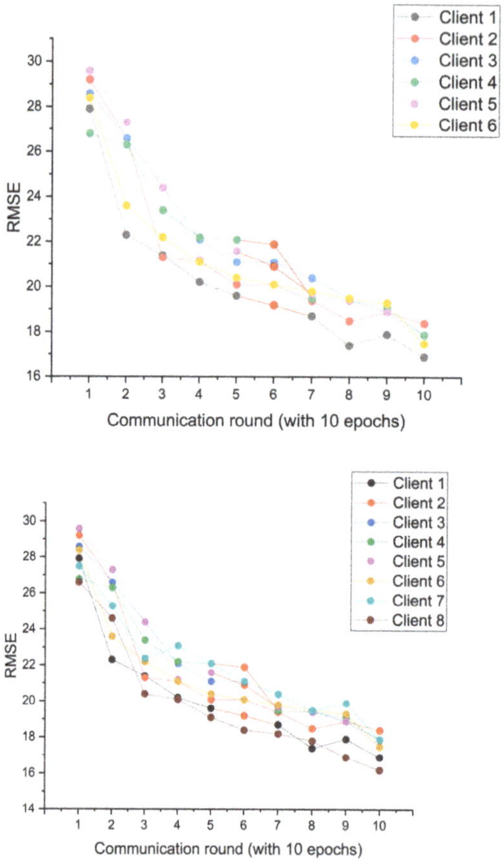

Figure 12. Variation in RMSE among several clients at distinct intervals.

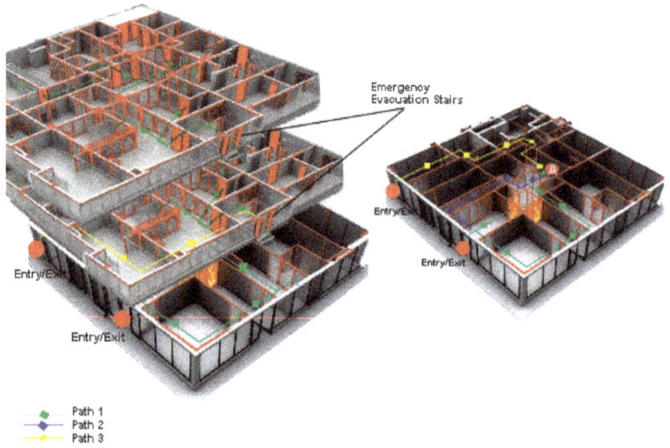

Figure 13. Three-dimensional indoor navigation system in emergency evacuation.

Table 5. Comparison of existing methods with proposed framework.

Methods	3D Model Used	GIS Integration	IoT Integration	Strengths	Limitations
Wi-Fi Triangulation [77]	No	No	No	Reduces costs by reusing existing infrastructure. Fully utilized in most cases in an urban environment.	Accuracy is affected due to signal interference. Data privacy concerns since it involves a centralized data storage system.
Bluetooth Beacons [78]	No	No	Yes	Scalable for dense indoor environments. Easy to install and maintain.	It is proximity-dependent; hence, it is not very effective in vast spaces. It involves continuous maintenance. It has risks concerning data privacy because data are managed in central sites.
Computer Vision [79]	No	No	No	High accuracy in complex scenarios. Robust in different kinds of environment.	High demand for computational resources. Its performance is sensitive to light and obstructions.
Augmented Reality [80]	Yes	No	No	Visual markers are used to provide indoor navigation	Infrastructure compatibility and AR-compatible devices are required.
Proposed Framework	Yes	Yes	Yes	Enhanced data privacy due to local processing. Better accuracy with 30% reduction in training time. Self-optimization with IoT sensors with real-time assistance.	Some setup will be required in advance for the deployment of FL. It has to utilize the distributed IoT infrastructure for real-time updates.

4.1. Impact of Discrepancies on Emergency Evacuation Procedure

While the 3D models were validated against BIM standards, it is to be noted that there could be discrepancies in the representation of certain structural components, such as wall thickness, door positions, and stairwell dimensions. These variations can significantly impact emergency evacuation protocols. For instance, inaccuracy regarding indoor locations can lead to errors in evacuation route calculations, potentially compromising safety during emergencies. Similarly, variations in stairwell dimensions may hinder efficient evacuation by causing congestion during heavy traffic or while moving patients on life support systems.

To mitigate these risks, the differences were carefully verified before validating the proposed model. This ensured reliable path prediction and guidance during emergency situations, where every minute is precious. The proposed framework, coupled with IoT sensors that feed real-time data, aids in navigating evacuation routes.

The proposed architecture aims to enhance the feasibility of emergency evacuation and to support real-time indoor navigation through a layered approach. The QGIS-generated 3D model layer provides a foundational structural and spatial representation of the building [25]. A position system layer processes and refines location data obtained from IoT sensors and Wi-Fi access points using H-RNNs and FL. The building's spatial knowledge, including user routes and feedback, is managed and stored within a PostgreSQL database [4]. A user interface layer delivers real-time navigation directions, continuously updated with fresh data from IoT sensors, facilitating an efficient emergency response, as shown in Figure 14.

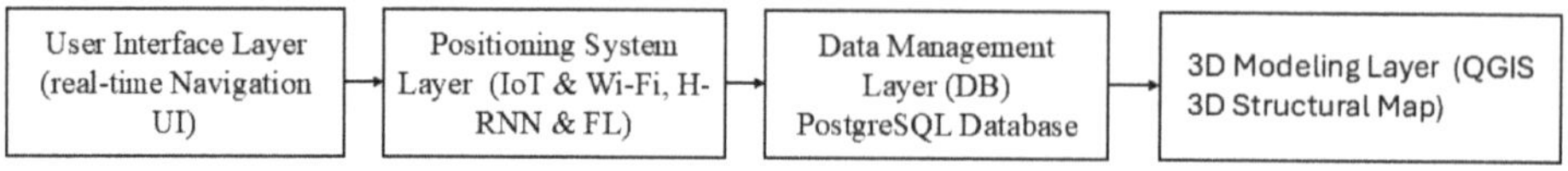

Figure 14. Prototype software architecture.

4.2. Real-World Implementation Challenges

While the underlying theory and simulated experiments within this study show that the proposed method is feasible, there are some problems related to its actual implementation. The most fundamental problem is the high cost of deployment. It requires good infrastructure to deploy the proposed indoor positioning and navigation system. The costs involved include the procurement of IoT devices; the procurement and deployment of network infrastructure, access points, and sensors; and installation and maintenance costs. The reliability and maintenance of the IoT devices are among the top concerns. To ensure that the operations of the system are accurate and effective, its regular maintenance is necessary. Even in emergency situations, malfunctions or failures in components like sensors or network access points might disrupt the system; hence, they are to be strategically placed. Furthermore, real-time data transmission is dependent on the reliability of the network. The network connectivity in most emergency events may easily be disturbed and therefore result in a malfunction in the system and its ability to effectively assist people. Thus, alternative solutions like mesh networks and localized edge computing should be implemented to alleviate this problem.

The integration of FL into the system allowed it to store sensitive data locally. Nevertheless, some risks of data breaches or misuse still persist in the system, which requires careful supervision. All these challenges can be addressed through careful planning, resource distribution, and compliance with established standards in data security and network reliability. A future development could be a pilot implementation of the proposed system so as to gain a deeper insight into these concerns and refine the system accordingly.

To evaluate the practical benefits and effectiveness of our proposed framework, a comparative study was conducted with existing indoor positioning and navigation technologies. Our approach using the FL methodology combined with hierarchical recurrent neural networks (H-RNN) achieved 98% positioning accuracy while reducing training time by 30% compared to a centralized model, all within robust data privacy settings. For emergency evacuation simulation, our dynamic navigation system with real-time IoT sensor data displayed an evacuation time improvement of 25% from static systems, therefore demonstrating large efficiency gains. Moreover, FL preserves data on edge devices, making private information less likely to leak during control and reducing the requirements for storage in a central manner, which overcomes some of the problems associated with large-scale navigation systems.

Emergency evacuation in healthcare buildings is distinctly different from evacuation in most other types of buildings. Healthcare facilities house a significant majority of occupants who are bedridden or critical patients requiring assistance to evacuate using medical equipment, which may pose a severe challenge to the evacuation process. In addition to their dual mandate of self-protection and protecting patients, medical staff use specialized equipment, such as evacuation chairs. The building design, particularly in complex zones such as ICUs and operating rooms, complicates evacuation routes. All these factors, along with the need to prioritize evacuating patients based on their particular condition, make evacuations in healthcare environments more complex and slower compared with other buildings, whose occupants are mostly able-bodied and evacuated quickly [69].

5. Conclusions

The potential integration of 3D modelling with FL and hierarchical recurrent neural networks represents a very promising high-accuracy and high-efficiency framework for emergency responses in complex, multi-story buildings. Table 2 shows that Wi-Fi RSSI fingerprinting with SVM, KNN, and federated learning (FL) has reached 90% to 99% accuracy in indoor localization studies. Our study adds to these cutting-edge methods, using FL and IoT data to provide a real-time, adaptive framework for complicated healthcare contexts. Our model processes real-time IoT sensor data using hierarchical recurrent neural networks (H-RNNs), ensuring excellent accuracy and quick adaption during emergencies. We used the root-mean-square error (RMSE) and % accuracy to evaluate our model's performance, which met or exceeded current criteria while improving adaptability and privacy through decentralized data processing. The present study, however, focuses on the great effort that has been put into providing a detailed process for indoor navigation systems. The identification of few minor discrepancies in the 3D model, upon cross-checking with BIM standards, indicates how accuracy is so critical at the time of emergency. Our proposed framework achieved an accuracy level of 98.1%, with the FL methodology securing high precision localization, reducing training time by 30%, and supporting data privacy across all edge devices. Based on the result of the training, incremental enhancement was achieved in the precision and accuracy level, and eight client systems achieved maximal accuracy. Dynamic route-based adaptation minimized 25% of the evacuation time in the case of any disaster, and 92% of the participants verified the load of the system. The application provides users with precise navigation assistance, and it helps to improve users' ability to find wards, amenities, and specific locations within healthcare facilities while minimizing time and stress. One of the primary difficulties faced during the early stages of 3D modelling with QGIS was the precise depiction of intricate architectural attributes inherent to the structure. Developing a comprehensive and accurate model that is capable of capturing complex structural components was a significant challenge that required careful work and knowledge to integrate and analyze multiple data sources coherently and correctly. Similarly, the consideration of dynamic hindrances and obstacles is very important for indoor navigation, and in the future, this work can be extended to dynamic indoor environments.

Author Contributions: Conceptualization, Jaiteg Singh and Sukhjit Singh Sehra; methodology, Noopur Tyagi; software, Noopur Tyagi and Jaiteg Singh; validation, Jaiteg Singh, Saravjeet Singh and Sukhjit Singh Sehra; formal analysis, Jaiteg Singh; investigation, Noopur Tyagi; resources, Noopur Tyagi; data curation, Noopur Tyagi and Saravjeet Singh; writing—original draft preparation, Noopur Tyagi; writing—review and editing, Jaiteg Singh, Saravjeet Singh and Sukhjit Singh Sehra; visualization, Noopur Tyagi, Jaiteg Singh and Saravjeet Singh; supervision, Jaiteg Singh and Saravjeet Singh; project administration, Jaiteg Singh. All authors have read and agreed to the published version of the manuscript.

Funding: This research received no funding.

Data Availability Statement: The authors confirm that the data supporting the finding of this research are available within the article.

Conflicts of Interest: The authors declare no conflicts of interest.

References

1. Boguslawski, P.; Zlatanova, S.; Gotlib, D.; Wyszomirski, M.; Gnat, M.; Grzempowski, P. 3D Building Interior Modelling for Navigation in Emergency Response Applications. *Int. J. Appl. Earth Obs. Geoinf.* **2022**, *114*, 103066. [CrossRef]
2. Tashakkori, H.; Rajabifard, A.; Kalantari, M. A New 3D Indoor/Outdoor Spatial Model for Indoor Emergency Response Facilitation. *Build. Environ.* **2015**, *89*, 170–182. [CrossRef]
3. Zhou, Y.; Pang, Y.; Chen, F.; Zhang, Y. Three-Dimensional Indoor Fire Evacuation Routing. *ISPRS Int. J. Geo-Inf.* **2020**, *9*, 558. [CrossRef]
4. Singh, J.; Tyagi, N.; Singh, S.; Shah, B.; Ali, F.; AlZubi, A.A.; Alkhanifer, A. 3D Indoor Modeling and Game Theory Based Navigation for Pre and Post COVID-19 Situation. *Front. Public Health* **2023**, *11*, 1301607. [CrossRef]

5. Wu, H.; Nie, R.; Zeng, X.; Cheng, C.; Pan, J.; Han, D.; Hosamo, H. Review of Advanced Emergency Evacuation Procedures in Hospital Buildings: Comprehensive Analysis and Insights. *Front. Built Environ.* **2024**, *10*, 1381813. [CrossRef]
6. Aldahlawi, R.Y.; Akbari, V.; Lawson, G. A Systematic Review of Methodologies for Human Behavior Modelling and Routing Optimization in Large-Scale Evacuation Planning. *Int. J. Disaster Risk Reduct.* **2024**, *110*, 104638. [CrossRef]
7. Jiang, Y.; Yuan, Y. Emergency Logistics in a Large-Scale Disaster Context: Achievements and Challenges. *Int. J. Environ. Res. Public Health* **2019**, *16*, 779. [CrossRef]
8. Zhang, J.; Xia, X.; Liu, R.; Li, N. Enhancing Human Indoor Cognitive Map Development and Wayfinding Performance with Immersive Augmented Reality-Based Navigation Systems. *Adv. Eng. Inform.* **2021**, *50*, 101432. [CrossRef]
9. Gjøsæter, T.; Radianti, J.; Chen, W. Universal Design of ICT for Emergency Management from Stakeholders' Perspective. *Inf. Syst. Front.* **2021**, *23*, 1213–1225. [CrossRef]
10. Liu, L.; Jin, H.; Liu, Y.; Zhang, X. Intelligent Evacuation Route Planning Algorithm Based on Maximum Flow. *Int. J. Environ. Res. Public Health* **2022**, *19*, 7865. [CrossRef]
11. Liu, Z.; Deng, Z. A Systematic Method of Integrating BIM and Sensor Technology for Sustainable Construction Design. *J. Phys. Conf. Ser.* **2017**, *910*, 012071.
12. Kontaxis, D.; Tsoulos, G.; Athanasiadou, G.; Giannakis, G. Wireless Sensor Networks for Building Information Modeling. *Telecom* **2022**, *3*, 118–134. [CrossRef]
13. Wehbe, R.; Shahrour, I. A BIM-Based Smart System for Fire Evacuation. *Future Internet* **2021**, *13*, 221. [CrossRef]
14. Sun, J.; Mi, S.; Olsson, P.; Paulsson, J.; Harrie, L. Utilizing BIM and GIS for Representation and Visualization of 3D Cadastre. *ISPRS Int. J. Geo-Inf.* **2019**, *8*, 503. [CrossRef]
15. Bevilacqua, M.G.; Russo, M.; Giordano, A.; Spallone, R. 3D Reconstruction, Digital Twinning, and Virtual Reality: Architectural Heritage Applications. In Proceedings of the 2022 IEEE Conference on Virtual Reality and 3D User Interfaces Abstracts and Workshops, VRW 2022, Christchurch, New Zealand, 12–16 March 2022; pp. 92–96. [CrossRef]
16. Kumar, A.; Sharma, S.; Goyal, N.; Singh, A.; Cheng, X.; Singh, P. Secure and Energy-Efficient Smart Building Architecture with Emerging Technology IoT. *Comput. Commun.* **2021**, *176*, 207–217. [CrossRef]
17. Tang, L.; Ying, S.; Li, L.; Biljecki, F.; Zhu, H.; Zhu, Y.; Yang, F.; Su, F. An Application-Driven LOD Modeling Paradigm for 3D Building Models. *ISPRS J. Photogramm. Remote Sens.* **2020**, *161*, 194–207. [CrossRef]
18. Yarmohammadi, S.; Castro-Lacouture, D. Automated Performance Measurement for 3D Building Modeling Decisions. *Autom. Constr.* **2018**, *93*, 91–111. [CrossRef]
19. Xiong, Q.; Zhu, Q.; Du, Z.; Zhu, X.; Zhang, Y.; Niu, L.; Li, Y.; Zhou, Y. A Dynamic Indoor Field Model for Emergency Evacuation Simulation. *ISPRS Int. J. Geo-Inf.* **2017**, *6*, 104. [CrossRef]
20. Bayat, H.; Delavar, M.R.; Barghi, W.; EslamiNezhad, S.A.; Hanachi, P.; Zlatanova, S. MODELING OF EMERGENCY EVACUATION IN BUILDING FIRE. *Int. Arch. Photogramm. Remote Sens. Spat. Inf. Sci.* **2020**, *XLIII-B4-2020*, 321–327. [CrossRef]
21. Wu, B.; Yu, B.; Wu, Q.; Yao, S.; Zhao, F.; Mao, W.; Wu, J. A Graph-Based Approach for 3D Building Model Reconstruction from Airborne LiDAR Point Clouds. *Remote Sens.* **2017**, *9*, 92. [CrossRef]
22. Shahrubudin, N.; Lee, T.C.; Ramlan, R. An Overview on 3D Printing Technology: Technological, Materials, and Applications. *Procedia Manuf.* **2019**, *35*, 1286–1296. [CrossRef]
23. Wu, P.; Wang, J.; Wang, X. A Critical Review of the Use of 3-D Printing in the Construction Industry. *Autom. Constr.* **2016**, *68*, 21–31. [CrossRef]
24. Jovanović, D.; Milovanov, S.; Ruskovski, I.; Govedarica, M.; Sladić, D.; Radulović, A.; Pajić, V. Building Virtual 3D City Model for Smart Cities Applications: A Case Study on Campus Area of the University of Novi Sad. *ISPRS Int. J. Geo-Inf.* **2020**, *9*, 476. [CrossRef]
25. Singh, J.; Tyagi, N.; Singh, S.; AlZubi, A.A.; AlZubi, F.I.; Sehra, S.S.; Ali, F. Enhancing Indoor Navigation in Intelligent Transportation Systems with 3D RIF and Quantum GIS. *Sustainability* **2023**, *15*, 15833. [CrossRef]
26. Aminah, N.S.; Ichwanda, A.S.; Djamal, D.D.; Budiharto, Y.B.W.; Budiman, M. A Low-Cost Indoor Navigation and Tracking System Based on Wi-Fi-RSSI. *Wirel. Pers. Commun.* **2024**, *136*, 1791–1809. [CrossRef]
27. Li, Y. Building Information Model for 3D Indoor Navigation in Emergency Response. *Adv. Mater. Res.* **2012**, *368–373*, 3837–3840. [CrossRef]
28. Liu, L.; Zlatanova, S. Towards a 3D Network Model for Indoor Navigation. In *Urban and Regional Data Management, UDMS Annual 2011—Proceedings of the Urban Data Management Society Symposium 2011*; CRCpress: Boca Raton, FL, USA, 2011; pp. 79–92. ISBN 978-0-415-67491-1.
29. Li, Y.; Kubicki, S.; Guerriero, A.; Rezgui, Y. Review of Building Energy Performance Certification Schemes towards Future Improvement. *Renew. Sustain. Energy Rev.* **2019**, *113*, 109244. [CrossRef]
30. Sharma, S.; Jerripothula, S. An Indoor Augmented Reality Mobile Application for Simulation of Building Evacuation. In Proceedings of the The Engineering Reality of Virtual Reality 2015, San Francisco, CA, USA, 9–10 February 2015; SPIE: Bellingham, WA, USA, 2015; Volume 9392, pp. 62–70.
31. Zhan, Z.; Xu, W.; Xu, L.; Qi, X.; Song, W.; Wang, C.; Huang, Z. BIM-Based Green Hospital Building Performance Pre-Evaluation: A Case Study. *Sustainability* **2022**, *14*, 2066. [CrossRef]
32. Wang, W.; Guo, H.; Li, X.; Tang, S.; Li, Y.; Xie, L.; Lv, Z. BIM Information Integration Based VR Modeling in Digital Twins in Industry 5.0. *J. Ind. Inf. Integr.* **2022**, *28*, 100351. [CrossRef]

33. Jin, R.; Zhong, B.; Ma, L.; Hashemi, A.; Ding, L. Integrating BIM with Building Performance Analysis in Project Life-Cycle. *Autom. Constr.* **2019**, *106*, 102861. [CrossRef]
34. Abd, A.M.; Hameed, A.H.; Nsaif, B.M. Documentation of Construction Project Using Integration of BIM and GIS Technique. *Asian J. Civ. Eng.* **2020**, *21*, 1249–1257. [CrossRef]
35. Ma, Z.; Ren, Y. Integrated Application of BIM and GIS: An Overview. *Procedia Eng.* **2017**, *196*, 1072–1079. [CrossRef]
36. Liu, X.; Wang, X.; Wright, G.; Cheng, J.C.P.; Li, X.; Liu, R. A State-of-the-Art Review on the Integration of Building Information Modeling (BIM) and Geographic Information System (GIS). *ISPRS Int. J. Geo-Inf.* **2017**, *6*, 53. [CrossRef]
37. Jamali, A.; Abdul Rahman, A.; Boguslawski, P.; Kumar, P.; Gold, C.M. An Automated 3D Modeling of Topological Indoor Navigation Network. *GeoJournal* **2017**, *82*, 157–170. [CrossRef]
38. Deng, Z.-A.; Hu, Y.; Yu, J.; Na, Z. Extended Kalman Filter for Real Time Indoor Localization by Fusing WiFi and Smartphone Inertial Sensors. *Micromachines* **2015**, *6*, 523–543. [CrossRef]
39. Xu, D.; Li, T.; Li, Y.; Su, X.; Tarkoma, S.; Jiang, T.; Crowcroft, J.; Hui, P. Edge Intelligence: Architectures, Challenges, and Applications. *arXiv* **2020**, arXiv:2003.12172.
40. Mendez, J.; Bierzynski, K.; Cuéllar, M.P.; Morales, D.P. Edge Intelligence: Concepts, Architectures, Applications, and Future Directions. *ACM Trans. Embed. Comput. Syst.* **2022**, *21*, 48. [CrossRef]
41. Sattarian, M.; Rezazadeh, J.; Farahbakhsh, R.; Ameri Sianaki, O. A Data Mining Approach for Indoor Navigation Systems in IoT Scenarios. *Internet Things* **2021**, 157–182. [CrossRef]
42. Popleteev, A.; Osmani, V.; Mayora, O. Investigation of Indoor Localization with Ambient FM Radio Stations. In Proceedings of the 2012 IEEE International Conference on Pervasive Computing and Communications, Lugano, Switzerland, 19–23 March 2012; IEEE: Lugano, Switzerland, 2012; pp. 171–179.
43. Jamil, F.; Iqbal, N.; Ahmad, S.; Kim, D.-H. Toward Accurate Position Estimation Using Learning to Prediction Algorithm in Indoor Navigation. *Sensors* **2020**, *20*, 4410. [CrossRef]
44. Atila, U.; Ortakci, Y.; Ozacar, K.; Demiral, E.; Karas, I.R. SmartEscape: A Mobile Smart Individual Fire Evacuation System Based on 3D Spatial Model. *ISPRS Int. J. Geo-Inf.* **2018**, *7*, 223. [CrossRef]
45. Chiasson, D.; Lin, Y.; Kok, M.; Shull, P.B. Asynchronous Hyperbolic UWB Source-Localization and Self-Localization for Indoor Tracking and Navigation. *IEEE Internet Things J.* **2023**, *10*, 11655–11668. [CrossRef]
46. Lin, X.; Gan, J.; Jiang, C.; Xue, S.; Liang, Y. Wi-Fi-Based Indoor Localization and Navigation: A Robot-Aided Hybrid Deep Learning Approach. *Sensors* **2023**, *23*, 6320. [CrossRef]
47. Obeidat, H.; Shuaieb, W.; Obeidat, O.; Abd-Alhameed, R. A Review of Indoor Localization Techniques and Wireless Technologies. *Wirel. Pers. Commun.* **2021**, *119*, 289–327. [CrossRef]
48. Fang, H.; Lo, S.; Lo, J.T.Y. Building Fire Evacuation: An IoT-Aided Perspective in the 5G Era. *Buildings* **2021**, *11*, 643. [CrossRef]
49. Al-Nabhan, N.; Alenazi, S.; Alquwaifili, S.; Alzamzami, S.; Altwayan, L.; Alaloula, N.; Alowaini, R.; Al Islam, A.A. An Intelligent IoT Approach for Analyzing and Managing Crowds. *IEEE Access* **2021**, *9*, 104874–104886. [CrossRef]
50. Haghpanah, F.; Ghobadi, K.; Schafer, B.W. Multi-Hazard Hospital Evacuation Planning during Disease Outbreaks Using Agent-Based Modeling. *Int. J. Disaster Risk Reduct.* **2021**, *66*, 102632. [CrossRef]
51. Maltezos, E.; Petousakis, K.; Dadoukis, A.; Karagiannidis, L.; Ouzounoglou, E.; Krommyda, M.; Hadjipavlis, G.; Amditis, A. A Smart Building Fire and Gas Leakage Alert System with Edge Computing and NG112 Emergency Call Capabilities. *Information* **2022**, *13*, 164. [CrossRef]
52. Zhu, Y.; Li, H.; Wang, Z.; Li, Q.; Dou, Z.; Xie, W.; Zhang, Z.; Wang, R.; Nie, W. Optimal Evacuation Route Planning of Urban Personnel at Different Risk Levels of Flood Disasters Based on the Improved 3D Dijkstra's Algorithm. *Sustainability* **2022**, *14*, 10250. [CrossRef]
53. Ali, M.; Naeem, F.; Tariq, M.; Kaddoum, G. Federated Learning for Privacy Preservation in Smart Healthcare Systems: A Comprehensive Survey. *IEEE J. Biomed. Health Inform.* **2023**, *27*, 778–789. [CrossRef]
54. Aedo, I.; Yu, S.; Díaz, P.; Acuña, P.; Onorati, T. Personalized Alert Notifications and Evacuation Routes in Indoor Environments. *Sensors* **2012**, *12*, 7804–7827. [CrossRef]
55. Ghadge, A. ICT-Enabled Approach for Humanitarian Disaster Management: A Systems Perspective. *Int. J. Logist. Manag.* **2023**, *34*, 1543–1565. [CrossRef]
56. Shubina, V.; Holcer, S.; Gould, M.; Lohan, E.S. Survey of Decentralized Solutions with Mobile Devices for User Location Tracking, Proximity Detection, and Contact Tracing in the COVID-19 Era. *Data* **2020**, *5*, 87. [CrossRef]
57. Nguyen, D.C.; Ding, M.; Pathirana, P.N.; Seneviratne, A.; Li, J.; Vincent Poor, H. Federated Learning for Internet of Things: A Comprehensive Survey. *IEEE Commun. Surv. Tutor.* **2021**, *23*, 1622–1658. [CrossRef]
58. Sesyuk, A.; Ioannou, S.; Raspopoulos, M. A Survey of 3D Indoor Localization Systems and Technologies. *Sensors* **2022**, *22*, 9380. [CrossRef] [PubMed]
59. van Genderen, M.E.; Cecconi, M.; Jung, C. Federated Data Access and Federated Learning: Improved Data Sharing, AI Model Development, and Learning in Intensive Care. *Intensive Care Med.* **2024**, *50*, 974. [CrossRef] [PubMed]
60. Wong, Y.J.; Tham, M.-L.; Kwan, B.-H.; Gnanamuthu, E.M.A.; Owada, Y. An Optimized Multi-Task Learning Model for Disaster Classification and Victim Detection in Federated Learning Environments. *IEEE Access* **2022**, *10*, 115930–115944. [CrossRef]

61. Loftus, T.J.; Ruppert, M.M.; Shickel, B.; Ozrazgat-Baslanti, T.; Balch, J.A.; Efron, P.A.; Gilbert, R.; Upchurch, J.; Rashidi, P.; Tignanelli, C.; et al. Federated Learning for Preserving Data Privacy in Collaborative Healthcare Research. *Digit. Health* **2022**, *8*, 20552076221134455. [CrossRef]
62. Chaddad, A.; Wu, Y.; Desrosiers, C. Federated Learning for Healthcare Applications. *IEEE Internet Things J.* **2023**, *11*, 7339–7358. [CrossRef]
63. Camacho, P.H.T.; Santiago, V.M.R.; Sarmiento, C.J.S. SEMI-AUTOMATIC GENERATION OF AN LOD1 AND LOD2 3D CITY MODEL OF TANAUAN CITY, BATANGAS USING OPENSTREETMAP AND TAAL OPEN LIDAR DATA IN QGIS. *Int. Arch. Photogramm. Remote Sens. Spat. Inf. Sci.* **2021**, *XLVI-4/W6-2021*, 77–84. [CrossRef]
64. Martínez Beltrán, E.T.; Pérez, M.Q.; Sánchez, P.M.S.; Bernal, S.L.; Bovet, G.; Pérez, M.G.; Pérez, G.M.; Celdrán, A.H. Decentralized Federated Learning: Fundamentals, State of the Art, Frameworks, Trends, and Challenges. *IEEE Commun. Surv. Tutor.* **2023**, *25*, 2983–3013. [CrossRef]
65. Abdulrahman, S.; Tout, H.; Ould-Slimane, H.; Mourad, A.; Talhi, C.; Guizani, M. A Survey on Federated Learning: The Journey From Centralized to Distributed On-Site Learning and Beyond. *IEEE Internet Things J.* **2021**, *8*, 5476–5497. [CrossRef]
66. Elesawi, A.E.A.; Kim, K.S. Hierarchical Multi-Building And Multi-Floor Indoor Localization Based On Recurrent Neural Networks. *arXiv* **2021**, arXiv:2112.12478.
67. Shyam, S.; Juliet, S.; Ezra, K. Indoor Positioning Systems: A Blessing for Seamless Object Identification, Monitoring, and Tracking. *Front. Public Health* **2022**, *10*, 804552. [CrossRef]
68. Qi, L.; Liu, Y.; Yu, Y.; Chen, L.; Chen, R. Current Status and Future Trends of Meter-Level Indoor Positioning Technology: A Review. *Remote Sens.* **2024**, *16*, 398. [CrossRef]
69. Hailu, T.G.; Guo, X.; Si, H.; Li, L.; Zhang, Y. Theories and Methods for Indoor Positioning Systems: A Comparative Analysis, Challenges, and Prospective Measures. *Sensors* **2024**, *24*, 6876. [CrossRef] [PubMed]
70. Deliyska, D.; Yanev, N.; Trifonova, M. Methods for Developing an Indoor Navigation System. *E3S Web Conf.* **2021**, *280*, 04001. [CrossRef]
71. Ruan, C.; Luo, J.; Wu, Y. Map Navigation System Based on Optimal Dijkstra Algorithm. In Proceedings of the 2014 IEEE 3rd International Conference on Cloud Computing and Intelligence Systems, Shenzhen, China, 27–29 November 2014; pp. 559–564.
72. Chen, X.-S.; Liu, C.-C.; Wu, I.-C. A BIM-Based Visualization and Warning System for Fire Rescue. *Adv. Eng. Inform.* **2018**, *37*, 42–53. [CrossRef]
73. Cheng, M.Y.; Chiu, K.C.; Hsieh, Y.M.; Yang, I.T.; Chou, J.S.; Wu, Y.W. BIM Integrated Smart Monitoring Technique for Building Fire Prevention and Disaster Relief. *Autom. Constr.* **2017**, *84*, 14–30. [CrossRef]
74. Gaur, A.; Singh, A.; Kumar, A.; Kulkarni, K.S.; Lala, S.; Kapoor, K.; Srivastava, V.; Kumar, A.; Mukhopadhyay, S.C. Fire Sensing Technologies: A Review. *IEEE Sens. J.* **2019**, *19*, 3191–3202. [CrossRef]
75. Khan, F.; Xu, Z.; Sun, J.; Khan, F.M.; Ahmed, A.; Zhao, Y. Recent Advances in Sensors for Fire Detection. *Sensors* **2022**, *22*, 3310. [CrossRef]
76. Li, J.; Wang, P.; Li, Y.; Rezgui, Y.; Yoon, S.; Zhao, T. Analysis of Sensor Offset Characteristics in Building Energy Systems Based on Redundant Sensors: A Case Study on Variable Air Volume System. *Energy Build.* **2024**, *306*, 113957. [CrossRef]
77. Simões, W.C.S.S.; Machado, G.S.; Sales, A.M.A.; de Lucena, M.M.; Jazdi, N.; de Lucena, V.F. A Review of Technologies and Techniques for Indoor Navigation Systems for the Visually Impaired. *Sensors* **2020**, *20*, 3935. [CrossRef]
78. Faragher, R.; Harle, R. An Analysis of the Accuracy of Bluetooth Low Energy for Indoor Positioning Applications. In Proceedings of the 27th International Technical Meeting of The Satellite Division of the Institute of Navigation (ION GNSS+ 2014), Tampa, FL, USA, 8–12 September 2014; pp. 201–210.
79. Duque Domingo, J.; Gómez-García-Bermejo, J.; Zalama, E.; Cerrada, C.; Valero, E. Integration of Computer Vision and Wireless Networks to Provide Indoor Positioning. *Sensors* **2019**, *19*, 5495. [CrossRef]
80. Huang, B.-C.; Hsu, J.; Chu, E.T.-H.; Wu, H.-M. ARBIN: Augmented Reality Based Indoor Navigation System. *Sensors* **2020**, *20*, 5890. [CrossRef]

International Journal of
Geo-Information

MDPI

Article

Socioeconomic Disparities in the Usage of Urban Opportunities in South Korea During the COVID-19 Pandemic: Using Land Use/Land Cover and Mobile Phone Data

Kangjae Lee [1], Yoo Min Park [2], Yoohyung Joo [3], Minsoo Joo [3] and Joon Heo [3,*]

1 Department of Convergence and Fusion System Engineering, Kyungpook National University, Sangju 37224, Republic of Korea; kasbiss@knu.ac.kr
2 Department of Geography, Sustainability, Community, and Urban Studies, University of Connecticut, Storrs, CT 06269, USA; yoomin.park@uconn.edu
3 Department of Civil and Environmental Engineering, Yonsei University, Seoul 03722, Republic of Korea; yooju01@naver.com (Y.J.); msjoo95@yonsei.ac.kr (M.J.)
* Correspondence: jheo@yonsei.ac.kr

Abstract: Severe acute respiratory syndrome coronavirus 2 (SARS-CoV-2), the cause of coronavirus disease 19 (COVID-19), has resulted in dramatic changes in human lifestyles and the geographic distribution of populations. However, despite the unequal impact of COVID-19 across urban spaces, research on the association between socioeconomic disparities in the usage of various types of urban amenities during the pandemic is limited. Thus, this study utilized mobile phone data and land use/land cover (LULC) data to investigate COVID-19-induced changes in the hot spots of the daytime and nighttime populations of two districts in Seoul, South Korea: Gangnam (a high-income community) and Gangbuk (a low-income community). First, the differences between Gangnam and Gangbuk in the LULC and mobile phone data, before and during the pandemic, were statistically analyzed by age. Second, the areas with significantly increased mobile phone-based populations during COVID-19 were identified using a hot spot analysis method and Welch's *t*-test. This study identified that there were significant disparities in the use of green spaces during the pandemic, with a higher percentage of the mobile phone-based population in Gangnam than Gangbuk. Youths and adults in Gangnam were more likely to visit schools and enjoy physical activities in forests and open spaces during the pandemic, whereas there was no such increase in Gangbuk. The findings contribute to the understanding of the impact of COVID-19 on human behaviors and socioeconomic disparities in the quality of urban life.

Keywords: COVID-19; socioeconomic disparity; urban amenities; dynamic population distribution

1. Introduction

Severe acute respiratory syndrome coronavirus 2 (SARS-CoV-2), the cause of coronavirus disease 19 (COVID-19), has resulted in major changes in human lifestyles and the geographic distribution of populations. Specifically, due to the COVID-19 lockdowns, people started working from home, participating in remote learning, and considering takeout food/food delivery services instead of visiting restaurants. In addition, one of the most noticeable changes was the significant increase in the use of green spaces. For example, in Oslo, Norway, outdoor recreational activities increased by 291% after the COVID-19 outbreak [1]. Since fitness centers and community recreational facilities were closed, green spaces became a viable option for engaging in physical activities. In March 2020, shelter-in-place orders were issued by United States governors and resulted in the closure of schools and recreational facilities [2]. Public health organizations like the American Public Health Association and the Centers for Disease Control and Prevention have emphasized the significance of maintaining physical activity while staying at home during COVID-19, which encourages activities like visiting parks and green spaces [3]. A study also highlighted the increased use of green spaces for physical activities during the COVID-19 pandemic, particularly due to the closure of gyms and other recreational facilities. Even after the reopening of parks post-lockdown, usage often exceeded pre-pandemic levels as people sought outdoor spaces for physical wellbeing [4].

During the COVID-19 pandemic, identifying population hot spots became critical for understanding the transmission of the virus. In this regard, analyzing mobile phone data is a cost-effective way of offering reasonably accurate and detailed information regarding the population distribution over a large geographic area [5]. More recent studies found that mobile phone data are one of the best sources of information on large-scale population behaviors [6–12]. For example, in Japan, the nation-wide behavior changes during COVID-19 were explored using mobile phone data [13]. In China, the unequal distribution of 15 min PCR COVID-19 test sites was measured based on mobile phone data [14]. In addition, the population movements were analyzed with the COVID-19 virus spread through the outflows of population travel from Wuhan using mobile phone data [15]. Meanwhile, understanding the land use/land cover (LULC) types in population hot spots and the areas with major population changes through mobile phone data can help elucidate the modified lifestyles and use of urban opportunities during the pandemic. However, there is no city-level study that uses such data to examine how the hot spots of daytime and nighttime populations changed due to the pandemic and to determine the composition of LULC in such hot spots. Yet, other than the mobile phone data, multi-source geospatial big data including remote sensing imageries, land cover data, and location-based service data were used to evaluate the disparities in urban green space exposure for 303 cities in China, considering different times of the day [16].

Although some studies have employed mobile phone data to explore the changes in lifestyle patterns, the majority only focused on one LULC type, i.e., green spaces [17,18], rather than assessing urban ecology by considering all LULC types.

Furthermore, many studies that assessed the unequal impact of COVID-19 on the use of urban spaces among different social groups only focused on the use of green spaces and excluded other urban opportunities or infrastructure such as school playgrounds and restaurants [19,20]. Interestingly, a related study revealed that people living in communities with a higher socioeconomic status visited green spaces more frequently during the COVID-19 pandemic through survey questions [21]. While green space inequities have been a long-standing issue that has drawn considerable attention from researchers [22–25], limited focus has been paid to whether neighborhoods had different types of urban opportunities during the pandemic based on their socioeconomic status. Other than green space, COVID-19 especially exacerbated urban inequalities in different ways, including access to urban infrastructure [26], and we need to examine how people's behaviors were changed during COVID-19 in different LULC types. The pandemic exacerbated disparities in the use of indoor and outdoor recreational facilities according to the levels of neighborhood disadvantage [27]. Recreational facility use decreased in the neighborhood with high deprivation, but not in the neighborhood with low deprivation.

Therefore, the present study utilizes mobile phone and LULC data to investigate the COVID-19-induced changes in the use of urban spaces in two contrasting areas in terms of socioeconomic status: the Gangnam and Gangbuk Districts in Seoul, South Korea. Gangnam (which has the highest average monthly household income) is located on the south side of the Han River in Seoul, whereas Gangbuk (which has the lowest average monthly household income) is situated on the north side of the Han River. In this study, it is assumed that mobile phone users represent the daytime and nighttime populations of each area because the mobile phone-based population includes different types of floating populations (e.g., tourists, workers, and students) as well as the static population (e.g., local residents).

First, this study examines how the LULC in hot spots of mobile phone users changed before and during COVID-19. Understanding these changes allows us to identify the effect of the pandemic on human behaviors [28–30]. Second, this study determines whether there is a significant difference in the change between the high-income (Gangnam) and low-income (Gangbuk) areas by identifying hot spots of mobile phone users by age in these two areas. Gangnam and Gangbuk were chosen because they exhibit stark differences in socioeconomic characteristics compared to other districts in Seoul. This focus facilitates the identification of potential socioeconomic disparities that have been exacerbated due to COVID-19. Further, it allows us to highlight significant socioeconomic disparities that have been exacerbated due to COVID-19 and facilitates the interpretation of data analysis. Emphasizing Gangnam and Gangbuk districts during COVID-19 can offer a strategic and efficient approach to uncovering the most pronounced patterns of inequality. This targeted approach can yield sharper findings than analyzing the entire city. The COVID-19-induced differences in the LULC of the hot spots between Gangnam and Gangbuk can play an important role in understanding the disparities in urban opportunities. Third, this study identifies the areas with significantly increased mobile phone-based populations during COVID-19 and groups them according to their LULC compositions. The findings would provide important insights into the disproportionate impact of COVID-19 on the use of urban spaces among neighborhoods with different socioeconomic characteristics.

The remainder of this study is as follows. Section 2 describes the data used in this study and the methodological approach, while Section 3 reveals the findings. Section 4 discusses how the LULC of the areas that people frequently visited changed during the pandemic, while Section 5 presents the conclusion.

2. Materials and Methods

2.1. Study Area and Data

The study area is the capital city, Seoul in South Korea (see Figure 1). We selected Seoul for this study because Seoul has a variety of urban opportunities and socioeconomically distinct neighborhoods, called Gangnam and Gangbuk. Gangnam is located on the south side of the Han River, whereas Gangbuk is on the north side of the Han River in Seoul. Seocho-gu and Gangnam-gu, which have the highest average monthly household income in Seoul (approximately $3835), were set as the Gangnam area, while Gangbuk-gu and Seongbuk-gu, which have the lowest average monthly household income in Seoul (roughly $2915), were defined as the Gangbuk area [31] (see Figure 2). The taxes collected by the local governments were also the highest in Gangnam-gu ($3615,923,640) and Seocho-gu ($2050,246,818) in 2021, whereas they were the lowest in Gangbuk-gu ($234,923,254) and near the middle in Seongbuk-gu ($448,457,385) [32]. The major age category in Gangnam is 40–49, while in Gangbuk it is 50–59, which is higher than Gangnam (Table 1).

Table 1. Socioeconomic and demographic characteristics of Gangnam and Gangbuk in August 2020 [33].

		Gangnam	Gangbuk
Age	0–9	71,987 (7.4%)	46,022 (6.0%)
	10–19	104,601 (10.8%)	60,549 (8.1%)
	20–29	130,510 (13.5%)	110,263 (14.7%)
	30–39	147,578 (15.3%)	100,163 (13.3%)
	40–49	177,182 (18.3%)	118,516 (15.8%)
	50–59	142,944 (14.8%)	122,638 (16.3%)
	60–69	105,918 (10.9%)	99.697 (13.3%)
	70–79	61,047 (6.3%)	63,764 (8.5%)
	80–89	21,103 (2.2%)	25,195 (3.4%)
	90–99	4003 (0.4%)	3514 (0.5%)
	Over 100	512 (0.1%)	629 (0.1%)

Table 1. *Cont.*

		Gangnam	Gangbuk
Sex	Male	462,687 (47.8%)	363,935 (48.5%)
	Female	504,698 (52.2%)	387,015 (51.5%)
Household income		$3835	$2915

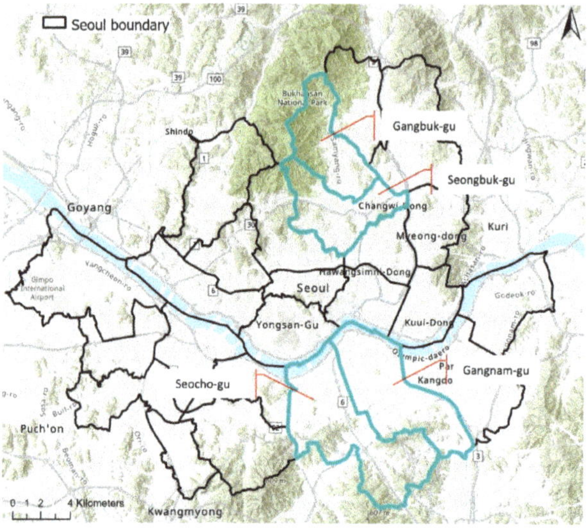

Figure 1. Gangnam (Gangnam-gu and Seocho-gu) and Gangbuk (Gangbuk-gu and Seongbuk-gu) districts.

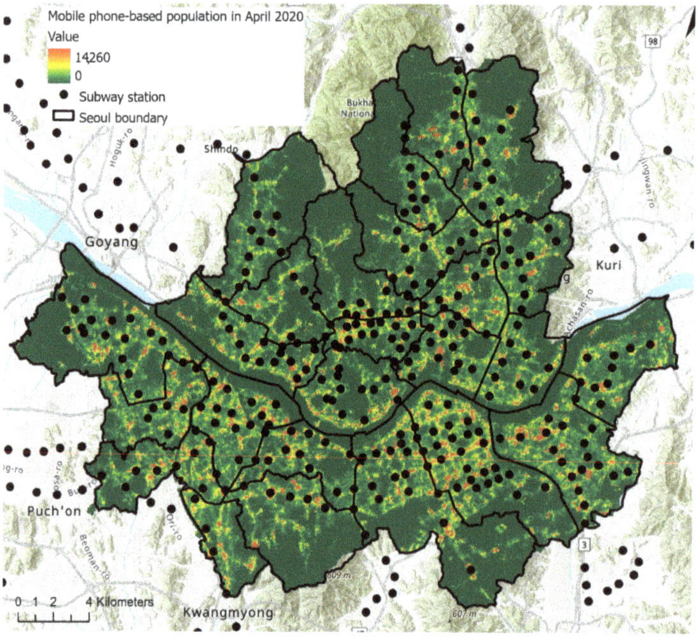

Figure 2. Distribution of the mobile phone-based population of Seoul in April 2020 and the locations of subway stations.

Gangnam is a major business area in Seoul, where a large number of startups and various information technology (IT) companies are located. It is also a hot spot to which many travelers visit, due to its great public transportation, as well as an area with a large daytime and nighttime population. Within this area, Gangnam-gu is recognized as South Korea's largest affluent village with the highest housing prices and the highest average standard of living. In addition, the financial and service industries have been well developed, and there are many high-rise office buildings. Although Gangbuk-gu includes a relatively low population density, Bukhansan National Park occupies a large portion of the area. In Seongbuk-gu, there is a combination of old 20th-century landscapes and modern high-tech urban landscapes, with many cultural assets and attractions.

This study used two types of datasets: mobile phone and LULC data. The mobile phone data was provided by SK Telecom, one of the largest mobile operators in South Korea. In fact, the total number of SK Telecom users accounts for 44.4% of the population in South Korea [8]. According to a report by Pew Research Center, South Korea had 100% mobile phone ownership and the highest smartphone penetration rate of 95% [34]. The data included the time-weighted monthly average number of mobile phone users in Seoul, which was estimated according to the aggregated locations of the mobile phones as well as other attributes such as gender, age, weekdays/weekend days, and time (see Table 2). Specifically, the averages were calculated by using the monthly average number of people positioned within a 50 m grid and the time that they remained there [8]. For instance, if two people stayed in a specific grid cell for a total of 72 h (3 days) within a 30-day month, then the monthly average value for the cell for that month is two people * 3 days/30 days, or 0.2. Figure 1 presents the mobile phone-based population in April 2020. It should be noted that this study focused on the data in April and August 2019 (before the pandemic) and April and August 2020 (during the pandemic) to determine any differences immediately right after the COVID-19 outbreak (April) and during the following summer (August). Specifically, we can see where people spent their time in the summer break or vacation in August during the COVID-19 pandemic compared to April.

Table 2. Description of the mobile phone dataset.

Attribute	Description	Example
X_COORD	Longitude	126.9780
Y_COORD	Latitude	37.5665
GNDR_CD	Gender code (1 or 2)	1
AGE_GR_SCTN_CD	Age group (0–4, 5–9, 10–14, 15–19, 20–24, . . ., 95–99)	2024
WKDY_CD	Weekday/weekend day code (1, 2, 3, 4, 5, 6, 7)	1
TMST_CD	Time slot code (0, 1, 2, . . ., 23)	7
FLOW_POP_CNT	Time-weighted monthly average of mobile phone-based population	0.01

This study used LULC data (released every five years) by the Ministry of Environment in South Korea (see Figure 3). Specifically, we used LULC data from 2020, which initially included 11 LULC types. However, in this study, the LULC types with low percentages (<5%) were merged with similar LULC types with higher percentages, resulting in a total of seven categories. Specifically, Gangnam had higher percentages of industrial and public facilities (10.2%), transportation facilities (10.9%), commercial and business areas (8.1%), mixed residential and business areas (10.3%), and river and lake areas (7.4%), compared to Gangbuk. However, Gangbuk had higher percentages of forest and open spaces (45.0%) and residential areas (29.1%) compared to Gangnam (see Table 3). When we downloaded the LULC data, we selected more grids and a larger coverage than Seoul to avoid the edge effect that might exist near the boundaries of Gangnam and Gangbuk.

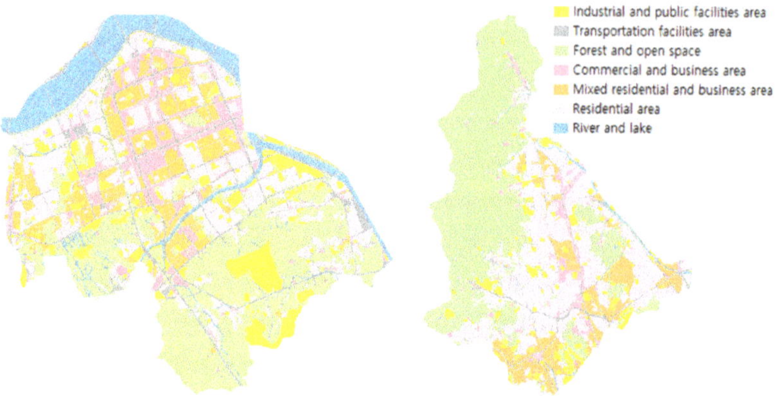

(a) Gangnam (b) Gangbuk

Figure 3. LULC in Gangnam and Gangbuk in 2020.

Table 3. Types of LULC and percentages in Gangnam and Gangbuk.

LULC Types	Percentage in Gangnam (%)	Percentage in Gangbuk (%)
Industrial and public facilities area	10.2	5.7
Transportation facilities area	10.9	6.1
Forest and open space	33.2	45.0
Commercial and business area	8.1	4.0
Mixed residential and business area	10.3	9.5
Residential area	19.9	29.1
River and lake	7.4	0.6

2.2. Data Analysis

Hot spots can be used to identify the areas with a significantly increased mobile phone-based population, especially during the COVID-19 pandemic. After subtracting the 2019 population from the 2020 population, only the top 0.5% (z-score: 2.58) of the hot spots were used to identify the differences in LULC types between Gangnam and Gangbuk. Focusing on the top 0.5% of hot spots for the LULC analysis can help identify emerging trends or patterns regarding the use of urban opportunities during the pandemic that may not be apparent when examining larger areas. It can help explore more extreme patterns in the use of urban opportunities that emerged during COVID-19, which better contrast with pre-pandemic trends. Additionally, it highlights areas with the greatest impact, potentially revealing critical insights about the concentration of activity, mobility patterns, and exposure to the pandemic. The Getis-Ord G_i^* statistic [35,36] was also used to identify the increase in the mobile phone-based population in 2020, compared to 2019. The equation of the G_i^* statistic is as follows:

$$G_i^* = \frac{\sum_{j=1}^{n} w_{ij}x_j - \overline{X}\sum_{j=1}^{n} w_{ij}}{S\sqrt{\frac{\left[n\sum_{j=1}^{n} w_{ij}^2 - \left(\sum_{j=1}^{n} w_{ij}\right)^2\right]}{n-1}}} \quad (1)$$

$$\overline{X} = \frac{\sum_{j=1}^{n} x_j}{n} \quad (2)$$

$$S = \sqrt{\frac{\sum_{j=1}^{n} x_j^2}{n} - \left(\overline{X}\right)^2} \quad (3)$$

where G_i^* is the statistic that describes the spatial dependency of location i over all n locations, w_{ij} is the symmetric spatial weight between locations i and j, and x_j is the value of the variable x of location j. The spatial weight was calculated based on the first order Queen's contiguity method to define adjacent neighbors because Queen's contiguity provides a more inclusive understanding of spatial relationships regarding hot spots, which considers all adjacent cells, including diagonally touching ones. In the Queen's contiguity, the spatial weight is set to 1 if the location pair shares either a common edge or a vertex and 0 otherwise. In this study, each location indicates a grid cell in Seoul, while the variable is the time-weighted monthly average mobile phone-based population and is the subtraction of the 2019 population from the 2020 population. Hot spots are calculated over the entire Seoul area; however, we focus only on Gangnam and Gangbuk.

The differences in the percentages of LULC types in hot spots were also statistically analyzed. Welch's t-test was used in this study since it was assumed that the variances in the percentages of LULC types in the hot spots between Gangnam and Gangbuk were not equal because there were LULC types with unequal variances found by using Levene's test ($p < 0.05$). As for Welch's t-test, it is a two-sample t-test that can determine the mean of the percentage of each LULC type in hot spots. The equation for Welch's t-test is as follows:

$$t = \frac{\overline{x}_1 - \overline{x}_2}{\sqrt{\frac{s_1^2}{n_1} + \frac{s_2^2}{n_2}}} \quad (4)$$

where x is the mean of the percentage of each LULC type in hot spots, s is the standard deviation, and n is the group size of hot spots. Mobile phone-based populations of different ages, including children (0–14), youths (15–24), adults (25–59), and seniors (60–99), were also considered to identify the hot spots of different population groups. We used R (v.4.2.2, R Foundation for Statistical Computing, Vienna, Austria) programming language for all the analyses.

3. Results

3.1. The Differences Between Gangnam and Gangbuk Based on the Percentages of LULC Types in Hot Spots for Children and Youths

In this study, the differences between Gangnam and Gangbuk according to LULC types in hot spots of the mobile phone-based population during the COVID-19 were statistically analyzed by using Welch's t-test and considering different age groups. Table 3 presents the statistically significant differences ($p < 0.05$). Additionally, a positive t-value indicates a larger percentage of a particular LULC type in Gangnam, whereas a negative t-value represents a larger percentage in Gangbuk.

In Table 4, the differences between hot spots in Gangnam and Gangbuk in April can be seen in the percentages of forest and open spaces ($t = 3.717$, $p < 0.001$), mixed residential and business areas ($t = 6.289$, $p < 0.001$), and residential areas ($t = -5.738$, $p < 0.001$) used by the children. Overall, many children in Gangnam spent a significant amount of time in forest and open spaces and mixed residential and business areas, while those in Gangbuk mainly stayed in residential areas. In particular, mixed residential and business areas had the highest t-value ($t = 6.289$, $p < 0.001$), whereas residential areas had the lowest ($t = -5.738$, $p < 0.001$). Regarding youths, many in Gangnam stayed in mixed residential and business areas ($t = 3.953$, $p < 0.001$), whereas those in Gangbuk spent much time in commercial and business areas ($t = -2.871$, $p = 0.006$).

In Table 5, in August, the differences between the hot spots in Gangnam and Gangbuk can be seen in the percentages of industrial and public facilities areas ($t = 3.671$, $p < 0.001$), forest and open spaces ($t = 5.162$, $p < 0.001$), mixed residential and business areas ($t = 5.426$, $p < 0.001$), and residential areas ($t = -3.850$, $p < 0.001$) used by the children. Overall, many children in Gangnam spent much time in industrial and public facilities areas, forest and open spaces, and mixed residential and business areas, while those in Gangbuk mainly stayed in residential areas. In particular, forest and open spaces and mixed residential and business areas in Gangnam had the highest t-values. Among the youths, industrial and public facilities areas (t = 5.015, $p < 0.001$), forest and open spaces (t = 3.084, p = 0.002), and mixed residential and business areas (t = 7.990, $p < 0.001$) had higher percentages in Gangnam than in Gangbuk, whereas residential areas (t = −2.481, p = 0.019) had a higher percentage in Gangbuk. Mixed residential and business areas had the highest t-value. Meanwhile, there were no hot spots in industrial and public facilities areas, forest and open spaces, and mixed residential and business areas in Gangbuk. Figures 4 and 5 show the hot spots of the increased population of children and youths in Gangbuk and Gangnam in April and August during COVID-19.

Table 4. Statistically significant differences in the percentages of LULC types in hot spots among the children and youths in April.

Category	LULC	t	p-Value	Percentages in Gangnam Hot Spots	Percentages in Gangbuk Hot Spots
Children	Industrial and public facilities area	0.291	0.771	8.51 ± 24.52	8.02 ± 23.22
	Transportation facilities area	1.530	0.126	11.91 ± 20.40	9.90 ± 16.45
	Forest and open space	**3.717**	**<0.001**	3.22 ± 15.45	0.28 ± 3.32
	Commercial and business area	−0.826	0.409	11.28 ± 27.49	12.95 ± 29.47
	Mixed residential and business area	**6.289**	**<0.001**	21.33 ± 37.08	7.39 ± 23.99
	Residential area	**−5.738**	**<0.001**	43.73 ± 45.43	61.47 ± 41.47
	River and lake	1.000	0.318	0.02 ± 0.40	0.00 ± 0.00
Youths	Industrial and public facilities area	0.842	0.402	6.08 ± 22.67	3.32 ± 13.51
	Transportation facilities area	−1.024	0.310	14.96 ± 23.62	19.78 ± 23.52
	Forest and open space	1.000	0.320	0.04 ± 0.34	0.00 ± 0.00
	Commercial and business area	**−2.871**	**0.006**	16.42 ± 30.71	37.72 ± 39.17
	Mixed residential and business area	**3.953**	**<0.001**	23.63 ± 37.82	4.36 ± 17.20
	Residential area	0.496	0.622	38.88 ± 43.69	34.83 ± 39.81
	River and lake	NA	NA	0.00 ± 0.00	0.00 ± 0.00

Bold font: statistically significant.

Table 5. Statistically significant differences in the percentages of LULC types in hot spots among the children and youths in August.

Category	LULC	t	p-Value	Percentages in Gangnam Hot Spots	Percentages in Gangbuk Hot Spots
Children	Industrial and public facilities area	**3.671**	**<0.001**	10.12 ± 26.71	3.45 ± 16.63
	Transportation facilities area	0.061	0.952	13.89 ± 22.09	13.77 ± 20.23
	Forest and open space	**5.162**	**<0.001**	3.22 ± 15.25	0.25 ± 1.95
	Commercial and business area	−1.971	0.051	15.57 ± 31.21	22.29 ± 34.70
	Mixed residential and business area	**5.426**	**<0.001**	21.49 ± 37.25	7.57 ± 23.61
	Residential area	**−3.850**	**<0.001**	35.70 ± 43.69	52.67 ± 44.40
	River and lake	1.432	0.153	0.02 ± 0.47	0.00 ± 0.00
Youths	Industrial and public facilities area	**5.015**	**<0.001**	9.98 ± 26.25	0.00 ± 0.00
	Transportation facilities area	0.500	0.620	21.26 ± 27.19	18.76 ± 23.65
	Forest and open space	**3.084**	**0.002**	3.83 ± 16.39	0.00 ± 0.00
	Commercial and business area	−2.029	0.051	20.31 ± 33.69	36.37 ± 38.91
	Mixed residential and business area	**7.990**	**<0.001**	22.04 ± 36.39	0.00 ± 0.00
	Residential area	**−2.481**	**0.019**	22.58 ± 38.07	44.87 ± 44.23
	River and lake	1.000	0.319	0.00 ± 0.03	0.00 ± 0.00

Bold font: statistically significant.

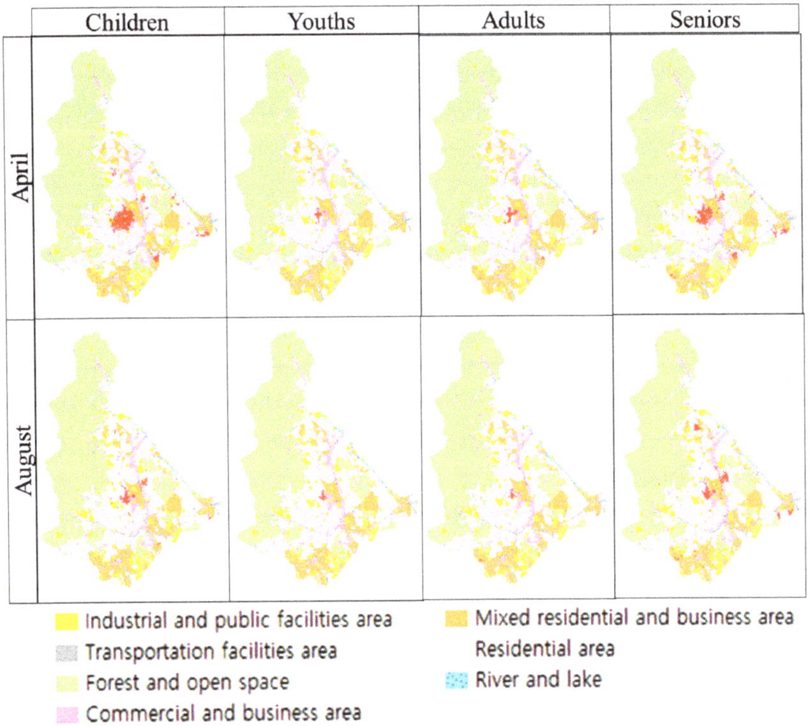

Figure 4. Hot spots (red) of the increased population of all age groups in Gangbuk in April and August during COVID-19.

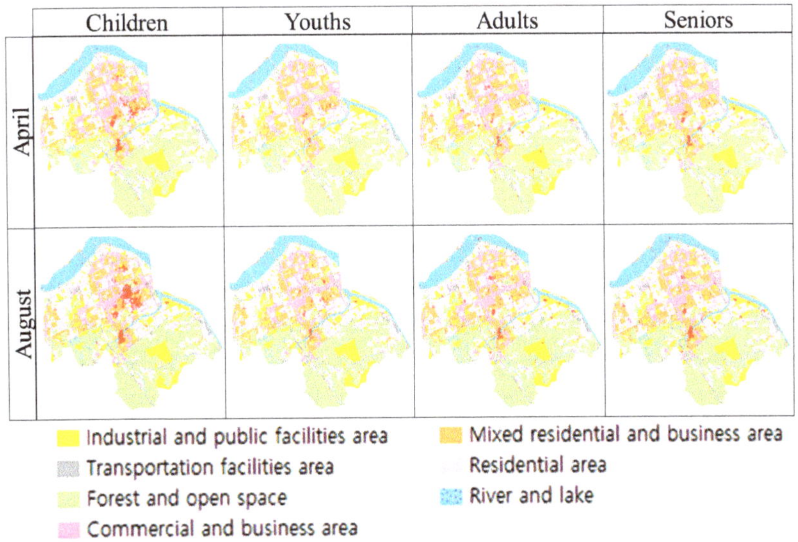

Figure 5. Hot spots (red) of the increased population of all age groups in Gangnam in April and August during COVID-19.

3.2. The Differences Between Gangnam and Gangbuk Based on the Percentages of LULC Types in Hot Spots for Adults and Seniors

In Table 6, the differences between the hot spots in Gangnam and Gangbuk can be seen in the percentages of forest and open spaces ($t = 4.040$, $p < 0.001$), commercial and business areas ($t = -2.101$, $p = 0.038$), and mixed residential and business areas ($t = 2.102$, $p = 0.037$) used by the adults. Overall, many adults in Gangnam spent much time in forest and open spaces and mixed residential and business areas, while there were no hot spots in forest and open spaces in Gangbuk, since many adults mostly stayed in commercial and business areas. Regarding the seniors in Gangnam, they stayed in transportation facilities areas ($t = 2.513$, $p = 0.012$), forest and open spaces ($t = 3.144$, $p = 0.002$), and mixed residential and business areas ($t = 2.243$, $p = 0.025$), whereas those in Gangbuk spent much time in residential areas ($t = -4.180$, $p < 0.001$). Figures 4 and 5 show the hot spots of the children, youths, adults, and seniors in Gangbuk and Gangnam in April, respectively, which were used to identify the differences in LULC. In both Gangbuk and Gangnam, most of the hot spots were located on tall apartment buildings due to the lockdown during COVID-19 in April. Gangbuk showed a few hot spot areas where the tall apartment buildings are located, whereas the hot spots in Gangnam were dispersed because apartment areas are located all over Gangnam.

Table 6. Statistically significant differences in the percentages of LULC types in hot spots among the adults and seniors in April.

Category	LULC	*t*	*p*-Value	Percentages in Gangnam Hot Spots	Percentages in Gangbuk Hot Spots
Adults	Industrial and public facilities area	0.921	0.358	10.83 ± 27.86	7.88 ± 22.31
	Transportation facilities area	0.504	0.615	20.56 ± 27.28	18.95 ± 22.35
	Forest and open space	**4.040**	**<0.001**	4.94 ± 18.08	0.00 ± 0.00
	Commercial and business area	**−2.101**	**0.038**	22.52 ± 35.71	33.18 ± 38.40
	Mixed residential and business area	**2.102**	**0.037**	18.78 ± 35.89	10.53 ± 26.57
	Residential area	−1.391	0.167	22.37 ± 37.61	29.46 ± 38.00
	River and lake	1.000	0.318	0.00 ± 0.02	0.00 ± 0.00
Seniors	Industrial and public facilities area	1.479	0.140	9.95 ± 25.98	6.77 ± 21.15
	Transportation facilities area	**2.513**	**0.012**	16.34 ± 23.33	11.602 ± 17.62
	Forest and open space	**3.144**	**0.002**	4.27 ± 16.09	0.69 ± 6.54
	Commercial and business area	−0.611	0.542	15.31 ± 30.69	17.06 ± 32.80
	Mixed residential and business area	**2.243**	**0.025**	17.80 ± 34.56	11.27 ± 29.34
	Residential area	**−4.180**	**<0.001**	36.30 ± 43.63	52.58 ± 42.70
	River and lake	−0.104	0.917	0.04 ± 0.53	0.04 ± 0.47

Bold font: statistically significant.

In August, among the adults, industrial and public facilities areas ($t = 6.450$, $p < 0.001$) and forest and open spaces ($t = 5.401$, $p < 0.001$) had higher percentages in Gangnam than in Gangbuk, whereas commercial and business areas ($t = -2.105$, $p = 0.042$) had a higher percentage in Gangbuk. Industrial and public facilities areas also had the highest t-value, indicating that this type of LULC in Gangnam and Gangbuk had the largest difference among the adults in August (see Table 7). There were also no hot spots in industrial and public facilities areas and forest and open spaces. As for the seniors, many stayed in industrial and public facilities areas ($t = 4.171$, $p < 0.001$), transportation facilities areas ($t = 3.006$, $p = 0.003$), forest and open spaces ($t = 2.905$, $p = 0.004$), and mixed residential and business areas ($t = 3.435$, $p = 0.001$) in Gangnam, whereas those in Gangbuk spent much time in residential areas ($t = -7.361$, $p < 0.001$), indicating the lowest t-value.

Table 7. Statistically significant differences in the percentages of LULC types in hot spots among the children and youths in August.

Category	LULC	t	p-Value	Percentages in Gangnam Hot Spots	Percentages in Gangbuk Hot Spots
Adults	Industrial and public facilities area	**6.450**	**<0.001**	8.85 ± 24.84	0.00 ± 0.00
	Transportation facilities area	1.012	0.317	21.89 ± 28.07	17.52 ± 23.20
	Forest and open space	**5.401**	**<0.001**	5.87 ± 19.70	0.00 ± 0.00
	Commercial and business area	**−2.105**	**0.042**	21.72 ± 34.53	36.61 ± 39.14
	Mixed residential and business area	0.896	0.376	19.12 ± 34.76	13.90 ± 31.63
	Residential area	−1.329	0.192	22.24 ± 38.23	31.98 ± 40.29
	River and lake	1.290	0.198	0.31 ± 4.34	0.00 ± 0.00
Seniors	Industrial and public facilities area	**4.171**	**<0.001**	7.97 ± 23.11	1.62 ± 10.41
	Transportation facilities area	**3.006**	**0.003**	20.17 ± 25.96	14.03 ± 19.46
	Forest and open space	**2.905**	**0.004**	5.66 ± 19.68	1.76 ± 10.12
	Commercial and business area	0.697	0.486	21.02 ± 34.32	18.86 ± 33.05
	Mixed residential and business area	**3.435**	**0.001**	22.31 ± 36.95	12.26 ± 27.99
	Residential area	**−7.361**	**<0.001**	22.84 ± 38.60	51.28 ± 43.92
	River and lake	−0.919	0.359	0.03 ± 0.60	0.19 ± 2.26

Bold font: statistically significant.

Figure S1 in the supplementary material shows the changes in the t-values among the different age groups in April and August. The t-values for all of the age groups were mostly positive in industrial and public facilities, transportation facilities areas, forest and open spaces, and mixed residential and business areas, while those were mostly negative in commercial and business areas and residential areas. The most noticeable change between April and August was that the t-values in the industrial and public facilities areas increased in August, compared to April.

4. Discussion

This study evaluated the disparities in urban opportunities between socioeconomically different neighborhoods, while considering the differences in age groups. Based on the findings, there were clear disparities in the usage of green spaces between the high- and low-income communities. The results also indicated that, in both April and August, forest and open spaces accounted for a higher percentage in the hot spots of the children, youths, adults, and seniors in Gangnam than in Gangbuk. In other words, more people spent time in green and open spaces in Gangnam, while there was no hot spot of the mobile phone-based population in forest and open spaces in Gangbuk during April and August. This means that more green spaces that people prefer for relaxing or those that have better access were located in Gangnam during the COVID-19 pandemic, even though the percentage of forest and open spaces was higher in Gangbuk (see Table 2). In particular, since Gangnam includes more offices and a better transportation network than Gangbuk, many people working in or visiting Gangnam might have utilized a nearby green space. According to previous studies, low-income people have less access to green space [37], and individuals with low incomes are less likely to secure stable employment, a situation that may have worsened due to COVID-19, resulting in reduced leisure time for them [38]. In addition, one study also found out that people in low-income communities have difficulties accessing green spaces due to the lack of transportation, whereas those in high-income communities have much easier access [39]. Inequalities in access to green spaces have been a major concern in many countries [40–43]. In related research, during the COVID-19 pandemic, green spaces have played a critical role in preventing mental health problems caused by social distancing and lockdowns [2]. This may worsen the health disparities in low-and high-income communities. In this regard, any disproportionate access to green spaces between low- and high-income neighborhoods during the pandemic must be taken seriously.

Socioeconomic disparities were also identified in industrial and public facilities areas. There is a very small percentage of industrial areas in Gangnam and Gangbuk, and the hot spots were over public facilities, including schools and recreational facilities. In all of the age groups, the population hot spots only had a higher percentage in such facilities in Gangnam during August. In particular, adults had the highest t-value ($t = 6.450$, $p < 0.001$). We also found that there were some hot spots in elementary, middle, and high schools in Gangnam, which were more than those in Gangbuk (not present). Moreover, it was revealed that not only the children or youths, but also the adults and seniors, visited schools for purposes other than education. This finding is contrary to the previous study that the COVID-19 pandemic was associated with a 46% and 62% decrease in the number of female and male children at school playgrounds outside of school hours in the U.S. [44]. In addition, children spent 27 min less in playgrounds than they used to before the pandemic in Turkey [45]. Nevertheless, the play and learning value of school playgrounds became important during COVID-19, and adaptive playground design was studied to promote the general wellbeing of students and outside learning space [46].

In South Korea, people mostly used public sports facilities to engage in physical activities, and among the facilities, playgrounds were used the most (57.4%) during the COVID-19 pandemic [47]. This was different from the finding in the U.S. that the popular locations for physical activity in emerging adults during the pandemic period were on roads/sidewalks (87.5% of survey participants) and at/around the home (85.7% of survey participants) [48]. For comparison, the percentage of the use of playgrounds was 47.0% in 2019 before the pandemic [49], but it increased by more than 10% after the COVID-19 outbreak. In this regard, there is a possibility that many people enjoyed physical activities in playgrounds near schools during the pandemic. Meanwhile, the pandemic decreased recreational walking outdoors in the communities with a low socioeconomic status, whereas it increased in the communities with a high socioeconomic status [50]. This indicates that the percentage of industrial and public facilities areas was higher in Gangnam. However, this pattern was only found in August, since playgrounds were open to residents during the summer break. For policy implications, policymakers should promote physical activities, such as educational and social events, in deprived neighborhoods, and provide better accessibility to locations where people in disadvantaged communities can engage in such activities.

One of the interesting findings in this study was the higher percentage of commercial and business areas in Gangbuk in April for the youths and in August for the adults. This result may be related to increased sales of businesses in some areas of Gangbuk and the significant decrease in sales in some areas of Gangnam [51]. According to its press release, there was the largest decrease in sales in the apparel industry and department stores in Gangnam. However, this is contrary to the finding that older adult workers became loyal customers who significantly contributed to the high sales of nearby commercial and business areas during the COVID-19 pandemic [50]. Hence, how the youths and adults were able to contribute to the increased sales in Gangbuk and what specific sectors they contributed to remain unclear.

In April and August, the hot spots of the children and seniors had a higher percentage of mixed residential and business areas in Gangnam, whereas in Gangbuk, the children and seniors had a higher percentage of residential areas. Since these age groups do not typically work in offices, this pattern suggests that many children and seniors in Gangnam and Gangbuk remained at home due to the social distancing and lockdowns. Due to the lockdown, children stayed at home, and parent–child activities at home became important during COVID-19 [52]. Further, older adults were vulnerable to COVID-19, and one of the protective mechanisms was an isolation at home, which led to unforeseen physical, mental, emotional, social, and financial repercussions [53]. Additionally, since Gangnam includes more offices and buildings for residential and commercial purposes than Gangbuk, the mixed residential and business areas showed a higher percentage. Conversely, since Gangbuk has fewer offices and buildings for residential and commercial purposes, a significant difference was shown in residential areas. In August, the only age group that did not have a higher percentage of mixed residential and business areas in Gangnam was the adults, indicating that many still went to work in person and did not remain at home for remote work. Although this is in line with the low percentage of remote work in South Korea before the COVID-19 pandemic, continuous policy efforts have been made to improve the inflexible employment culture. In fact, the utilization of remote work in South Korea was much lower (4.5%) than other countries (U.S.: 43%; France: 29%; England, 27%; and Japan: 13%) before the pandemic [54], and it was most likely to remain low after the outbreak of COVID-19. However, the situation did not improve during the pandemic because the proportion of remote workers (which was less than 0.5% until 2019) only increased to 2.5% in 2020 [55]. Moreover, the percentage of jobs that allowed remote work was relatively low in the manufacturing, wholesale, and retail industries [56]. However, more data are necessary to support the finding that the percentage of remote work was relatively low in South Korea during the pandemic.

The concept of a 15 min city, where all essential services are accessible within a 15 min walk or bike ride, gained new relevance during COVID-19 [57]. The pandemic highlighted the importance of local accessibility and the need for safe and nearby options for working, shopping, and recreation. As people attempted to minimize travel and maintain social distancing, the idea of living in a community where amenities are close at hand became increasingly appealing. Additionally, the focus on public health and outdoor spaces emphasized the value of walkable neighborhoods in supporting both physical and mental wellbeing during lockdowns and beyond [58]. Particularly, researchers revealed disadvantaged neighborhoods for 15 min green and blue space accessibility in Hong Kong [59]. In Italy, regarding the 15 min city concept, researchers found disparities in access to services of general interest including the areas for housing, water and energy supply, public transport, health, and culture [60].

At this point, several limitations in this study should be noted. First, this study focused only on two months (April and August) due to budget constraints for data purchase. However, we believe that the two months that we selected can be representative because in Korea, April is a month with no special holidays and is representative of a month focused on work, while August is representative of a month when people take the most vacations away from work. In addition, we have observed that several previous studies focusing on COVID-19 used short-term data given the time-sensitive nature of the pandemic-related topic, and produced sound and meaningful results [61–64]. For example, among those studies, Mustafa et al. (2023) conducted analyses of the accessibility and perceptions of urban green space based on survey data from 13 May to 15 June 2020, and the authors found that the size of urban green space had a significant effect on its visitation and usage during the pandemic [61]. However, future research could utilize data from other months during the COVID-19 pandemic when more funds are available to identify the consistency in findings. Moreover, while the data from these two months were sufficient for our analysis, examining longer-term data in the future could help reveal seasonal changes in hot spots and identify disparities in urban opportunities that may occur during specific seasons. Second, while this study focused on the usage of urban opportunities, including green space, future research can evaluate not only the usage but also the accessibility to those amenities by considering transportation options and travel distance from populations (e.g., grid cells or centroids of an administrative unit). This may help further highlight socioeconomic disparities in the quality of urban life. Third, an edge effect could have influenced the results. Because the LULC data this study had access to were made only for Seoul, we could not obtain the data for surrounding areas and thus could not consider the potential influences of LULC near the boundaries of the two districts. Fourth, as the mobile phone data did not provide the exact number of people tracked, we could not explain whether the hot spots indicated people spending more time and/or more people crowded there. We interpreted the patterns in both ways; however, it needs to be clearer with the increased number of people and time usage for future research. Fifth, the SK Telecom mobile phone data do not include sociodemographic information about its users, which makes it challenging to identify data representativeness. However, we believe that SK Telecom mobile phone users are reasonably representative of the general population in

South Korea as 44.4% of the population in South Korea uses SK Telecom, which is one of the two major mobile carriers in South Korea, alongside KT Corporation. It is generally considered that the two mobile carriers offer similar quality of service and pricing. Lastly, since this study only explored urban settings in South Korea, people's modified behaviors in other settings during the pandemic might have differed from the findings of this study. More studies are needed to explore the impact of the pandemic in other settings.

5. Conclusions

This study investigated the changes in the use of urban spaces in Seoul, South Korea, before and during the COVID-19 pandemic, by using mobile phone and LULC data. It also identified how socioeconomic status influenced the changes by comparing two contrasting areas (i.e., Gangnam and Gangbuk) in Seoul in terms of income and the amount of taxes. Additionally, this study contributed to advancing the understanding of the impact of COVID-19 on human behaviors and inequalities in urban opportunities by using geographical methods and mobile phone data.

Overall, this study revealed that disparities in green space usage between high- and low-income communities became greater during the COVID-19 pandemic for all age groups. In particular, there were significant differences in the forest and open spaces among the adults in April and August, with no hot spots of increased population in Gangbuk. There were also socioeconomic disparities in the industrial and public facilities areas in all age groups. For example, people in Gangnam were more likely to visit schools (as an industrial and public facility) and enjoy physical activities, whereas there were no hot spots in industrial and public facilities among the youths and adults in Gangbuk.

The findings of this study shed new light on how the COVID-19 pandemic has exacerbated the socioeconomic disparities in the usage of and variety of urban opportunities between communities with different income levels. This study also proposes the provision of preferable green spaces with better transportation networks in order to relieve the inequalities in usage of green spaces between high- and low-income communities. Moreover, policies that promote health in low-income communities should be developed, which should differ from those in high-income communities. Specifically, future policies should not solely focus on the equal provision of playgrounds to promote physical activities in low-income communities, but they should be more about education and awareness regarding the benefits of physical activities. Furthermore, finding accessible locations in which people in low-income communities can visit for physical activities should be another policy goal.

Supplementary Materials: The following supporting information can be downloaded at: https://www.mdpi.com/article/10.3390/ijgi13120421/s1, Figure S1: The t-values of the different LULC types among the children, youths, adults, and seniors.

Author Contributions: Conceptualization, Kangjae Lee; methodology, Kangjae Lee, Yoo Min Park, Yoohyung Joo, Minsoo Joo and Joon Heo; software, Kangjae Lee and Minsoo Joo; validation, Kangjae Lee; formal analysis, Kangjae Lee and Minsoo Joo; investigation, Kangjae Lee; resources, Kangjae Lee; data curation, Kangjae Lee and Minsoo Joo; writing—original draft preparation, Kangjae Lee; writing—review & editing, Kangjae Lee, Yoo Min Park, Yoohyung Joo, Minsoo Joo and Joon Heo; visualization, Kangjae Lee; supervision, Joon Heo; project administration, Joon Heo; funding acquisition, Joon Heo. All authors have read and agreed to the published version of the manuscript.

Funding: This work was supported by the National Research Foundation of Korea (NRF) grant funded by the Korean government (MSIT) (No. 2021R1A2C2009636).

Data Availability Statement: This can be provided upon request.

Conflicts of Interest: The authors declare no conflicts of interest.

References

1. Venter, Z.S.; Barton, D.N.; Gundersen, V.; Figari, H.; Nowell, M. Urban Nature in a Time of Crisis: Recreational Use of Green Space Increases during the COVID-19 Outbreak in Oslo, Norway. *Environ. Res. Lett.* **2020**, *15*, 104075. [CrossRef]
2. Slater, S.J.; Christiana, R.W.; Gustat, J. Recommendations for Keeping Parks and Green Space Accessible for Mental and Physical Health During COVID-19 and Other Pandemics. *Prev. Chronic Dis.* **2020**, *17*, 200204. [CrossRef] [PubMed]
3. Centers for Disease Control and Prevention. Visiting Parks and Recreational Facilities. Available online: https://stacks.cdc.gov/view/cdc/88255/cdc_88255_DS1.pdf (accessed on 22 May 2024).
4. Volenec, Z.M.; Abraham, J.O.; Becker, A.D.; Dobson, A.P. Public Parks and the Pandemic: How Park Usage Has Been Affected by COVID-19 Policies. *PLoS ONE* **2021**, *16*, e0251799. [CrossRef] [PubMed]
5. Deville, P.; Linard, C.; Martin, S.; Gilbert, M.; Stevens, F.R.; Gaughan, A.E.; Blondel, V.D.; Tatem, A.J. Dynamic Population Mapping Using Mobile Phone Data. *Proc. Natl. Acad. Sci. USA* **2014**, *111*, 15888–15893. [CrossRef]
6. Grantz, K.H.; Meredith, H.R.; Cummings, D.A.T.; Metcalf, C.J.E.; Grenfell, B.T.; Giles, J.R.; Mehta, S.; Solomon, S.; Labrique, A.; Kishore, N.; et al. The Use of Mobile Phone Data to Inform Analysis of COVID-19 Pandemic Epidemiology. *Nat. Commun.* **2020**, *11*, 4961. [CrossRef]
7. Wesolowski, A.; Buckee, C.O.; Engø-Monsen, K.; Metcalf, C.J.E. Connecting Mobility to Infectious Diseases: The Promise and Limits of Mobile Phone Data. *J. Infect. Dis.* **2016**, *214*, S414–S420. [CrossRef]
8. Yun, S.B.; Kim, S.; Ju, S.; Noh, J.; Kim, C.; Wong, M.S.; Heo, J. Analysis of Accessibility to Emergency Rooms by Dynamic Population from Mobile Phone Data: Geography of Social Inequity in South Korea. *PLoS ONE* **2020**, *15*, e0231079. [CrossRef]
9. Lim, H.; Kim, S.; Heo, J. Graph Analyses of Phone-Based Origin-Destination Data for Understanding Urban Human Mobility in Seoul, Korea. In Proceedings of the 3rd ACM SIGSPATIAL International Workshop on Prediction of Human Mobility, Chicago, IL, USA, 5 November 2019; pp. 62–65.
10. Lee, W.K.; Sohn, S.Y.; Heo, J. Utilizing Mobile Phone-Based Floating Population Data to Measure the Spatial Accessibility to Public Transit. *Appl. Geogr.* **2018**, *92*, 123–130. [CrossRef]
11. Ma, J.W.; Ju, S.; Nguyen, H.M.; Yun, S.B.; Yoon, S.; Heo, J. Spatio-Temporal Factor Analysis of Characterizing Mass Protest Events Using Taxi Trajectory in Seoul, Korea. In Proceedings of the 1st ACM SIGSPATIAL Workshop on Analytics for Local Events and News, Redondo Beach, CA, USA, 7 November 2017; pp. 1–7.
12. Yun, S.B.; Hieu, N.M.; Park, S.Y.; Lim, H.; Heo, J. Implementation of Floating Population Analysis for Smart Cities: A Case Study in Songdo Incheon South Korea. In Proceedings of the 2nd ACM SIGSPATIAL Workshop on Prediction of Human Mobility, Seattle, WA, USA, 6 November 2018; pp. 32–36.
13. Hara, Y.; Yamaguchi, H. Japanese Travel Behavior Trends and Change under COVID-19 State-of-Emergency Declaration: Nationwide Observation by Mobile Phone Location Data. *Transp. Res. Interdiscip. Perspect.* **2021**, *9*, 100288. [CrossRef]
14. Wang, J.; Kwan, M.-P.; Liu, D.; Peng, X. Assessing the Spatial Distribution of and Inequality in 15-Minute PCR Test Site Accessibility in Beijing and Guangzhou, China. *Appl. Geogr.* **2023**, *154*, 102925. [CrossRef]
15. Lu, X.; Tan, J.; Cao, Z.; Xiong, Y.; Qin, S.; Wang, T.; Liu, C.; Huang, S.; Zhang, W.; Marczak, L.B.; et al. Mobile Phone-Based Population Flow Data for the COVID-19 Outbreak in Mainland China. *Health Data Sci.* **2021**, *2021*, 9796431. [CrossRef] [PubMed]
16. Song, Y.; Chen, B.; Ho, H.C.; Kwan, M.-P.; Liu, D.; Wang, F.; Wang, J.; Cai, J.; Li, X.; Xu, Y.; et al. Observed Inequality in Urban Greenspace Exposure in China. *Environ. Int.* **2021**, *156*, 106778. [CrossRef] [PubMed]
17. Heo, S.; Lim, C.C.; Bell, M.L. Relationships between Local Green Space and Human Mobility Patterns during COVID-19 for Maryland and California, USA. *Sustainability* **2020**, *12*, 9401. [CrossRef]
18. Zhai, W.; Yue, H.; Deng, Y. Examining the Association between Social Characteristics of Urban Green Space Visitors and the Early Outbreak of COVID-19. *Appl. Geogr.* **2022**, *147*, 102768. [CrossRef]
19. de Freitas, R.S.G.; Stedefeldt, E. COVID-19 Pandemic Underlines the Need to Build Resilience in Commercial Restaurants' Food Safety. *Food Res. Int.* **2020**, *136*, 109472. [CrossRef]
20. Saragih, J.F.B.; Subroto, T.Y.W. Child-Friendly School: Female Students' Strategies for Equality in Accessibility of School Playground. *J. Asian Archit. Build. Eng.* **2022**, *22*, 2047–2057. [CrossRef]
21. Pipitone, J.M.; Jović, S. Urban Green Equity and COVID-19: Effects on Park Use and Sense of Belonging in New York City. *Urban For. Urban Green.* **2021**, *65*, 127338. [CrossRef]
22. Liu, D.; Kwan, M.-P.; Kan, Z. Analysis of Urban Green Space Accessibility and Distribution Inequity in the City of Chicago. *Urban For. Urban Green.* **2021**, *59*, 127029. [CrossRef]
23. Sharifi, F.; Nygaard, A.; Stone, W.M.; Levin, I. Accessing Green Space in Melbourne: Measuring Inequity and Household Mobility. *Landsc. Urban Plan.* **2021**, *207*, 104004. [CrossRef]
24. Shen, Y.; Sun, F.; Che, Y. Public Green Spaces and Human Wellbeing: Mapping the Spatial Inequity and Mismatching Status of Public Green Space in the Central City of Shanghai. *Urban For. Urban Green.* **2017**, *27*, 59–68. [CrossRef]
25. Williams, T.G.; Logan, T.M.; Zuo, C.T.; Liberman, K.D.; Guikema, S.D. Parks and Safety: A Comparative Study of Green Space Access and Inequity in Five US Cities. *Landsc. Urban Plan.* **2020**, *201*, 103841. [CrossRef]
26. Boza-Kiss, B.; Pachauri, S.; Zimm, C. Deprivations and Inequities in Cities Viewed Through a Pandemic Lens. *Front. Sustain. Cities* **2021**, *3*, 645914. [CrossRef]
27. Lee, S.; Lee, C.; Xu, M.; Li, W.; Ory, M. People Living in Disadvantaged Areas Faced Greater Challenges in Staying Active and Using Recreational Facilities during the COVID-19 Pandemic. *Health Place* **2022**, *75*, 102805. [CrossRef]

28. Ashraf, K.; Park, Y.M.; Browning, M.H.E.M.; Wang, J.; Wang, R.; Lee, K. Examining the Joint Effect of Air Pollution and Green Spaces on Stress Levels in South Korea: Using Machine Learning Techniques. *Int. J. Digit. Earth* **2024**, *17*, 2372321. [CrossRef]
29. Karurung, W.S.; Lee, K.; Lee, W. Comparison of Different Green Space Measures and Their Impact on Dementia Cases in South Korea: A Spatial Panel Analysis. *ISPRS Int. J. Geo-Inf.* **2024**, *13*, 126. [CrossRef]
30. Lee, K. Association between Depression and Green Space before and after the COVID-19: Panel Data Evidence in South Korea. *Korean J. Geomatics* **2022**, *40*, 459–467. [CrossRef]
31. Herald. Monthly Household Income by Districts in Seoul. Available online: http://biz.heraldcorp.com/view.php?ud=20180330000760 (accessed on 22 May 2024).
32. Seoul Metropolitan Government Seoul Metropolitan City Local Tax Collection. Available online: https://data.seoul.go.kr/dataList/177/S/2/datasetView.do# (accessed on 22 May 2024).
33. Seoul. Statistics on the Registered Population of Seoul. Available online: https://data.seoul.go.kr/dataList/10718/S/2/datasetView.do# (accessed on 22 May 2024).
34. KBS World. S. Korea's Smartphone Penetration Highest in the World at 95%. Available online: https://world.kbs.co.kr/service/news_view.htm?lang=e&Seq_Code=142787#:~:text=According%20to%20a%20report%20published,100%20percent%20mobile%20phone%20ownership (accessed on 22 May 2024).
35. Getis, A.; Ord, J.K. The Analysis of Spatial Association by Use of Distance Statistics. *Geogr. Anal.* **2010**, *24*, 189–206. [CrossRef]
36. Ord, J.K.; Getis, A. Local Spatial Autocorrelation Statistics: Distributional Issues and an Application. *Geogr. Anal.* **2010**, *27*, 286–306. [CrossRef]
37. Yu, S.; Zhu, X.; He, Q. An Assessment of Urban Park Access Using House-Level Data in Urban China: Through the Lens of Social Equity. *Int. J. Environ. Res. Public Health* **2020**, *17*, 2349. [CrossRef]
38. Gao, S.; Zhai, W.; Fu, X. Green Space Justice amid COVID-19: Unequal Access to Public Green Space across American Neighborhoods. *Front. Public Health* **2023**, *11*, 1055720. [CrossRef]
39. Marquet, O.; Aaron Hipp, J.; Alberico, C.; Huang, J.-H.; Fry, D.; Mazak, E.; Lovasi, G.S.; Floyd, M.F. Park Use Preferences and Physical Activity among Ethnic Minority Children in Low-Income Neighborhoods in New York City. *Urban For. Urban Green.* **2019**, *38*, 346–353. [CrossRef]
40. Lindsey, G.; Maraj, M.; Kuan, S. Access, Equity, and Urban Greenways: An Exploratory Investigation. *Prof. Geogr.* **2001**, *53*, 332–346. [CrossRef]
41. Matthew McConnachie, M.; Shackleton, C.M. Public Green Space Inequality in Small Towns in South Africa. *Habitat Int.* **2010**, *34*, 244–248. [CrossRef]
42. Wright Wendel, H.E.; Zarger, R.K.; Mihelcic, J.R. Accessibility and Usability: Green Space Preferences, Perceptions, and Barriers in a Rapidly Urbanizing City in Latin America. *Landsc. Urban Plan.* **2012**, *107*, 272–282. [CrossRef]
43. Wüstemann, H.; Kalisch, D.; Kolbe, J. Access to Urban Green Space and Environmental Inequalities in Germany. *Landsc. Urban Plan.* **2017**, *164*, 124–131. [CrossRef]
44. Lanza, K.; Durand, C.P.; Alcazar, M.; Ehlers, S.; Zhang, K.; Kohl, H.W. School Parks as a Community Health Resource: Use of Joint-Use Parks by Children before and during COVID-19 Pandemic. *Int. J. Environ. Res. Public Health* **2021**, *18*, 9237. [CrossRef]
45. Bozkurt, M. Locked-down!: How Children's Access and Use of Urban Green Spaces and Playgrounds Changed after COVID 19 Outbreak. *Adnan Menderes Üniv. Ziraat Fakültesi Derg.* **2021**, *18*, 303–310. [CrossRef]
46. Quinn, A.; Russo, A. Adaptive School Grounds Design in Response to COVID-19: Findings from Six Primary Schools in South East England. *Build. Environ.* **2022**, *215*, 108946. [CrossRef]
47. Ministry of Culture, Sports and Tourism. National Living Sports Survey. 2021. Available online: https://policy.nl.go.kr/search/searchDetail.do?rec_key=SH2_PLC20220283455 (accessed on 22 May 2024).
48. Yi, L.; Wang, S.D.; Chu, D.; Ponnada, A.; Intille, S.S.; Dunton, G.F. Examining Whether Physical Activity Location Choices Were Associated with Weekly Physical Activity Maintenance Across 13 Months of the COVID-19 Pandemic in Emerging Adults. *J. Phys. Act. Health* **2022**, *19*, 446–455. [CrossRef]
49. Ministry of Culture, Sports and Tourism. National Living Sports Survey. 2019. Available online: https://www.mcst.go.kr/kor/s_policy/dept/deptView.jsp?pSeq=1297&pDataCD=0417000000&pType=07 (accessed on 22 May 2024).
50. Lee, K. Analysis of Changes in Geographical Factors Affecting Sales in Commercial Alleys after COVID-19 Using Machine Learning Techniques. *Heliyon* **2022**, *8*, e10708. [CrossRef]
51. Seoul Metropolitan Government Smart City Policy Bureau. *Impact of COVID-19 Varies Greatly by Regions for Living Population and by Industries for Store Sales*; Seoul Metropolitan Government Smart City Policy Bureau: Seoul, Republic of Korea, 2020.
52. Lu, J.; Zhang, M.; Yuan, M. Parenting and Parent–Child Home Practice during the COVID-19 Pandemic: A Case in Central China. *Sci. Rep.* **2023**, *13*, 18655. [CrossRef] [PubMed]
53. Cocuzzo, B.; Wrench, A.; O'Malley, C. Effects of COVID-19 on Older Adults: Physical, Mental, Emotional, Social, and Financial Problems Seen and Unseen. *Cureus* **2022**, *14*, e29493. [CrossRef] [PubMed]
54. Ministry of Employment and Labor. Comprehensive Manual for Working from Home. Available online: https://www.moel.go.kr/common/downloadFile.do?file_seq=20201000322&bbs_seq=20200900802&bbs_id=29&file_ext=pdf (accessed on 22 May 2024).
55. Son, Y.-J. Changes in the Way We Work after COVID-19 and Employment Impact Analysis. *Employ. Impact Assess. Brief.* **2022**, *28*, 1–8.

56. Choi, S. Characteristics and Distribution of Teleworkable Jobs Based on Physical Working Conditions. *J. Econ. Geogr. Soc. Korea* **2020**, *23*, 276–291. [CrossRef]
57. Moreno, C.; Allam, Z.; Chabaud, D.; Gall, C.; Pratlong, F. Introducing the "15-Minute City": Sustainability, Resilience and Place Identity in Future Post-Pandemic Cities. *Smart Cities* **2021**, *4*, 93–111. [CrossRef]
58. Weng, M.; Ding, N.; Li, J.; Jin, X.; Xiao, H.; He, Z.; Su, S. The 15-Minute Walkable Neighborhoods: Measurement, Social Inequalities and Implications for Building Healthy Communities in Urban China. *J. Transp. Health* **2019**, *13*, 259–273. [CrossRef]
59. Liu, D.; Kwan, M.-P.; Kan, Z.; Wang, J. Toward a Healthy Urban Living Environment: Assessing 15-Minute Green-Blue Space Accessibility. *Sustainability* **2022**, *14*, 16914. [CrossRef]
60. Murgante, B.; Annunziata, A. Application of the 15-Minute City Criteria to a Metropolitan Area: The Case Study of the Metropolitan City of Cagliari, Italy. In Proceedings of the Computational Science and Its Applications—ICCSA 2024 Workshops, Hanoi, Vietnam, 1–4 July 2024; Gervasi, O., Murgante, B., Garau, C., Taniar, D., Rocha, A.M.A.C., Faginas Lago, M.N., Eds.; Lecture Notes in Computer Science. Springer Nature: Cham, Switzerland, 2024; Volume 14817, pp. 218–233, ISBN 978-3-031-65237-0.
61. Mustafa, A.; Kennedy, C.; Lopez, B.; McPhearson, T. Perceived and Geographic Access to Urban Green Spaces in New York City during COVID-19. *Cities* **2023**, *143*, 104572. [CrossRef]
62. Mollalo, A.; Vahedi, B.; Rivera, K.M. GIS-Based Spatial Modeling of COVID-19 Incidence Rate in the Continental United States. *Sci. Total Environ.* **2020**, *728*, 138884. [CrossRef]
63. Martellucci, C.A.; Sah, R.; Rabaan, A.A.; Dhama, K.; Casalone, C.; Arteaga-Livias, K.; Sawano, T.; Ozaki, A.; Bhandari, D.; Higuchi, A.; et al. Changes in the Spatial Distribution of COVID-19 Incidence in Italy Using GIS-Based Maps. *Ann. Clin. Microbiol. Antimicrob.* **2020**, *19*, 30. [CrossRef]
64. Nasiri, R.; Akbarpour, S.; Zali, A.R.; Khodakarami, N.; Boochani, M.H.; Noory, A.R.; Soori, H. Spatio-Temporal Analysis of COVID-19 Incidence Rate Using GIS: A Case Study—Tehran Metropolitan, Iran. *GeoJournal* **2022**, *87*, 3291–3305. [CrossRef]

International Journal of *Geo-Information*

MDPI

Article

Examining Spatial Accessibility and Equity of Public Hospitals for Older Adults in Songjiang District, Shanghai

Mirkamiljan Mahmut [1], Pei Yin [1], Bozhezi Peng [1], Jiani Wu [1], Tao Wang [1], Shengqiang Yuan [2] and Yi Zhang [1,3,*]

[1] State Key Laboratory of Ocean Engineering, School of Ocean and Civil Engineering, Shanghai Jiao Tong University, Shanghai 200240, China; mirkamil_mok@sjtu.edu.cn (M.M.); yp9901@sjtu.edu.cn (P.Y.); bozhezi.peng@sjtu.edu.cn (B.P.); jianizi@sjtu.edu.cn (J.W.); wangtao127@sjtu.edu.cn (T.W.)
[2] Shanghai Municipal Engineering Design Institute (Group) Co., Ltd., Shanghai 200092, China; yuanshengqiang@smedi.com
[3] Institute of Healthy Yangtze River Delta, Shanghai Jiao Tong University, Shanghai 200240, China
* Correspondence: darrenzhy@sjtu.edu.cn

Abstract: In developing countries, aging is rapid and new towns in suburban and rural districts are emerging. However, the spatial accessibility and equity of healthcare services for older adults in new towns is rarely examined. This study is among the earliest attempts to evaluate the spatial accessibility and equity of public hospitals for older adults, using data from Songjiang District, Shanghai, China. A modified Gaussian Huff-based three-step floating catchment area (GH3SFCA) method was adopted based on the real-time travel costs of public transit, driving, cycling, and walking. The Gini coefficient and Bivariate Moran's Index were integrated to estimate spatial equity. The results showed that the spatial accessibility of high-tier hospitals decreases from the central areas to the outskirts for older adults in Songjiang. Meanwhile, the accessibility of low-tier hospitals varies substantially across areas. Although the low-tier hospitals are distributed evenly, their Gini coefficient showed less equitable spatial accessibility than the high-tier hospitals. Furthermore, driving and cycling lead to more equitable spatial accessibility than public transit or walking. Finally, communities with a low-supply–high-demand mismatch for public hospitals were suggested to be improved preferentially. These findings will facilitate planning strategies for public hospitals for older adults in developing new towns.

Keywords: public hospitals; spatial accessibility; equity; older adults; floating catchment area

1. Introduction

As aging is becoming more rapid globally, around 20% of people are expected to be 60 years or older by 2050 [1]. In China, the population has aged significantly in recent decades, and it is expected to boom in the future [2–4]. By the end of 2023, the aging population in China reached 296 million, covering 21.1% of the general population. This percentage is expected to rise to 35.1% in 2050 [5]. By the end of 2021, older adults over 60 took up 36.3% of the total population in Shanghai, and the proportions were 25.9% for over age 65, 16.6% for over age 70, and 5.6% for over age 80. There is a constant and growing need for healthcare services in rural, suburban, and urban areas, particularly during population growth and aging [6,7]. Age-related chronic diseases, such as cancer, arthritis, heart disease, and stroke, are more likely to occur as people get older [8]. Accessibility to healthcare is recognized as essential to the general health and quality of life of older adults. Examining spatial variations in older adults' access to public hospitals can help identify inequity and suggest resource allocation [9,10]. Spatial barriers for older adults to reach public hospitals result in their reduced satisfaction with disease-prevention services and lower utilization of public hospitals [11,12]. More significantly, compared to their younger counterparts, older adults experience worsening inequities in healthcare access. They are more likely to have worse health conditions and fewer options for mobility, such as difficulty walking and reduced or stopped driving [13]. Equity in spatial accessibility has received growing attention among researchers, who are using spatial accessibility to evaluate inequity [14–16]. A study in India found that the utilization of public health facilities increased with age among older adults, but health-seeking behavior decreased with age among them [17]. In addition to enhancing spatial accessibility, planning and investments in public healthcare services should prioritize the needs of the dependent and vulnerable, such as older people and those with disabilities.

New towns in western industrialized countries were gradually brought under local government supervision in the mid–late 1980s, slowing planning and construction [18]. Conversely, with the acceleration of economic globalization, new towns are emerging in suburban and rural areas of developing countries. New town development became an important concept in Chinese urban planning at the beginning of the 21st century. Shanghai launched its new town project as early as 2000, and this project has since been replicated by other Chinese cities. In 2017, Shanghai planned to cultivate five new towns, including Songjiang, Jiading, Qingpu, Fengxian, and Nanhui, into comprehensive node towns with a radiation-driving role in the Yangtze River Delta urban agglomeration [19]. The new generation of new towns are more comprehensively planned in terms of land use profile and urban functions, focusing on not only economic development but also livability [20]. Today, more than 3800 new towns in China occupy nearly 30,000 km^2 of land and provide shelters for about 150 million residents [21]. Before the media used the term "ghost cities" to describe new town developments with few residents, neither the public nor researchers paid much attention to the insufficient planning of new towns [22]. An important part of making these new towns more livable is to understand and improve the accessibility and equity of healthcare for their residents.

The concept of accessibility has evolved in many ways since it was brought up in 1959 [23]. Accessibility can, in short, be defined as the relative ease by which certain locations can be reached from other locations [24]. The accessibility of health services can be measured using the space between the population demand for and the available healthcare supply, which is influenced by the travel impedance in between [25,26]. According to earlier research, access and proximity are highly correlated with the use of healthcare services [27–31]. Therefore, policy making and urban planning are necessary to enable people access these services easily [32]. To that end, it is necessary to be able to assess the current state of the healthcare accessibly. An essential advantage of the accessibility approach is the analysis of spatial and social inequalities [33,34]. The value of the methods for spatial health research is becoming more and more recognized, with the ultimate goal to uncover social disparities in spatial access to healthcare [35,36]. Spatial accessibility to healthcare services is generally measured with GIS-based tools. It focuses on the role of spatial distances in the interactions between populations' medical demands and healthcare supply [37,38]. Several methods have been applied to measure the spatial accessibility of healthcare services, with common methods including the two-step floating catchment area (2SFCA) method, potential model, and gravity model. The 2SFCA method is the most widely used in the evaluation of the spatial accessibility of public hospitals. It incorporates the interaction between supply, demand, and minimum cost into the measure of accessibility. This method has advantages in the equity measurement of medical resources [39].

The traditional 2SFCA accessibility measurement was improved from different aspects. In order to solve the defects of the dichotomous method of the 2SFCA method to deal with distance, many studies introduced the distance decay function in the original model, mainly in the form of exponential function [35], Gaussian function [40], and kernel density function [41]. As an extension of demand or supply competition, the enhanced 2SFCA method aims to include the distance decay effect into the original 2SFCA method by incorporating different weights for different time zones [42]. Considering the competition effect between facilities when multiple facilities exist within the search radius of a demand point, 3SFCA is proposed by adding a third step to the search including all demand points and facilities [43]. The Enhanced 3SFCA (E3SFCA) method proposed by Luo aims to overcome the problem of overestimation in the 2SFCA and E2SFCA methods [44,45]. As an extension of travel modes, Tao and Wang (2022) aimed to measure transportation-induced healthcare inequity by comparing the accessibility of hospitals under different transportation situations [46]. Xing and Ng (2022) adopted the modal accessibility gap (MAG) Index to reveal the spatial disparities in accessibility between the public transport and private car modes [47]. As for demand data in FCA methods, some researchers used detailed information on individual household addresses as medical demand points [48]. In other studies, due to statistical reasons, populations were aggregated to larger spatial units. The choice of data aggregation method is crucial in accessibility analyses, as different approaches can introduce spatial biases. Kowalski (2022) demonstrated the influence of population data aggregation methods on walking accessibility results, and suggested that reducing aggregated data to more precise levels can reduce aggregation errors [49].

Spatial accessibility is vital for older adults in seeking healthcare services in primary hospitals and specialty care [50,51]. Uneven spatial distribution of populations, healthcare facilities, and the transport system connecting them can cause many healthcare disparities [52]. Transportation policies are established to reduce spatial barriers for the aging population, such as public transit services, pedestrian environments, car or van rides, and social support [53–57]. For example, Zainab described the importance of public transit for older adults in Sydney to the greater usage of dental care [50]. Loo and Lam highlighted the importance of a walkable pedestrian environment around healthcare facilities in order to promote active aging [55].

An increasing number of studies have focused on the spatial equity of older adults' access to healthcare services. Health policies need to include the supply of more accessible health services, especially for the aging population, who use healthcare facilities more frequently and intensively than other age groups [58,59]. Researchers found that there is an negative correlation between patients' physical location (usually residential) and their use of healthcare services [60]. Tao and Cheng showed the uneven distribution of spatial accessibility to hospitals for older adults in Beijing, where the level of accessibility decreases significantly from the central area outwards. Their findings indicated that older adults were disadvantaged in the competition with their younger counterparts for healthcare services [61]. Spatial accessibility and inequity indices were used to evaluate disparities in senior community care services. The results suggested that policymakers should not only measure overall accessibility but also aim for a more equitable distribution [62]. Moreover, spatial accessibility can help to identify healthcare service shortage areas and inform the equitable allocation of resources [63].

Various approaches have been explored to measure equity in healthcare accessibility, with simple economic indicators and complicated spatial models. The Gini coefficient has been used in recent research to assess transport equity from a social justice perspective [15,48,64,65]. For instance, the spatial disparity between the population and physicians in Japan was analyzed using Lorenz curves and Gini coefficients [66]. The disparity in the geographical distribution of clinics in the metropolitan city of Daejeon, South Korea, was measured by hot-spot analysis [67]. The spatiotemporal disparity in public healthcare resources across China in the period of 2003–2015 was analyzed using Moran's Index model and the dynamic spatial Durbin panel model [68].

However, there are still research gaps in the existing literature. Firstly, few studies have focused on new towns in developing countries. Compared with urban areas, the policies for new towns will boost population size in the future, causing low accessibility and equity with regard to healthcare facilities, especially for older adults [69]. Secondly, although accessibility-related equity studies are emerging, there is a lack of consideration of the hierarchical characteristics of hospitals. Hospitals of higher tiers could provide basic medical services like primary or specialty hospitals. Considering all medical facilities to be the same may result in a biased understanding of accessibility [48]. Thirdly, many previous accessibility studies estimated the actual travel time based on the grade and average speed of road sections, neglecting the impact of actual traffic conditions on the time cost. In morning peak hours, the travel time to publics hospitals would be longer, and it is natural for older adults to go to hospitals early to receive medical services sooner.

In view of the above research gaps, this study evaluates the spatial accessibility and equity of public hospitals for older adults in Songjiang District, Shanghai, China. The research objectives are as follows: (1) to adopt a modified Gaussian Huff-based three-step floating catchment area (GH3SFCA) method that focuses on measuring the spatial accessibility associated with public hospitals; (2) to explore the spatial inequity of public hospitals in Songjiang and identify the spatial disparity patterns for older adults; and (3) to identify the priority of the locations where older adult public hospital accessibility improvements are most needed in Songjiang.

The contributions of this study are three-fold. First, the modified GH3SFCA method adopted in this study incorporated the Gaussian distance decay function and Huff probability model, which are more linked to travel behaviors during public hospital trips and enhance the accuracy in calculating spatial accessibility and equity. Second, real-time travel time costs were obtained to reflect the actual situation at peak hour for four prevailing travel modes, making the results better suited for the circumstances compared to traditional road network analysis. Third, instead of choosing large administrative units (e.g., subdistricts or districts), this study employed small administrative units (i.e., communities and villages). This helps to discover fine-grained variability in the spatial accessibility and equity of public hospitals and derive targeted planning strategies in different communities.

The research framework of this paper includes three parts (Figure 1). Firstly, we collect and preprocess data on the older population, public hospitals and travel time cost. Secondly, we adopted a modified GH3SFCA method and calculate accessibility with the supply (public hospitals) and demand (older population) data and travel time cost data. Finally, the spatial equity of the public hospitals is analyzed using a Lorenz curve, the Gini coefficient, and Bivariate global and local Moran's Indices.

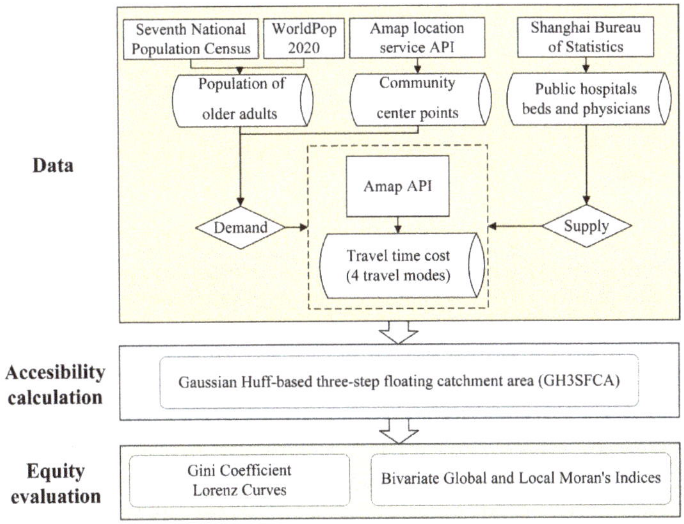

Figure 1. Research framework.

2. Research Data

2.1. Study Area

In this research, we chose Songjiang District as the study area. In the 2001 Shanghai One City Nine Towns Planning, Songjiang became the one of the first new towns in Shanghai. As the experimental site for Shanghai's new town project, Songjiang pioneered a new mode of outer suburban development and became the role model for other towns [69]. In 2000, the population of Songjiang was 0.64 million, and there were 18 hospitals with 2846 hospital beds and 3018 physicians. As the most populated new town in Shanghai, the population in Songjiang tripled to 1.9 million in 2021. Nevertheless, the number of hospitals only increased to 22 (+22%), with 3991 hospital beds (+40%) and 6318 physicians (+109%). Therefore, Songjiang would be a good case for studying the spatial accessibility and equity of healthcare services in developing countries' new towns during rapid urbanization.

Songjiang is in the southwest of Shanghai, with a total area of 604.64 km^2. The administrative division of Chinese cities has four levels: city–district (county, new towns)–subdistrict–community (village). There are 17 subdistricts in Songjiang, and a total of 356 communities (villages) under these subdistricts. The locations of the study area is shown in Figure 2.

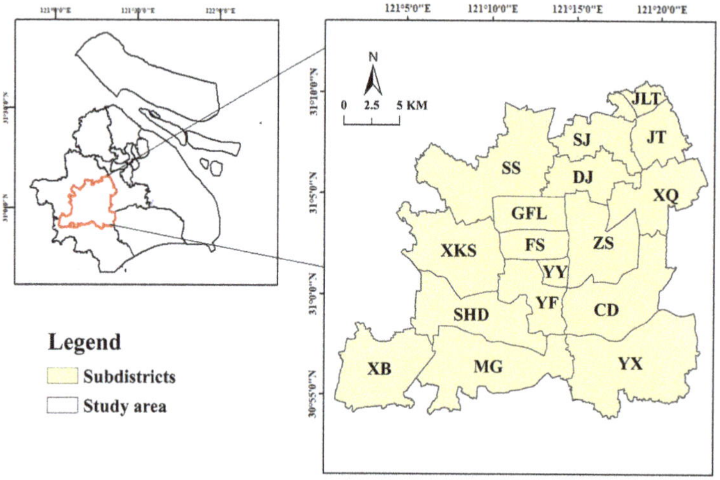

Figure 2. Study area and spatial distribution of community centers.

2.2. Data

2.2.1. Public Hospitals

In China, hospitals are categorized into three tiers–primary, secondary, and tertiary–providing different qualities and types of services [70,71]. Primary hospitals in China provide diagnoses and treatments for common diseases and serve the basic public health needs of residents in adjacent communities. Secondary hospitals offer more services than primary ones and provide outpatient, emergency, and surgery services. Tertiary hospitals have the largest scale and are equipped with sufficient medical facilities and highly skilled staff to diagnose and treat difficult diseases. However, hospital services are not delivered through this multi-tier system in line with a gatekeeping and two-directional referral network [71,72]. High-tier (secondary and tertiary) hospitals also provide primary care, and residents have the freedom to access high-tier hospitals to receive first diagnosis and treatment services. They serve nearby residents and also attract those from a further distance. There are a total of 22 public hospitals in Songjiang: primary (15), secondary (6), and tertiary (1) (Table 1). The locations of public hospitals were obtained through the Amap location service API. The distribution of public hospitals and community centers is shown in Figure 3. Secondary and tertiary hospitals are more spatially aggregated in the center of Songjiang than primary hospitals.

Table 1. Service capacity of different public hospitals in Songjiang (2021).

Characteristics	Primary	Secondary	Tertiary
Number of hospitals	15	6	1
Hospital beds (mean)	138	252	805
Physicians and staff (mean)	206	358	1577
Annual diagnosis and treatment sessions (mean, in 2021)	264,333	360,680	1,491,291

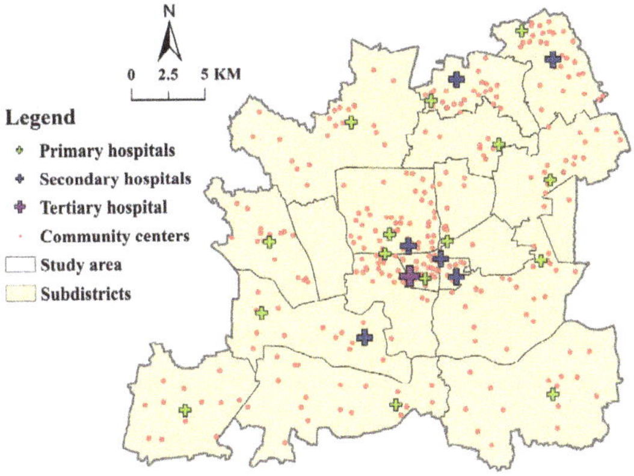

Figure 3. The distribution of public hospitals and community centers.

In this study, we combined secondary and tertiary hospitals into one category, and primary hospitals formed another. There are two reasons for this: (1) primary hospitals are called community healthcare centers or clinics, while secondary and tertiary hospitals are general or specialized hospitals and overlap in their functions [73]; (2) there is only one tertiary hospital in the study area, which could not be analyzed because it lacked attraction competition in the FCA methods.

2.2.2. Older Population Distribution

In the Law of the PRC on the Protection of the Rights and Interests of Older Adults, citizens over 60 years of age are called older adults. According to the Seventh National Population Census in 2021, the aging population (60 and above) in Songjiang accounts for 302,000 people, 16% of the general population. In China, city administrative division has four levels: city–district (county, new towns)–subdistrict–community (village). Many current studies on the accessibility of medical facilities were conducted at the subdistrict level, taking the mass center of the subdistrict as the population demand point [74]. In this study, we set the 356 community administration centers (hereafter referred to as community centers) as the demand point for health services. We obtained the coordinates of all community centers through the Amap API service. Then, the entirety of Songjiang was divided into 306 community areas by the ArcGIS 10.7 Thiessen Polygons tool, based on the current 356 community centers. Some community centers were automatically merged by the ArcGIS Thiessen Polygons tool due to geographical proximity.

Firstly, we obtained a 100 m × 100 m resolution population raster dataset of China from the WorldPop website for the year 2020, and clipped the Songjiang raster data from it. Secondly, the WorldPop population raster data were divided into the community areas outlined above. We modified the population of each community under each subdistrict by proportion according to the population of the 17 subdistricts in the 2020 Seventh National Population Census in Songjiang District. The total population of Songjiang District in the raster data was adjusted from 1.4 m in WorldPop to 1.9 m in the Seventh National Census. Lastly, the proportion of the older population in each subdistrict in the Census was used to calculate the average of the older population raster data in each community. The population density of older people in Songjiang is shown in Figure 4. In terms of spatial distribution, the older population in Songjiang is densely represented in central and northeastern subdistricts (>1000 persons/km^2). On the contrary, the population density of older people in most other subdistricts is lower than 500 persons/km^2. The significant variation in the population density of older people (S.D. = 756 persons/km^2) requires a sensible allocation of public hospitals.

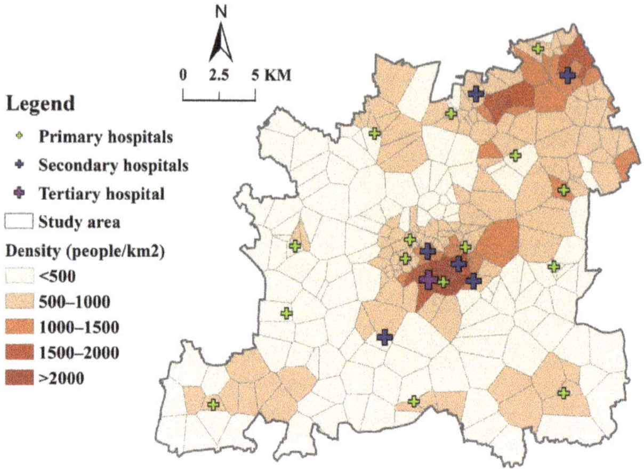

Figure 4. Population density of older people of Songjiang District.

2.2.3. Travel Time Cost

Determining the threshold is an important part of floating catchment area analysis. A small threshold can polarize the distributional pattern, while a large one would flatten the geographical pattern and mask local clusters with high values [75]. Generally, different tiers of hospitals have different searching thresholds due to the varied service capacity and attraction to residents. Shanghai commenced 15 min life circle planning in 2014. One of the aims is to ensure access to community (or primary) hospitals within a 15 min walking or cycling distance [76]. Therefore, we set a 15 min time threshold for primary hospitals for walking or cycling. For driving, we set it at 15 min, and for public transit, to 30 min considering time loss due to waiting and transferring. Since secondary and tertiary hospitals have higher service capacities, the time threshold for walking was set at 30 min, which is the maximum walking endurance time [77]. Similarly, cycling, driving, and public transit for secondary and tertiary hospitals were set at 30, 30, and 45 min.

The peak hour is another key factor in understanding accessibility to public hospitals, and it was provided by hospitals in Songjiang. Our study focused on regular medical services and general departments in hospital medical services, and emergency services and emergency rooms were not taken into consideration. The service hour begins at 8 A.M. according to the public hospital appointment schedule for general medical departments. Public hospitals offer a number of appointments for one time period, and every patient appointed in a certain time period (say 8:00–9:00 A.M.) waits in line in order of arrival. The hospitals, especially secondary and tertiary, are often crowded in China, and patients tend to arrive early to reduce their waiting time [78]. The peak hour is around 8–9 A.M. for primary hospitals, and is between 7:30 and 8:30 A.M. for secondary and tertiary hospitals as residents arrive early to line up. Peak hour travel time data were obtained and averaged for weekdays during a week (4–8 December 2023) through the Amap API. Using 306 community centers as the origin and 22 public hospitals as the destination, we collected the actual travel time cost for four travel modes: public transit, driving, cycling, and walking.

According to our field research at Songjiang Central Hospital on 27 November 2023, patients would prefer electric bikes to bicycles to go to hospitals. This aligns with the finding that the preferred transportation mode of Chinese nonmotor vehicle users is shifting from bicycles to electric bikes [79]. Private electric bikes are commonly-used in China [80]. They can be accessed in the majority of cities and almost all suburban and rural areas. Field research in rural and suburban areas in China shows that, unless they have a critical illness, residents are willing to go to medical facilities by themselves or with their family members by electric bike. This is consistent with the travel options in rural and suburban areas of China, where the terrain is flat and travel distances are moderate [81]. There are also some studies about older riders of electric bikes [82]. Therefore, we considered travel time by electric bike to represent cycling.

The peak hour travel time was recorded as the passage of time from the community to the public hospital for a specific travel mode. The travel times in this study were provided directly by Amap and captured by us through an API. The estimated travel times were returned based on actual conditions, including traffic jams in driving and public transportation, as well as pedestrian crossings, overpasses, and the speed of travel modes. The time is based on a huge amount of actual travel data from users, of all age groups. However, the cycling (electric bikes) time of older adults, even with a family member driving, would be longer than that of younger adults [79]. Walking speed can also be expected to be reduced in adults of older age [83]. Therefore, we multiplied the cycling and walking times of older adults by factors of 1.15 and 1.3, respectively. A total of $306 \times 22 \times 4$ travel time cost datapoints were obtained from Amap, and example data for walking mode are shown in Table 2.

Table 2. Example of obtained travel time data from community to public hospital by walking (in seconds).

Community ID /Hospital ID	0	1	2	……	20	21	22
0	1619	4297	2632	……	3831	5747	3603
1	1113	4255	2054	……	3904	6213	3524
2	868	4178	2011	……	3535	6399	3514
……	……	……	……	……	……	……	……
304	2939	4414	2177	……	4770	5508	3749
304	4578	3742	4752	……	6246	8754	2633
305	4041	6334	3434	……	5423	5151	5656

These results show that for all tiers of hospitals, driving and cycling have a lower mean travel time, followed by public transit. Notably, walking has an average travel time that is more than six times longer than that of driving (see Table 3).

Table 3. Statistical characteristics of travel time cost (in minutes).

Hospital Tier and Travel Mode	Max	Min	Mean	S.D.
Primary hospitals				
Public transit	251	0	85.34	30.92
Driving	81	0	33.30	12.92
Cycling	185	0	60.21	31.91
Walking	669	0	223.82	119.36
Secondary and tertiary hospitals				
Public transit	196	0	71.45	28.11
Driving	76	3	33.30	13.74
Cycling	180	1	51.00	29.29
Walking	697	3	195.89	114.85

3. Methods

3.1. Evaluation of Spatial Accessibility

Since Luo and Wang developed the two-step floating catchment area (2SFCA) method to measure spatial access, it has been widely used [26,31,84]. It defines the service area of a healthcare provider by a threshold while accounting for the capability of the provider to satisfy its nearby demands. The calculation takes two steps, and is formulated as Equations (1) and (2).

$$R_j = \frac{S_j}{\sum_{k\in\{d_{kj}<d_0\}} P_k} \tag{1}$$

$$A_i = \sum_{j\in\{d_{kj}<d_0\}} R_j \tag{2}$$

where R_j is the supply-to-demand ratio of facility j; S_j is the capacity of facility j; P_k is the population at location k; d_{kj} is the distance between k and j; and d_0 is the threshold travel distance.

3.2. Gaussian Huff-Based Three-Step Floating Catchment Area Method (GH3SFCA)

In this study, a modified Gaussian Huff-based 3SFCA was adopted to evaluate the spatial accessibility of public hospitals for the older adults in each community area inside the study area with different travel modes. It consisted of the following three steps.

Step 1: The demand probability of each community was calculated with regard to every service provider, taking into account the supply competition. The Huff probability model can overcome the problems of both over- and under-estimating population demand and adopts a more comprehensive service competition scheme which includes both travel cost and service capacity [44]. The calculation made according to the Huff model [44] was as follows:

$$Huff_{ij} = \frac{S_j f(d_{ij})}{\sum_{j\in\{d_{ij}<d_0\}} S_j f(d_{ij})} \tag{3}$$

The demand probability $Huff_{ij}$ for community i seeking healthcare at hospital j increases with the service capacity S_j of hospital j and decreases with distance according to the decay function $f(d_{ij})$ applied. In this study, we use hospital beds as the service capacity S_j indicator [74,85,86]. In the model, d_{ij} refers to the actual peak hour travel time from community i to hospital j, and d_0 is the travel time threshold. Furthermore, the demand probability depends on alternative health service providers and therefore is calculated in relation to the capacities and distances to all locations within the maximal relevant catchment expressed by the sum $\sum_{k\in\{d_{ij}<d_0\}} S_j f(d_{ij})$ in the dominator. The maximal relevant catchment size d_0 is assessed individually with reference to each hospital's type and travel modes.

In FCA methods, a distance weight is attributed to every subzone according to a distance decay function:

$$f(d_{ij}) = \begin{cases} G(d_{ik}) & d_{ij} < d_0 \\ 0 & d_{ij} \geq d_0 \end{cases} \tag{4}$$

Various functions have been used so far: the Gaussian function, gravity function, exponential function, inverse power function, or logistic-based function [87].We adopted the widely used Gaussian Function as the decay function, as it tends to choose the nearest destination points [88]. In case studies of healthcare accessibility, especially by low-speed travel modes, the Gaussian decay function would be more appropriate in choosing the closest services [49]. The Gaussian decay function is as follows:

$$G(d_{ij}) = \frac{exp\left(-\frac{1}{2}\left(\frac{d_{ij}}{d_0}\right)^2\right) - exp(-\frac{1}{2})}{1 - exp(-\frac{1}{2})}, \quad d_{ij} < d_0 \tag{5}$$

Step 2: The Huff probability was calculated in step 1, and a supply ratio was determined for each hospital j as follows:

$$R_j = \frac{S_j}{\sum_{k\in\{d_{ij}<d_0\}} Huff_{ij} P_i} \quad (6)$$

The supply ratio R_j is given by the service capacity S_j of hospital j divided by the sum of population P_i of all communities i within the maximum catchment size d_0 multiplied by their probability $Huff_{ij}$ of seeking service from hospital j.

The second step of the GH3SFCA incorporates the strengths by accounting for the absolute differences in distances. Unlike the previous method, this is accomplished by eliminating a distance weight from the denominator rather than adding one more distance weight to the numerator. This can be carried out because the impact of distance is taken into account in both the first and last steps, having already been taken into account within the Huff probability.

Step 3: The accessibility value A_i is calculated for each community i as the sum of the supply ratios R_j of all hospitals j reachable for community i within the maximum catchment size d_0, multiplied by the corresponding Huff probabilities $Huff_{ij}$ and the distance decay function $f(d_{ij})$:

$$A_i = \sum_{j\in\{d_{ij}<d_0\}} Huff_{ij} R_j f(d_{ij}) \quad (7)$$

3.3. Lorenz Curve and Gini Coefficient

In this study, the Gini Index was used to evaluate the inequality associated with accessibility value when different travel modes are used. It was also used to measure the medical demand of older adults at the community level. A higher Gini coefficient indicates a more uneven accessibility distribution for older adults. The Gini coefficient was calculated as follows:

$$Gini = 1 - \sum_{i=1}^{n} (X_i - X_{i-1})(Y_i - Y_{i-1}) \quad (8)$$

where $Gini$ is the Gini coefficient, $X_i (i = 1, 2, \ldots n)$ is the cumulative percentage of the older population in the community area, and $Y_i (i = 1, 2, \ldots n)$ is the cumulative ratio of resources in the community area. The Lorenz curve, plotted to obtain the Gini coefficient, denotes the rank-ordered cumulative distribution of accessibility for residents in different communities across Songjiang.

3.4. Spatial Inequity Analysis

Geospatial analysis was performed by calculating the global Moran's Index, an inferential statistic which estimates spatial autocorrelation and falls between −1 and +1. More positive or negative values correspond to greater spatial clustering or competitive dispersion, respectively. To test the null hypothesis of random spatial distribution, empiric significance is computed through permutation to yield a pseudo-p-value. A pseudo-p-value is a summary of the results of the reference distribution and is dependent on the number of permutations used [89].

To visualize spatial clustering, local indicators of spatial autocorrelation (LISA) maps were created using local Moran's Index calculations. This statistic identifies significant locations as high–high or low–low spatial clusters and high–low or low–high spatial outliers relative to neighboring regions [90]. Furthermore, the bivariate global Moran's Index measures the spatial autocorrelation between a variable in one geographic area and another variable in a neighboring area, and in this study, the local Moran's Index was mapped with bivariate LISA (BiLISA) maps.

GeoDa version 1.22 was used for geospatial analyses. All global and local bivariate Moran's indices and BiLISA maps were permuted 999 times. The default significance level was set at 0.05.

4. Results

4.1. Accessibility to Public Hospitals

The statistical results of accessibility to public hospitals by different travel modes for the GH3SFCA and 2SFCA methods are shown in Table 4. In the GH3SFCA results, primary hospitals have lower average accessibility than secondary and tertiary hospitals across all four travel modes, while they have the highest maximum accessibility values. Among the four travel modes, cycling has the highest average accessibility value for all tiers of hospitals, followed by driving, public transit, and walking. A possible reason for this is that cycling is less influenced by peak hour traffic congestion, and public transit takes longer due to waiting and transfers. Noticeably, the standard deviations of driving accessibility are the lowest, followed by public transit, cycling, and walking, which is the highest. This indicates that high-speed travel modes lead to less of a distribution discrepancy in accessibility, regardless of the tier of the hospital. In the 2SFCA model, the accessibility values are significantly larger. It is noticeable that the standard deviations of the GH3SFCA accessibility results are lower than those of the 2SFCA results, indicating less of a distribution discrepancy in accessibility using the adopted modified GH3SFCA method.

Table 4. Statistical characteristics of accessibility value.

Method and Hospital Tier	Travel Mode	Max	Min	Average	S.D.
GH3SFCA					
Primary	Public transit	0.1080	0	0.0050	0.0127
	Driving	0.0348	0	0.0093	0.0083
	Cycling	0.0775	0	0.0110	0.0150
	Walking	0.3854	0	0.0111	0.0430
Secondary and Tertiary	Public transit	0.0474	0	0.0093	0.0126
	Driving	0.0297	0	0.0112	0.0080
	Cycling	0.0415	0	0.0134	0.0137
	Walking	0.1704	0	0.0106	0.0271
2SFCA					
Primary	Public transit	4.9769	0	0.2991	0.5736
	Driving	9.4824	0	0.8113	1.1271
	Cycling	6.3342	0	0.6578	0.9218
	Walking	3.2168	0	0.0960	0.3560
Secondary and Tertiary	Public transit	36.8257	0	2.5231	4.9714
	Driving	44.7585	0	5.1939	6.6275
	Cycling	38.6620	0	3.7520	5.9968
	Walking	9.3154	0	0.5243	1.4736

The distribution of spatial accessibility to primary hospitals for older adults is presented in Figure 5. The results show that primary hospitals are more accessible in the outskirts, while tertiary hospitals have better accessibility in areas surrounding the new town center. The level of accessibility to secondary and tertiary hospitals is unevenly distributed, decreasing significantly from the new town center outwards. This result is due to the concentration of tertiary and secondary hospitals in central areas of Songjiang, reflecting the unfavorable inter-area disparities. On the contrary, the high accessibility levels for primary hospitals are not so pronounced in the new town center. Primary hospitals are more accessible in wider areas and several highly accessible clusters on the outskirts. This overall picture of accessibility is consistent with a pattern of concentrated secondary and tertiary hospitals and more dispersed locations of primary hospitals in new towns. The central area has a high accessibility value due to its developed economy, convenient transportation service, and rich medical facilities. However, there are some communities in the central area that have low accessibility to primary hospitals, caused by the high population density of older people compared to the outskirts. The areas underserved by public transit and walking are significantly larger in number than those underserved by driving and cycling. This indicates that it is hard for residents to access public hospitals by public transit or walking within an acceptable time threshold. The number of areas underserved is the least for driving mode. Even in traffic jams, the speed of cars helps them to access hospitals more quickly than any other travel mode.

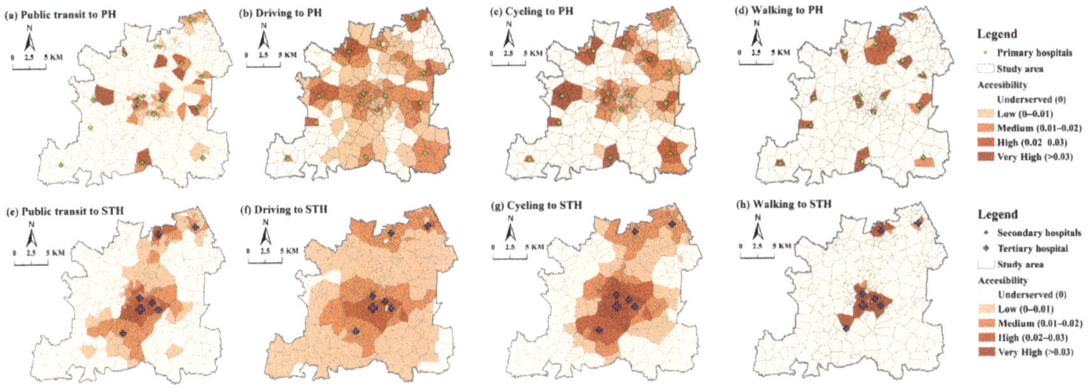

Figure 5. Accessibility distribution with GH3SFCA (PH = primary hospitals; STH = secondary and tertiary hospitals).

The accessibility distribution patterns to public hospitals with the 2SFCA method are shown in Figure 6. The distribution pattern and number of underserved areas are close to the results of the GH3SFCA method. However, the areas of high and very high accessibility are more numerous with the 2SFCA method, especially in the central area of Songjiang. In addition, the quantiles we use for 2SFCA have a higher value, to show a clear distribution level. This means 2SFCA overestimates the accessibility values in high-value area.

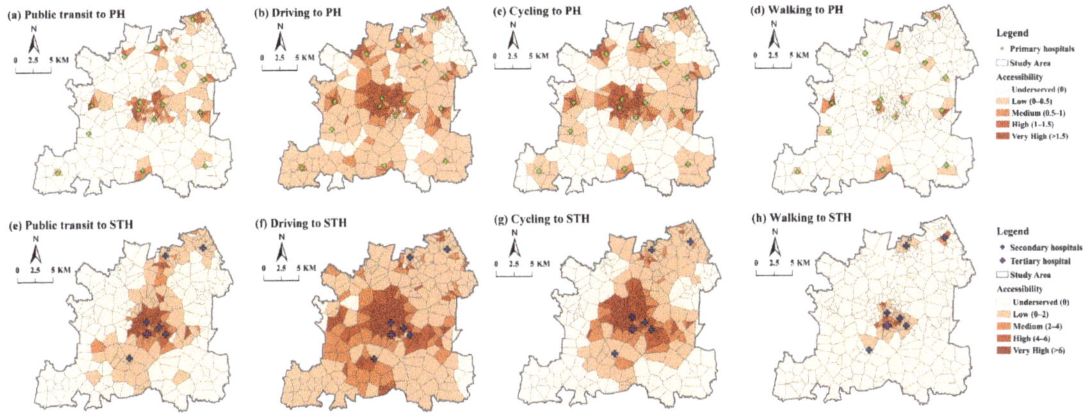

Figure 6. Accessibility distribution with 2SFCA (PH = primary hospitals; STH = secondary and tertiary hospitals).

To further explore the differences in the accessibility distribution for public hospitals across travel modes, we compared the number of communities with accessibility at various levels (see Figure 7). Combining all four travel modes, the number of communities with high and very high levels of accessibility for secondary and tertiary hospitals is 239, higher than that for primary hospitals (152). Considering specific travel modes, the accessibility to different tiers of public hospitals shows varied characteristics. For cycling, the number of communities with high and very high accessibility to hospitals at all levels is the highest out of the four travel modes. For public transit, primary hospitals have larger underserved areas than secondary and tertiary hospitals. On the contrary, the number of communities with more than medium accessibility to all tiers of hospitals by driving is close, while the number of areas with very high accessibility is very low for all tiers. Walking trips have a much better distribution of accessibility, with the highest number of very-high-accessibility neighborhoods, but also the highest percentage of underserved communities.

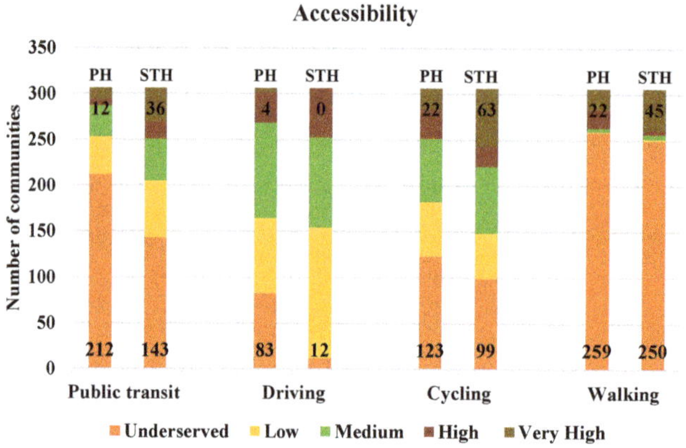

Figure 7. Number of communities with different levels of accessibility to public hospitals, with very high on top and underserved on bottom (PH = primary hospitals; STH = secondary and tertiary hospitals).

4.2. Gini Coefficient Analysis

The accessibility inequity across public hospitals and different travel modes is shown by the Lorenz curve in Figure 8 and the Gini coefficient in Figure 9. The value of the Gini coefficient ranges from 0 to 1. A lower Gini coefficient indicates more equal access to public hospitals by older adults, with 1 being completely unequal.

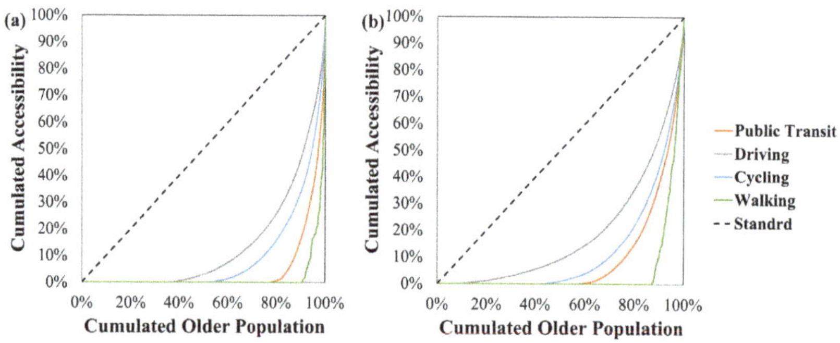

Figure 8. Lorenz curve of public hospitals in different travel modes. (**a**) Primary hospitals. (**b**) Secondary and tertiary hospitals.

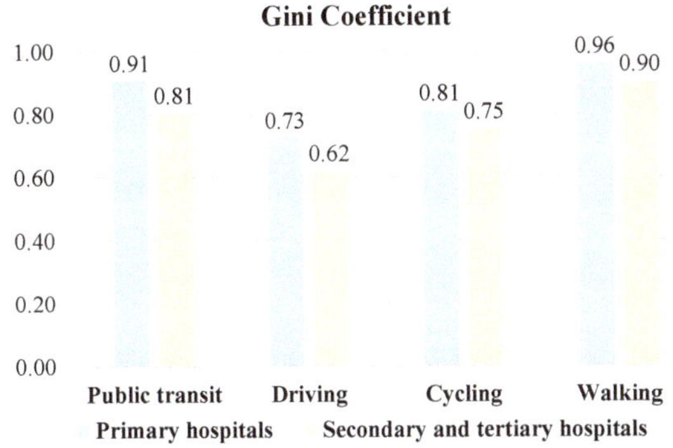

Figure 9. Gini coefficient of accessibility to public hospitals by four travel modes.

Most communities in Songjiang showed more unequal accessibility by public transit and walking than by driving and cycling (Figure 8). At all tiers of public hospitals, accessibility by driving had the lowest Gini coefficient (0.73 for primary hospitals and 0.62 for secondary and tertiary hospitals) (Figure 9). This suggested that older adults driving to public hospitals obtained more spatially equal medical services than those traveling by other travel modes in Songjiang. In contrast, walking (0.96 and 0.90) and public transit (0.91 and 0.81) resulted in the highest Gini coefficients. These results indicated that older adults who walk or use public transit to access public hospitals had the largest spatial disparity between different communities. With Gini coefficients of 0.81 and 0.75, accessibility by cycling was slightly more equal across communities than by public transit or walking. Moreover, the Gini coefficients for all travel modes in primary hospitals were higher than those in secondary and tertiary hospitals. These findings demonstrated that older adults visiting primary hospitals experienced more unequal accessibility than those visiting secondary and tertiary hospitals, regardless of travel mode.

4.3. Spatial Relationships Between Population Density of Older People and Accessibility Distribution

Accessibility measures the overall availability of public hospitals within a certain time threshold, but the service efficiency of public hospitals is also highly related to the population density of older people. Therefore, we used Bivariate Global and Local Moran's Indices to conduct a spatial correlation analysis between the population density of older people and accessibility distribution.

As shown in Table 5, the bivariate global Moran's Index values are close to zero for primary hospitals among all four modes (first row). This result shows no significant global spatial correlation between accessibility and the population density of older people for primary hospitals. However, for secondary and tertiary hospitals, the bivariate global Moran's Index values for the four modes are 0.672, 0.608, 0.584, and 0.496, respectively. They all pass the 5% significance level test, suggesting a positive spatial correlation between accessibility and the population density of older people across different travel modes.

Table 5. Bivariate Moran's Index values for public hospitals using different travel modes.

Tier of Hospital	Statistics	Public Transit	Driving	Cycling	Walking
Primary	Moran's Index	0.051	−0.011	−0.030	−0.018
	Pseudo-p-value	0.030	0.333	0.115	0.241
Secondary and Tertiary	Moran's Index	0.672	0.608	0.584	0.496
	Pseudo-p-value	0.001	0.001	0.001	0.001

By using the bivariate local Moran's Index, the spatial relationships between the population density of older people (medical service demand) and public hospital accessibility (medical service supply) are divided into five types, namely, high–high (HH) cluster, high–low (HL) outlier, low–high (LH) outlier, low–low (LL) cluster, and non-significant. The first 'High (or Low)' stands for the demand for medical services by older adults. The second 'High (or Low)' represents the supply of medical services by public hospitals across four travel modes. Both the HH and LL clusters mean spatial match. The HH cluster indicates a positive spatial match (high demand and supply) and the LL cluster means a negative spatial match (low demand and supply). Both the HL outlier and LH outlier indicate a spatial mismatch between public hospital accessibility and the population density of older people. The LH outlier means a positive spatial mismatch in which supply outweighs demand, while the HL outlier means a negative spatial mismatch in which demand outweighs supply. Notably, communities belonging to the HL outliers need special attention as they lack the medical services of public hospitals when traveling by at least one of the four travel modes. The non-significant type means the spatial relationships between population densities and public hospitals are not significant in the area.

The clusters and outliers for primary hospitals are shown in the BiLISA maps in Figure 10. The distribution patterns are differentiable across the four travel modes, and most communities have non-significant spatial relationships for public transit and walking. The number of communities in HH clusters (deep red areas in Figure 10) is small among all four travel modes (1, 6, 0, and 2, respectively). Most of the communities in the LL clusters (deep blue areas) and LH clusters (light blue areas) are related to driving (54 LL and 46 LH) and cycling (54 LL and 32 LH). The LL communities are generally distributed in the southwestern part of Songjiang, whereas the LH communities are scattered inside the entire district. Regarding the HL outliers (light red areas), communities travel significantly more by walking (43) than by the other three modes. These communities, which are experiencing a shortfall of medical services from primary hospitals, are densely located in northeast Songjiang, including subdistricts of JT, JLT, SJ, and XQ. It is noticeable that northeast Songjiang has all five types of spatial relationships, demonstrating the complexity of the correlations between the population density of older people and primary hospital accessibility in these areas.

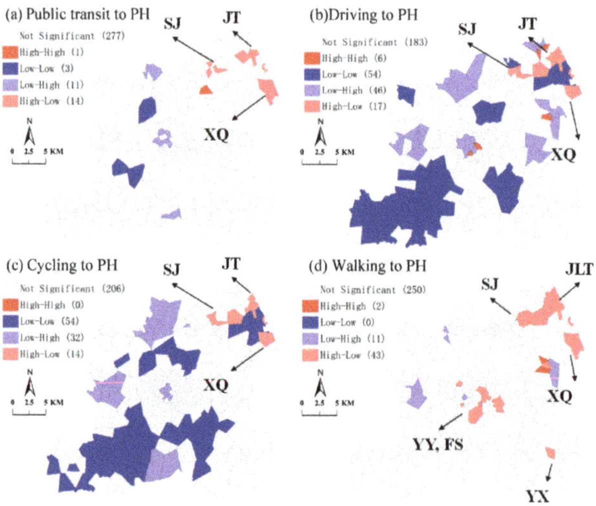

Figure 10. BiLISA map between population density of older people and accessibility to primary hospitals (PH = primary hospitals).

For secondary and tertiary hospitals (Figure 11), the spatial clusters and outlier patterns are similar across four travel modes, except for walking. The numbers of LL communities are high for public transit (80), driving (76), and cycling (91), while there are none for walking. The LL communities are mostly distributed around the outskirts of Songjiang. On the contrary, the HH communities are located in the central areas of Songjiang and surrounded by the LH communities. These two types of communities possess most of the secondary and tertiary hospitals, which provide sufficient medical services for older adults. As for the HL outliers, there are 22 communities related to walking and 10, 6, and 7 to public transit, driving, and cycling, respectively. The HL communities are mainly located in the XQ and JLT subdistricts in northeast Songjiang, where secondary and tertiary hospitals are scarce, but population densities high.

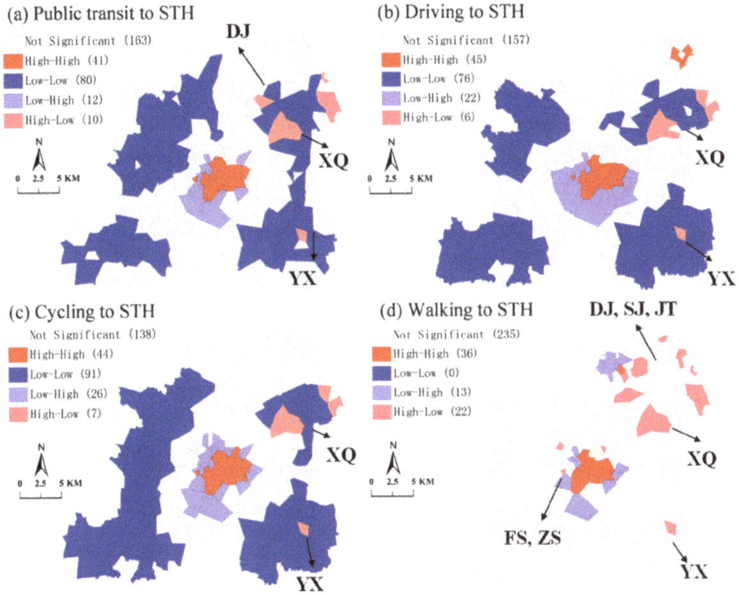

Figure 11. BiLISA map between population density of older people and accessibility to primary hospitals (STH = secondary and tertiary hospitals).

5. Discussion

5.1. Spatial Accessibility to Public Hospitals

The differences in GH3SFCA and 2SFCA occur for a few reasons. One major limitation of 2SFCA is that it defines a supply facility as being accessible or inaccessible by a threshold distance, while the generalized 2SFCA incorporates distance decay in the supply–demand interaction [91]. A stronger distance decay function like Gaussian, which we used in our study, is more likely to result in a decentralized polycentric structure of accessibility. Our results align with some studies which state that while it has a minor impact on most accessible areas, it tends to identify more areas with the poorest accessibility [92]. On the other hand, the major advantage of introducing Huff probability is that it adopts a more comprehensive service competition scheme which includes both travel time and service capacity, but without overestimating distance effects [44].

These results suggest an insufficient healthcare service supply from public hospitals in Songjiang. For primary hospitals, the spatial accessibility decreases with the distance between surrounding communities and hospitals. This result makes sense, as each subdistrict in Songjiang is equipped with one primary hospital, except for JT. In geographically large or densely populated subdistricts, low spatial accessibility to primary hospitals is found among older adults, especially when traveling by public transit or walking. Regarding geographically large subdistricts, this study identified the SS and XKS subdistricts in northwest Songjiang, and the MG and XB subdistricts in southwest Songjiang. The subdistricts with a dense population of older people include the YY, FS, and ZS subdistricts in central Songjiang and the SJ and JT subdistricts in the northeast. Another study showed great disparity in accessibility to primary healthcare services in rural and suburban areas [73]. Therefore, the number of hospital beds and doctors should be increased in order to improve the provision of primary hospital services. It is also possible to set up another primary hospital in a subdistrict according to special circumstances.

The spatial accessibility to secondary and tertiary hospitals, however, declines from the central areas to outskirts of the entirety of Songjiang, regardless of travel mode. Some studies have found that the accessibility to secondary and tertiary hospitals in urban areas in developing countries is generally higher than that to primary hospitals [93], which is consistent with the average data in the new town area in our study. This may also be related to the higher threshold set for secondary and tertiary hospitals.

The seven secondary and tertiary hospitals in Songjiang are situated in the densely populated areas, with five in the central areas and the remaining two in the northeast. Consequently, these hospitals are not fully accessible to older adults from communities in other areas, albeit to varying degrees. Regarding different travel modes, driving is the most accessible, followed by electric bikes. Consistent with previous literature, this finding is due to the speed and mobility of these two modes. Additionally, the majority of communities are underserved in terms of hospitals service with the public transit and walking modes, particularly in the outskirts of Songjiang. Thus, new branches of tertiary hospitals should be built in areas with low accessibility, or some secondary hospitals of appropriate size should be established.

Moreover, the development of public transit should be accelerated in underserved areas. Public transportation is considered to be more environmentally friendly and more sustainable than private vehicles. Driving is still a choice for some residents, but quite a lot of families do not own private cars in Shanghai [94]. It has become a consensus to prioritize the development of public transit in China. Public transport interchanges can be optimized, and additional routes and frequencies can be established. The accessibility of healthcare facilities can be significantly improved by eliminating underserved areas of healthcare facilities through public transport.

In addition, the efficiency of the referral system should be improved in order to achieve an overall balance between the supply and demand of public hospital services. Different tiers of hospitals have different service capacities, and their attractiveness to older adults varies. Patients usually have a higher preference for higher-tier hospitals. An efficient referral system can guide patients' hospital preferences and increase the equity of public hospitals [95].

5.2. Equity Analysis and Planning Suggestion

Considering the medical service supply (i.e., number of hospital beds) and demand (population density of older people), this study further examined the spatial equity of public hospitals by four travel modes. No global spatial correlation was found between the population density of older people and the spatial equity of primary hospitals. Nevertheless, a significant global spatial correlation was detected for secondary and tertiary hospitals. These results indicate more unequitable accessibility of primary hospitals than secondary and tertiary hospitals, especially by public transit and walking. A possible reason for this surprising finding is that the medical service supply of a primary hospitals is, on average, around 60% lower than that of a secondary or tertiary hospital. Meanwhile, some studies have found that the accessibility of secondary and tertiary hospitals in the central urban area of Shanghai is generally higher than that of primary hospitals, which is consistent with the average data in the suburbs of Shanghai in our study. As primary hospitals provide basic diagnoses and treatments to older adults in adjacent communities, they are more frequently visited than secondary and tertiary hospitals. Presumably, communities with a dense population of older people are more often underserved by primary hospitals than by secondary or tertiary hospitals. The BiLISA map further visualized the community-level distributions of spatial matches and mismatches between the population density of older people and medical service from public hospitals for the four travel modes. The typical 'high-demand–low-supply' communities are located in northeast Songjiang, including the JT, JLT, SJ, and XQ subdistricts. The YX subdistrict also has communities with 'high-demand–low-supply'.

In future planning, these communities with 'high-demand–low-supply' should be prioritized in order to increase their capacity to supply healthcare services. Figure 12 depicts this study's suggested sites for newly established primary and secondary hospitals. The JT subdistrict lacks primary hospitals due to previous planning reasons. At the same time, there are many communities with high populations of older people and a scarcity of primary hospitals located both within and around JT. Therefore, a primary hospital should be established in the JT subdistrict with 170 beds, higher than the average number of beds in primary hospitals. For high-tier hospitals, there are communities with 'high-demand–low-supply' in the YX subdistrict, along with communities with 'low-demand–low-supply' in the surrounding area. Therefore, only one secondary hospital is suggested, with the average number of beds of a secondary hospital (252).

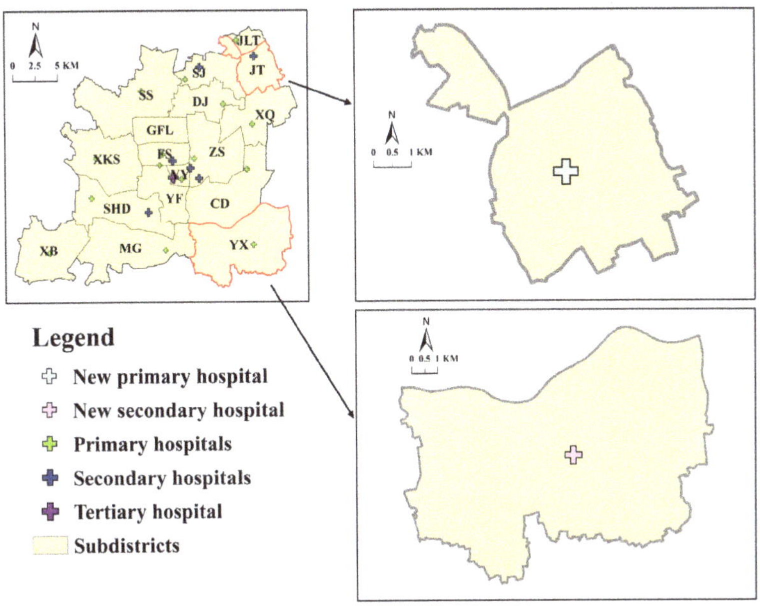

Figure 12. Suggested sites for newly planned hospitals in Songjiang.

6. Conclusions

Developing countries are experiencing a tremendous increase in their aging populations, and are also witnessing the emergence of new towns. Nevertheless, the spatial accessibility and equity of healthcare services for older adults in new towns is rarely studied. This study is one of the early attempts to assess the spatial accessibility and equity of public hospitals for older adults, with data from Songjiang District, Shanghai, China. A Gaussian Huff-based three-step floating catchment area (GH3SFCA) method was adopted based on the real-time travel costs of public transit, driving, cycling, and walking. The results demonstrated the uneven spatial distribution patterns of public hospital services for different travel modes. Our findings will facilitate planning strategies and policies for public hospitals for older adults in new towns.

The advantages in this paper are as follows: (1) the real-time peak hour travel time of four travel modes, obtained by Amap API, echoes older adults' travel conditions during actual public hospital visits; (2) the community-level analysis yields more accurate results than a subdistrict-level analysis, alleviates unnecessary deviation in travel time estimation, and discovers fine-grained variability in spatial accessibility and equity; and (3) by examining older adults' accessibility and equity for different tiers of public hospital services, areas where improvement should be prioritized were found and plans suggested for them.

This study focused on the overall accessibility of different tiers of hospitals, as in some previous studies [48,96]. However, due to data limitations, different medical services in different departments were not discussed, such as emergencies and specialized diagnoses. On the demand side, because of the lack of detailed demographic data for older adults, we could not examine spatial accessibility related to specified medical needs and travel behaviors. Older adults in different age groups may have different medical needs, like chronic diseases, and travel mode options, like car ownership or mobility; these factors could affect healthcare accessibility. Also, our results did not consider medical demand and supply around the borders of the study area. The majority of the studies on this subject did not consider population and hospital services outside of the study area. A few studies considered a buffer zone outside of the study area, but still used the data and discussed the results inside the study area [97].

Based on our findings, we suggest some future research directions. As we focus on older adults, factors such as gender, income, and social status, which may have important influences on older adults' access to hospitals, are not considered. Furthermore, the different choices of travel mode are a complicated problem with many factors that need to be considered. These require a large number of detailed studies and could be investigated in the future.

Author Contributions: Conceptualization, Mirkamiljan Mahmut, Pei Yin and Yi Zhang; Methodology, Mirkamiljan Mahmut and Pei Yin; Software, Mirkamiljan Mahmut and Pei Yin; Validation, Mirkamiljan Mahmut, Bozhezi Peng and Tao Wang; Formal Analysis, Mirkamiljan Mahmut, Bozhezi Peng and Yi Zhang; Investigation, Mirkamiljan Mahmut; Resources, Shengqiang Yuan; Data Curation, Mirkamiljan Mahmut, Pei Yin and Bozhezi Peng; Writing—Original Draft Preparation, Mirkamiljan Mahmut and Pei Yin; Writing—Review and Editing, Pei Yin, Tao Wang and Yi Zhang; Visualization, Mirkamiljan Mahmut and Jiani Wu; Supervision, Yi Zhang; Funding Acquisition, Shengqiang Yuan, Tao Wang and Yi Zhang. All authors have read and agreed to the published version of the manuscript.

Funding: This study was supported by the National Social Science Foundation (No. 22AZD082), Shanghai Social Science Foundation (Nos. 2023BSH003, 22Z350204369, and 2022BSH005), Shanghai Scientific Research Foundation (Nos. 23DZ1202900, 23DZ1203200, 23DZ1202400, 22DZ1203200, 21Z510203259, and 21DZ1200800), Special Project of Healthy Shanghai Action (No. JKS-HZX_2022-13), and Scientific Research Fund (No. K2015K017).

Data Availability Statement: Some data used in this study are confidential and can only be provided with restrictions.

Conflicts of Interest: Author Shengqiang Yuan is a Shanghai Municipal Engineering Design Institute (Group) Co., Ltd., Shanghai 200092, China employee. The remaining authors declare that the research was carried out in the absence of any commercial or financial relationships that could be construed as a potential conflict of interest, by providing the disclosure form of potential conflict of interest.

References

1. Fatima, K.; Moridpour, S.; De Gruyter, C.; Saghapour, T. Elderly Sustainable Mobility: Scientific Paper Review. *Sustainability* **2020**, *12*, 7319. [CrossRef]
2. Peng, B.; Wang, L.; Wu, J.; Li, C.; Wang, T.; Yuan, S.; Zhang, Y. Association between Built Environment and Bus Usage among Older Adults: Urban–Rural Differences in the Nonlinearities. *ISPRS Int. J. Geo-Inf.* **2024**, *13*, 316. [CrossRef]
3. Cheng, L.; Chen, X.; Yang, S.; Cao, Z.; De Vos, J.; Witlox, F. Active travel for active ageing in China: The role of built environment. *J. Transp. Geogr.* **2019**, *76*, 142–152. [CrossRef]

4. World Health Organization. *China Country Assessment Report on Ageing and Health*; WHO: Geneva, Switzerland, 2015.
5. United Nations. *World Population Ageing*; Department of Economic and Social Affairs: New York City, NY, USA, 2017.
6. Murray, A.T.; Grubesic, T.H. Locational planning of health care facilities. In *Spatial Analysis in Health Geography*; Routledge: London, UK, 2016; pp. 243–260.
7. Xiaohelaiti, X.; Liu, X.; Li, C.; Wang, T.; Wu, J.; Peng, B.; Zhang, Y. Neighborhood environment and body mass index in community-dwelling older adults in China: The mediating role of transport-related physical activity. *Geriatr. Nurs.* **2024**, *55*, 304–310. [CrossRef]
8. Prince, M.J.; Wu, F.; Guo, Y.; Gutierrez Robledo, L.M.; O'Donnell, M.; Sullivan, R.; Yusuf, S. The burden of disease in older people and implications for health policy and practice. *Lancet* **2015**, *385*, 549–562. [CrossRef]
9. Dewulf, B.; Neutens, T.; De Weerdt, Y.; Van de Weghe, N. Accessibility to primary health care in Belgium: An evaluation of policies awarding financial assistance in shortage areas. *BMC Fam. Pract.* **2013**, *14*, 122. [CrossRef]
10. Widener, M.J.; Hatzopoulou, M. Contextualizing research on transportation and health: A systems perspective. *J. Transp. Health* **2016**, *3*, 232–239. [CrossRef]
11. Cvitkovich, Y.; Wister, A. The importance of transportation and prioritization of environmental needs to sustain well-being among older adults. *Environ. Behav.* **2001**, *33*, 809–829. [CrossRef]
12. Hiscock, R.; Pearce, J.; Blakely, T.; Witten, K. Is neighborhood access to health care provision associated with individual-level utilization and satisfaction? *Health Serv. Res.* **2008**, *43*, 2183–2200. [CrossRef]
13. Satariano, W.A.; Guralnik, J.M.; Jackson, R.J.; Marottoli, R.A.; Phelan, E.A.; Prohaska, T.R. Mobility and aging: New directions for public health action. *Am. J. Public Health* **2012**, *102*, 1508–1515. [CrossRef]
14. Cheng, L.; Caset, F.; De Vos, J.; Derudder, B.; Witlox, F. Investigating walking accessibility to recreational amenities for elderly people in Nanjing, China. *Transp. Res. Part D Transp. Environ.* **2019**, *76*, 85–99. [CrossRef]
15. Lucas, K.; Van Wee, B.; Maat, K. A method to evaluate equitable accessibility: Combining ethical theories and accessibility-based approaches. *Transportation* **2016**, *43*, 473–490. [CrossRef]
16. Ricciardi, A.M.; Xia, J.C.; Currie, G. Exploring public transport equity between separate disadvantaged cohorts: A case study in Perth, Australia. *J. Transp. Geogr.* **2015**, *43*, 111–122. [CrossRef]
17. Roopani; Dumka, N.; Ahmad, T.; Hannah, E.; Kotwal, A. Health facility utilization and Healthcare-seeking behaviour of the elderly population in India. *J. Fam. Med. Prim. Care* **2023**, *12*, 902–916. [CrossRef] [PubMed]
18. Charney, I. Re-planning an edge city: Tysons in the post-suburban era. *Cities* **2020**, *106*, 102919. [CrossRef]
19. Gu, X.; Zhou, H.; Zhang, L. Spatial Accessibility Assessment of Healthcare Services and Governance Optimization in New Urban Areas of Megacity: The Case of Five New Towns in Shanghai. *Urban Stud.* **2022**, *29*, 20–26.
20. Wang, L.; Kundu, R.; Chen, X. Building for what and whom? New town development as planned suburbanization in China and India. In *Suburbanization in Global Society*; Emerald Group Publishing Limited: Bradford, UK, 2010; Volume 10, pp. 319–345.
21. Wang, K.L.J.; Wang, H. *China's New Town and New District 40 Years: Process, Evaluation, and Prospect*; China Architecture & Building Press: Beijing, China, 2021.
22. Powell, B. Inside China's runaway building boom. *Time Magazine*, 5 April 2010.
23. Hansen, W.G. How accessibility shapes land use. *J. Am. Inst. Plan.* **1959**, *25*, 73–76. [CrossRef]
24. Morris, J.M.; Dumble, P.L.; Wigan, M.R. Accessibility indicators for transport planning. *Transp. Res. Part A Gen.* **1979**, *13*, 91–109. [CrossRef]
25. Penchansky, R.; Thomas, J.W. The concept of access: Definition and relationship to consumer satisfaction. *Med. Care* **1981**, *19*, 127–140. [CrossRef]
26. Luo, W.; Wang, F. Measures of spatial accessibility to health care in a GIS environment: Synthesis and a case study in the Chicago region. *Environ. Plan. B Plan. Des.* **2003**, *30*, 865–884. [CrossRef]
27. Abernathy, W.J.; Hershey, J.C. A spatial-allocation model for regional health-services planning. *Oper. Res.* **1972**, *20*, 629–642. [CrossRef]
28. Alegana, V.A.; Wright, J.A.; Pentrina, U.; Noor, A.M.; Snow, R.W.; Atkinson, P.M. Spatial modelling of healthcare utilisation for treatment of fever in Namibia. *Int. J. Health Geogr.* **2012**, *11*, 6. [CrossRef] [PubMed]
29. Mayhew, L.D.; Leonardi, G. Equity, efficiency, and accessibility in urban and regional health-care systems. *Environ. Plan. A* **1982**, *14*, 1479–1507. [CrossRef]
30. Tanser, F.; Gething, P.; Atkinson, P. Location-allocation Planning. In *A Companion to Health and Medical Geography*; Wiley: Hoboken, NJ, USA, 2009; pp. 540–566.
31. Wang, F. Measurement, optimization, and impact of health care accessibility: A methodological review. *Ann. Assoc. Am. Geogr.* **2012**, *102*, 1104–1112. [CrossRef]
32. Wang, F. *Quantitative Methods and Socio-Economic Applications in GIS*; CRC Press: Boca Raton, FL, USA, 2014.
33. Kwan, M.P.; Weber, J. Individual accessibility revisited: Implications for geographical analysis in the twenty-first century. *Geogr. Anal.* **2003**, *35*, 341–353.
34. Neutens, T.; Schwanen, T.; Witlox, F.; De Maeyer, P. Equity of urban service delivery: A comparison of different accessibility measures. *Environ. Plan. A* **2010**, *42*, 1613–1635. [CrossRef]
35. Guagliardo, M.F. Spatial accessibility of primary care: Concepts, methods and challenges. *Int. J. Health Geogr.* **2004**, *3*, 3. [CrossRef]

36. Neutens, T. Accessibility, equity and health care: Review and research directions for transport geographers. *J. Transp. Geogr.* **2015**, *43*, 14–27. [CrossRef]
37. Langford, M.; Higgs, G. Measuring potential access to primary healthcare services: The influence of alternative spatial representations of population. *Prof. Geogr.* **2006**, *58*, 294–306. [CrossRef]
38. Mao, L.; Nekorchuk, D. Measuring spatial accessibility to healthcare for populations with multiple transportation modes. *Health Place* **2013**, *24*, 115–122. [CrossRef]
39. Rauch, S.; Stangl, S.; Haas, T.; Rauh, J.; Heuschmann, P.U. Spatial inequalities in preventive breast cancer care: A comparison of different accessibility approaches for prevention facilities in Bavaria, Germany. *J. Transp. Health* **2023**, *29*, 101567. [CrossRef]
40. Dai, D. Black residential segregation, disparities in spatial access to health care facilities, and late-stage breast cancer diagnosis in metropolitan Detroit. *Health Place* **2010**, *16*, 1038–1052. [CrossRef] [PubMed]
41. Dai, D.; Wang, F. Geographic disparities in accessibility to food stores in southwest Mississippi. *Environ. Plan. B Plan. Des.* **2011**, *38*, 659–677. [CrossRef]
42. Luo, W.; Qi, Y. An enhanced two-step floating catchment area (E2SFCA) method for measuring spatial accessibility to primary care physicians. *Health Place* **2009**, *15*, 1100–1107. [CrossRef]
43. Wan, N.; Zou, B.; Sternberg, T. A three-step floating catchment area method for analyzing spatial access to health services. *Int. J. Geogr. Inf. Sci.* **2012**, *26*, 1073–1089. [CrossRef]
44. Luo, J. Integrating the huff model and floating catchment area methods to analyze spatial access to healthcare services. *Trans. GIS* **2014**, *18*, 436–448. [CrossRef]
45. Luo, J. Analyzing potential spatial access to primary care services with an enhanced floating catchment area method. *Cartogr. Int. J. Geogr. Inf. Geovisualization* **2016**, *51*, 12–24. [CrossRef]
46. Tao, Z.; Wang, Q. Facility or Transport Inequality? Decomposing Healthcare Accessibility Inequality in Shenzhen, China. *Int. J. Environ. Res. Public Health* **2022**, *19*, 6897. [CrossRef] [PubMed]
47. Xing, J.; Ng, S.T. Analyzing spatiotemporal accessibility patterns to tertiary healthcare services by integrating total travel cost into an improved E3SFCA method in Changsha, China. *Cities* **2022**, *122*, 103541. [CrossRef]
48. Cheng, L.; Yang, M.; De Vos, J.; Witlox, F. Examining geographical accessibility to multi-tier hospital care services for the elderly: A focus on spatial equity. *J. Transp. Health* **2020**, *19*, 100926. [CrossRef]
49. Lechowski, Ł. Effects of choice of data aggregation method to a point on walking accessibility results using the G2SFCA method. *Pr. Kom. Geogr. Komun. PTG* **2022**, *25*, 74–93. [CrossRef]
50. Zainab, U.I.; Kruger, E.; Tennant, M. Major metropolis rail system access to dental care for the retired and elderly: A high-resolution geographic study of Sydney, Australia. *Gerodontology* **2015**, *32*, 302–308. [CrossRef]
51. Evans, R.; Larkins, S.; Cheffins, T.; Fleming, R.; Johnston, K.; Tennant, M. Mapping access to health services as a strategy for planning: Access to primary care for older people in regional Queensland. *Aust. J. Prim. Health* **2017**, *23*, 114–122. [CrossRef] [PubMed]
52. Messinger-Rapport, B. Disparities in long-term healthcare. *Nurs. Clin. N. Am.* **2009**, *44*, 179–185. [CrossRef] [PubMed]
53. Yuan, Y.; Yang, M.; Wu, J.; Rasouli, S.; Lei, D. Assessing bus transit service from the perspective of elderly passengers in Harbin, China. *Int. J. Sustain. Transp.* **2019**, *13*, 761–776. [CrossRef]
54. Cheng, L.; Chen, X.; Yang, S.; Wu, J.; Yang, M. Structural equation models to analyze activity participation, trip generation, and mode choice of low-income commuters. *Transp. Lett.* **2019**, *11*, 341–349. [CrossRef]
55. Loo, B.P.; Lam, W.W.Y. Geographic accessibility around health care facilities for elderly residents in Hong Kong: A microscale walkability assessment. *Environ. Plan. B Plan. Des.* **2012**, *39*, 629–646.
56. Jin, Z.; Northridge, M.E.; Metcalf, S.S. Modeling the influence of social ties and transportation choice on access to oral healthcare for older adults. *Appl. Geogr.* **2018**, *96*, 66–76. [CrossRef]
57. Zhang, Q.; Northridge, M.E.; Jin, Z.; Metcalf, S.S. Modeling accessibility of screening and treatment facilities for older adults using transportation networks. *Appl. Geogr.* **2018**, *93*, 64–75. [CrossRef]
58. Hudson, E.; Nolan, A. Public healthcare eligibility and the utilisation of GP services by older people in Ireland. *J. Econ. Ageing* **2015**, *6*, 24–43. [CrossRef]
59. Wu, J.; Li, C.; Zhu, L.; Liu, X.; Peng, B.; Wang, T.; Yuan, S.; Zhang, Y. Nonlinear and threshold effects of built environment on older adults' walking duration: Do age and retirement status matter? *Front. Public Health* **2024**, *12*, 1418733. [CrossRef] [PubMed]
60. Kelly, C.; Hulme, C.; Farragher, T.; Clarke, G. Are differences in travel time or distance to healthcare for adults in global north countries associated with an impact on health outcomes? A systematic review. *BMJ Open* **2016**, *6*, e013059. [CrossRef]
61. Tao, Z.; Cheng, Y. Modelling the spatial accessibility of the elderly to healthcare services in Beijing, China. *Environ. Plan. B Urban Anal. City Sci.* **2019**, *46*, 1132–1147. [CrossRef]
62. Wu, H.-C.; Tseng, M.-H. Evaluating disparities in elderly community care resources: Using a geographic accessibility and inequality index. *Int. J. Environ. Res. Public Health* **2018**, *15*, 1353. [CrossRef]
63. Cheng, Y.; Wang, J.; Rosenberg, M.W. Spatial access to residential care resources in Beijing, China. *Int. J. Health Geogr.* **2012**, *11*, 32. [CrossRef]
64. Cao, M.; Zhang, Y.; Zhang, Y.; Li, S.; Hickman, R. Using different approaches to evaluate individual social equity in transport. In *A Companion to Transport, Space and Equity*; Edward Elgar Publishing: Cheltenham, UK, 2019; pp. 209–228.

65. Guzman, L.A.; Oviedo, D. Accessibility, affordability and equity: Assessing 'pro-poor'public transport subsidies in Bogotá. *Transp. Policy* **2018**, *68*, 37–51. [CrossRef]
66. Shinjo, D.; Aramaki, T. Geographic distribution of healthcare resources, healthcare service provision, and patient flow in Japan: A cross sectional study. *Soc. Sci. Med.* **2012**, *75*, 1954–1963. [CrossRef]
67. Lee, K.-S. Disparity in the spatial distribution of clinics within a metropolitan city. *Geospat. Health* **2013**, *7*, 199–207. [CrossRef] [PubMed]
68. Song, X.; Wei, Y.; Deng, W.; Zhang, S.; Zhou, P.; Liu, Y.; Wan, J. Spatio-temporal distribution, spillover effects and influences of China's two levels of public healthcare resources. *Int. J. Environ. Res. Public Health* **2019**, *16*, 582. [CrossRef]
69. Shen, J.; Wu, F. The suburb as a space of capital accumulation: The development of new towns in Shanghai, China. *Antipode* **2017**, *49*, 761–780. [CrossRef]
70. Pan, J.; Zhao, H.; Wang, X.; Shi, X. Assessing spatial access to public and private hospitals in Sichuan, China: The influence of the private sector on the healthcare geography in China. *Soc. Sci. Med.* **2016**, *170*, 35–45. [CrossRef] [PubMed]
71. Zhang, S.; Song, X.; Wei, Y.; Deng, W. Spatial equity of multilevel healthcare in the metropolis of Chengdu, China: A new assessment approach. *Int. J. Environ. Res. Public Health* **2019**, *16*, 493. [CrossRef] [PubMed]
72. Yu, W.; Li, M.; Ye, F.; Xue, C.; Zhang, L. Patient preference and choice of healthcare providers in Shanghai, China: A cross-sectional study. *BMJ Open* **2017**, *7*, e016418. [CrossRef] [PubMed]
73. Yang, T.; Luo, W.; Tian, L.; Li, J. Integrating Spatial and Non-Spatial Dimensions to Evaluate Access to Rural Primary Healthcare Service: A Case Study of Songzi, China. *ISPRS Int. J. Geo-Inf.* **2024**, *13*, 142. [CrossRef]
74. Liu, L.; Zhao, Y.; Lyu, H.; Chen, S.; Tu, Y.; Huang, S. Spatial Accessibility and Equity Evaluation of Medical Facilities Based on Improved 2SFCA: A Case Study in Xi'an, China. *Int. J. Environ. Res. Public Health* **2023**, *20*, 2076. [CrossRef]
75. Luo, W.; Whippo, T. Variable catchment sizes for the two-step floating catchment area (2SFCA) method. *Health Place* **2012**, *18*, 789–795. [CrossRef]
76. Qian, Z.; Liu, Q.; Huang, D. Three Scales and Planning Trends of 15-Minute Life Circle. *Urban Plan. Int.* **2022**, *37*, 63–70.
77. Wu, W.; Zheng, T. Establishing a "dynamic two-step floating catchment area method" to assess the accessibility of urban green space in Shenyang based on dynamic population data and multiple modes of transportation. *Urban For. Urban Green.* **2023**, *82*, 127893. [CrossRef]
78. Hu, Y.; Zhang, Z. Skilled doctors in tertiary hospitals are already overworked in China. *Lancet Glob. Health* **2015**, *3*, e737. [CrossRef]
79. Weinert, J.X.; Ma, C.; Yang, X. *The Transition to Electric Bikes in China and Its Effect on Travel Behavior, Transit Use, and Safety*; UC Davis: Institute of Transportation Studies: Davis, CA, USA, 2006.
80. Peng, B.; Zhang, Y.; Li, C.; Wang, T.; Yuan, S. Nonlinear, threshold and synergistic effects of first/last-mile facilities on metro ridership. *Transp. Res. Part D Transp. Environ.* **2023**, *121*, 103856. [CrossRef]
81. Zhang, J.; Lin, D.; Zhou, X.; Li, F.; Zhou, Y.M.; Cheng, Y.Q.; Wang, P. Spatial accessibility and equality of public medical facilities in rural areas based on the improved 3SFCA: A case of Haikou City. *Prog. Geogr.* **2022**, *41*, 636–647. [CrossRef]
82. Li, Y.; Chen, Q.; Ma, Q.; Yu, H.; Huang, Y.; Zhu, L.; Zhang, H.; Li, C.; Lu, G. Injuries and risk factors associated with bicycle and electric bike use in China: A systematic review and meta-analysis. *Saf. Sci.* **2022**, *152*, 105769. [CrossRef]
83. Bohannon, R.W. Comfortable and maximum walking speed of adults aged 20–79 years: Reference values and determinants. *Age Ageing* **1997**, *26*, 15–19. [CrossRef]
84. Zhang, F.; Li, D.; Ahrentzen, S.; Zhang, J. Assessing spatial disparities of accessibility to community-based service resources for Chinese older adults based on travel behavior: A city-wide study of Nanjing, China. *Habitat Int.* **2019**, *88*, 101984. [CrossRef]
85. Jin, T.; Cheng, L.; Wang, K.; Cao, J.; Huang, H.; Witlox, F. Examining equity in accessibility to multi-tier healthcare services across different income households using estimated travel time. *Transp. Policy* **2022**, *121*, 1–13. [CrossRef]
86. Li, C.; Wang, J. A hierarchical two-step floating catchment area analysis for high-tier hospital accessibility in an urban agglomeration region. *J. Transp. Geogr.* **2022**, *102*, 103369. [CrossRef]
87. Bauer, J.; Groneberg, D.A. Measuring spatial accessibility of health care providers–introduction of a variable distance decay function within the floating catchment area (FCA) method. *PLoS ONE* **2016**, *11*, e0159148. [CrossRef]
88. Del Conte, D.E.; Locascio, A.; Amoruso, J.; McNamara, M.L. Modeling multimodal access to primary care in an urban environment. *Transp. Res. Interdiscip. Perspect.* **2022**, *13*, 100550. [CrossRef]
89. Anselin, L. *An Introduction to Spatial Data Science with GeoDaVolume 1: Exploring Spatial Data*; CRC Press: Boca Raton, FL, USA, 2024.
90. Anselin, L. Local indicators of spatial association—LISA. *Geogr. Anal.* **1995**, *27*, 93–115. [CrossRef]
91. Wang, F. Inverted Two-Step Floating Catchment Area Method for Measuring Facility Crowdedness. *Prof. Geogr.* **2018**, *70*, 251–260. [CrossRef]
92. Wang, C.; Leitner, M.; Paulus, G. Multiscale Analysis of Spatial Accessibility to Acute Hospitals in Carinthia, Austria. *ISPRS Int. J. Geo-Inf.* **2023**, *12*, 491. [CrossRef]
93. Cheng, M.; Tao, L.; Lian, Y.; Huang, W. Measuring Spatial Accessibility of Urban Medical Facilities: A Case Study in Changning District of Shanghai in China. *Int. J. Environ. Res. Public Health* **2021**, *18*, 9598. [CrossRef] [PubMed]
94. Gu, X.; Zhang, L.; Tao, S.; Xie, B. Spatial Accessibility to Healthcare Services in Metropolitan Suburbs: The Case of Qingpu, Shanghai. *Int. J. Environ. Res. Public Health* **2019**, *16*, 225. [CrossRef] [PubMed]

95. Siegel, M.; Koller, D.; Vogt, V.; Sundmacher, L. Developing a composite index of spatial accessibility across different health care sectors: A German example. *Health Policy* **2016**, *120*, 205–212. [CrossRef] [PubMed]
96. Liu, T.Y.; Deng, Q.T.; Wang, S.Y.; Wang, G.B. Equity Evaluation of Multilevel Medical Facility Allocation Based on Ga2SFCA. *J. Urban Plan. Dev.* **2023**, *149*, 04023041. [CrossRef]
97. Shao, Y.; Luo, W. Supply-demand adjusted two-steps floating catchment area (SDA-2SFCA) model for measuring spatial access to health care. *Soc. Sci. Med.* **2022**, *296*, 114727. [CrossRef]

International Journal of
Geo-Information

MDPI

Article

Space–Time Analysis of the COVID-19 Pandemic and Its Relationship with Socioeconomic and Demographic Variables in the Metropolitan Region of São Paulo, Brazil

Keila Valente de Souza de Santana [1,*], Aluízio Marino [1], Gabriela Rosa Martins [2], Pedro Henrique Barbosa Muniz Lima [1], Pedro Henrique Rezende Mendonça [3] and Raquel Rolnik [1]

[1] Faculty of Architecture and Urban Planning, University of São Paulo, São Paulo 05508-080, Brazil; aluizio.marino@usp.br (A.M.); pedro.barbosa.lima@usp.br (P.H.B.M.L.); raquelrolnik@usp.br (R.R.)
[2] Faculty of Philosophy, Literature and Human Sciences, University of São Paulo, São Paulo 05508-080, Brazil; gmartins@usp.br
[3] Institute of Mathematics and Statistics, University of São Paulo, São Paulo 05508-090, Brazil; pedro.rezende.mendonca@alumni.usp.br
* Correspondence: keilla@usp.br

Abstract: This study sought to identify clusters of a high and low risk of incidence and mortality from COVID-19 throughout the pandemic period, from 2020 to 2022, in the Metropolitan Region of São Paulo (MRSP), analyzing their relationship with socioeconomic and demographic variables. Spatiotemporal and temporal variations in the clusters were determined using scan statistics, a multidimensional point process that performs multiple tests for each geographic point analyzed, in SaTScan v10.0. Socioeconomic and demographic differences were analyzed using the nonparametric Mann–Whitney and Kruskal–Wallis tests. Temporal clusters of high incidence and high mortality were observed in May 2020 and March to June 2021. In the spatiotemporal analysis, the clusters of high incidence and high mortality were concentrated in the city of São Paulo and neighboring cities, indicating that the capital was an area of influence and convergence at all times during the COVID-19 pandemic. Clusters of low mortality were found in the central region of the capital, which concentrates the highest incomes and the lowest percentages of Black, mixed-race, and Indigenous people in the MRSP. All clusters were identified in densely occupied areas and point to a pattern of disease spread that is related to income and ethnicity, as well as to the circulation dynamics of a metropolitan region.

Keywords: COVID-19; space–time cluster; Metropolitan Region of São Paulo; population density; socioeconomic variables

1. Introduction

The COVID-19 (coronavirus disease 2019) pandemic, an infectious disease caused by the highly transmissible coronavirus SARS-CoV-2 (Severe Acute Respiratory Syndrome—Coronavirus-2), was first detected in December 2019 in the People's Republic of China [1]. In Brazil, at the national level, measures such as social distancing, lockdowns, and extensive testing to track the disease were severely hampered by political bias. The number of deaths and people infected by COVID-19 increased steadily in the first months of the pandemic [2], and the rapid spread of the virus triggered heterogeneous health and social repercussions across Brazil's states and municipalities [3].

São Paulo, Brazil's most populous state (45 million inhabitants), was severely affected by COVID-19, leading the state government to declare the closure of businesses, schools, and other non-essential services. Initially, the virus spread rapidly in the capital, also called São Paulo, and its metropolitan region, where the first case of the disease was identified in Brazil. Although the capital was a hotspot for the disease, with the highest number of cases at the beginning of the pandemic, cases quickly spread to neighboring municipalities and the interior of the state, which had the highest rate in the country during this period [3,4].

Without a country-wide policy, measures to restrict the movement of people were adopted by some states and others by municipalities, which generated different epidemiological scenarios. The strategies adopted to control the COVID-19 pandemic in the Metropolitan Region of São Paulo (MRSP), such as social isolation, were sometimes established independently by the municipalities that comprise it, without taking into account territorial specificities and the links between them. MRSP, with 20 million inhabitants, is the largest city in the country and is characterized by a high level of interdependence between the municipalities and high levels of circulation density in the public transportation system, with millions of commuters using buses, trains, and the subway daily [5]. Jobs, businesses, and economic opportunities are highly concentrated in the capital, the center of MRSP, where a higher-income population lives. The combination of a high degree of internal circulation density with exclusively municipal restrictions, which did not consider this metropolitan area's territorial dynamics, may have contributed to the ineffectiveness in controlling the spread of the disease.

The inclusion of the territorial dimension as a non-pharmacological action to combat the COVID-19 pandemic is still essential today, given the risk of the emergence and re-emergence of diseases. Therefore, the spatial analysis of the spread of the disease, through geographic information systems (GIS), not only contributes to the elaboration of territorial scenarios that could have guided and enabled strategic actions but can also guide current policies that mitigate the effects of socio-territorial inequalities on health [6]. Therefore, this study sought to identify areas with a high and low risk of incidence and mortality from COVID-19 throughout the pandemic period, from 2020 to 2022, in the MRSP, analyzing their relationship with socioeconomic and demographic variables and considering the urban territorial dynamics of a metropolis. Our hypothesis is that the use of a congested public transportation system which had not put in place any protection measures by inhabitants of peripheral regions may have influenced the dynamics of contamination of the local population through community transmission of COVID-19.

Through the development of geoinformation technologies, detailed analyses and visualizations of the propagation patterns of the COVID-19 pandemic still play an important role in understanding spatial clusters and trends in SARS-CoV-2 transmission. This article used the free software SaTScan (an abbreviation for Space and Time Scan Statistics) that can detect increased disease activity without a priori specification of the time period, geographic location, or size. As a recognized surveillance tool, the detection of "active" and "emerging" spatiotemporal clusters of COVID-19 in Brazil was mainly carried out at the municipal scale during the COVID-19 pandemic [4,7,8]. Through prospective spatiotemporal scanning analysis of the disease, they assessed whether the mortality rate, the GINI index, and social inequality were predictors of the relative risk of each cluster through a Generalized Linear Model (GLM) among Brazilian municipalities [8]. Our study is the first in Brazil to detect spatial–temporal clusters of COVID-19 cases and deaths on a more detailed scale, in areas of the São Paulo Metropolitan Region, and to assess the socioeconomic and demographic differences between them throughout the pandemic period. Despite being a retrospective study, we seek to disseminate a viable method of health surveillance that can be carried out during health emergencies and that considers the particularities of a metropolitan urban territory in local decision-making, where regional dynamics are sometimes disregarded.

2. Study Site

The MRSP is the largest city in South America and the sixth largest in the world, according to a 2014 United Nations (UN) report [5]. The MRSP is made up of 39 municipalities (Figure 1), including São Paulo, the capital of the state of São Paulo and the MRSP's center. The municipalities in this region, which are distributed into five sub-regions, are listed below:

i. North: Caieiras, Cajamar, Francisco Morato, Franco da Rocha, and Mairiporã.

ii. East: Arujá, Biritiba-Mirim, Ferraz de Vasconcelos, Guararema, Guarulhos, Itaquaquecetuba, Mogi das Cruzes, Poá, Salesópolis, Santa Isabel, and Suzano.
iii. Southeast: Diadema, Mauá, Ribeirão Pires, Rio Grande da Serra, Santo André, São Bernardo do Campo, and São Caetano do Sul.
iv. Southwest: Cotia, Embu, Embu-Guaçu, Itapecerica da Serra, Juquitiba, São Lourenço da Serra, Taboão da Serra, and Vargem Grande Paulista.
v. West: Barueri, Carapicuíba, Itapevi, Jandira, Osasco, Pirapora do Bom Jesus, and Santana de Parnaíba.

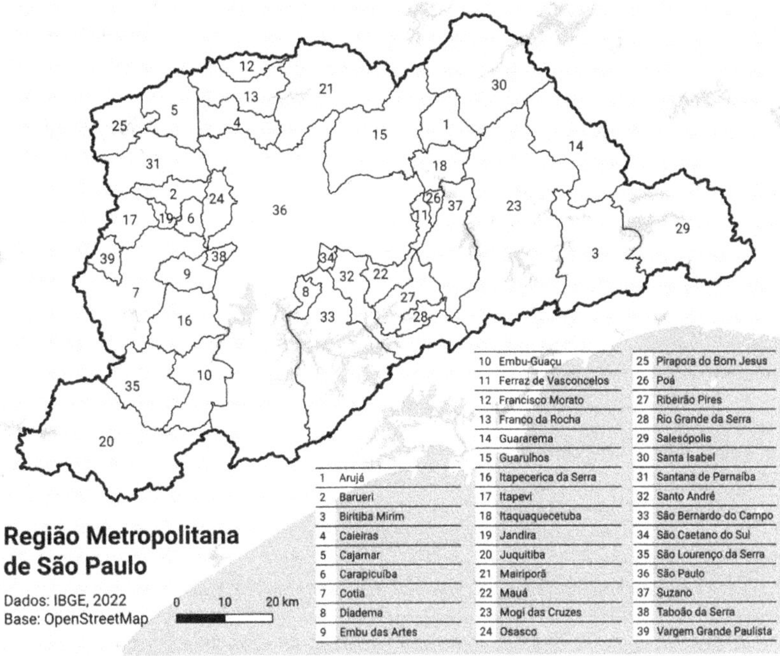

Figure 1. Map showing the municipalities of the MRSP. Source: IBGE.

The capital is home to 12,330,000 inhabitants; it is the economic epicenter of the country and is a global city. In addition to São Paulo, the municipalities of Guarulhos, São Bernardo, Santo André, and Osasco have significant populations exceeding 700,000 inhabitants. Two cities in the region have the highest population densities in Brazil: Taboão da Serra and Diadema, with 13,400 and 12,800 inhabitants per km^2, respectively [6].

It is worth noting that population and economic activity are not evenly distributed throughout the metropolitan area. The MRSP is home to municipalities with a very complex economy, such as São Paulo, Guarulhos, Osasco, Barueri and the municipalities of ABC (santo André, Sao Bernardo, São Caetano, Mauá and Diadema), as well as municipalities with less economic weight, such as Francisco Morato, and mostly ones like Juquitiba. Most of those more densely populated municipalities also have the highest numbers of daily commuters to the capital [9].

3. Materials and Methods

This is an ecological and descriptive study assessing secondary data about the incidence and mortality of COVID-19 in the 633 weighting areas of the 39 municipalities that comprise the MRSP. Weighting areas (WA) are territorial units identified by sets of contiguous census sectors belonging to the same district, for the purpose of weighting the results of the population census sample questionnaire. A census sector is a territorial unit established for survey control purposes, comprising a continuous area located in a single urban or rural block, with a size and number of households that allow the survey by a census agent [10].

Information from the period March 2020 to February 2022 about the date of notification, sex, age, disease progression, and postal code of each patient with COVID-19 who recovered or died was accessed through a partnership with the Data Center of the State of São Paulo (CDESP), which provided data from the Epidemiological Surveillance System (SIVEP-Gripe) of the State Epidemiological Surveillance Center. These data were grouped by postal code (first five digits of the postal code) and georeferenced using the postal code database of the Centro de Estudos da Metrópole (Center for Metropolitan Studies) [11]. Linear geometries of the postal code grouping system were intersected with the weighting areas from the 2010 IBGE Census, with cases assigned proportionally to the length of the intersected lines. This study was approved by the Research Ethics Committee of the School of Psychology, Universidade de São Paulo, report number CAAE: 71605223.2.0000.5561, 14 August 2023.

The socioeconomic variables—per capita income, persons per household, and percentage of Black, Brown (mixed-race), and Indigenous people (BBIP)—by WA were built based on data from the Brazilian Institute of Geography and Statistics (IBGE), according to the 2010 census, the most recent census available. The variables were selected according to bibliographic references that analyzed the relationship between COVID-19 spread and socioeconomic factors [6–8].

Dasymetric mapping techniques were used to analyze the population density, which subdivide areas of origin into smaller spatial units so that there is greater internal consistency of the variable being mapped [12]. In this study, the variable of population density was calculated by dividing the number of inhabitants in WA by the total area built for residential purposes in that area. This analysis used Google Open Buildings, a large-scale open dataset that contains the vectorization of building roof contours generated from a deep learning model that was trained to determine building areas from high-resolution satellite images. Data are available under the Creative Commons Attribution license (CC BY-4.0) and the Open Data Commons Open Database License (ODbL) v1.0 [13].

The analyses were performed using the incidence and mortality rates for COVID-19 obtained for the 633 weighted areas of the 39 municipalities of the MRSP from March 2020 to February 2021, Year 1, and from March 2021 to February 2022, Year 2. To detect spatiotemporal clusters, the SaTScan v10.0 software was used, which uses a scanning window that varies in both space and time. This window spans examining different geographic regions and periods to identify where there is an anomalous concentration of the event [14]. Thus, the scanning window is an interval in time, a circle or an ellipse in space, or a cylinder with a circular or elliptical base in space–time, as in our study in which multiple different window sizes were used. The Poisson probability distribution model was used, which counts cases and deaths in space and time [15]. The cluster analysis model was built with the following conditions: COVID-19 cases and deaths were grouped by month, without cluster overlap, with circular clusters; the proportion of the population considered was 10% for the spatial scanning window, calculated by the Gini index in SatScan for purely spatial analysis. This option encourages the search for smaller true clusters and can be characterized as a coefficient of population inequality [14]. We also calculated the RR (relative risk) of COVID-19 occurrence and mortality, considering each WA and clusters in relation to the surrounding areas.

In SaTScan, the expected number of cases is estimated based on the spatial and temporal distribution of the population. In our study, no population adjustment was necessary, since the population did not vary substantially in the territory and period analyzed. However, the rates were adjusted for sex and age, as they are potential confounders for the outcome analyzed. Thus, the software calculated the expected cases in each location, taking into account the expected cases and deaths in each demographic group. This means that the expected number of cases was adjusted to reflect the age and gender structure of the population in each location, by comparing the proportion of observed cases with those that would be expected for that demographic composition. In the case of COVID-19, the risk catching of the disease was higher among the elderly, and the software adjusted the expected cases to take this into account when a location has a predominantly elderly population. This type of adjustment ensures that the clusters identified reflect a real risk, and not just differences in the demographic structure of the population [14,15].

Statistical tests were calculated using the likelihood ratio. The null hypothesis (H0) is that the observed number of cases is the same as the expected number. The alternative hypothesis (H1) is that the number of observed cases and deaths exceeds the expected number of cases derived from the null model. The window with the maximum likelihood is the most likely cluster, meaning that the observed data are more likely under the hypothesis that a cluster exists, indicating a possible focus of concentration of cases. SaTScan uses this measure to assess whether the number of events in a region or period is higher than expected, taking into account the overall incidence rate outside the scanning window. The likelihood ratio therefore serves as the criterion for identifying where and when clusters are present, with the cluster with the highest likelihood ratio being identified as the most likely. A *p*-value is assigned to the cluster. Results with a *p*-value < 0.05 using 999 Monte Carlo simulations were considered significant [15].

After identifying the space–time clusters, we statistically compared the values of the demographic and socioeconomic variables of the group of WAs belonging to high-mortality clusters to low-mortality clusters and between high-incidence clusters. Then, we compared the values of the groups for variables using the Mann–Whitney and Kruskal–Wallis non-parametric tests for the non-normal distribution of data. The null hypothesis was that the medians and interquartile ranges for the same variable were equal, with a significance level of 5%.

SaTScan™ version 10.0.1 (Kulldorff, Harvard Medical School, Boston, MA, USA), which uses geographical coordinates [14], was used to identify cases grouped in space–time and time. Maps with significant clusters and their relative risks from the space–time analyses were generated in QGIS 3.28. Temporal trends were obtained in SatScan. The significance level was set at $p = 0.05$. R 4.3.2 for Mac was used for database manipulation and statistical analysis.

4. Results

A total of 191,083 cases of COVID-19 were reported in the MRSP between March 2020 and February 2022. According to the progression of the patient's condition, the notifications were either recovery or death. This study was conducted in two periods, from March 2020 to February 2021 and from March 2021 to February 2022. In the first period of the pandemic, 100,587 cases were reported, with an annual rate of 512.9 cases per 100,000 inhabitants. In the second period of the pandemic, 89,783 cases were reported, with an annual rate of 457.8 cases per 100,000 inhabitants.

4.1. Incidence Clusters

In temporal terms (Figure 2A), a high-incidence cluster was identified in the first period of the pandemic in May (relative risk [RR] = 3.07), while a low-incidence cluster was present from August to October 2020 (RR = 0.47). The high-incidence cluster interval identified in the second period of the pandemic was from March to June, with RR ranging from 1.78 to 3.58. A low-incidence period was also identified, beginning in July (RR = 0.87) (Figure 2B).

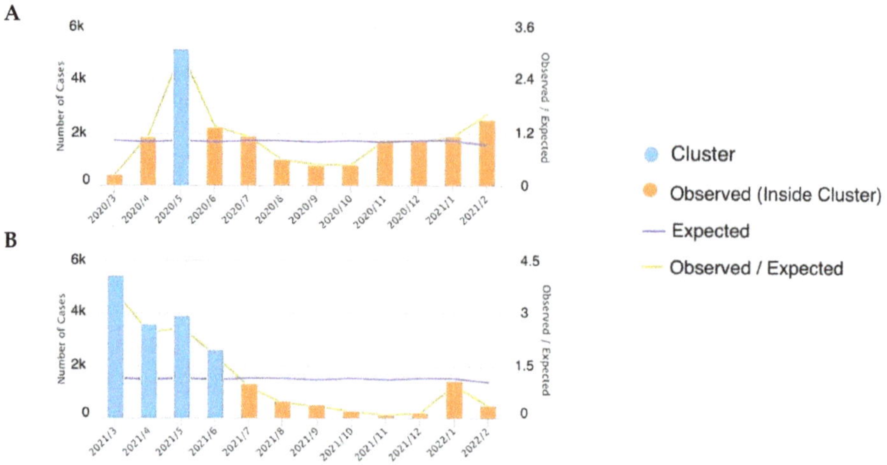

Figure 2. Distribution of COVID-19 cases in the MRSP. (**A**) Seasonal analysis showing the months of low and high risk in Year 1 (March 2020 to February 2021). (**B**) Seasonal analysis showing the months of low and high risk in Year 2 (March 2021 to February 2022).

In the first period of the pandemic, three significant high-incidence clusters were identified using the space–time scan statistics of the total number of cases (Figure 3A). All were located in the capital, the municipality of São Paulo, and neighboring cities, particularly in May 2020. Cluster 1, located in the south region of the city of São Paulo and including the cities of Taboão, Embu, Itapecerica da Serra, Embu-Guaçu, Diadema, and São Bernardo do Campo, showed the highest relative risk (RR = 3.2; p-value < 0.001), followed by cluster 3 (RR = 2.2; p-value < 0.001), located in the northwest region of the capital and including part of the cities of Cajamar and Osasco, and cluster 2 (RR = 2; p-value < 0.001), located in the northeast region of the capital and including part of the city of Guarulhos and a smaller part of the city of Ferraz de Vasconcelos. No low-risk cluster was identified in this period.

In the second period of the pandemic, three space–time clusters located in the capital São Paulo and neighboring municipalities were also observed, from March to June 2021 (Figure 3B). Cluster 1, located in the south region of São Paulo and including the entire municipality of Diadema and part of Embu, Itapecerica da Serra, Embu-Guaçu and São Bernardo do Campo, displayed a high relative risk (RR = 2.9; p-value < 0.001), followed by cluster 2 (RR = 2.9; p-value < 0.001), in the east region of the capital and including part of Guarulhos and a small portion of Ferraz de Vasconcelos, and cluster 3 (RR = 2.6; p-value < 0.001), located in the northwest region of the capital, including all municipalities of Barueri, Carapicuíba, and Osasco in this period, as well as a large part of Cajamar, Santana de Parnaíba, and Taboão da Serra, and to a smaller extent, the cities of Cotia and Itapevi.

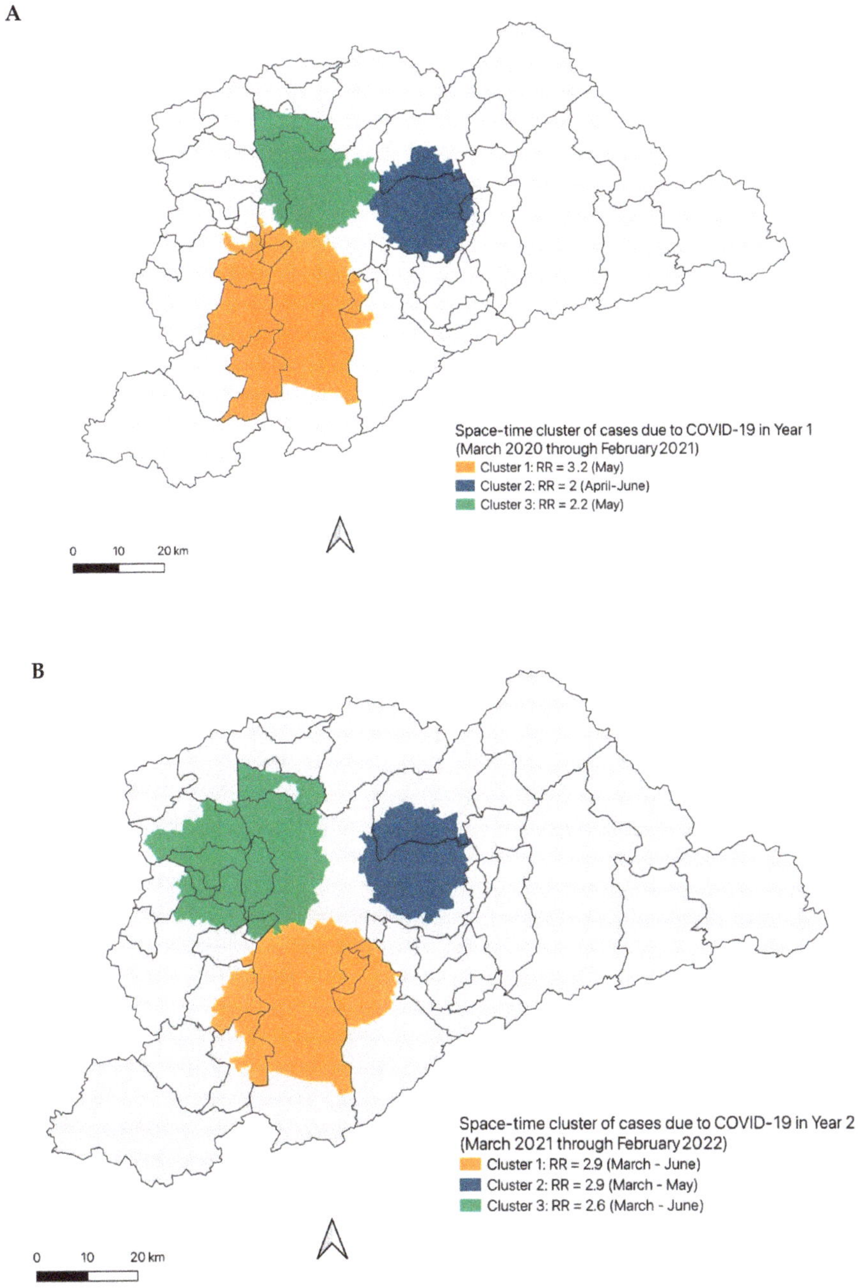

Figure 3. (**A**) Space–time clusters of COVID-19 incidence in Year 1 of the pandemic, from March 2020 to February 2021. (**B**) Space–time clusters of COVID-19 incidence in Year 2 of the pandemic, from March 2021 to February 2022.

The statistical comparison of the demographic and socioeconomic variables from the weighting areas presented in the space–time high-incidence clusters showed important differences between the three groups (Table 1). In the first period of the pandemic, all analyses resulted in significant *p*-values, except for population density. The areas in clusters 1 and 2 had a lower per capita income, a higher percentage of BBIP, and a higher number of people per household. The median per capita income of cluster 3 was more than 50% higher than those of clusters 1 and 2. The interquartile range of cluster 3 was also much higher than the first and especially the third quartile of clusters 1 and 2.

Table 1. Median and interquartile range of socioeconomic indicators of the space–time clusters of COVID-19 incidence in Year 1 (March 2020 to February 2021) and Year 2 (March 2021 to February 2022). Method: Kruskal–Wallis. Median (25^0, 75^0 percentile). * p Value < 0.001.

Variable	High-Incidence Cluster in Year 1			High-Incidence Cluster in Year 2		
	1	2	3	1	2	3
Per capita income	551 (461–881)	559 (442–719)	989 (611–1918) *	567 (469–892)	661 (513–867)	739 (521–1179) *
BBIP (%)	52 (40–56)	45 (35–54)	29 (18–42) *	50 (37–56)	40 (30–49.3)	43 (28.3–50) *
People per household	3.4 (3.2–3.5)	3.4 (3.3–3.5)	3.1 (2.8–3.4) *	3.3 (3.2–3.4)	3.3 (3.2–3.3)	3.3 (3.1–3.4)
Population density	328 (253–405)	297 (260–346)	324 (238–411)	334 (255–407)	283 (251–329)	318 (220–379) *

In the second period of the pandemic, all analyses resulted in significant *p*-values, except for the number of people per household. The areas in clusters 1 and 2 had lower per capita income when compared to cluster 3. The median per capita income in cluster 3 remained higher than those of clusters 1 and 2, by just over 10%.

4.2. Mortality Clusters

In temporal terms (Figure 4A), a high-mortality cluster was identified in the first year of the pandemic in May (relative risk [RR] = 3.7), while a low-risk cluster was present from August 2020 to January 2021 (RR = 0.53). The high-mortality interval identified in the second period of the pandemic was in March and April, with RR ranging from 5.47 to 2.77. A low-mortality period was also identified, beginning in July (RR = 0.67) (Figure 3B).

In the first year of the pandemic, seven significant high-mortality clusters were identified using the space–time scan statistics of total deaths (Figure 5A). All clusters were located in the capital or neighboring cities, in particular in May 2020. In all high-mortality clusters, the relative risk was higher than 2.7. Two low-mortality clusters were identified in the capital, one in the central area (RR = 0.33; *p*-value < 0.001), and one in the north region of the capital, near Guarulhos, from July to December 2020 (RR = 0.35; *p*-value < 0.001).

In the second year of the pandemic, four space–time high-mortality clusters were observed in the capital and neighboring cities, from March to May 2021 (Figure 5B). In all high-mortality clusters, the relative risk was higher than 3.4. A low-mortality cluster was identified in the central-south region of the capital from July to December 2021.

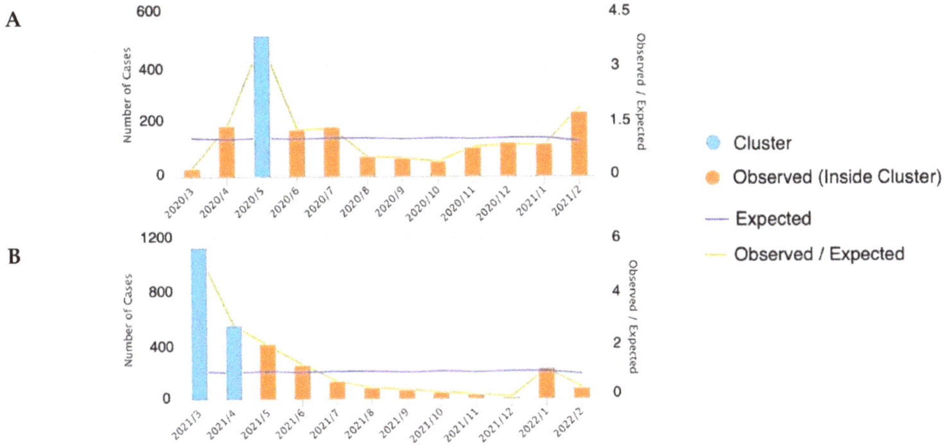

Figure 4. Distribution of deaths due to COVID-19 in the MRSP. (**A**) Seasonal analysis showing the months of the low- and high-mortality clusters in Year 1 (March 2020 to February 2021). (**B**) Seasonal analysis showing the months of low- and high-mortality clusters in Year 2 (March 2021 to February 2022).

The statistical comparison of the demographic and socioeconomic variables of the weighting areas included in the space–time high-mortality clusters for COVID-19 mortality showed important differences between the high- and low-risk groups (Table 2). In the first year of the pandemic, all analyses resulted in significant *p*-values, except for the variable of population density. The areas in the high-mortality clusters had lower per capita income, a higher percentage of BBIP, and a higher number of people per household. The median per capita income of low-risk clusters was three times higher than that of the high-mortality clusters.

In the second year of the pandemic, all analyses resulted in significant *p*-values. The areas in the high-mortality clusters had a lower per capita income than the low-mortality clusters. High-mortality clusters also had a higher percentage of BBIP and a higher number of people per household. There was no significant difference between the clusters in terms of population density in the first period of the study. In the second period of the study, the low-mortality cluster appeared to have a lower population density than the high-mortality cluster. In this case, both the internal variability of the cluster and the urban dynamics of the greater concentration of buildings in central areas need to be assessed.

Table 2. Median and interquartile range of socioeconomic indicators of the space–time clusters of COVID-19 deaths in Year 1 (March 2021 to February 2022) and Year 2 (March 2021 to February 2022). Method: Kruskal–Wallis. Median (25^0, 75^0 percentile). * p Value < 0.001.

Variable	COVID-19 Death Clusters in Year 1		COVID-19 Death Clusters in Year 2	
	High-Mortality	**Low-Mortality**	**High-Mortality**	**Low-Mortality**
Per capita income	548 (452–745)	1943 (989–3490) *	558 (454–718)	3362 (2223–3956) *
BBIP (%)	49 (38–54)	18 (9–20) *	47 (38–45)	12 (9–20) *
People per household	3.4 (3.3–3.5)	2.6 (2.4–3.1) *	3.4 (3.3–3.5)	2.5 (2.3–2.7) *
Population density	314 (243–396)	349 (268–424)	300 (238–361)	355 (256–440) *

A

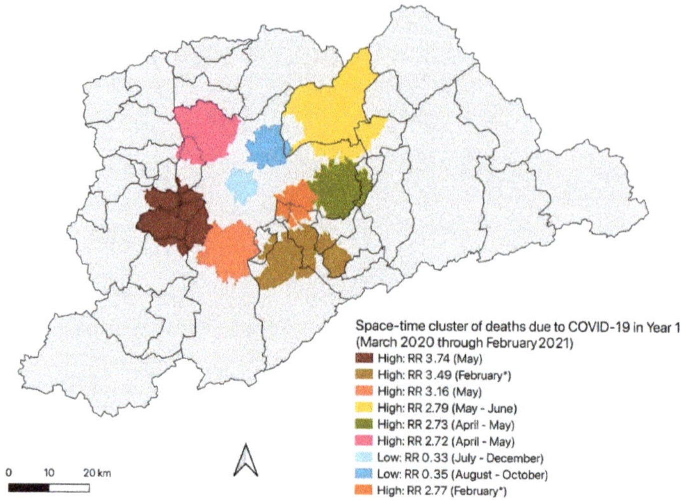

B

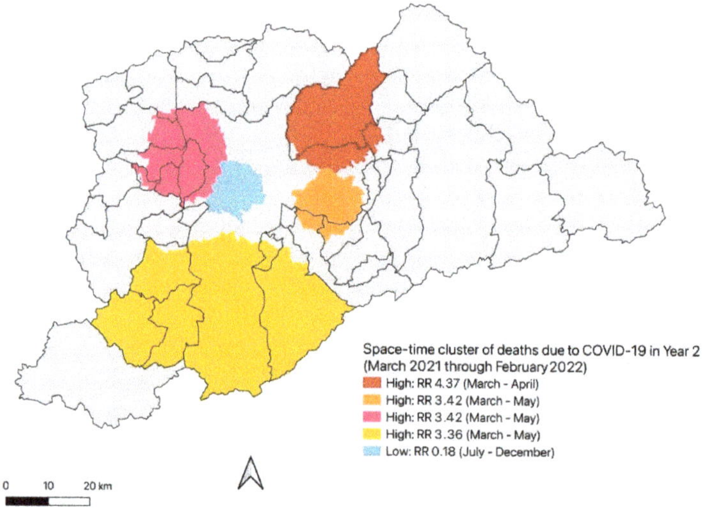

Figure 5. (**A**) Space–time clusters of COVID-19 deaths in Year 1 of the pandemic, from March 2020 to February 2021. * Year: 2021. (**B**) Space–time clusters of COVID-19 deaths in Year 2 of the pandemic, from March 2021 to February 2022.

5. Discussion

Using the multidimensional point scanning method, we identified temporal and spatiotemporal clusters of case and death notifications that demonstrated that the spread of the COVID-19 pandemic did not occur randomly or homogeneously in the MRSP. Based on surveillance data, we found that a spatiotemporal pattern of incidence and risk of death from COVID-19 during the pandemic was related to social and demographic factors and to the insertion of specific locations in the dynamics of metropolitan circulation of people and goods. The significant socioeconomic differences between the clusters express that in addition to sex, age, and comorbidities, widely discussed in the literature as mortality risk variables in relation to COVID-19, social determinants and territorial relations are also variables that can explain such an impact [4,7,8].

In the purely temporal analysis, four notable moments were identified during the two periods analyzed. In the first half of both 2020 and 2021, high-incidence clusters were identified, followed by the second half of each year, displaying low-risk clusters. In the first period (March 2020 to February 2021), after just over 2 months from the first recorded case, in May 2020, a high-incidence cluster with RR > 3 was detected, followed by a prominent decrease in risk, leading to a greater relaxation of control measures in the second half of 2020 [16].

In Brazil, although with the mandatory use of masks, crowds were promoted in the pre-election and election periods in November, in addition to the reopening of businesses and the permitting of travel in the second half of 2020 [16]. These measures, combined with the circulation of the Alpha, Gamma and Delta variants, influenced the high rate of transmission of COVID-19 in the population in early 2021 [17]. The present study reinforces this premise by identifying that the months of March to June 2021 stood out with the highest risk of incidence and mortality from the disease. The decrease in the number of cases and deaths in the region occurred from the second half of 2021, when a first dose of the vaccine had been administered to more than 50% of the population [17].

Vaccination began in February 2021, but as there were few doses available, priority was given to people with comorbidities and elderly people and did not consider socioeconomic and professional aspects, with the exception of prioritizing health professionals [18]. The poorest people who live in peripheral municipalities and needed to be at work in person and made greater use of public transportation, even though they were territorially more vulnerable and exposed to the virus, were not prioritized in the vaccination process.

In the spatiotemporal analysis, this study demonstrated that the high-incidence and high-mortality clusters were concentrated in the WA of São Paulo and neighboring municipalities, indicating that the capital was an area of influence and convergence at all times during the pandemic. Studies have already shown that COVID-19 cases began in the capital, São Paulo, and that they dispersed due to spatial contiguity, shortly after the start of the pandemic in March 2020. However, the scale of analysis in these studies was intra-urban, only in the municipality of São Paulo or inter-municipal, analyzing the dispersion throughout the state of São Paulo [3,4,6,7,19]. Our study was the first to analyze the spatiotemporal dynamics of the COVID-19 pandemic on a more detailed scale of the MRSP, WA, which is an accessible scale of spatial analysis for the entire Brazilian territory. This method pointed to a dynamic of virus dispersion that appears to be associated with an urban dynamic of regional circulation axes that involve the capital and certain neighboring municipalities.

The high-incidence spatial-temporal cluster identified between April and June 2020 in the area where Guarulhos International Airport is located, in a city neighboring São Paulo, corroborates studies that demonstrate the influence of mobility on the spread of the SARS-CoV-2 virus [3,4,8]. São Paulo/Guarulhos International Airport is the largest airport in Brazil and the second busiest in Latin America in terms of the number of passengers transported and the transportation of goods [20]. The other incidence clusters identified are in locations with a high density of people using public transportation [21].

The public transportation system in the SPMR follows a highly radial model, structured to transport passengers from the outskirts to the center, or from the neighborhoods to the radial transportation axes [21]. The areas with the highest mobility rates are located in the central region of the capital, while the areas with the highest immobility rates are located in the outskirts and in neighboring municipalities [22]. These peripheral areas of the capital and neighboring municipalities are home to the majority of the population that still needed to use public transportation to attend essential services that continued to operate in person even during the implementation of control and social distancing measures [22].

Only essential services such as food, supplies, health, banking, cleaning, and security services continued to operate in person during the pandemic [16,17]. Because of this, there was a reduction in the number of public transportation services to avoid economic losses for the companies providing these services [23]. This measure was adopted to respond to the drop in the number of passengers, which accompanied the migration of activities to remote work. However, for those whose work did not allow them to stay at home, the reduction in the number of vehicles increased waiting times for trips and, at times, increased crowding, which may have favored the transmission of the novel coronavirus [23,24].

Our study indicates that social determinants related to income and race influenced the incidence and mortality rates of the disease and need to be considered in the continuation of studies on the relationship between the territorial process of spread of the COVID-19 pandemic and urban mobility. Social behaviors, often managed by economic subsistence needs, were decisive for the pattern of virus transmission [25]. In the present analysis of the spatiotemporal clusters of disease incidence, there were statistically significant differences in the socioeconomic variables per capita income and percentage of BBIP among the three spatiotemporal clusters with the highest risk of incidence that were detected in the same period. This reflects a concentration of areas with a high risk of disease incidence also in an area of lower social vulnerability.

Despite the limitations of the analysis that considered the average of an area with widely fragmented social and economic conditions, this result expresses the need for analyses that seek to deepen the understanding of how complex socioeconomic dynamics intertwine with territorial dynamics and interfere in the spread of diseases. We understand that analyses of the relationship between health and social vulnerabilities need to be carried out spatially, as this relationship does not materialize homogeneously throughout the territory. Regarding COVID-19, although there were other municipalities that were equally or more vulnerable in the metropolitan region, they were not as affected as those where daily interaction with the capital was more frequent. In our study, clusters were identified in densely occupied areas and point to a pattern of disease spread that is related to income and ethnicity, as well as to the circulation dynamics of a metropolitan region.

Regarding COVID-19 mortality, our study reveals low- and high-mortality clusters at different times during the pandemic in the MRSP, in addition to significant differences in income and ethnicity between these clusters. It was shown that low-risk mortality clusters had a higher average per capita income, a lower BBIP percentage, and fewer people per household. The capital of São Paulo is very segregated along ethnic–racial lines. Although 36% of the capital population is Black, some high-income districts are almost 95% white [26]. Generally speaking, there has been a consolidation of the districts, places, and positions of the white social classes in the most developed, rich, and urbanized areas in the center southwest quadrant of the city, while in the distant outskirts, in the favelas and in low-income housing complexes, the Black population has become increasingly concentrated [27].

Studies show a correlation between COVID-19 mortality and socioeconomic indicators, suggesting that living conditions directly affected vulnerability to the disease, as evidenced by the impact on impoverished and Black populations [28,29]. In Brazil, despite the cash transfer policy adopted, called "Emergency Aid", studies show that mortality rates increased as formal remuneration decreased, highlighting the differentiated impact of the pandemic [30]. This situation may be a reflection of limited access to quality health services in impoverished areas [28].

In our study, we observed that there were no low-incidence clusters in the center southwest region of the city of São Paulo, but there was a low-mortality cluster, in an area with a concentration of the highest incomes in the MRSP. In contrast, high-mortality clusters were observed in the most peripheral region of the capital São Paulo, as well as in neighboring municipalities. By integrating epidemiological models with georeferenced data and socioeconomic indicators, we analyzed how the virus spread in a complex urban environment, characterizing significant territorial disparities in incidence and mortality risk. The method employed in the present study has been widely used to detect statistically significant spatiotemporal clusters of diseases, as well as to calculate relative risks, contributing to the real-time geographic surveillance of diseases and early detection of epidemics and retrospective analysis [3,7,8,25]. We highlight the role of social inequalities interwoven with the spatial dynamics of COVID-19, detailing mortality risks in the 633 weighted areas of the MRSP. Additionally, we provide insights into how urban mobility and specific variables contributed to the spread of coronavirus infection.

The limitations of this study include the use of aggregated data from the corresponding areas, without controlling for individual patient conditions, such as chronic disease conditions. There are also inherent biases in the dataset used due to differentiated access to healthcare, as there was no mass testing to track the disease and, at times, the tests were not accessible throughout the outpatient network, which led to underreporting of cases [31]. Another limitation was the use of information on per capita income, BBIP, and people per household from the 2010 census. Data from the 2022 census have not yet been made available on an WA scale and, therefore, our study probably underestimates changes in the socioeconomic structure even if no such changes occurred in urban aspects in the territories analyzed during this period.

The choice of analysis period influences SaTScan's ability to detect clusters [32]. The choice of parameters, such as the maximum temporal window for cluster detection, the Poisson distribution, and the shape of the cluster (circular or elliptical), can have a greater or lesser impact on the sensitivity of the model to detect clusters [14]. In the COVID-19 pandemic, the temporal distribution of cases was very heterogeneous and there were outbreaks concentrated in certain months during 2020 and 2021. Our study was intentionally carried out in two periods, Year 1 and Year 2, because clusters that are evident in shorter periods may be diluted in longer periods of analysis. The incidence of COVID-19 decreased significantly in the second half of 2021, with lower rates and a more homogeneous distribution, and the software can interpret that the data are closer to what was expected, reducing the chance of identifying significant clusters.

Even though health actions are strongly associated with medical measures, the spread of the pandemic exposed the need for a territorialized reading of health problems in order to design public policies. The use of geotechnologies during the COVID-19 pandemic, both in academic publications and on information panels of health institutions, highlights the importance of such analyses in public health management. However, access to maps as an efficient means of communicating about the spread of diseases is still a challenge due to the difficulty in incorporating urban complexity and limitations in access to data and qualified labor. This study sought an epidemiological investigation model accessible to public health surveillance management and a subsequent statistical analysis of social variables to contribute to the prioritization of policies and actions to mitigate the spread and impacts of diseases.

6. Conclusions

This study detected temporal and spatiotemporal clusters of WA in the MRSP in the first two years of the COVID-19 pandemic, as well as the respective RR calculated by the incidence within the cluster in relation to the incidence outside the cluster. The method employed can facilitate additional targeted interventions at more detailed spatial scales. In addition, carrying out tests for the set of areas that form the cluster, detecting areas with low and high rates within the cluster, reduces the possibility of detecting a cluster with only one unit of analysis.

Since public health policies to contain the spread of COVID-19 at the beginning of the pandemic relied mainly on non-pharmacological measures, a better understanding of the effectiveness of these measures through spatial analysis would allow for targeted interventions that could have mitigated the effects of the pandemic in the urban environment. However, the analyses performed here may also contribute to better outcomes in controlling future outbreaks. This is because this approach has proven useful for infectious disease surveillance and identifying statistically significant clusters of cases and deaths. However, it needs to be strengthened by adjusting efforts to analyze relevant covariates, such as poverty levels and access to healthcare. Even so, mapping spatiotemporal clusters of different outcomes can support public health policies and contribute to the advancement of epidemiological studies with ecological designs, also allowing for analyses of the relationship between health risks and social and economic indicators.

Author Contributions: Conceptualization, Keila Valente de Souza de Santana, Pedro Henrique Rezende Mendonça, Pedro Henrique Barbosa Muniz Lima, Aluízio Marino and Raquel Rolnik; methodology, Keila Valente de Souza de Santana, Pedro Henrique Rezende Mendonça, Gabriela Rosa Martins and Pedro Henrique Barbosa Muniz Lima; software, Keila Valente de Souza de Santana, Pedro Henrique Rezende Mendonça, Gabriela Rosa Martins and Pedro Henrique Barbosa Muniz Lima; formal analysis, Keila Valente de Souza de Santana; resources, Raquel Rolnik; writing—original draft preparation, Keila Valente de Souza de Santana; writing—review and editing, Pedro Henrique Rezende Mendonça and Raquel Rolnik; visualization, Pedro Henrique Rezende Mendonça, Pedro Henrique Barbosa Muniz Lima, Gabriela Rosa Martins, Aluízio Marino and Raquel Rolnik; supervision, Raquel Rolnik; project administration, Aluízio Marino and Raquel Rolnik; funding acquisition, Raquel Rolnik All authors have read and agreed to the published version of the manuscript.

Funding: This research was funded by São Paulo State Research Support Foundation (Fapesp). Funding number: 2023/03355-6, and 2021/08276-1.

Data Availability Statement: Data are contained within this article.

Conflicts of Interest: The authors declare no conflicts of interest.

References

1. World Health Organization. Coronavirus Disease 2019 (COVID-19): Situation Report, 73. 2020. Available online: https://www.who.int/emergencies/diseases/novel-coronavirus-2019 (accessed on 8 January 2024).
2. UNASUS. Coronavírus: Brasil Confirma Primeiro Caso da Doença. Available online: https://www.unasus.gov.br/noticia/coronavirus-brasil-confirma-primeiro-caso-da-doenca (accessed on 28 January 2024).
3. Palasio, R.G.S.; Lorenz, C.; Lucas, P.C.; Nielsen, L.; Masuda, E.T.; Trevisan, C.M. Spatial, spatio-temporal, and origin-destination flow analyses of patients with severe acute respiratory syndrome hospitalized for COVID-19 in Southeastern Brazil, 2020–2021. *Rev. Do Inst. De Med. Trop. De São Paulo* **2023**, *65*, e6.
4. Ferreira, R.V.; Martines, M.R.; Toppa, R.H.; Assunção, L.M.; Desjardins, M.R.; Delmelle, E. Utilizing prospective space-time scan statistics to discover the dynamics of coronavirus disease 2019 clusters in the State of São Paulo, Brazil. *Rev. Da Soc. Bras. De Med. Trop.* **2022**, *55*, e0607.
5. São Paulo. Plano de Desenvolvimento Urbano Integrado da Região Metropolitana de São Paulo. Available online: https://rmsp.pdui.sp.gov.br/ (accessed on 8 May 2024).
6. Barrozo, L.V. Desigualdades na mortalidade infantil no Município de São Paulo: Em busca do melhor indicador. *Confins* **2018**. [CrossRef]
7. Gomes, D.S.; Andrade, L.A.; Ribeiro, C.J.N. Risk clusters of COVID-19 transmission in northeastern Brazil: Prospective space-time modeling. *Epidemiol. Infect.* **2020**, *148*, e188. [CrossRef] [PubMed]
8. Martines, M.R.; Ferreira, R.V.; Toppa, R.H.; Assunção, L.M.; Desjardins, M.R.; Delmelle, E.M. Detecting space–time clusters of COVID-19 in Brazil: Mortality, inequality, socioeconomic vulnerability, and the relative risk of the disease in Brazilian municipalities. *J. Geogr. Syst.* **2021**, *23*, 7–36. [CrossRef] [PubMed]
9. Gaspar, R.C.; Aparício, C.A.; Bessa, V. A metrópole de São Paulo: Desenvolvimento econômico recente e configuração interna. In *São Paulo: Transformações na Ordem Urbana*; Bógus, L., Pasternak, S., Eds.; Eds.; Letra Capital: Rio de Janeiro, Brazil, 2015.
10. IBGE. Censo Populacional. Available online: https://cidades.ibge.gov.br/brasil/sp/araraquara/panorama (accessed on 8 February 2024).
11. Metrópole Cded. Base Cartográfica Digital Georreferenciada de Logradouros da Região Metropolitana de São Paulo—Edicão. 2020. Available online: https://centrodametropole.fflch.usp.br/pt-br/node/9838 (accessed on 8 March 2024).
12. Research Google. Open Buildings: A Dataset of Buildings Footprint to Support Social Good Applications. Available online: https://sites.research.google/gr/open-buildings/ (accessed on 1 February 2024).
13. Petrov, A. One hundred years of dasymetric mapping: Back to the origin. *Cartogr. J.* **2012**, *49*, 256–264. [CrossRef]
14. Kulldorff, M. SaTScanTM User Guide. 2018. Available online: https://www.satscan.org/SaTScan_TM_Manual_do_Usu%C3%A1rio_Portugues.pdf (accessed on 1 March 2024).
15. Kulldorff, M. A spatial scan statistic. *Commun. Stat.-Theory Methods* **1997**, *26*, 1481–1496. [CrossRef]
16. São Paulo. Governo de SP Reforça Controle de Pandemia e Põe Estado na Fase Amarela. São Paulo: Governo do Estado 2020. Available online: https://www.saopaulo.sp.gov.br/noticias-coronavirus/governo-de-sp-reforca-controle-de-pandemia-e-poe-estado-na-fase-amarela-2/ (accessed on 8 July 2024).
17. Brasil. Ministério da Saúde. Boletim Epidemiológico Especial: Doença Pelo Novo Coronavírus—COVID-19. Semana epidemiológica 39. Brasília, DF: Ministério da Saúde. 2021. Available online: https://www.gov.br/saude/pt-br/centrais-

de-conteudo/publicacoes/boletins/epidemiologicos/covid-19/2021/boletim_epidemiologico_covid_83.pdf (accessed on 3 October 2024).
18. São Paulo (Município). Secretaria Municipal da Saúde. Instrutivos Para priorização de doses da Vacina de COVID-19 no Município de São Paulo e Documentos Técnicos. São Paulo: Secretaria Municipal da Saúde. 2024. Available online: https://capital.sp.gov.br/web/saude/w/vigilancia_em_saude/doencas_e_agravos/coronavirus/315208 (accessed on 3 October 2024).
19. Demenech, L.M.; Dumith, S.d.C.; Vieira, M.E.C.D.; Silva, L.N. Desigualdade econômica e risco de infecção e morte por COVID-19 no Brasil. *Rev. Bras. De Epidemiol.* **2020**, *23*, e200095. [CrossRef] [PubMed]
20. OGLOBO. Entre os Maiores do Mundo, Aeroporto de Guarulhos é o Segundo Mais Pontual. 2017. Available online: https://oglobo.globo.com/boa-viagem/entre-os-maiores-do-mundo-aeroporto-de-guarulhos-o-segundo-mais-pontual-20728827 (accessed on 6 June 2024).
21. Rolnik, R.; Klintowitz, D. Mobilidade na cidade de São Paulo. *Estud. Avançados* **2011**, *25*, 89–108. [CrossRef]
22. Pilotto, A.S.; Novaski, M.A.M. Indicadores de mobilidade urbana na RMSP a partir da pesquisa OD-Metrô. *Cad. Metrópole* **2022**, *25*, 229–254. [CrossRef]
23. Mendonça, P.H.R.; Rolnik, R.; Yeuw, T.T.; Marino, A. *Mobilidade na Cidade de São Paulo: Lições das Transformações Durante a Pandemia de COVID-19*; Enanpur: Belém, Brazil, 2023.
24. Silva, R.B. Vidas no sufoco nos transportes na pandemia: Um App de mapeamento colaborativo para alerta de lotação na Região Metropolitana de São Paulo (RMSP). *Confin. Rev. Fr.-Brésilienne De Géographie/Rev. Fr.-Bras. De Geogr.* **2023**, *58*, 1–24.
25. Barrozo, L.V.; Serafim, M.B.; Moraes, S.L.; Mansur, G. Monitoramento espaço-temporal das áreas de alto risco de COVID-19 nos municípios do Brasil. *Hygeia Rev. Bras. De Geogr. Médica E Da Saúde* **2020**, *16*, 417. [CrossRef]
26. IBGE. Instituto Brasileiro de Geografia e Estatística. Censo Demográfico. 2022. Available online: https://www.ibge.gov.br/estatisticas/sociais/trabalho/22827-censo-demografico-2022.html (accessed on 8 May 2024).
27. Oliveira, R.J.; Oliveira, R.M.S. São Paulo cidade negra no século XXI. *Rev. Da ABPN* **2020**, *12*, 489–515. [CrossRef]
28. Oliveira, R.; Cunha, A.; Santos Gadelha, A.; Carpio, C.; Oliveira, R.; Corrêa, R. Desigualdades raciais e a morte como horizonte: Considerações sobre a COVID-19 e o racismo estrutural. *Cad. De Saúde Pública* **2020**, *36*, e00150120. [CrossRef] [PubMed]
29. Barreto, W.L.; Pereira, F.H.; Perez, Y.; Schimit, P.H.T. Spatial dynamics of COVID-19 in São Paulo: A cellular automata and GIS approach. *Spat. Spatio-Temporal Epidemiol.* **2024**, *50*, 100674. [CrossRef] [PubMed]
30. Rede Nossa São Paulo. A COVID-19 e as Desigualdades:O Que os Dados nos Contam Após um ano de Pandemia. 2021. Available online: https://www.nossasaopaulo.org.br/wp-content/uploads/2021/09/Mapa-da-Desigualdade-Especial-Covid-2021.pdf (accessed on 8 October 2024).
31. FIOCRUZ. MonitoraCOVID-19 Avalia Cobertura dos Testes em Massa no Controle da Epidemia no Brasil. MonitoraCOVID-19, Fundação Oswaldo Cruz (Fiocruz). 2021. Available online: https://portal.fiocruz.br/noticia/monitoracovid-19-avalia-cobertura-dos-testes-em-massa-no-controle-da-epidemia-no-brasil (accessed on 8 October 2024).
32. Levin-Rector, A.; Kulldorff, M.; Peterson, E.R.; Hostovich, S.; Greene, S.K. Prospective Spatiotemporal Cluster Detection Using SaTScan: Tutorial for Designing and Fine-Tuning a System to Detect Reportable Communicable Disease Outbreaks. *JMIR Public Health Surveill* **2024**, *10*, e50653. [CrossRef] [PubMed]

International Journal of
Geo-Information

MDPI

Article

Mining Spatiotemporal Mobility Patterns Using Improved Deep Time Series Clustering

Ziyi Zhang [1,*], Diya Li [2], Zhe Zhang [1,2] and Nick Duffield [1,3]

1 Department of Electrical and Computer Engineering, Texas A&M University, College Station, TX 77843, USA; zhezhang@tamu.edu (Z.Z.); duffieldng@tamu.edu (N.D.)
2 Department of Geography, Texas A&M University, College Station, TX 77843, USA; diya.li@tamu.edu
3 Texas A&M Institute of Data Science, Texas A&M University, College Station, TX 77843, USA
* Correspondence: zyzhang@tamu.edu

Abstract: Mining spatiotemporal mobility patterns is crucial for optimizing urban planning, enhancing transportation systems, and improving public safety by providing useful insights into human movement and behavior over space and time. As an unsupervised learning technique, time series clustering has gained considerable attention due to its efficiency. However, the existing literature has often overlooked the inherent characteristics of mobility data, including high-dimensionality, noise, outliers, and time distortions. This oversight can lead to potentially large computational costs and inaccurate patterns. To address these challenges, this paper proposes a novel neural network-based method integrating temporal autoencoder and dynamic time warping-based K-means clustering algorithm to mutually promote each other for mining spatiotemporal mobility patterns. Comparative results showed that our proposed method outperformed several time series clustering techniques in accurately identifying mobility patterns on both synthetic and real-world data, which provides a reliable foundation for data-driven decision-making. Furthermore, we applied the method to monthly county-level mobility data during the COVID-19 pandemic in the U.S., revealing significant differences in mobility changes between rural and urban areas, as well as the impact of public response and health considerations on mobility patterns.

Keywords: spatiotemporal data mining; mobility patterns; time series clustering; deep learning

1. Introduction

Spatiotemporal mobility pattern mining is a crucial area of data mining that focuses specifically on identifying and analyzing movement patterns within mobility data as they shift over time and across different locations. These patterns have provided useful insights in a wide range of applications, such as urban planing [1–5], traffic management [6–8], and disaster reduction [9–12]. With advancements in data storage and processing capabilities, real-world applications now have the capacity to store and retain data over extended periods [13]. Consequently, mobility data across various domains are increasingly being preserved in the form of time series data, facilitating more comprehensive analysis and long-term insights.

Researchers have developed various methods leveraging time series data to perform related analysis such as classification [14,15], clustering [10,16–19], forecasting [20–24], and causal inference [25–27]. Among these tasks, time series clustering is particularly challenging but important. Time series clustering has gained significant attention for its effectiveness across diverse fields, including climate [28–30], energy [31,32], and the environment [33,34]. Despite the advances in time series clustering, several challenges persist, including high dimensionality, noise, outliers, and time distortions. These issues often lead to increased computational costs and reduced accuracy in clustering outcomes.

An appropriate representation can help mitigate high dimensionality, noise, and outliers, and reduce computational costs, leading to more efficient and accurate time series clustering. Many studies have been carried out with a focus on dimensionality reduction (DR) techniques. For example, principal component analysis (PCA)-based K-means algorithm [16,35,36] has been proposed to achieve faster and more accurate time series clustering. This method constructs common projection axes as the prototype for each cluster, enabling more efficient clustering by reducing dimensionality while preserving essential data characteristics. Non-negative matrix factorization (NMF) is also employed as a DR technique prior to applying the K-Means clustering algorithm [37,38].

With the advancement of neural networks (NNs), deep representation learning [39] has focused on constructing meaningful and compact data representations. This approach aims to capture essential features from raw data, enabling more efficient processing and improving the performance of downstream tasks such as classification, clustering, and forecasting. Deep time series clustering [40] exemplifies how deep representation learning can be used to analyze time series data. In this approach, temporal representations are first learned through advanced deep representation learning techniques, and then clustering algorithms are applied to temporal representations to extract meaningful clusters. Researchers have devoted considerable effort to improving deep time series clustering. For example, the authors in [40–45] employed the convolutional autoencoder (CAE) for extracting representations and K-means as the clustering algorithm. To better capture temporal information, some studies developed a temporal autoencoder (TAE) by integrating a recurrent neural network (RNN) into the convolutional autoencoder, which resulted in improved performance [46–49].

However, we found that existing methods often overlook several critical characteristics of mobility datasets, making it challenging to apply these methods directly to mobility data. These challenges include determining whether the extracted temporal representations are suitable for downstream clustering algorithms, as well as addressing issues related to high dimensionality, noise, outliers, and time distortions in their methods. In an effort to overcome these obstacles within a comprehensive framework, we introduce a novel method that combines a neural network-based temporal autoencoder with a dynamic time warping-based K-means clustering algorithm. Additionally, we propose an optimization strategy to improve the quality of generated temporal representations, making them more suitable for the downstream K-means clustering algorithm. This approach not only mitigates the impact of high dimensionality, noise, outliers, and time distortions but also ensures that the features extracted are well-suited for specific applications. The efficiency of our proposed algorithm is demonstrated through extensive experiments on synthetic and real-world spatiotemporal mobility data, proving its exceptional ability to precisely identify spatiotemporal mobility patterns. The significant contributions of this work are outlined as follows:

- We formalize the task of mining spatiotemporal mobility patterns using a deep time series clustering approach and introduce a comprehensive framework that integrates a neural network-based temporal autoencoder with a dynamic time warping-based K-means clustering algorithm.
- We propose an optimization strategy to enhance the generated temporal representations, making them more suitable for the downstream K-means clustering algorithm.
- Extensive experiments on both synthetic and real-world mobility datasets demonstrate that our proposed approach outperforms existing time series clustering techniques, especially when dealing with data characterized by high dimensionality, noise, outliers, and time distortions.
- We reveal significant differences in mobility changes between rural and urban areas, as well as the influence of public response and health considerations on mobility in the U.S. by applying our method to mobility data during the COVID-19 pandemic.

We have organized our paper as follows: Section 2 presents the data used in this study and our proposed methodology; Section 3 presents the comparative performance evaluation, module contribution analysis, and a case study on mining spatiotemporal mobility patterns during the COVID-19 pandemic in the U.S.; Section 4 discusses the limitations and provides directions for future research, while Section 5 concludes the study.

2. Materials and Methods

2.1. Data

We used three distinct real-world time series datasets to thoroughly evaluate the effectiveness of our method in identifying and analyzing spatiotemporal mobility patterns. The first, Melbourne Pedestrian Time Series Data, consists of detailed hourly pedestrian counts collected from 10 distinct locations across Melbourne, Australia, throughout the entirety of 2017. These data originate from an automated system (Figure 1) designed to monitor pedestrian activity in the city, with the goal of providing valuable insights into pedestrian movement patterns. By analyzing these data, urban planners can better understand the flow of people through different parts of the city, enabling more informed decisions about urban infrastructure and planning. The placement of sensors in various locations allows for the analysis of spatial variations in pedestrian traffic, while the continuous data collection across a full year enables a comprehensive temporal analysis, taking into account seasonal changes, holidays, and other factors that influence pedestrian behavior.

Similarly, the second, Chinatown Pedestrian Time Series Data, offers monthly pedestrian counts for Chinatown-Swanston Street (North) in Melbourne, Australia, also for the year 2017. This dataset is categorized based on whether the counts were collected on regular weekdays or weekends, providing a granular view of temporal variations in pedestrian activity. By examining these data, we were able to evaluate our method's capability to recognize not only spatial patterns but also temporal variations, such as differences in pedestrian traffic between weekdays and weekends. This level of detail is crucial for understanding how different times of the week influence foot traffic in specific areas, which is valuable for businesses, city planners, and local authorities.

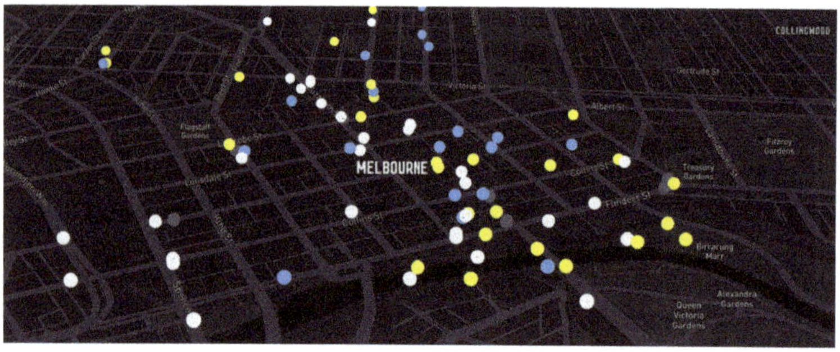

Figure 1. The pedestrian counting system in the city of Melbourne is a network of sensors, represented in various colors, located throughout key areas of the city to count pedestrian movements in real time. This system helps monitor foot traffic trends, providing valuable insights into urban mobility, crowd behavior, and the impact of major events such as festivals and public holidays, as well as changes in mobility patterns.

The third, COVID-19 Mobility Time Series Data, is derived from the Trips by Distance datasets published by the Bureau of Transportation Statistics in the United States. This dataset provides county-level mobility information for the COVID-19 pandemic, tracking the average distance people traveled from their homes across 3142 counties between March 2020 and May 2020. This period is particularly significant as it coincides with the early stages of the pandemic when policies such as lockdowns, social distancing measures, and travel restrictions were being rapidly implemented and modified across the country. The dataset offers a unique opportunity to examine how these dynamic policies influenced human mobility patterns on a large scale. By using these data as a case study, we aimed to identify spatiotemporal mobility patterns under rapidly changing conditions, providing insights into how public health interventions and shifting regulations impacted movement across different regions. This analysis helps to illustrate the broader applicability of our method to real-world phenomena influenced by both spatial and temporal factors.

In addition to real-world data, we used a synthetic dataset to evaluate the performance of our proposed method in handling noise, outliers, and time distortions, as visualized in Figure 2. We followed the model presented by [50] and then generated these time series with different trends as follows:

$$\begin{aligned} f_1(t) &= (5+\alpha) \cdot g_{[a,b]}(t) + \epsilon, \\ f_2(t) &= (5+\alpha) \cdot g_{[a,b]}(t) \cdot \frac{t-a}{b-a} + \epsilon, \\ f_3(t) &= (5+\alpha) \cdot g_{[a,b]}(t) \cdot \frac{b-t}{b-a} + \epsilon. \end{aligned} \tag{1}$$

In this context, t ranges from 1 to 128, and a is defined as an integer-valued uniform random variable within the range from 16 to 32. The difference $b-a$ follows an integer-valued uniform distribution with bounds from 32 to 96. Both α and ϵ are variables drawn from a standard normal distribution $\mathcal{N}(0,1)$. Additionally, $g_{[a,b]}$ represents the indicator function defined over the interval $[a,b]$, which can be expressed as follows:

$$g_{[a,b]}(t) = \begin{cases} 1 & a \le t \le b \\ 0 & \text{otherwise} \end{cases} \tag{2}$$

where $f_1(t), f_2(t)$, and $f_3(t)$ represent the generation functions for the time series with different trends.

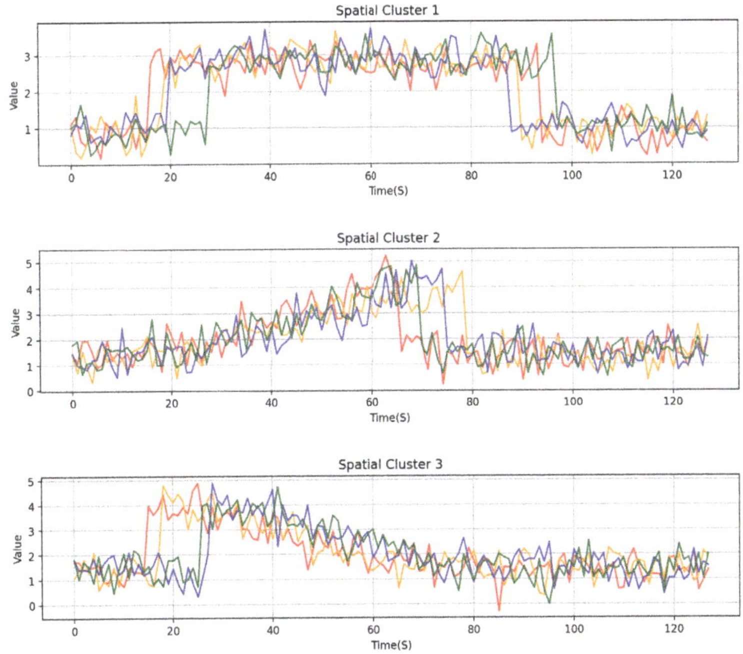

Figure 2. This synthetic time series data includes noise, outliers, and time distortions. We assume the presence of three distinct spatial clusters. Locations within the same spatial cluster, represented by different colors, typically exhibit similar patterns or trends in time series data.

2.2. Methods

This section details our two-stage, improved deep time series clustering (I-DTSC) method for uncovering spatiotemporal mobility patterns. The first stage is a neural network-based temporal autoencoder for learning the temporal representations. The second stage is to utilize a dynamic time warping-based K-means clustering algorithm on learned temporal representations to generate k spatial clusters. After generating k spatial clusters, we visualize them on a map and explore the spatiotemporal patterns. The framework is illustrated in Figure 3, and we discuss our proposed method in the following parts.

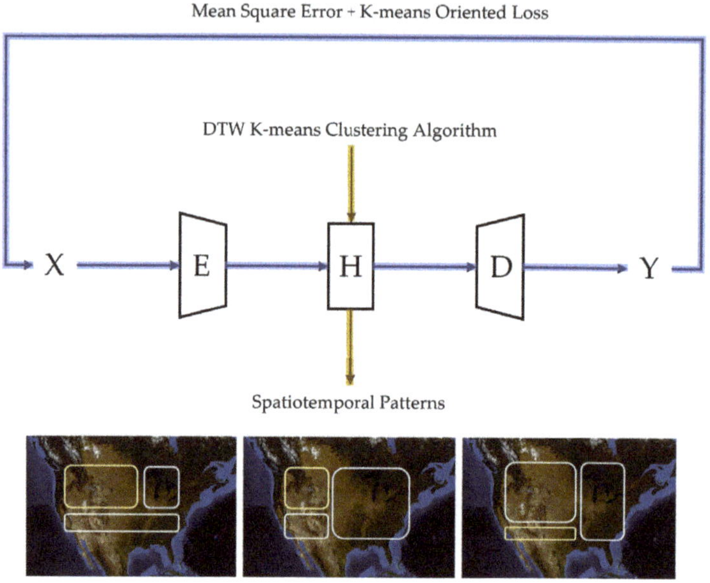

Figure 3. The workflow of our proposed method. X represents the input time series data with location coordinates, E denotes the encoding process, and H is the latent space where temporal representations are learned. D is the decoding process, which maps the temporal representations to Y. After generating the temporal representations in H, apply the dynamic time warping-based K-means (DTW K-means) clustering algorithm to produce spatiotemporal patterns and visualize them on the map using location coordinates. Exploring dynamic spatiotemporal mobility patterns, represented by squares in different colors, enables better decision-making.

Given a collection of time series data from n locations, denoted by $\mathcal{X} = (x_1, x_2, ..., x_n)$, where each time series $x_i \in \mathbb{R}^T$. We introduce a non-linear mapping function $E(\cdot) : x_i \rightarrow h_i$ for encoding, and another non-linear mapping function $D(\cdot) : h_i \rightarrow y_i$ for decoding. Specifically, we design the non-linear mapping $E(\cdot)$ by employing the initial two layers as a one-dimensional convolutional neural network (1D-CNN) layer followed by a max-pooling layer, aimed at capturing short-term patterns within the data. A 1D-CNN is a specialized type of neural network designed for processing sequential data. Unlike their 2D counterparts, which are well-suited for image data, 1D-CNNs are ideal for analyzing time series data, audio signals, and any form of data that unfold over time or space. A latent representation of the n-th feature map of the existing layer is given by the following form:

$$h_i^n = \sigma(x_i \times W^n + b^n), \tag{3}$$

where W represents the filters, b is the corresponding bias for the n-th feature map, and σ denotes the activation function (e.g., sigmoid, ReLU), and $\times$ indicates the 1D convolution operation. The next two layers are Bi-directional Long Short-Term Memory (Bi-LSTM) layers, which are for learning temporal changes in two directions of time. A Bi-LSTM network is a special type of recurrent neural network that learns from sequences of data, like sentences or time series. Unlike a regular recurrent neural network that only looks at data from the beginning to the end, Bi-directional LSTMs extend the standard LSTM models by utilizing two LSTMs applied to the input data. In the first pass, an LSTM processes the input sequence in its original order (i.e., the forward layer). In the second pass, the input sequence is reversed and fed into another LSTM (i.e., the backward layer). This bi-directional approach enhances the model's ability to learn long-term dependencies, thereby improving its overall accuracy. For each element in the input sequence, each layer of standard LSTMs performs the following computations:

$$\begin{aligned} i_t &= \sigma(W_{ii}x_t + b_{ii} + W_{hi}h_{t-1} + b_{ii}), \\ f_t &= \sigma(W_{if}x_t + b_{if} + W_{hf}h_{t-1} + b_{hf}), \\ g_t &= \tanh(W_{ig}x_t + b_{ig} + W_{hg}h_{t-1} + b_{hg}), \\ o_t &= \sigma(W_{io}x_t + b_{io} + W_{ho}h_{t-1} + b_{ho}), \\ c_t &= f_t \odot c_{t-1} + i_t \odot g_t, \\ h_t &= o_t \odot \tanh(c_t). \end{aligned} \tag{4}$$

Here, h_t represents the hidden state at time t, c_t is the cell state at time t, and x_t denotes the input at time t. The term h_{t-1} refers to the hidden state from the previous time step or the initial hidden state at $t = 0$. The variables i_t, f_t, g_t, and o_t correspond to the input, forget, cell, and output gates, respectively. σ is the sigmoid function, tanh is the hyperbolic tangent function, and $\odot$ denotes the Hadamard (element-wise) product.

After the non-linear mapping $E(\cdot)$, the original temporal sequence $x_i \in \mathbb{R}^T$ is encoded into a considerably reduced representation $h_i \in \mathbb{R}^d$, where d represents the dimensionality of the temporal representation. The selection of d may vary, being either larger or smaller than T. In our experiments, we opt for $d < T$, aiming to preserve the most significant information in a lower-dimensional space, while enhancing computational efficiency when processing high-dimensional datasets. The decoding process $D(\cdot)$ is facilitated by a fully-connected neural network, which reconstructs the temporal representations back into a new time series $y_i \in \mathbb{R}^T$. In the optimization process, the mean square error (MSE) is employed as the metric to quantify reconstruction loss, as demonstrated by the subsequent formula:

$$\mathcal{L}_{MSE} = \frac{1}{n}\sqrt{\sum_{i=1}^{n} ||y_i - x_i||_2}. \tag{5}$$

Beyond merely preserving the most informative representation through the reconstruction loss expressed in Equation (5), we incorporate an additional K-means oriented loss. This facilitates the formation of cluster structures within the learned temporal representations, yielding representations that are particularly amenable to the K-means clustering algorithm. Specifically, by considering a static matrix $H \in \mathbb{R}^{n\times d}$, the challenge of finding the optimal solution in K-means clustering is reinterpreted as a problem of maximizing the trace in the context of the Gram matrix. By employing spectral relaxation, the K-means objective is transformed into a formulation that sidesteps local minima, thereby promising optimal solutions:

$$\mathcal{L}_{K-means} = Tr(H^T H) - Tr(F^T H^T H F), \tag{6}$$

where Tr denotes the matrix trace. The close-form solution for F is derived by assembling the first k singular vectors of H, following the principles outlined in the Ky Fan theorem [17]. Unlike static matrices, in our approach, the latent temporal representation H is dynamically learned within the network. This dynamic learning process effectively serves as a regularization term for H; the overall objective is to minimize the below equation:

$$\min_H \mathcal{L}_{MSE} + \lambda \mathcal{L}_{K-means}, \tag{7}$$

where λ is a balancing factor that regulates the trade-off between the mean squared error and the K-means oriented loss.

After generating temporal representations, we apply a dynamic time warping-based K-means clustering algorithm to these representations. Dynamic time warping can be seen as an extension of Euclidean distance, which offers local (non-linear) alignment. The calculating procedure of dynamic time warping can be illustrated as follows: given two temporal sequences $P \in \mathbb{R}^n$ and $Q \in \mathbb{R}^n$, formulate an $n \times n$ matrix, with the element at intersection i, j quantifying the Euclidean between p^i and q^j; the goal of dynamic time warping distance is to identify the path of minimum cumulative distance across this matrix. Define this path by $M = \{m_1, m_2, ..., m_k\}$, where the dynamic time warping distance is determined as the smallest sum of Euclidean distance along the path M:

$$M^* = \arg\min_M (\sqrt{\sum_{i=1}^{k} m_i}). \tag{8}$$

This whole process can be summarized in Algorithm 1.

Algorithm 1 Dynamic Time Warping

```
procedure INPUT(P, Q)        ▷ Time Series P with length n; Time Series Q with length n.
    for i = 1 to n do
        for j = 1 to n do
            Matrix(i, j) ← sqrt((p^i − q^j)^2)
    Define a path through the matrix: M = m_1, m_2, ..., m_k, k ≥ n
    DTW ← argmin_M( sqrt( Σ_{m=1}^{K} m_k ) )
    return DTW
```

The detailed procedure of applying a dynamic time warping-based K-means clustering algorithm to these representations is outlined in Algorithm 2, which operates on temporal representations $H \in \mathbb{R}^{n \times d}$, where n is the number of locations and d is the dimension of temporal latent representations. The algorithm starts by selecting k central temporal representations from H at random to serve as initial centroids. Subsequently, each temporal representation is assigned to the nearest centroid, determined by the smallest dynamic time warping distance. The next step involves updating the centroids by recalculating the mean position of the temporal representations assigned to each centroid, followed by a re-evaluation of the dynamic time warping distances between each temporal representation and the new centroids. This iterative process continues until the assignments of temporal representation to centroids stabilize and no further reassignments occur.

Algorithm 2 Dynamic Time Warping-based K-means on Temporal Representations

1: **procedure** INPUT(H, k) ▷ n-size temporal representations: $H \in \mathbb{R}^{n \times d}$; number of clusters: $k < n$.
2: Randomly initialize k centroids $(c_1, c_2, ..., c_k) \in H$.
3: Calculate dynamic time warping distance between each temporal representation in $H = (h_1, h_2, ..., h_n)$ and each centroid in $(c_1, c_2, ..., c_k) \in H$.
4: Assign the temporal representation in H to the centroid c_i by selecting the one with the smallest dynamic time warping distance from it among all k centroids, and finally form k spatial clusters: $C = (c_1, c_2, ..., c_k)$.
5: Recalculate the new k central temporal representations in $C = (c_1, c_2, ..., c_k)$.
6: Stop until C will not change; otherwise, repeat from Step 3.
7: **return** C

The final step involves visualizing and interpreting the spatial clusters. The generated k spatial clusters are represented as $C = (c_1, c_2, ..., c_k)$, where each c_i consists of a set of geographic locations that exhibit similar trends or patterns. These locations are then projected onto a map using their coordinates, allowing us to explore spatiotemporal patterns. To quantify the spatial clusters, we introduce a metric called the average travel distance of a cluster, defined as follows:

$$Average\ Travel\ Distance\ (ATD) = \frac{1}{N}\sum_{n=1}^{N}\sum_{t=1}^{T} dist_{n,t}, \tag{9}$$

where N represents the number of locations within a cluster, T denotes the number of time steps, and $dist_{n,t}$ is the travel distance in the n-th location at time step t.

The ATD reflects the average distance traveled within a cluster over a specified number of time steps. It quantifies how much movement occurs, on average, within the geographic locations of a cluster over time. This can provide insights into the mobility patterns of the regions in the cluster, indicating whether certain areas have high or low travel activity. By comparing ATD across clusters, we can assess the relative mobility within different geographic areas, potentially linking these patterns to underlying socioeconomic or environmental factors.

3. Results

3.1. Comparative Performance Evaluation

To evaluate the effectiveness of our proposed method in identifying mobility patterns, we first formulate the problem as follows: consider a set of n geographic locations, each represented by a time series $\mathcal{X} = \{x_1, x_2, ..., x_n\}$, where each time series $x_i \in \mathbb{R}^T$, where x_i^t denotes the observation at time t for location i, and T is the total number of time steps. The goal is to group these time series into k spatial clusters, denoted by $\{c_1, c_2, \ldots, c_k\}$, such that locations within the same cluster exhibit similar temporal patterns. The objective can be formulated as finding a partition $\{c_1, c_2, \ldots, c_k\}$ of the set of time series $\{x_1, x_2, ..., x_n\}$ that minimizes within-cluster variance while maximizing between-cluster variance. This can be expressed as follows:

$$\min_{\{c_1,c_2,...,c_k\}} \sum_{j=1}^{k}\sum_{x_j \in c_j} dist(x_j, z_j), \tag{10}$$

where z_j is the centroid of cluster c_j, and $\mathrm{dist}(x_j, z_j)$ is a distance measure between the time series x_j and the cluster centroid z_j.

To verify the clustering, time series classification can be applied to the clusters. Given a set of labels $\{l_1, l_2, \ldots, l_k\}$ corresponding to known categories, the classification task assigns each time series x_i to one of the labels based on its cluster assignment. The accuracy of this classification provides a measure of how well the clustering captures meaningful, discriminative patterns in the data. We have access to ground truth information, allowing us to evaluate the cluster results against these ground truth locations. Therefore, we choose to employ the Rand Index, which can be expressed as follows:

$$Rand\ Index = \frac{2 \cdot (TP + TN)}{n(n-1)}. \tag{11}$$

In this context, true positives (TP) represent the count of time series pairs accurately grouped within the same spatial cluster. Conversely, true negatives (TN) refer to the count of time series pairs accurately assigned to distinct spatial clusters, while n denotes the size of the spatiotemporal dataset.

We compared our proposed method with some widely used methods and present the results in Table 1. Our proposed method demonstrates superior performance by achieving the highest average rand index. The synthetic dataset, characterized by noise, outliers, and time distortions, presents significant challenges for traditional K-means clustering methods. These traditional methods fail primarily due to their reliance on Euclidean distance, which lacks robustness to time distortions.

Although our proposed temporal autoencoder and dynamic time warping-based K-means clustering algorithm without K-means oriented loss (I-DTSC w/o KL) shows improvement over most clustering algorithms, its performance is close to that of the DTW-based K-means (DTW K-Means) approach. We acknowledge that the efficient computation is due to the advantage brought by the dimensionality reduction of the temporal autoencoder, but the potential of the temporal autoencoder has not been fully realized, leading to the neglect of some important information in the original time series.

The complete framework of I-DTSC exhibited exceptional robustness to noise, outliers, and time distortions. This approach guides the generation of more reliable and informative representations, thereby facilitating superior performance. In the case of the Melbourne dataset, our analysis indicates an absence of time distortions in this dataset, allowing traditional K-means to perform adequately; thus, the advantages of DTW K-means clustering algorithms are less pronounced in this context. Despite this, our proposed method outperforms other time series clustering techniques in identifying spatial clusters from time series collected in different locations. For the Chinatown dataset, which aims to differentiate between weekday and weekend time series collected at the same location, most methods fail to discern this distinction. This failure is often due to the subtlety of the differences; for instance, weekend mobility may still exceed typical levels during the evening and overnight periods. Conversely, our proposed method effectively identifies these critical differences, distinguishing between weekday and weekend patterns. Consequently, our method exhibits the highest performance in this context.

Table 1. Comparative results on synthetic and real-world mobility data. (Metric: Rand Index).

Category	Methods	Synthetic Mobility Data	Melbourne Mobility Data	Chinatown Mobility Data
Variants of K-means	K-means	0.6824 ± 0.0094	0.8767 ± 0.0064	0.5414 ± 0.0008
	DTW K-means	0.8836 ± 0.0124	0.8584 ± 0.0054	0.5714 ± 0.0094
DR-based K-means	NMF + K-means	0.5898 ± 0.0068	0.8514 ± 0.0075	0.5036 ± 0.0008
	PCA + K-means	0.7259 ± 0.0003	0.8699 ± 0.0046	0.5376 ± 0.0047
NN-based K-means	CAE + K-means	0.6575 ± 0.0012	0.8612 ± 0.0049	0.6712 ± 0.0075
	TAE + K-means	0.6891 ± 0.0021	0.8718 ± 0.0163	0.7088 ± 0.0035
Ours	I-DTSC w/o KL	0.8804 ± 0.0071	0.8601 ± 0.0049	0.6932 ± 0.0154
	I-DTSC	0.9117 ± 0.0036	0.8834 ± 0.0013	0.9055 ± 0.0099

3.2. Module Contribution Analysis

To better understand our proposed method, we first examined the role of the temporal autoencoder, as depicted in Figure 4. By employing our designed architecture and focusing on minimizing the mean square error between the original and reconstructed time series, we ensured that the temporal representations preserved essential characteristics, such as trends, while simultaneously reducing data dimensionality and mitigating noise and outliers. However, we found that only using the temporal autoencdoer does not address time distortions. This observation is also supported by performance comparisons, demonstrating that traditional K-means clustering methods struggle with datasets characterized by significant time distortions.

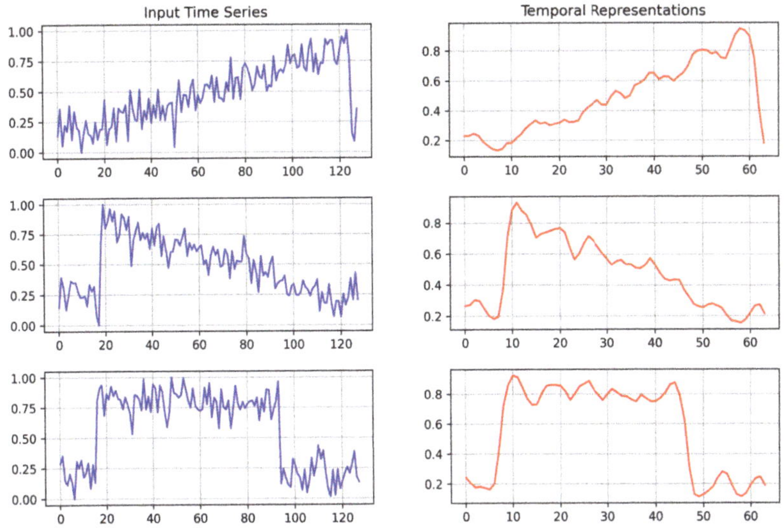

Figure 4. The temporal representations (**right**; red), with a reduced dimensionality of 64 compared to the original input time series dimension of 128 (**left**; blue), successfully preserved essential characteristics, such as trends. This reduction in dimensionality not only retained critical information but also helped mitigate noise and outliers.

Time distortions are a prevalent issue, particularly in real-world time series datasets. The traditional K-means clustering algorithm, which employs Euclidean distance as the similarity metric, is efficient and requires low computational resources, with a complexity of $O(n)$. However, this method often fails when confronted with time distortions, as the utilization of Euclidean distance cannot adequately align time points affected by distortions. A more suitable solution is to employ a DTW K-means clustering algorithm, which can yield more accurate results. Nonetheless, this strategy significantly increases computational demands, with a time complexity of $O(n^2)$. In our proposed method, we aim to achieve accurate results while also reducing time complexity. By compressing the original time series of length n to temporal representation with a shorter length m, where $m < n$, we apply the DTW K-means clustering algorithm not on the original series but on the temporal representations. This adjustment lowers the time complexity to $O(m^2)$. Our experimental findings suggest that the temporal autoencoder and DTW K-means clustering algorithm can mutually enhance each other's performance, achieving a balance between accuracy and computational efficiency.

In our experiments, we also analyzed the role of K-means oriented loss illustrated in Equation (6) for optimization. We conducted experiments on the Chinatown time series dataset to compare learning temporal representations with and without the K-means oriented loss. Figure 5 illustrates the results: without the K-means oriented loss, the representations appear scattered and chaotic; however, integrating the K-means oriented loss guides the process of learning temporal representations, resulting in structured temporal representations.

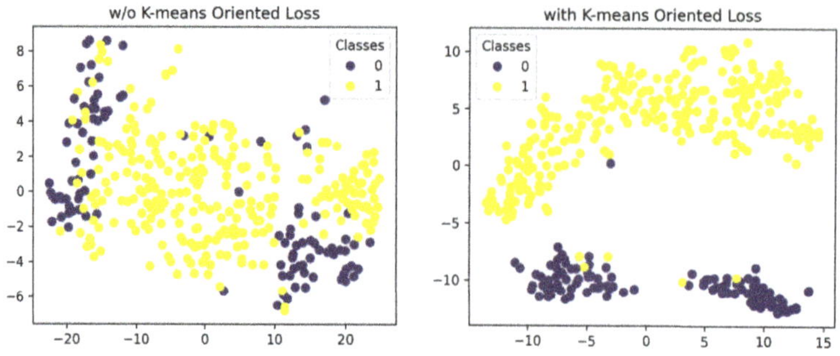

Figure 5. The visualization using t-SNE on the Chinatown time series dataset compares temporal representations without K-means oriented loss (**left**) and temporal representations with K-means oriented loss (**right**).

3.3. *Case Study: Mining Spatiotemporal Mobility Patterns During COVID-19 Pandemic*

The COVID-19 pandemic has caused a substantial negative impact on public health, infected more than 704 million people, and caused 7.01 million deaths worldwide as of September 2024. The United States government had issued social distancing measures to restrict gatherings, domestic and international travel, and business activities to reduce the COVID-19 cases and mortality rate. In response to the crisis, researchers developed various spatial models to analyze the distributions of the disease patterns and their dependency on factors such as mobility [11,51–53], social [54,55], economic [56,57], and demographic factors [31,58]. Furthermore, some existing methods were focused on spatiotemporal data modeling in COVID-19-related research to improve decision-making [59–64].

As detailed in this section, we applied our proposed method to uncover spatiotemporal patterns hidden in the COVID-19 mobility data. We adopted the elbow method to identify the optimal cluster number. Specifically, the elbow method is a widely used heuristic in mathematical optimization, which involves selecting a point-referred to as the "Elbow" or "Knee of the curve" beyond which the benefits of further improvements do not justify the additional cost [65]. In clustering, this approach suggests choosing a number of clusters such that adding more clusters does not significantly enhance the model's accuracy. We conducted several experiments with different values of k across three months. Based on the results, we selected $k = 4$ as the optimal number of clusters. In other words, we categorized the 3142 counties into 4 groups, indicating that counties within the same group exhibit similar mobility patterns.

Figure 6 presents the spatiotemporal mobility patterns derived from our proposed method using four distinct colors to represent varying levels of mobility, where lighter shades indicate higher mobility. The results offer granular insights into mobility patterns during the three key phases of the COVID-19 pandemic: before the implementation of stay-at-home orders, during the stay-at-home period, and throughout the reopening phase. In the following sections, we delve into detailed observations of spatiotemporal mobility patterns, along with potential factors that contribute to these patterns.

Before the national pandemic response fully ramped up, the Midwest and Southern regions of the U.S. exhibited relatively high mobility levels, as indicated by the green and yellow shades across counties in states like Iowa, Kansas, Missouri, and Texas. These areas, being more rural in nature, likely saw higher movement due to daily activities such as agricultural work and commuting over larger distances. Additionally, many of these regions did not implement early restrictions, contributing to sustained levels of mobility during the initial phase of the pandemic. In contrast, coastal and urban areas, such as those on the East Coast (New York, New Jersey, Massachusetts) and the West Coast (California, Washington), displayed more moderate mobility levels. While formal restrictions had yet to be implemented in these areas, voluntary reductions in movement may have already begun as media coverage of the pandemic intensified. Urban centers, which typically rely more on public transportation and have higher population densities, experienced a shift in mobility patterns as non-essential travel was curtailed earlier compared to more rural areas.

During the stay-at-home period, the map reveals a significant nationwide reduction in mobility, with most counties shaded in deep purple, indicating low movement across both urban and rural areas. These widespread declines reflect the effectiveness of stay-at-home orders, which kept the majority of the population indoors except for essential activities like grocery shopping and medical appointments. However, there were notable exceptions in states such as Wyoming, Nebraska, and parts of Texas, where mobility remained relatively higher, as indicated by green and yellow shades. This can be attributed to essential industries, particularly in rural and agricultural regions, that required continued operation, looser restrictions in states with lower population densities, and localized outbreak responses where fewer COVID-19 cases were reported, resulting in less urgency to limit movement [66].

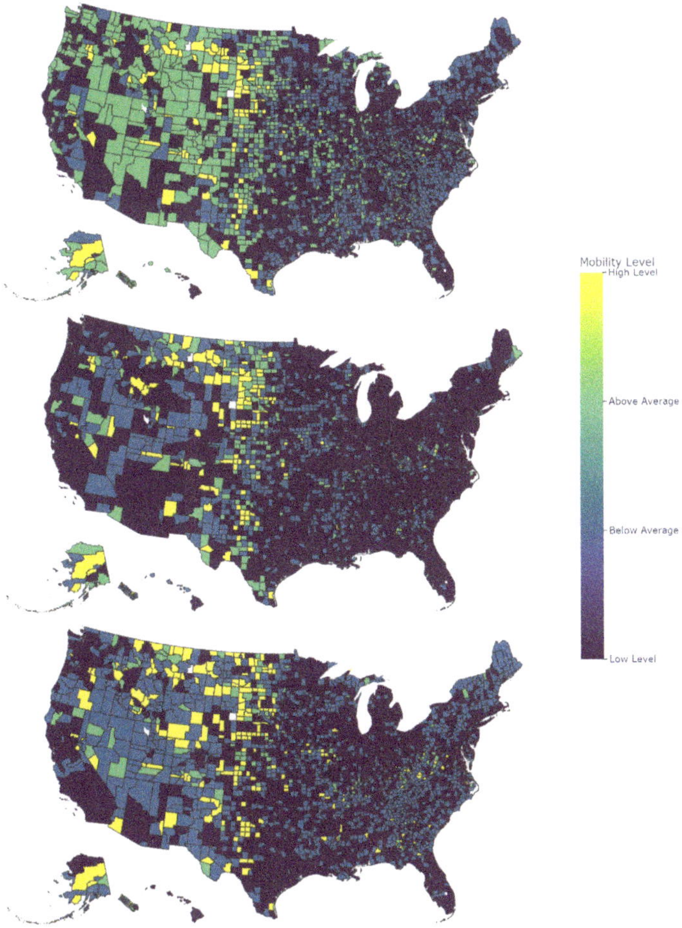

Figure 6. Spatiotemporal mobility patterns during the COVID-19 pandemic in three phases: before stay-at-home, during stay-at-home, and reopening (**top** to **bottom**). Mobility is categorized into four levels: high, above average, below average, and low, reflecting different movement trends across regions.

The bottom map reflects the reopening period when states began to relax restrictions and reopen their economies, leading to a partial recovery in mobility. In regions like the Midwest (Nebraska, Iowa, Kansas) and the South (Texas, Florida, Georgia), mobility levels noticeably increased, as indicated by the green and yellow shades. These states were among the first to prioritize economic recovery, allowing residents to return to work, shopping, and other activities, even amid rising COVID-19 cases. In contrast, coastal and urban areas, particularly on the East Coast (New York, New Jersey, Massachusetts) and the West Coast (California, Oregon, Washington), experienced slower mobility recovery, as shown by the persistent purple areas [52]. This slower rebound can be attributed to several factors, including ongoing caution and phased reopening strategies, especially in regions hit hardest early in the pandemic, where sectors operated under strict guidelines to avoid a second wave. Additionally, many large companies in cities like New York and San Francisco continued to enforce work-from-home policies, reducing the need for commuting and contributing to lower mobility. In states like Florida and Texas, the increased mobility may also reflect the reopening of tourist destinations and leisure activities, alongside higher traffic to commercial centers as restrictions on dining, retail, and entertainment venues were eased.

Across all three maps, clear differences emerge between rural and urban regions in terms of mobility patterns. Rural areas consistently show higher mobility both before and during the pandemic, likely due to the essential nature of agricultural and logistical work, which required continued movement. In contrast, urban areas experienced more significant reductions in mobility during the stay-at-home orders, likely due to stricter enforcement and the widespread ability to transition to remote work [67]. Mobility trends also closely align with state and local policy decisions regarding stay-at-home orders and reopening strategies. States in the Midwest and South, which reopened earlier, saw a quicker return to higher mobility, while states that adopted more cautious approaches experienced more gradual increases. Additionally, public response and health considerations influenced mobility. In areas with higher COVID-19 case rates or where perceived risk was greater, residents may have voluntarily reduced movement even during the reopening phase, as seen in lower mobility levels in states like New York and California.

Figure 7 presents the *ATD* across the stages: before the stay-at-home policies, during the stay-at-home orders, and during the reopening phase, categorized by high, above average, below average, and low mobility levels. The analysis reveals a significant reduction in mobility patterns immediately following the implementation of social distancing policies in March, with a gradual increase observed in May as reopening orders were enacted. This trend underscores the direct relationship between mobility shifts and the stringency of social distancing measures enforced by states. The results also highlight that some states were slower to curtail mobility in response to the pandemic, likely due to a combination of less severe outbreaks, more lenient local regulations, or lower levels of public concern and awareness. Overall, the result demonstrates that mobility across most states declined sharply in response to the onset of COVID-19 and the corresponding implementation of public health guidelines [68].

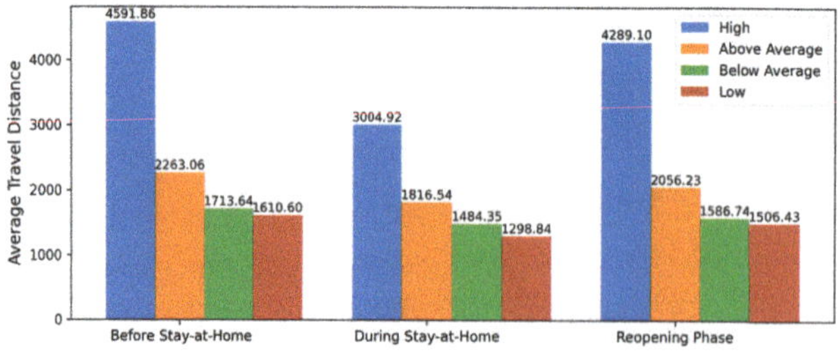

Figure 7. Average travel distance (*ATD*) across different stages from March to May 2020 (in meters).

4. Discussion

4.1. Limitations

It is important to point out some limitations of our work. First, although we used data from several locations, including Melbourne, Australia, and the United States, they are not enough to represent global mobility patterns, as our analysis might have miss important variations, particularly in underrepresented regions like developing countries. A wider geographical area needs to be considered to better understand a broader range of spatiotemporal patterns.

Second, through extensive experiments, we found that the choice of method should be tailored to the specific dataset. For datasets with minimal noise, outliers, or time distortions, or where these factors do not significantly impact the results, applying K-means with Euclidean distance directly can be both efficient and effective. However, in our study, we operated under the assumption of uncertain data quality and consider the worst-case scenario, where high-dimensionality, noise, outliers, and time distortions are present. Under these conditions, we developed a method that balances both accuracy and efficiency to handle these challenges effectively. Additionally, we used the elbow method to determine the optimal number of spatial clusters. However, in practical situations, where ground truth about spatial clusters is unavailable, the number of clusters may need to be adjusted based on specific applications, with the primary goal being to support better decision-making.

Third, we acknowledge that mobility is influenced by various factors, and understanding how mobility patterns evolve on their own may not be sufficient for informed decision-making. Thus, a deeper exploration into how specific socioeconomic conditions, such as economic status and population density, affect mobility patterns would enhance the analysis. Additionally, this study primarily focused on short-term mobility changes using only three months of mobility data from the COVID-19 pandemic in the U.S. Long-term analysis is necessary to gain a more comprehensive understanding of spatiotemporal mobility patterns.

4.2. Future Work

Here, we propose two future directions that should be explored. First, using more advanced neural network architectures, such as hybrid models combining convolutional, recurrent, or attention-based networks, along with improved optimization strategies, could better capture the relationships between multiple inputs and support long-term analysis. These enhanced architectures would provide a deeper understanding of the intricate dynamics within mobility data. Additionally, employing more suitable clustering algorithms, such as density-based or hierarchical methods, could enhance both the efficiency and accuracy of clustering the generated representations, leading to more nuanced insights into mobility patterns.

Second, we need to address more challenging situations, such as handling time series data with missing values, irregular sampling, and incomplete location information. In many real-world mobility datasets, data collection may be incomplete due to sensor failures, communication errors, or irregular intervals in reporting. Developing robust methods to impute missing values or work effectively with irregular time intervals is essential. Techniques such as interpolation, time series imputation models, and incorporating probabilistic methods could help mitigate the effects of missing data. Additionally, extending the models to handle irregularly spaced data points could improve their applicability and reliability in real-world scenarios, ensuring more accurate analysis and pattern detection.

5. Conclusions

This study proposes an improved deep time series clustering method for effectively mining spatiotemporal mobility patterns. By integrating a neural network-based temporal autoencoder with a dynamic time warping-based K-means clustering algorithm, we successfully address challenges such as high dimensionality, noise, outliers, and time distortions in mobility data, resulting in a more robust clustering approach. Extensive experiments on both synthetic and real-world datasets demonstrated the effectiveness of our method. Applying our approach to mobility data of the COVID-19 pandemic in the U.S. revealed significant differences in mobility patterns between rural and urban areas. Rural areas consistently exhibited higher mobility, both before and during the pandemic, likely due to the essential nature of agricultural and logistical work that required continued movement. In contrast, urban areas experienced more substantial reductions in mobility during stay-at-home orders, likely due to stricter enforcement and the widespread adoption of remote work. Additionally, public response and health considerations influenced mobility patterns. In regions with higher COVID-19 case rates or greater perceived risk, residents voluntarily reduced movement, even during reopening phases, as observed in lower mobility levels in states like New York and California. This application highlights the broader implications of our proposed method in potential fields such as public health, epidemiology, transportation analysis, urban planning, smart cities, and environmental monitoring.

Author Contributions: Conceptualization, Ziyi Zhang, Zhe Zhang, and Nick Duffield; methodology, Ziyi Zhang; software, Ziyi Zhang and Diya Li; validation, Ziyi Zhang; formal analysis, Ziyi Zhang; investigation, Diya Li; resources, Diya Li; data curation, Diya Li; writing—original draft preparation, Ziyi Zhang; writing—review and editing, Zhe Zhang; visualization, Ziyi Zhang; supervision, Zhe Zhang and Nick Duffield; project administration, Zhe Zhang and Nick Duffield; funding acquisition, Zhe Zhang and Nick Duffield. All authors have read and agreed to the published version of the manuscript.

Funding: This research was funded by U.S. National Science Foundation (NSF) Grant #2339174 CAREER: A Cyberinfrastructure Enabled Hybrid Spatial Decision Support System for Improving Coastal Resilience to Flood Risks and #2321069 Collaborative Research: CyberTraining: Implementation: Small: Broadening Adoption of Cyberinfrastructure and Research Workforce Development for Disaster Management.

Data Availability Statement: The Melbourne Pedestrian Time Series Data and the Chinatown Pedestrian Time Series Data (https://www.cs.ucr.edu/~eamonn/time_series_data/, accessed on 15 January 2024), as well as the COVID-19 Mobility Time Series Data (https://data.bts.gov/Research-and-Statistics/Trips-by-Distance/w96p-f2qv, accessed on 10 September 2021), were utilized in this study.

Conflicts of Interest: The authors declare no conflicts of interest.

Abbreviations

The following abbreviations are used in this manuscript:

ATD	Average Travel Distance
BiLSTM	Bi-directional Long Short-Term Memory
CAE	Convolutional Autoencoder
DR	Dimensionality Reduction
DTW	Dynamic Time Warping
I-DTSC	Improved Deep Time Series Clustering
KL	K-means oriented Loss
MSE	Mean Square Error
NN	Neural Network
NMF	Non-negative Matrix Factorization
PCA	Principal Component Analysis
RI	Rand Index
ReLU	Rectified Linear Unit
RNN	Recurrent Neural Network
TAE	Temporal Autoencoder
TN	True Negative
TP	True Positive
1D-CNN	One-Dimensional Convolutional Neural Network

References

1. Hasan, S.; Schneider, C.M.; Ukkusuri, S.V.; González, M.C. Spatiotemporal patterns of urban human mobility. *J. Stat. Phys.* **2013**, *151*, 304–318. [CrossRef]
2. Alessandretti, L.; Sapiezynski, P.; Lehmann, S.; Baronchelli, A. Multi-scale spatio-temporal analysis of human mobility. *PLoS ONE* **2017**, *12*, e0171686. [CrossRef] [PubMed]
3. Caldeira, A.M.; Kastenholz, E. Spatiotemporal tourist behaviour in urban destinations: A framework of analysis. *Tour. Geogr.* **2020**, *22*, 22–50. [CrossRef]
4. Zhai, H.; Gu, B.; Wang, Y. Evaluation of policies and actions for nature-based solutions in nationally determined contributions. *Land Use Policy* **2023**, *131*, 106710. [CrossRef]
5. Zhai, H.; Gu, B.; Zhu, K.; Huang, C. Feasibility analysis of achieving net-zero emissions in China's power sector before 2050 based on ideal available pathways. *Environ. Impact Assess. Rev.* **2023**, *98*, 106948. [CrossRef]
6. Mao, F.; Ji, M.; Liu, T. Mining spatiotemporal patterns of urban dwellers from taxi trajectory data. *Front. Earth Sci.* **2016**, *10*, 205–221. [CrossRef]
7. Neves, F.; Finamore, A.C.; Madeira, S.C.; Henriques, R. Mining actionable patterns of road mobility from heterogeneous traffic data using biclustering. *IEEE Trans. Intell. Transp. Syst.* **2021**, *23*, 6430–6445. [CrossRef]
8. Xiao, G.; Wang, Y.; Wu, R.; Li, J.; Cai, Z. Sustainable maritime transport: A review of intelligent shipping technology and green port construction applications. *J. Mar. Sci. Eng.* **2024**, *12*, 1728. [CrossRef]
9. Song, X.; Zhang, Q.; Sekimoto, Y.; Shibasaki, R. Prediction of human emergency behavior and their mobility following large-scale disaster. In Proceedings of the 20th ACM SIGKDD International Conference on Knowledge Discovery and Data Mining, New York, NY, USA, 24–27 August 2014; pp. 5–14.
10. Zhang, Z.; Li, D.; Zhang, Z.; Duffield, N. A time-series clustering algorithm for analyzing the changes of mobility pattern caused by COVID-19. In Proceedings of the 1st ACM SIGSPATIAL International Workshop on Animal Movement Ecology And Human Mobility, Beijing, China, 2 November 2021; pp. 13–17.
11. Hu, N.; Zhang, Z.; Duffield, N.; Li, X.; Dadashova, B.; Wu, D.; Yu, S.; Ye, X.; Han, D.; Zhang, Z. Geographical and temporal weighted regression: Examining spatial variations of COVID-19 mortality pattern using mobility and multi-source data. *Comput. Urban Sci.* **2024**, *4*, 6. [CrossRef]
12. Li, D.; Zhang, Z.; Alizadeh, B.; Zhang, Z.; Duffield, N.; Meyer, M.A.; Thompson, C.M.; Gao, H.; Behzadan, A.H. A reinforcement learning-based routing algorithm for large street networks. *Int. J. Geogr. Inf. Sci.* **2024**, *38*, 183–215. [CrossRef]
13. Aghabozorgi, S.; Shirkhorshidi, A.S.; Wah, T.Y. Time-series clustering—A decade review. *Inf. Syst.* **2015**, *53*, 16–38. [CrossRef]
14. Zhao, B.; Lu, H.; Chen, S.; Liu, J.; Wu, D. Convolutional neural networks for time series classification. *J. Syst. Eng. Electron.* **2017**, *28*, 162–169. [CrossRef]
15. Zhang, Z.; Li, D.; Song, Z.; Duffield, N.; Zhang, Z. Location-Aware social network recommendation via temporal graph networks. In Proceedings of the 7th ACM SIGSPATIAL Workshop on Location-Based Recommendations, Geosocial Networks and Geoadvertising, Hamburg, Germany, 13 November 2023; pp. 58–61.
16. Li, L.; Prakash, B.A. Time series clustering: Complex is simpler! In Proceedings of the 28th International Conference on Machine Learning (ICML-11), Bellevue, WA, USA, 28 June–2 July 2011; pp. 185–192.
17. Ma, Q.; Zheng, J.; Li, S.; Cottrell, G.W. Learning representations for time series clustering. In Proceedings of the Advances in Neural Information Processing Systems 32, Vancouver, BC, Canada, 8–14 December 2019.
18. Xu, K.; Chen, L.; Wang, S. Data-driven kernel subspace clustering with local manifold preservation. In Proceedings of the 2022 IEEE International Conference on Data Mining Workshops (ICDMW), Orlando, FL, USA, 28 November–1 December 2022; IEEE: Piscataway, NJ, USA, 2022; pp. 876–884.
19. Xu, K.; Chen, L.; Wang, S. A multi-view kernel clustering framework for categorical sequences. *Expert Syst. Appl.* **2022**, *197*, 116637. [CrossRef]
20. Rasul, K.; Seward, C.; Schuster, I.; Vollgraf, R. Autoregressive denoising diffusion models for multivariate probabilistic time series forecasting. In Proceedings of the International Conference on Machine Learning, Virtual, 18–24 July 2021; PMLR; pp. 8857–8868.
21. Zhou, T.; Ma, Z.; Wen, Q.; Wang, X.; Sun, L.; Jin, R. Fedformer: Frequency enhanced decomposed transformer for long-term series forecasting. In Proceedings of the International Conference on Machine Learning, Baltimore, MD, USA, 17–23 July 2022; PMLR; pp. 27268–27286.
22. Zhang, Z.; Ren, S.; Qian, X.; Duffield, N. Towards invariant time series forecasting in smart cities. In Proceedings of the Companion Proceedings of the ACM on Web Conference 2024, Singapore, 13–17 May 2024; pp. 1344–1350.
23. Xu, K.; Chen, L.; Patenaude, J.M.; Wang, S. Rhine: A regime-switching model with nonlinear representation for discovering and forecasting regimes in financial markets. In Proceedings of the 2024 SIAM International Conference on Data Mining (SDM), Houston, TX, USA, 18–20 April 2024; SIAM: Philadelphia, PA, USA, 2024; pp. 526–534.
24. Xu, K.; Chen, L.; Patenaude, J.M.; Wang, S. Kernel representation learning with dynamic regime discovery for time series forecasting. In Proceedings of the Pacific-Asia Conference on Knowledge Discovery and Data Mining, Taiwan, China, 7–10 May 2024; Springer: Berlin/Heidelberg, Germany, 2024; pp. 251–263.
25. Pamfil, R.; Sriwattanaworachai, N.; Desai, S.; Pilgerstorfer, P.; Georgatzis, K.; Beaumont, P.; Aragam, B. Dynotears: Structure learning from time-series data. In Proceedings of the International Conference on Artificial Intelligence and Statistics, Online, 26–28 August 2020; PMLR; pp. 1595–1605.

26. Tank, A.; Covert, I.; Foti, N.; Shojaie, A.; Fox, E.B. Neural granger causality. *IEEE Trans. Pattern Anal. Mach. Intell.* **2021**, *44*, 4267–4279. [CrossRef]
27. Zhang, Z.; Ren, S.; Qian, X.; Duffield, N. Learning Flexible Time-windowed Granger Causality Integrating Heterogeneous Interventional Time Series Data. In Proceedings of the 30th ACM SIGKDD Conference on Knowledge Discovery and Data Mining, Barcelona, Spain, 25–29 August 2024; pp. 4408–4418.
28. Steinbach, M.; Tan, P.N.; Kumar, V.; Klooster, S.; Potter, C. Discovery of climate indices using clustering. In Proceedings of the Ninth ACM SIGKDD International Conference on Knowledge Discovery and Data Mining, Washington, DC, USA, 24–27 August 2003; pp. 446–455.
29. Ji, M.; Xie, F.; Ping, Y. A dynamic fuzzy cluster algorithm for time series. In *Abstract and Applied Analysis*; Wiley Online Library: Hoboken, NJ, USA, 2013; Volume 2013, p. 183410.
30. Elangasinghe, M.; Singhal, N.; Dirks, K.; Salmond, J.; Samarasinghe, S. Complex time series analysis of PM10 and PM2. 5 for a coastal site using artificial neural network modelling and k-means clustering. *Atmos. Environ.* **2014**, *94*, 106–116. [CrossRef]
31. Kontis, V.; Bennett, J.E.; Rashid, T.; Parks, R.M.; Pearson-Stuttard, J.; Guillot, M.; Asaria, P.; Zhou, B.; Battaglini, M.; Corsetti, G.; et al. Magnitude, demographics and dynamics of the effect of the first wave of the COVID-19 pandemic on all-cause mortality in 21 industrialized countries. *Nat. Med.* **2020**, *26*, 1919–1928. [CrossRef] [PubMed]
32. Iglesias, F.; Kastner, W. Analysis of similarity measures in times series clustering for the discovery of building energy patterns. *Energies* **2013**, *6*, 579–597. [CrossRef]
33. Shumway, R.H. Time-frequency clustering and discriminant analysis. *Stat. Probab. Lett.* **2003**, *63*, 307–314. [CrossRef]
34. Huang, X.; Li, Z.; Lu, J.; Wang, S.; Wei, H.; Chen, B. Time-series clustering for home dwell time during COVID-19: What can we learn from it? *ISPRS Int. J. Geo-Inf.* **2020**, *9*, 675. [CrossRef]
35. Yang, K.; Shahabi, C. A PCA-based similarity measure for multivariate time series. In Proceedings of the 2nd ACM International Workshop on Multimedia Databases, Washington, DC, USA, 13 November 2004; pp. 65–74.
36. Li, H. Multivariate time series clustering based on common principal component analysis. *Neurocomputing* **2019**, *349*, 239–247. [CrossRef]
37. Zhou, L.; Du, G.; Tao, D.; Chen, H.; Cheng, J.; Gong, L. Clustering multivariate time series data via multi-nonnegative matrix factorization in multi-relational networks. *IEEE Access* **2018**, *6*, 74747–74761. [CrossRef]
38. He, G.; Wang, H.; Liu, S.; Zhang, B. CSMVC: A multiview method for multivariate time-series clustering. *IEEE Trans. Cybern.* **2021**, *52*, 13425–13437. [CrossRef]
39. Bengio, Y.; Courville, A.; Vincent, P. Representation learning: A review and new perspectives. *IEEE Trans. Pattern Anal. Mach. Intell.* **2013**, *35*, 1798–1828. [CrossRef]
40. Alqahtani, A.; Ali, M.; Xie, X.; Jones, M.W. Deep time-series clustering: A review. *Electronics* **2021**, *10*, 3001. [CrossRef]
41. Tavakoli, N.; Siami-Namini, S.; Adl Khanghah, M.; Mirza Soltani, F.; Siami Namin, A. An autoencoder-based deep learning approach for clustering time series data. *SN Appl. Sci.* **2020**, *2*, 1–25. [CrossRef]
42. Özgül, O.F.; Bardak, B.; Tan, M. A convolutional deep clustering framework for gene expression time series. *IEEE/ACM Trans. Comput. Biol. Bioinform.* **2020**, *18*, 2198–2207. [CrossRef]
43. Mousavi, S.M.; Zhu, W.; Ellsworth, W.; Beroza, G. Unsupervised clustering of seismic signals using deep convolutional autoencoders. *IEEE Geosci. Remote. Sens. Lett.* **2019**, *16*, 1693–1697. [CrossRef]
44. Karadayı, Y.; Aydin, M.N.; Öğrenci, A.S. A hybrid deep learning framework for unsupervised anomaly detection in multivariate spatio-temporal data. *Appl. Sci.* **2020**, *10*, 5191. [CrossRef]
45. Chadha, G.S.; Islam, I.; Schwung, A.; Ding, S.X. Deep convolutional clustering-based time series anomaly detection. *Sensors* **2021**, *21*, 5488. [CrossRef] [PubMed]
46. Madiraju, N.S. Deep Temporal Clustering: Fully Unsupervised Learning of Time-Domain Features. Master's Thesis, Arizona State University, Tempe, AZ, USA, 2018.
47. Trosten, D.J.; Strauman, A.S.; Kampffmeyer, M.; Jenssen, R. Recurrent deep divergence-based clustering for simultaneous feature learning and clustering of variable length time series. In Proceedings of the ICASSP 2019–2019 IEEE International Conference on Acoustics, Speech and Signal Processing (ICASSP), Brighton, UK, 12–17 May 2019; IEEE: Piscataway, NJ, USA, 2019; pp. 3257–3261.
48. Ienco, D.; Interdonato, R. Deep multivariate time series embedding clustering via attentive-gated autoencoder. In Proceedings of the Advances in Knowledge Discovery and Data Mining: 24th Pacific-Asia Conference, PAKDD 2020, Singapore, 11–14 May 2020; Proceedings, Part I 24; Springer: Berlin/Heidelberg, Germany, 2020; pp. 318–329.
49. Lafabregue, B.; Weber, J.; Gançarski, P.; Forestier, G. End-to-end deep representation learning for time series clustering: A comparative study. *Data Min. Knowl. Discov.* **2022**, *36*, 29–81. [CrossRef]
50. Saito, N. Local Feature Extraction and Its Applications Using a Library of Bases. Ph.D.Thesis, Yale University, New Haven, CT, USA, 1994.
51. Zhou, Y.; Liu, X.C.; Grubesic, T. Unravel the impact of COVID-19 on the spatio-temporal mobility patterns of microtransit. *J. Transp. Geogr.* **2021**, *97*, 103226. [CrossRef]
52. Gao, S.; Rao, J.; Kang, Y.; Liang, Y.; Kruse, J. Mapping county-level mobility pattern changes in the United States in response to COVID-19. *SIGSpatial Spec.* **2020**, *12*, 16–26. [CrossRef]

53. Nouvellet, P.; Bhatia, S.; Cori, A.; Ainslie, K.E.; Baguelin, M.; Bhatt, S.; Boonyasiri, A.; Brazeau, N.F.; Cattarino, L.; Cooper, L.V.; et al. Reduction in mobility and COVID-19 transmission. *Nat. Commun.* **2021**, *12*, 1–9. [CrossRef] [PubMed]
54. Bavel, J.J.V.; Baicker, K.; Boggio, P.S.; Capraro, V.; Cichocka, A.; Cikara, M.; Crockett, M.J.; Crum, A.J.; Douglas, K.M.; Druckman, J.N.; et al. Using social and behavioural science to support COVID-19 pandemic response. *Nat. Hum. Behav.* **2020**, *4*, 460–471. [CrossRef]
55. Clemente-Suárez, V.J.; Navarro-Jiménez, E.; Moreno-Luna, L.; Saavedra-Serrano, M.C.; Jimenez, M.; Simón, J.A.; Tornero-Aguilera, J.F. The impact of the COVID-19 pandemic on social, health, and economy. *Sustainability* **2021**, *13*, 6314. [CrossRef]
56. Brodeur, A.; Gray, D.; Islam, A.; Bhuiyan, S. A literature review of the economics of COVID-19. *J. Econ. Surv.* **2021**, *35*, 1007–1044. [CrossRef]
57. Padhan, R.; Prabheesh, K. The economics of COVID-19 pandemic: A survey. *Econ. Anal. Policy* **2021**, *70*, 220–237. [CrossRef]
58. Shah, P.; Owens, J.; Franklin, J.; Mehta, A.; Heymann, W.; Sewell, W.; Hill, J.; Barfield, K.; Doshi, R. Demographics, comorbidities and outcomes in hospitalized Covid-19 patients in rural southwest Georgia. *Ann. Med.* **2020**, *52*, 354–360. [CrossRef]
59. Li, D.; Chaudhary, H.; Zhang, Z. Modeling spatiotemporal pattern of depressive symptoms caused by COVID-19 using social media data mining. *Int. J. Environ. Res. Public Health* **2020**, *17*, 4988. [CrossRef]
60. Zhu, S.; Bukharin, A.; Xie, L.; Santillana, M.; Yang, S.; Xie, Y. High-resolution spatio-temporal model for county-level COVID-19 activity in the US. *ACM Trans. Manag. Inf. Syst. (TMIS)* **2021**, *12*, 1–20. [CrossRef]
61. Liu, L.; Hu, T.; Bao, S.; Wu, H.; Peng, Z.; Wang, R. The spatiotemporal interaction effect of COVID-19 transmission in the United States. *ISPRS Int. J. Geo-Inf.* **2021**, *10*, 387. [CrossRef]
62. Wang, Y.; Liu, Y.; Struthers, J.; Lian, M. Spatiotemporal characteristics of the COVID-19 epidemic in the United States. *Clin. Infect. Dis.* **2021**, *72*, 643–651. [CrossRef] [PubMed]
63. Maiti, A.; Zhang, Q.; Sannigrahi, S.; Pramanik, S.; Chakraborti, S.; Cerda, A.; Pilla, F. Exploring spatiotemporal effects of the driving factors on COVID-19 incidences in the contiguous United States. *Sustain. Cities Soc.* **2021**, *68*, 102784. [CrossRef] [PubMed]
64. Song, Z.; Zhang, Z.; Lyu, F.; Bishop, M.; Liu, J.; Chi, Z. From Individual Motivation to Geospatial Epidemiology: A Novel Approach Using Fuzzy Cognitive Maps and Agent-Based Modeling for Large-Scale Disease Spread. *Sustainability* **2024**, *16*, 5036. [CrossRef]
65. Liu, F.; Deng, Y. Determine the number of unknown targets in open world based on elbow method. *IEEE Trans. Fuzzy Syst.* **2020**, *29*, 986–995. [CrossRef]
66. Cuadros, D.F.; Branscum, A.J.; Mukandavire, Z.; Miller, F.D.; MacKinnon, N. Dynamics of the COVID-19 epidemic in urban and rural areas in the United States. *Ann. Epidemiol.* **2021**, *59*, 16–20. [CrossRef]
67. Huang, Y.; Li, R. The lockdown, mobility, and spatial health disparities in COVID-19 pandemic: A case study of New York City. *Cities* **2022**, *122*, 103549. [CrossRef]
68. Badr, H.S.; Du, H.; Marshall, M.; Dong, E.; Squire, M.M.; Gardner, L.M. Association between mobility patterns and COVID-19 transmission in the USA: A mathematical modelling study. *Lancet Infect. Dis.* **2020**, *20*, 1247–1254. [CrossRef]

International Journal of
Geo-Information

MDPI

Article

Investigating Spatial Effects through Machine Learning and Leveraging Explainable AI for Child Malnutrition in Pakistan

Xiaoyi Zhang [1], Muhammad Usman [2], Ateeq ur Rehman Irshad [3], Mudassar Rashid [4,*] and Amira Khattak [5]

1 College of Liberal Arts and Science, University of Illinois Urbana-Champaign, Urbana, IL 61801, USA; xiaoyi6@illinios.edu
2 Faculty of Economic Sciences, University of Warsaw, 00-927 Warszawa, Poland; m.usman@uw.edu.pl
3 Deanship of Educational Services, Prince Sultan University, Riyadh 11586, Saudi Arabia; airshad@psu.edu.sa
4 Department of Economics, COMSATS University Islamabad, Islamabad 45550, Pakistan
5 Department of Marketing, College of Business Administration, Prince Sultan University, Riyadh 11586, Saudi Arabia; akhattak@psu.edu.sa
* Correspondence: mudassar.rashid@comsats.edu.pk

Abstract: While socioeconomic gradients in regional health inequalities are firmly established, the synergistic interactions between socioeconomic deprivation and climate vulnerability within convenient proximity and neighbourhood locations with health disparities remain poorly explored and thus require deep understanding within a regional context. Furthermore, disregarding the importance of spatial spillover effects and nonlinear effects of covariates on childhood stunting are inevitable in dealing with an enduring issue of regional health inequalities. The present study aims to investigate the spatial inequalities in childhood stunting at the district level in Pakistan and validate the importance of spatial lag in predicting childhood stunting. Furthermore, it examines the presence of any nonlinear relationships among the selected independent features with childhood stunting. The study utilized data related to socioeconomic features from MICS 2017–2018 and climatic data from Integrated Contextual Analysis. A multi-model approach was employed to address the research questions, which included Ordinary Least Squares Regression (OLS), various Spatial Models, Machine Learning Algorithms and Explainable Artificial Intelligence methods. Firstly, OLS was used to analyse and test the linear relationships among selected variables. Secondly, Spatial Durbin Error Model (SDEM) was used to detect and capture the impact of spatial spillover on childhood stunting. Third, XGBoost and Random Forest machine learning algorithms were employed to examine and validate the importance of the spatial lag component. Finally, EXAI methods such as SHapley were utilized to identify potential nonlinear relationships. The study found a clear pattern of spatial clustering and geographical disparities in childhood stunting, with multidimensional poverty, high climate vulnerability and early marriage worsening childhood stunting. In contrast, low climate vulnerability, high exposure to mass media and high women's literacy were found to reduce childhood stunting. The use of machine learning algorithms, specifically XGBoost and Random Forest, highlighted the significant role played by the average value in the neighbourhood in predicting childhood stunting in nearby districts, confirming that the spatial spillover effect is not bounded by geographical boundaries. Furthermore, EXAI methods such as partial dependency plot reveal the existence of a nonlinear relationship between multidimensional poverty and childhood stunting. The study's findings provide valuable insights into the spatial distribution of childhood stunting in Pakistan, emphasizing the importance of considering spatial effects in predicting childhood stunting. Individual and household-level factors such as exposure to mass media and women's literacy have shown positive implications for childhood stunting. It further provides a justification for the usage of EXAI methods to draw better insights and propose customised intervention policies accordingly.

Keywords: regional health inequalities; childhood stunting; climate vulnerability; spatial hotspots; machine learning; explainable artificial intelligence

1. Introduction

In 2015, the United Nations declared the Sustainable Development Goals (Target 2.2), with an objective of "ending all forms of malnutrition by 2030". The first 1000 days of a child's life are considered crucial for mental and physical development. Good early days are proven to be key catalysts for the overall growth of a child [1]. Therefore, a gritty and realistic focus on reducing childhood stunting is required to comprehend the most critical period of children's development.

Globally, in 2019, 144 million children under the age of five years had stunted growth. Although there has been a consistent decline in the growth of stunting since 2000 (199.5 million were stunted), the progress seems insufficient to meet the 40% reduction target by 2025 set by World Health Assembly [2].

Africa and Asia are burdened with the highest number of stunted children with 54% and 40%, respectively. Specifically, in South Asia, Pakistan bears the third-highest childhood stunting rate followed by India. Childhood stunting has been a persistent threat to child growth in Pakistan. Historic data on child malnutrition reveals that childhood stunting has remained alarmingly high with minimal improvement over time. In the year 2011, the stunting rate was 44% and, despite some efforts, it only decreased slightly to 38% by 2018. Recent estimates on childhood stunting present a rather dismal picture as it increased to 40%. These historical data suggest that the country has been grappling with this enduring issue for an extended period of time [3].

Socioeconomic and environmental challenges such as high poverty, widespread food insecurity, poor quality of water and inadequate sanitation facilities and stagnating agricultural productivity are the major contributors to poor health outcomes and deteriorating human capital [4]. In Pakistan, 30% of households lack adequate sanitation facilities and more than approximately 2.1 million individuals are deprived of safe drinking water. It has been firmly established that if the current conditions such as high poverty are not improved, the lack of basic sanitation and safe drinking water and prevalence of diseases would further worsen in the coming years [5].

Several studies have elucidated that illiteracy, poor sanitation facilities, lack of improved drinking water, poverty and bigger household size may in part contribute to childhood stunting. Existing literature on Lower Middle Income Countries (LIMCs) has empathized household and individual factors as the significant contributors to childhood stunting. In [6] it was concluded that breast feeding practices, household wealth status, maternal nutrition and child food intake are crucial factors in determining childhood stunting. Similarly, using a mutually adjusted logistic regression, [7] determined that in children who were aged between 6 and 8 months, limited intake of complementary foods and short maternal stature were significantly linked with higher risk of childhood stunting. For children who were aged between 6 and 23 months, household wealth, maternal height, maternal education and age at marriage were found to be significant correlates of childhood stunting. The authors of [8] used the two recent most Indonesian Family Life Survey (IFLS) to examine the variations in prevalence of childhood stunting between 2007 and 2014. They revealed that household wealth status, mothers' education, place of delivery and the availability of sanitation facilities contribute most to childhood stunting. Furthermore, they found that improvement in health care access significantly contributed to reducing the stunting gap between richer and poorer children. Additionally, [9] asserted that children from poor households with unavailability of sanitation facilities and lack of safe drinking water were at more risk of having stunted growth.

Maternal stature and education play a crucial role in child's development. The authors of [10] used the fourth Indian National Family Health Survey to identify risk factors for chronic undernutrition in India. They calculated odds ratios using logistic regression. Based on their findings, they determined the five most vital factors for childhood stunting. They argued that illiterate mothers, poor households, short maternal stature, poor dietary intake and low maternal weight are the main contributing factors. These factors had a population-attributable risk of 67.2% for stunting. Similarly, using the latest available

Indian National Family Health Survey (2015–2016), [11] analysed the relative importance of 23 correlates of stunting. They estimated logistic regression models to evaluate the importance of selected predictors. Based on their results, they identified short maternal stature as the most important contributing factor to stunting. Other key factors were poor household status, poor air quality of households, lack of maternal education and low maternal BMI. Additionally, they found weaker associations for dietary intake, breastfeeding and parental factors.

Maternal caretaker behaviour and early female child marriage have been identified as risk factors for child development. The authors of [12] inspected the intergenerational effects of early child marriage on stunting and child development in Sub Saharan Africa. They concluded that the odds of being stunted are 29% higher for children born to women who married before the age 18 in comparison to those women who married later in their lives. They further examined the mechanisms through which risk of stunting increases. They added that early child marriage is not the sole path to stunting. However, contextual factors such as maternal education and household wealth matter for child development and health.

In recent years, researchers have assessed the role of environmental covariates such as rainfall, temperature, droughts and floods, etc., on stunting. A recent study by [13] revealed that along with socioeconomic features, high climate vulnerability exacerbates childhood stunting in comparison to low climate vulnerability. In sub-Saharan Africa the odds ratio for child health outcomes were higher in the presence of droughts and political instability [14]. Similarly, using multivariate regression models, authors assessed the relationship between exposure to climate variations (rainfall and temperature) in utero and early child development. They suggested that higher rainfall during early life bears a negative relationship with stunting. However, higher prenatal temperatures have negative repercussions during the early life of children and consequently lead to severe stunting. Additionally, they identified potential pathways such as heat stress, infectious diseases caused by climatic variations and more time devoted to work during pregnancies in dry seasons through which the odds of stunting increase [15]. In Indonesia, a similar study was conducted to detect the association between climate exposures and child undernutrition. They argued that delays in monsoon rainfall during the prenatal period had an adverse effect on child height during the early 2–4 years [16].

Lately, there has been growing recognition of integrating spatial data and geographic factors to uncover the multifaceted nature of childhood stunting. Numerous studies have illustrated that childhood stunting varies across regions, a term often used to describe this phenomenon being geographical heterogeneity. For instance, spatial hotspots were identified with high stunting rates amongst districts in the Upper West, Upper East and Western North regions in Ghana. These districts were characterised by low access to basic health services, high poverty levels and low educational attainment. On the other hand, clusters with low childhood stunting were observed in the Greater Accra, Volta and Bono regions [17]. Similarly, a study conducted in India identified 146 hot spots as high prevalence and 130 cold spots as low prevalence districts. Districts with high stunting rates were mostly concentrated in the states of Bihar, Jharkhand and Uttar Pradesh, while low prevalence districts were largely observed in the states of Himachal Pradesh, Kerala, Tamil Nadu and West Bengal. Factors such as large household size, open defecation, female illiteracy, household poverty and unavailability of improved drinking water were associated with higher stunting rates [18]. In Ethiopia, a similar study was conducted which revealed a spatial dependency in childhood stunting. Districts with the highest prevalence of childhood stunting were found in Northern Ethiopia. By leveraging logistic regression, the authors concluded that factors such as low level of female education, poor household wealth and older age were exacerbating stunting in the children under 5 years of age [19]. Similarly, in another study, spatial heterogeneity was observed in Ethiopia across locations suggesting a variation in childhood stunting. The estimates of logistic regression indicated that children who had anaemic history, malnourished mothers, low educational attainment and mothers with multiple births were most likely to be severely stunted [20]. A secondary spatial analysis of the RDHS 2014–15 cross sectional data revealed that low maternal education, non-optimal feeding practices, lack of improved water and belonging to poor households were significant contributors to childhood stunting [21].

It is evident from the existing literature that researchers have focused mainly either on household- or on individual-level factors. Furthermore, from the methodological perspective, there exists a vast amount of literature which has predominantly employed ordinary least squares or logistic regression. These methods are very well known for testing linear relationships [22]. Spatial studies are limited to the spatial distribution of child malnutrition rates. Rare usages of spatial models, the possible significant impact of spatial lag component on nearby districts, and integrated spatial machine learning approaches in the area of regional health inequalities have not yet been thoroughly explored. Additionally, as childhood stunting is influenced by a complex interaction of multiple factors, traditional linear models such as OLS may not adequately capture potential nonlinear relationships. In this regard, employing Explainable Artificial Intelligence (EXAI) methods such as LIME and SHAP could help us identify such intricate relationships, which are not identifiable with conventional approaches. Furthermore, to best of our knowledge, no study has been conducted to examine spatial correlates of childhood stunting for all the districts of Pakistan. Therefore, this study attempts to quantify the possible spatial correlates of childhood stunting for all the regions of Pakistan. This study is more comprehensive and inclusive. Moreover, the primary focus of this research is to provide a novel methodological perspective and implementation of spatial machine learning and EXAI methods for regional health economics in a spatial context.

Specifically, this research aims to address these aforementioned research gaps through (1) investigating the spatial distribution of childhood stunting in Pakistan, (2) spatial examination of the relationships between socioeconomic, climatic features and childhood stunting, (3) identification and validation of spatial lag using spatial machine learning algorithms and (4) examination of nonlinear relationships using EXAI techniques.

The present study brings novelty to the recognition and validation of the significance of spatial lag components (i.e., average value in the neighbourhood) and proposes a methodological approach using spatial machine learning. The integrated methodology provides additional insights to researchers and policymakers compared to conventional statistical methods, which typically assume that effects remain stationary. Additionally, the inclusion of climatic covariates along with other socioeconomic features could help address the issue of sparse determinants of stunting. Understanding the relationship between climate covariates and stunting would allow for the understanding of how climate change might shape childhood stunting in the future. Moreover, examination of nonlinear relationships will aid in developing targeted health intervention programs and policies for populations with significant needs.

2. Materials and Methods

This study covered all 145 districts from all provinces (Punjab, Sindh, Kpk, Gilgit-Baltistan), excluding ICT (Islamabad Capital Territory represented as white region), made available in the form of shapefiles. All districts were included in the analysis. Districts were mapped using shapefiles of Pakistan from DIV-GIS. All computations and estimations were performed in R Studio. The following Figure 1 is the official map of Pakistan portraying all the districts covered.

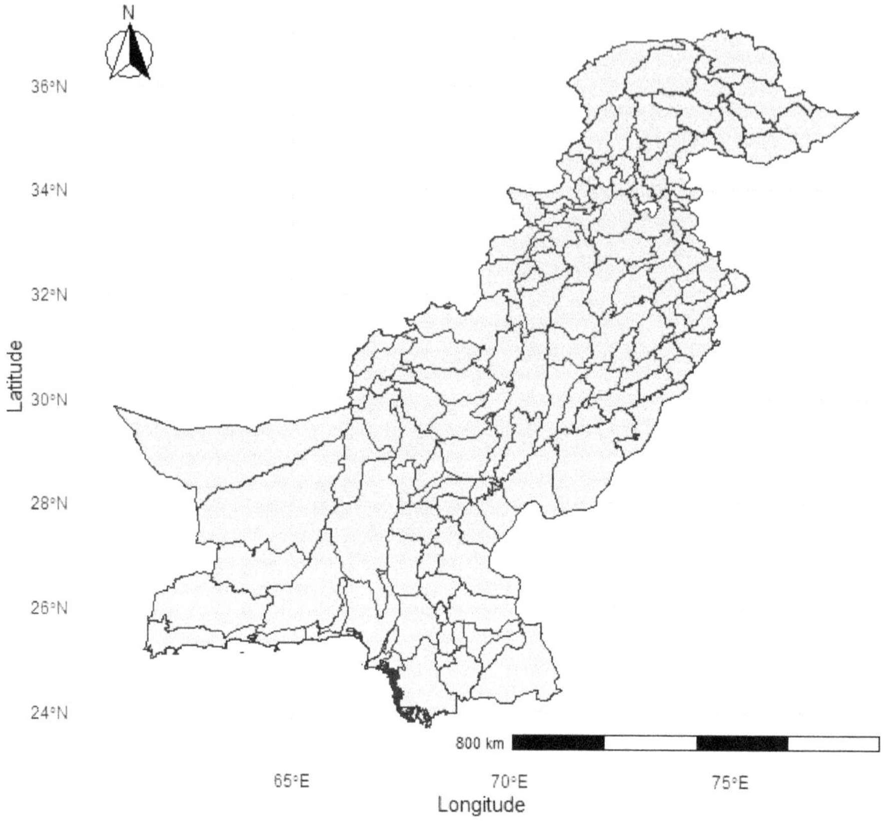

Figure 1. Regional map of Pakistan.

2.1. Sampling and Data Collection

The study uses a cross-sectional dataset from multiple sources, the Multiple Indicator Cluster Survey (MICS) and the Integrated Household Survey (ICA), which were matched accordingly at the district level. MICS (accessed on 13 December 2023) (https://mics.unicef.org/surveys) is an internationally recognized household survey that provides district level estimates of more than 125 key indicators related to demographic, socioeconomic, health, to assess the overall situation of women aged 14–49 years and children under five years of age. The latest available MICS survey from year 2017–2018 was used in this study. A two-stage standardized sampling approach was followed to select the survey samples from all regions. In the first step, enumeration areas were selected from the primary sampling units. In the second step, a household was selected from the chosen enumeration areas. The enumeration areas were selected with unequal probability means with probability proportional to size. The total sample was comprised of 53,480 households in 2692 cluster samples, with a response rate of approximately 98% across all regions [23].

2.2. Variables

In this study, the outcome variable was the percentage of stunted children under the age of five, defined by MICS as children whose height-for-age z-scores were below minus two standard deviations. Independent features were obtained from three different sources. Socioeconomic features, including female literacy, meaning the percentage of women who can read a short simple statement and also attended secondary school education; premature birth rate, representing the percentage of all children who were born before 37 weeks of pregnancy; marriage before age 15, showing the percentage of women who got married before reaching the age of 15; multidimensional poverty (MDP), entailing people of all age groups living in poverty; women's exposure to mass media, meaning the percentage of women who read a newspaper or watch any sort of electronic media at least once per week; and full immunization, meaning the percentage of vaccinated children, were retrieved from MICS 2018. All the abovementioned features were aggregated as percentages. Additionally, district-level climate vulnerability was retrieved from Integrated Contextual Analysis [24]. Climate vulnerability includes two primary hazards: (1) floods and (2) droughts. Flood hazard data were retrieved from the National Disaster Management Authority (NDMA). It reflects the total number of recorded flood events from 1950–2015. Drought data, obtained from the Pakistan Meteorological Department, are based on multiple factors such as soil moisture, precipitation, dependency on seasonal rainfall and drought frequency (based on Standardized Precipitation Index). All districts were categorized into a three-point scale—low, medium and high—according to their vulnerability to floods and droughts (https://reliefweb.int/report/pakistan/integrated-context-analysis-ica-vulnerability-food-insecurity-and-natural-hazards, (accessed on 10 November 2023)). Climate vulnerability was classified into three levels: low, medium and high. Each district was assigned a vulnerability classification based on its exposure to climate change.

2.3. Statistical Analysis

We started with an OLS estimation. In the second step, we calculated the variance inflation factor (VIF) for all our explanatory features to assess potential multicollinearity. The VIF value for all the independent features was below 7. In the next step, we performed spatial distribution and visualization of childhood stunting. In order to test spatial autocorrelation in childhood stunting, we used Moran's statistic as given by (1):

$$I = \frac{N}{\Sigma_i \Sigma_j \omega_{ij}} \frac{\Sigma_i \Sigma_j \omega_{ij} (X_i - X)(X_j - X)}{\Sigma_i (X_i - \overline{X})^2} \tag{1}$$

The computation of Moran's statistic is based on the famous spatial weights matrix. ω_{ij} in the above equation signifies the spatial weights matrix. Moran's value is in the range $[-1, 1]$. A positive value reveals a positive spatial autocorrelation and vice versa. A positive value suggests that districts exhibit similar values to their neighbours. Furthermore, Moran's scatter plot was generated, which is composed of four quadrants: Hotspots (regions with high values next to each other), Cold spots (regions with low values next to each other) and Spatial outliers (districts with high and low values next to each other and vice versa) [25,26].

In the presence of spatial autocorrelation in the error term, estimates from OLS are biased and inconsistent. This allows one to employ spatial models. Therefore, after confirming that errors were not random but spatially dependent, we employed the Spatial Durbin Error Model (SDEM). SDEM allows us to control for spatial dependence in error terms and examine the relationships between dependent and independent features with a reference to the average value of independent variables in the neighbourhood. Furthermore, it allows us to examine and evaluate whether the value from the neighbourhood matters. The model equations are given as follows:

$$\text{OLS Regression Model}: y = \alpha + \beta X + \varepsilon \tag{2}$$

$$\text{SDEM Model}: y = \beta_0 + \beta X + WX\theta + u, \text{where } u = \lambda W u + \varepsilon \tag{3}$$

where y depicts the dependent variable, i.e., childhood stunting, α and β_0 are both intercepts, β is the regression coefficient, X entails independent variables and ε represents the error term. In Equation (3), W is the spatial weights row standardized matrix, θ is known as the Durbin component, which consists of the spatial lag of explanatory features, and u is the spatial error term that is used to capture spatial autocorrelation in the error term.

The core of this study was to examine if the average value (spatial lag) of our selected independent features impacted childhood stunting in the nearby districts. To fulfill this objective, we implemented an integrated spatial machine learning approach, which represents a move from explainability to forecasting [27]. We incorporated the significant spatial lag component of Flood and Drought Vulnerability (average value from the neighbourhood) from the SDEM estimates and trained that feature value as an input variable into XGBoost and Random Forest machine learning algorithms. After estimating models, we extracted the most important features for childhood stunting. Both models have built in feature selection methods for identifying the most important features [28]. This step was performed to validate and identify the importance of spatial lag with the help of machine learning algorithms.

In the last step we leveraged EXAI methods to identify the existence of nonlinear relationships with our outcome variable. We employed these methods on the trained machine learning algorithms to extract the desired results. In general, the main purpose of EXAI is to offer more than the machine learning black box and explain why the algorithm is acting the way it does. There are two main categories of EXAI techniques: SHapley Additive exPlanations (SHAP) and Local Interpretable Model Agnostics Explanations (LIME). Compared to LIME, SHAP gives a more holistic explanation when it comes to the outcomes of the machine learning algorithm [29,30]. In this way, it employs a game theory approach to determine the extent of each feature in arriving at the final prediction. In addition, it reveals how much each feature contributes to the model and the influence of the features on the prediction. This is carried out by assessing the relevance of the feature in the range of all the features as opposed to the relevance of the feature in isolation. Therefore, SHAP can help to explain how the model leverages individual features to make predictions and consequently provide more insights into the functioning of the model [31–33].

3. Results

The spatial distribution clearly reveals patterns of local densification in childhood stunting in Pakistan. Districts belonging to Punjab province (light shaded regions) possess lower to moderate stunting rates. As one moves into the northeast (Kpk) and southwest (Sindh) regions, we find a clear and visible increase in childhood stunting ranging between 33.5% and 52.3%. Furthermore, the largest province by area, i.e., Baluchistan, on the western side of Pakistan exhibits severe childhood stunting. Figure 2 below clearly shows the district and regional spatial diversity in childhood stunting in Pakistan.

Descriptive statistics are summarized in Table 1, which presents the severity of the discussed issue. The average rate of childhood stunting in Pakistan (excluding ICT) was approximately 40% with an alarming maximum value of 78.60%. Furthermore, the mean values for other chosen measures such as multidimensional poverty stood at 40.98%, female literacy 38.48%, premature birth rate 11.37%, full immunization 42.56%, etc. Table 1 also depicts the corresponding maximum and minimum values for selected independent features.

Table 1. Descriptive statistics.

Variables	Mean	Std. Dev.	Min	Max
Stunting (%)	40.33	14.95	10.10	78.60
Mean household size	7.57	2.40	3.90	19.0
Premature birth rate (%)	11.37	11.48	0.10	75.30
Full immunization (%)	42.56	24.93	13.30	85.40
Multidimensional poverty (%)	40.98	21.53	2.0	87.80
Female literacy (%)	38.48	22.86	3.50	84.70
Women's exposure to mass media (%)	31.12	30.62	0.00	86.60
Marriage before 15 (%)	6.89	4.49	0.80	29.40

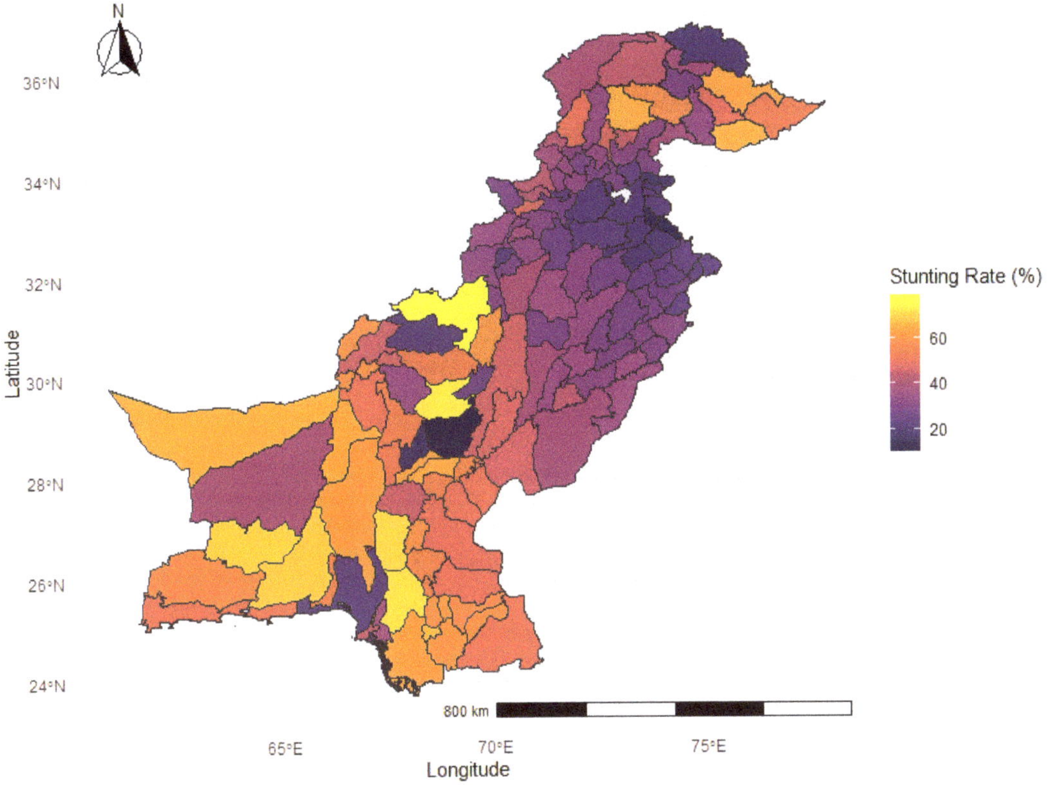

Figure 2. Spatial distribution of childhood stunting at the regional level in Pakistan.

In the next step we tested childhood stunting for spatial autocorrelation using Moran's statistic. The significant Moran's value of 0.56 ($p < 0.000001$) confirmed a positive spatial autocorrelation in childhood stunting, which negates spatial independence and suggests that similar problems exist in neighbouring regions. Figure 3 shows Moran's scatter plot and is composed of four quadrants. Districts with low similar values are grouped together in quadrant III. Districts with high positive values are grouped together in quadrant I. Quadrant II and quadrant IV contain spatial outliers where high and low values are grouped together.

Figure 4 illustrates the same thing as a scatter plot. It shows districts in green colour with low values surrounded by similar districts (low–low regions), light shaded districts possessing higher stunting rates and surrounded by similar districts (high–high regions) and in between a few outliers (low–high regions).

Table 2 below summarizes the estimation results. OLS results demonstrates that multidimensional poverty, women's exposure to mass media, marriage before age 15, and low and high climate vulnerability possess significant relationships with childhood stunting. Specifically, keeping all other factors constant, on average if we observe a percentage point (p.p) increase in multidimensional poverty, it may increase childhood stunting by 0.34 p.p. Additionally, on average high climate vulnerability increases childhood stunting by 0.5 p.p in comparison to medium climate vulnerability (base category). By contrast, on average, low climate vulnerability is negatively associated with childhood stunting. Furthermore, keeping other factors constant, if on average women's exposure to mass media increases by one p.p, we might observe a 0.13 p.p reduction in childhood stunting.

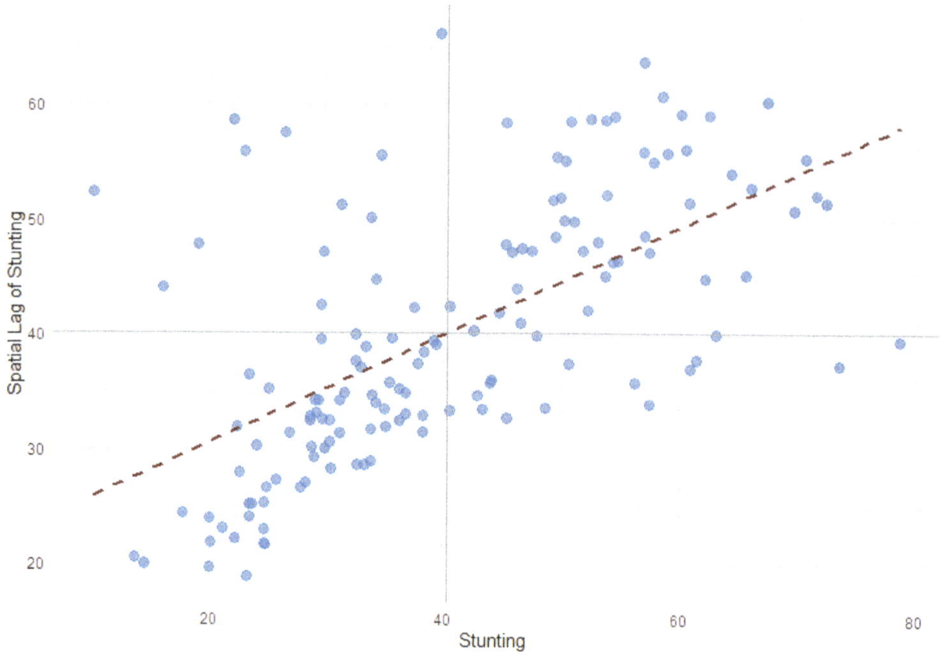

Figure 3. Moran's scatter plot.

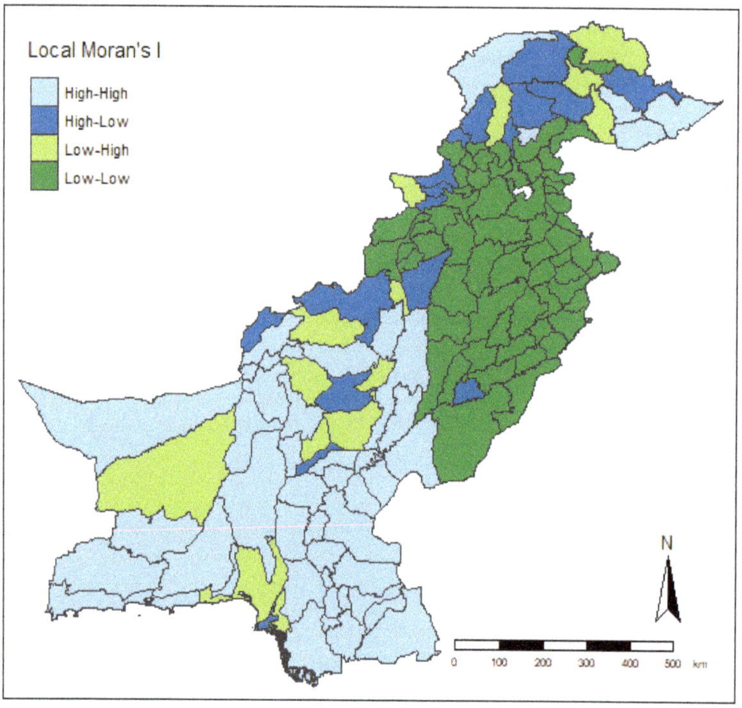

Figure 4. Moran's map.

Table 2. Estimation results.

Variables	OLS Model	SDEM Model
Female literacy	−0.07 (0.07)	−0.004 (0.08)
Multidimensional poverty	0.34 (0.08 ***)	0.24 (0.08 *)
Full immunization	−0.08 (0.05)	−0.01 (0.05)
Marriage before age 15	0.72 (0.227 **)	0.81 (0.21 **)
Women's exposure to mass media	−0.13 (0.04 **)	−0.01 (0.07)
Premature birth rate	0.07 (0.07)	0.06 (0.06)
Mean household size	0.15 (0.35)	−0.07 (0.32)
Flood and drought vulnerability Low	−0.41 (2.20 *)	−4.67 (2.32 *)
Flood and drought vulnerability High	0.51 (2.10 *)	2.08 (1.98 *)
Spatial lag		
Mass media exposure		−0.33 (0.09 **)
Flood and drought vulnerability High		7.06 (3.79 *)
Spatial lag-λ		0.09 (0.13)
Model diagnostics		
Adjusted R-square	0.58	0.71
AIC	1065.2	1063.1

Note: Standard errors in parentheses; *** $p < 0.001$; ** $p < 0.01$; * $p < 0.05$; $\dot{p} < 0.1$.

SDEM estimates show that marriage before age 15 and multidimensional poverty have significant relationships with childhood stunting. In contrast to OLS results, SDEM results demonstrate a severe impact of high climate vulnerability on childhood stunting. Furthermore, the significant λ value demonstrates the existence of spatial dependency in the error term. Additionally, significant values of spatial lag (women's exposure to mass media and high climate vulnerability) suggest a possible impact of these features on childhood stunting in nearby and neighbouring districts. These results confirm that the average value from the neighbourhood of these features (spatial lag) does impact childhood stunting not only in the given district but also in the neighbouring districts as well. In other words, the impact of spatial lag is not geographically bounded.

Model diagnostics show that SDEM outperformed OLS estimates, as the AIC value for SDEM is 1063 < 1065.2 (OLS AIC). The small difference in AIC values between OLS and SDEM demonstrates that both models fit the data well, with a slight advantage for the SDEM estimates. Additionally, it implies that spatial dependence may not improve the model performance. However, SDEM estimates are still preferable as they account for spatial autocorrelation, which OLS fails to capture, resulting in biased and inconsistent estimates. Furthermore, the value-adjusted R-square is also higher in the case of SDEM, which indicates the total variation in childhood stunting as explained by our independent variables.

Validation of Spatial Lag Component through XGBoost and Random Forest

This section involves the validation of significant spatial lag features as evident from SDEM results. We formulated an integrated approach in which we incorporated the spatial lag value of high climate vulnerability along with other independent features into XGBoost and Random Forest machine learning algorithms. These steps were performed to double-check and validate the significance of spatial lag. Both these machine learning algorithms follow a two-step methodology in extracting the most important features. Both use recursive feature elimination by measuring relative importance and ranking features in several ways such as the split method and average gain method. The most important features are used for building the final model and the remaining ones are used in minimizing residuals [34].

Figure 5 above shows the most important features as extracted by XGBoost and Random Forest. Both extracted the same features, and one noticeable thing is that both extracted the spatial lag of high climate vulnerability as one of the important features.

These results further confirm that the average value from the neighbourhood indeed plays an important role and its impacts are not geographically bounded.

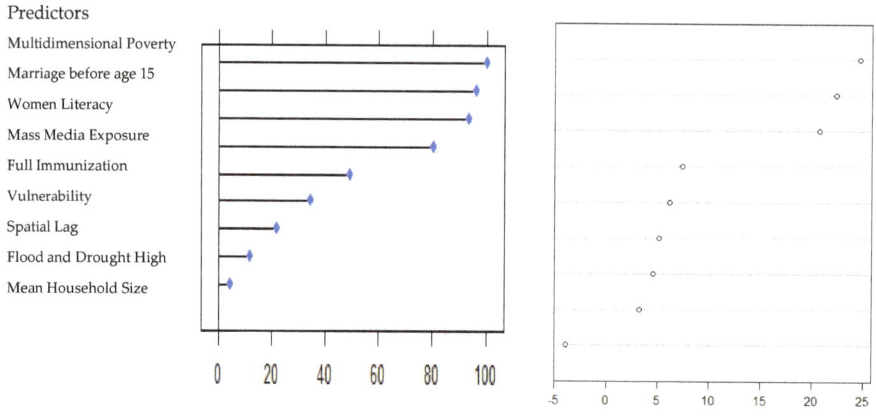

(a) XGBoost Variable Importance (b) Random Forest Variable Importance

Figure 5. Validation of spatial lag and variable importance via (**a**) XGBoost, (**b**) Random Forest.

Figure 6 below exhibits a partial dependency plot that indicates the existence of a nonlinear relationship between multidimensional poverty and childhood stunting, as identified by EXAI Random Forest. However, the ordinary least square regression shows a perfect linear relationship to represent the predicted value of childhood stunting for a random observation. It clearly shows that OLS predicts an approximate value of 54, while EXAI suggests the predicted value to be 57.23 (the real value was 60). This further shows the predictive performance of ML algorithms in comparison to traditional OLS regression.

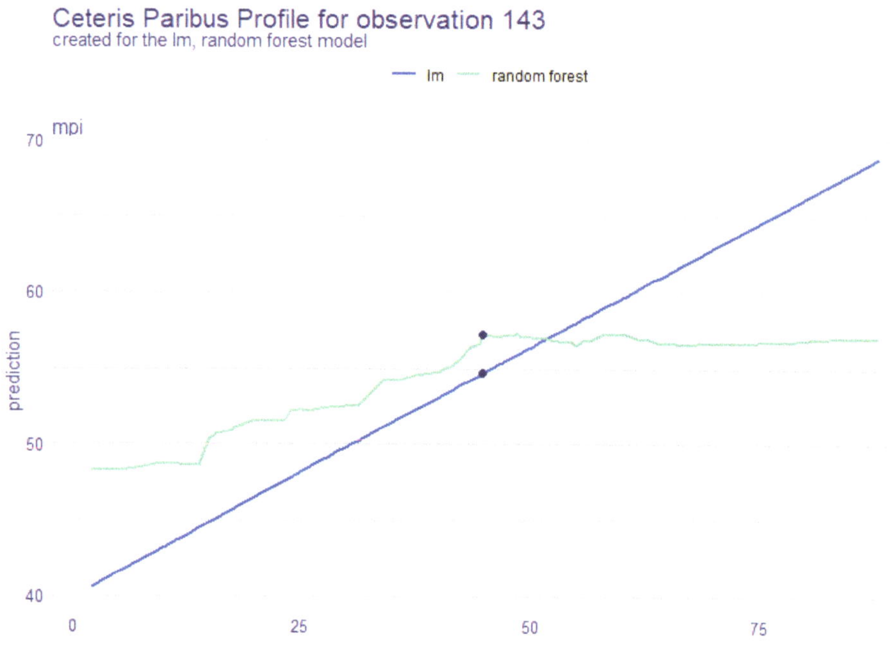

Figure 6. Partial dependency plot.

Figure 7 provides further explanation of local predictions using the SHapley method. It explains the contribution from each feature with positive large values, suggesting a large contribution from each specific feature. For this specific observation, it shows that marriage before age 15 contributes most to this predicted value.

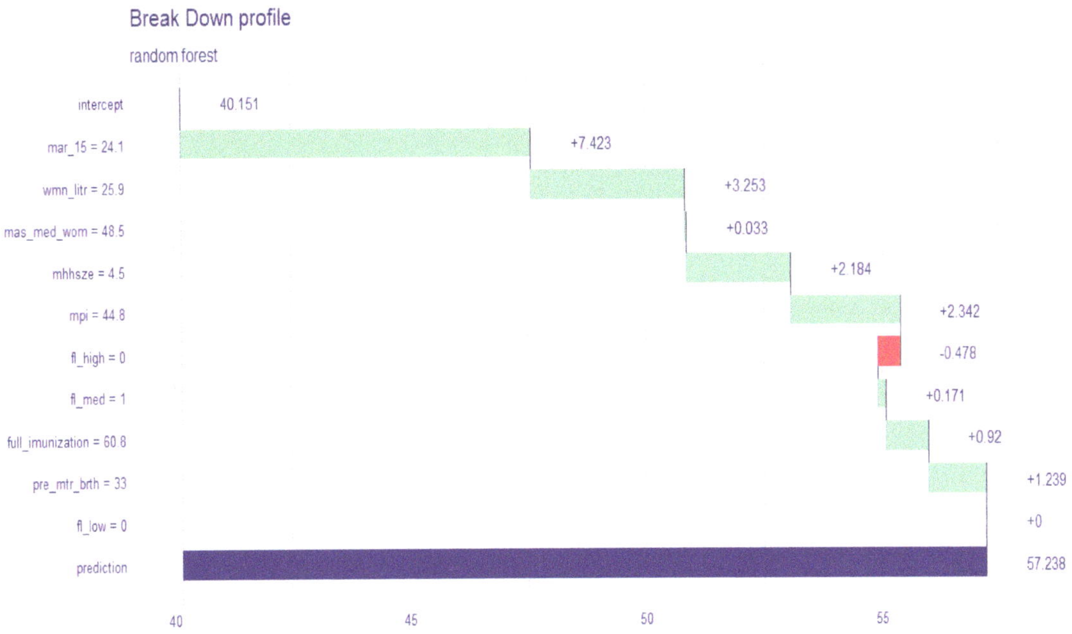

Figure 7. Breakdown profile for a local prediction.

4. Discussion

Child malnutrition remains a significant threat to the development prospects of low- and middle-income countries, including Pakistan. Addressing child malnutrition in all its forms is a key primary objective within the framework of Sustainable Development Goals (SDGs). The present study illustrated two crucial outcomes pertaining to the long-lasting issue of child malnutrition. The initial findings revealed significant spatial inequalities (clusters and spatial outliers) concerning childhood stunting across Pakistan. Moreover, the conducted study analyzed the impact of socioeconomic and climate factors on childhood stunting across all districts in Pakistan, specifying the importance of spatial spillover effects and the existence of nonlinear relationships between the studied features and childhood stunting.

The current study highlights the spatial dependence in childhood stunting across districts in Pakistan. Out of 144 districts examined, 46 exhibited childhood stunting rates exceeding 50%. Notably, the majority of these districts are clustered in southern Punjab Province, northern Kashmir and northwest Khyber Pakhtunkhwa. In contrast, regions in central Pakistan and Gilgit-Baltistan Province have low rates of childhood stunting.

The study investigated the impact of climate vulnerability on childhood stunting revealing significant spatial spillover effects. The findings reveal that high climate vulnerability not only influences childhood stunting within a district but also affects childhood stunting in nearby regions. This suggest the existence of a spatial spillover effect that is not bounded by geographical boundaries [35,36]. The study also found that multidimensional poverty exacerbates childhood stunting. Poor households lack access to fundamental health and other essential services, which consequently impacts children's growth and development. These results align with existing research on the nexus between poverty and child malnutrition [37,38].

The results show the presence of a nonlinear relationship between multidimensional poverty and childhood stunting, suggesting that childhood stunting does not increase proportionally with poverty. Poor households are financially constrained, limiting their access to essential services like education, health care and nutritious food, etc. Low- and middle-income countries bear the substantial burden of child malnutrition. Such existing nutritional disparities hamper productivity and human capital, making countries prone to vicious cycles of poverty where child malnutrition and poverty reinforce each other.

5. Conclusions

The study explored the spatial correlates of child malnutrition at a district level. The findings highlight the geographical variation in childhood stunting in Pakistan, with 46 districts facing an alarming rate of childhood stunting above 50%, concentrated in the west, northeast and south regions of Pakistan. Socioeconomic features and climate vulnerability both play an important role in determining childhood stunting. Additionally, the study found evidence of spatial spillover effects throughout the neighbourhood of high climate vulnerability and women's exposure to mass media, suggesting the potential significant impact of spatial lag in nearby locations.

The findings from this study clearly demonstrate the importance of considering climate vulnerability as a key determinant of childhood stunting. Pakistan has experienced devastating floods. According to the reports from World Health Organization, more than 116 districts were affected and declared as calamity-hit last year [39]. Not only that, more than 2000 health facilities were completely destroyed, leaving millions without access to health and medical treatment [40]. These events further exacerbate food insecurity and elevate waterborne diseases, thereby worsening child malnutrition and consequently childhood stunting. Integrated and context-based policies are necessary to tackle the alarming issue of childhood stunting. It is pertinent to consider the underlying contextual features and design and implement policies accordingly.

Author Contributions: Conceptualization, Muhammad Usman and Mudassar Rashid; methodology, Muhammad Usman, Ateeq ur Rehman Irshad and Amira Khattak; software, Xiaoyi Zhang and Muhammad Usman; validation, Muhammad Usman, Mudassar Rashid and Ateeq ur Rehman Irshad; formal analysis, Muhammad Usman and Xiaoyi Zhang; investigation, Ateeq ur Rehman Irshad; resources, Muhammad Usman and Amira Khattak; data curation, Muhammad Usman; writing—original draft, Xiaoyi Zhang and Muhammad Usman; writing—review and editing, Muhammad Usman, Ateeq ur Rehman Irshad and Amira Khattak; visualization, Muhammad Usman, Ateeq ur Rehman Irshad and Amira Khattak; supervision, Mudassar Rashid and Ateeq ur Rehman Irshad; project administration, Mudassar Rashid and Ateeq ur Rehman Irshad. All authors have read and agreed to the published version of the manuscript.

Funding: The authors Ateeq Ur Rehman Irshad and Aamira Khattak would like to thank Prince Sultan University for paying the APC and the support through TAS research laboratory.

Data Availability Statement: All data were collected from publicly open repositories and are available upon request.

Conflicts of Interest: The authors declare no conflicts of interest.

References

1. United Nations System Standing Committee on Nutrition (UNSCN). *Nutrition and the Post-2015 Sustainable Development Goals;* UNSCN: Geneva, Switzerland, 2014.
2. UNICEF. *Global Nutrition Report;* United Nations Global Marketplace: New York, NY, USA, 2018.
3. UNICEF. *National Nutrition Survey Pakistan;* United Nations Global Marketplace: New York, NY, USA, 2017.
4. Khan, A.Y.; Fatima, K.; Ali, M. Sanitation ladder and undernutrition among under-five children in Pakistan. *Environ. Sci. Pollut. Res.* **2021**, *28*, 38749–38763. [CrossRef] [PubMed]

5. Qamar, K.; Nchasi, G.; Mirha, H.T.; Siddiqui, J.A.; Jahangir, K.; Shaeen, S.K.; Islam, Z.; Essar, M.Y. Water sanitation problem in Pakistan: A review on disease prevalence, strategies for treatment and prevention. *Ann. Med. Surg.* **2022**, *82*, 104709. [CrossRef] [PubMed]
6. Smith, L.C.; Haddad, L. Reducing Child Undernutrition: Past Drivers and Priorities for the Post-MDG Era. *World Dev.* **2015**, *68*, 180–204. [CrossRef]
7. Kim, R.; Mejía-Guevara, I.; Corsi, D.J.; Aguayo, V.M.; Subramanian, S. Relative importance of 13 correlates of child stunting in South Asia: Insights from nationally representative data from Afghanistan, Bangladesh, India, Nepal, and Pakistan. *Soc. Sci. Med.* **2017**, *187*, 144–154. [CrossRef]
8. Rizal, M.F.; van Doorslaer, E. Explaining the fall of socioeconomic inequality in childhood stunting in Indonesia. *SSM Popul. Health* **2019**, *9*, 100469. [CrossRef]
9. Saaka, M.; Saapiire, F.N.; Dogoli, R.N. Independent and joint contribution of inappropriate complementary feeding and poor water, sanitation and hygiene (WASH) practices to stunted child growth. *J. Nutr. Sci.* **2021**, *10*, e109. [CrossRef]
10. Beal, T.; Le, D.T.; Trinh, T.H.; Burra, D.D.; Huynh, T.; Duong, T.T.; Truong, T.M.; Nguyen, D.S.; Nguyen, K.T.; de Haan, S.; et al. Child stunting is associated with child, maternal, and environmental factors in Vietnam. *Matern. Child Nutr.* **2019**, *15*, e12826. [CrossRef]
11. Kumar, P.; Chauhan, S.; Patel, R.; Srivastava, S.; Bansod, D.W. Prevalence and factors associated with triple burden of malnutrition among mother-child pairs in India: A study based on National Family Health Survey 2015–16. *BMC Public Health* **2021**, *21*, 391. [CrossRef]
12. Kim, R.; Rajpal, S.; Joe, W.; Corsi, D.J.; Sankar, R.; Kumar, A.; Subramanian, S. Assessing associational strength of 23 correlates of child anthropometric failure: An econometric analysis of the 2015–2016 National Family Health Survey, India. *Soc. Sci. Med.* **2019**, *238*, 112374. [CrossRef]
13. Efevbera, Y.; Bhabha, J.; Farmer, P.E.; Fink, G. Girl child marriage as a risk factor for early childhood development and stunting. *Soc. Sci. Med.* **2017**, *185*, 91–101. [CrossRef]
14. Usman, M.; Kopczewska, K. Spatial and Machine Learning Approach to Model Childhood Stunting in Pakistan: Role of Socio-Economic and Environmental Factors. *Int. J. Environ. Res. Public Health* **2022**, *19*, 10967. [CrossRef] [PubMed]
15. Kinyoki, D.K.; Berkley, J.A.; Moloney, G.M.; Odundo, E.O.; Kandala, N.-B.; Noor, A.M. Environmental predictors of stunting among children under-five in Somalia: Cross-sectional studies from 2007 to 2010. *BMC Public Health* **2016**, *16*, 654. [CrossRef] [PubMed]
16. Thiede, B.C.; Gray, C. Climate exposures and child undernutrition: Evidence from Indonesia. *Soc. Sci. Med.* **2020**, *265*, 113298. [CrossRef] [PubMed]
17. Johnson, F.A. Spatiotemporal clustering and correlates of childhood stunting in Ghana: Analysis of the fixed and nonlinear associative effects of socio-demographic and socio-ecological factors. *PLoS ONE* **2022**, *17*, e0263726.
18. Gupta, A.K.; Santhya, K.G. Proximal and contextual correlates of childhood stunting in India: A geo-spatial analysis. *PLoS ONE* **2020**, *15*, e0237661. [CrossRef] [PubMed]
19. Tamir, T.T.; Techane, M.A.; Dessie, M.T.; Atalell, K.A. Applied nutritional investigation spatial variation and determinants of stunting among children aged less than 5 y in Ethiopia: A spatial and multilevel analysis of Ethiopian Demographic and Health Survey 2019. *Nutrition* **2022**, *103–104*, 111786. [CrossRef]
20. Hailu, B.A.; Bogale, G.G.; Beyene, J. Spatial heterogeneity and factors influencing stunting and severe stunting among under-5 children in Ethiopia: Spatial and multilevel analysis. *Sci. Rep.* **2020**, *10*, 16427. [CrossRef]
21. Ndagijimana, A.; Nduwayezu, G.; Kagoyire, C.; Elfving, K.; Umubyeyi, A.; Mansourian, A.; Lind, T. Childhood stunting is highly clustered in Northern Province of Rwanda: A spatial analysis of a population-based study. *Heliyon* **2024**, *10*, e24922. [CrossRef]
22. Ahmad, D.; Afzal, M.; Imtiaz, A. Effect of socioeconomic factors on malnutrition among children in Pakistan. *Future Bus. J.* **2020**, *6*, 30. [CrossRef]
23. Multiple Indicator Cluster Survey 2017–2018—Punjab. (2018, November 1). UNICEF Pakistan. Available online: https://www.unicef.org/pakistan/reports/multiple-indicator-cluster-survey-2017-18-punjab (accessed on 13 December 2023).
24. Integrated Context Analysis (ICA): On Vulnerability to Food Insecurity and Natural Hazards—Pakistan, 2017. Available online: https://reliefweb.int/report/pakistan/integrated-context-analysis-ica-vulnerability-food-insecurity-and-natural-hazards (accessed on 10 November 2023).
25. Anselin, L. The Moran scatterplot as an ESDA tool to assess local instability in spatial association. In *Spatial Analytical Perspectives on GIS*; Routledge: Abingdon-on-Thames, UK, 2019; pp. 111–126.
26. Getis, A.; Ord, J.K. The Analysis of Spatial Association by Use of Distance Statistics. *Geogr. Anal.* **1992**, *24*, 189–206. [CrossRef]
27. Lundberg, S.M.; Lee, S.I. A unified approach to interpreting model predictions. *Adv. Neural Inf. Process. Syst.* **2017**, *30*, 4765–4774.
28. Li, X.; Du, M.; Chen, J.; Chai, Y.; Lakkaraju, H.; Xiong, H. M^4: A Unified XAI Benchmark for Faithfulness Evaluation of Feature Attribution Methods across Metrics, Modalities and Models. *Adv. Neural Inf. Process. Syst.* **2023**, *36*, 1630–1643.
29. Rothman, D. *Hands-On Explainable AI (XAI) with Python: Interpret, Visualize, Explain, and Integrate Reliable AI for Fair, Secure, and Trustworthy AI Apps*; Packt Publishing Ltd.: Birmingham, UK, 2020.
30. Naz, Z.; Khan MU, G.; Saba, T.; Rehman, A.; Nobanee, H.; Bahaj, S.A. An explainable AI-enabled framework for interpreting pulmonary diseases from chest radiographs. *Cancers* **2023**, *15*, 314. [CrossRef] [PubMed]

31. Shi, X.; Wong, Y.D.; Li, M.Z.-F.; Palanisamy, C.; Chai, C. A feature learning approach based on XGBoost for driving assessment and risk prediction. *Accid. Anal. Prev.* **2019**, *129*, 170–179. [CrossRef]
32. Akhtar, K.; Yaseen, M.U.; Imran, M.; Khattak SB, A.; Nasralla, M.M. Predicting inmate suicidal behavior with an interpretable ensemble machine learning approach in smart prisons. *PeerJ Comput. Sci.* **2024**, *10*, e2051. [CrossRef]
33. Rehman, A.; Haseeb, K.; Saba, T.; Lloret, J.; Sendra, S. An optimization model with network edges for multimedia sensors using artificial intelligence of things. *Sensors* **2021**, *21*, 7103. [CrossRef]
34. Mahapatra, B.; Walia, M.; Rao, C.A.R.; Raju, B.M.K.; Saggurti, N. Vulnerability of agriculture to climate change increases the risk of child malnutrition: Evidence from a large-scale observational study in India. *PLoS ONE* **2021**, *16*, e0253637. [CrossRef]
35. Okunlola, O.A.; Kassouri, Y. Empirical investigation of the agriculture–malnutrition nexus in Africa: Spatial clustering and spillover effects. *Rev. Dev. Econ.* **2023**, *27*, 685–709. [CrossRef]
36. Rahman, M.A.; Halder, H.R.; Rahman, M.S.; Parvez, M. Poverty and childhood malnutrition: Evidence-based on a nationally representative survey of Bangladesh. *PLoS ONE* **2021**, *16*, e0256235.
37. Siddiqui, F.; Salam, R.A.; Lassi, Z.S.; Das, J.K. The Intertwined Relationship Between Malnutrition and Poverty. *Front. Public Health* **2020**, *8*, 453. [CrossRef]
38. Adeyeye, S.A.O.; Ashaolu, T.J.; Bolaji, O.T.; Abegunde, T.A.; Omoyajowo, A.O. Africa and the Nexus of poverty, malnutrition and diseases. *Crit. Rev. Food Sci. Nutr.* **2023**, *63*, 641–656. [CrossRef] [PubMed]
39. United Nations. *Global Nutrition Overview*; United Nations: New York, NY, USA, 2022.
40. National Disaster Management Authority. *Pakistan (2022) Floods Response Plan: 1—Pakistan*; United Nations Office for the Coordination of Humanitarian Affairs: New York, NY, USA, 2022.

International Journal of
Geo-Information

MDPI

Article

Association between Autism Spectrum Disorder and Environmental Quality in the United States

Jianyong Wu [1,*], Alexander C. McLain [2], Paul Rosile [1] and Darryl B. Hood [1]

[1] Division of Environmental Health Sciences, College of Public Health, The Ohio State University, Columbus, OH 43210, USA
[2] Department of Epidemiology and Biostatistics, University of South Carolina, Columbia, SC 29208, USA
* Correspondence: wu.6255@osu.edu; Tel.: +1-614-292-2435

Abstract: Autism spectrum disorder (ASD) has become an emerging public health problem. The impact of multiple environmental factors on the prevalence of ASD remains unclear. This study examined the association between the prevalence of ASD and the environmental quality index (EQI), an indicator of cumulative environmental quality in five major domains, including air, water, land, built and sociodemographic variables in the United States. The results from Poisson regression models show that the prevalence of ASD has a positive association with the overall EQI with a risk ratio (RR) of 1.03 and 95% confidence intervals (CI) of 1.01–1.06, indicating that children in counties with poor environmental quality might have a higher risk of ASD. Additionally, the prevalence of ASD has a positive association with the air index (RR = 1.04, 95% CI: 1.01–1.06). These associations varied in different rural–urban groups and different climate regions. This study provided evidence for adverse effects of poor environmental quality, particularly air pollutants, on children's neurodevelopment.

Keywords: autism; environmental quality; air pollution; water quality; geographically weighted regression

1. Introduction

Autism spectrum disorder (ASD), also known as autism, is a group of neurodevelopmental disorders that are typically diagnosed in early childhood. The symptoms of ASD often become noticeable at age 2–3, though some signs may appear earlier or later. Children with ASD often have difficulties in social communication and interaction, such as body language and facial expressions, and also have restricted or repetitive behaviors, such as hand-flapping or a rigid adherence to routines [1]. In the recent few decades, the prevalence of ASD has increased rapidly in the United States and globally [2,3]. The latest report from the Centers for Disease Control and Prevention (CDC) estimated that the ASD prevalence was about 1 in 36 children aged 8 years in 2020, which is a drastic increase compared with the prevalence of 1 in 150 children in 2000 in the United States [3]. Additionally, it is estimated that over 5.4 million adults have ASD in the United States [4]. Children with ASD often face a lifetime of adverse consequences, posing significant challenges to individuals and their families. The lifelong nature of ASD often requires ongoing support and intervention, which can impose substantial financial and emotional burdens on families. The economic impact includes costs associated with medical care and special education, as well as indirect costs such as lost productivity and caregiver stress [5–7]. As a result, ASD has become an emerging public health problem.

The etiology of ASD is not fully understood. Generally, it is believed that ASD is caused by a combination of genetic and environmental factors [8–10]. The contribution of genetic factors to the etiology of ASD has been recognized in several studies, which have shown that the risk of ASD onset is disproportionately increased among first-degree relatives of probands [11,12] and that the onset of ASD highly coincides among monozygotic twins [13,

14]. However, genetic risk factors alone cannot explain the role of environmental factors in ASD.

In recent years, a large amount of evidence supports that exposure to environmental factors, including pesticides, phthalates, polychlorinated biphenyls (PCBs), solvents, toxic waste, heavy metals, and air pollution, have significantly contributed to the increase in the risk of autism [9,15–39]. Among these environmental risk factors, the effects of air pollutants have been widely investigated. However, no single environmental risk factor has been found to play a causal role in the onset of ASD [9,40]. In addition, some environmental factors may have beneficial effects. For example, Wu and Jackson found that greenspace was inversely associated with the risk of childhood autism in California public elementary school districts [41]. A cohort study in Metro Vancouver and Ontario, Canada found that exposure to greenspace during pregnancy was associated with a slight reduction in the likelihood of ASD [42]. The inverse association between greenspace and ASD has also been observed in case-control studies conducted in Shanghai, China and Ontario, Canada [43,44].

Children are likely to be exposed to multiple environmental factors, and different factors may have different effects on children's neurodevelopment. Therefore, it is necessary to understand the cumulative effects of multiple environmental factors. Although the associations between ASD and some single environmental factors or constructs have been recognized, the combined effects of environmental factors across multiple constructs on ASD are still unknown. To fill this gap, the connection between ASD prevalence and environmental quality index was investigated. The environmental quality index (EQI), developed by the United States Environmental Protection Agency (USEPA), represents the information across five environmental domains, facilitating a comprehensive evaluation of environmental quality based on over 100 variables and enhancing our comprehension of how environmental quality influences health outcomes [45–47]. Although the EQI has been used to study various health outcomes [48–52], its application to ASD has been limited. Understanding the association between environmental quality and ASD is important for several reasons. First, it can inform public health strategies to reduce exposure to harmful conditions and improving overall environmental quality. Additionally, it can guide the development of effective and focused interventions for at-risk communities.

The objective of this study is to examine the association between ASD and environmental quality in the US. First, the study examined the associations of ASD prevalence with the overall environmental quality index (EQI) and the domain-specific indices using Poisson regression models. Then the spatial variations in the associations were examined by stratification of urbanicity and climate regions. Furthermore, the local variations in the associations were determined by geographically weighted regression (GWR) models. Finally, sensitivity analyses examined whether urbanicity or climate had an impact on the associations between ASD and EQI. The flowchart of the method is shown in Figure 1. The findings from this study provide insight into understanding the combined effects of environmental factors on the risk of ASD, thus helping to find approaches to reducing its risk.

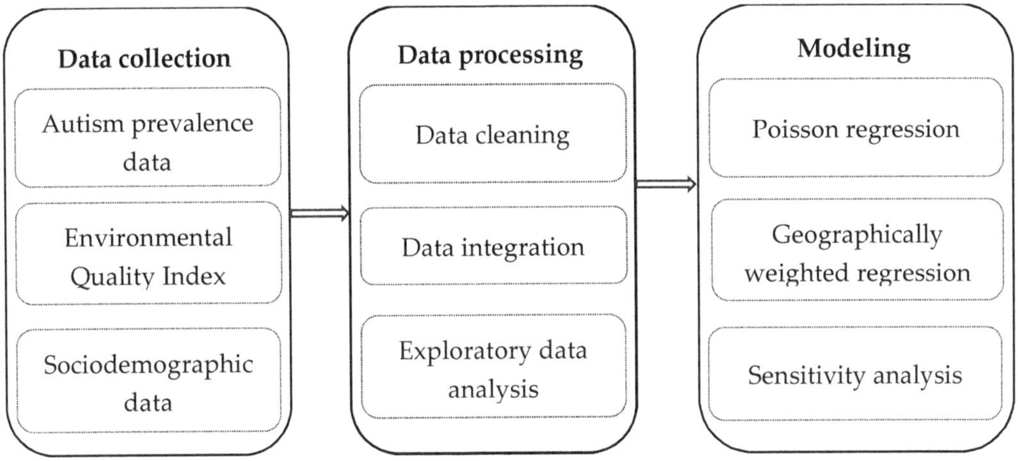

Figure 1. The flowchart of the methodology of this study.

2. Materials and Methods

2.1. ASD Prevalence Data

The prevalence of ASD at the county level in the United States was determined with the 2016–2018 National Survey of Children's Health (NSCH). The survey involves a sampling approach that selects an equal number of households from each state. Within these households, a child is randomly chosen, with a higher selection probability (80%) for those with special needs. The survey, managed by the US Census Bureau, was conducted via landline and cellular phones across all states and the District of Columbia, with responses collected from parents or guardians. The county-level prevalence of ASD was estimated from 70,913 children aged 5–17, using a model-based spatial small area estimation approach [53].

2.2. Environmental Quality Index

The EQI dataset, representing the ambient environmental quality in all counties in the United States during 2006–2010, was obtained from the USEPA (https://www.epa.gov/healthresearch/environmental-quality-index-eqi, accessed on 28 July 2024). The method to create the EQI was described elsewhere [45,46]. Briefly, 139 variables in different domains were collected and reduced to an overall EQI and five domain-specific EQIs, namely, air, water, land, built, and sociodemographics, using principal component analysis (PCA). The air domain includes data from monitoring, emissions, and modeled estimates to evaluate criteria and hazardous air pollutants. The water domain covers a range of data types—modeled, monitoring, reported, survey/study, and miscellaneous—to address water quality, contamination, domestic use, and other water-related factors. The land domain focuses on agriculture, pesticides, contaminants, facilities, and radon, reflecting land use and environmental contamination. The built environment domain assesses factors such as traffic, transit access, pedestrian safety, and access to essential services, including food, recreation, health care, education, and the presence of subsidized housing. Lastly, the sociodemographic domain evaluates crime and socioeconomic conditions to understand their impact on overall environmental quality and quality of life. A detailed list of these variables and the descriptive statistics are available in the EQI technical report [47].

2.3. Covariates

Considering environmental quality is different between urban and rural areas, we stratified the EQI into four groups based on the Rural–Urban Continuum codes (RUCC), including metropolitan urbanized (RUCC1), nonmetropolitan urbanized (RUCC2), less urbanized (RUCC3), and thinly populated (RUCC4) areas. The RUCC was developed by the US Department of Agriculture. Originally, it had 9 categories, but these were condensed into four categories in several studies [49,50,52].

To understand whether climate influences the association between ASD prevalence and EQI, we divided all counties into six climate regions following a previous study [50], including humid subtropical; Mediterranean; and three warm summer continental regions, dry continental, hot summer continental, and dry. These groups were derived from the original eighteen regions based on their monthly and annual average of precipitation and temperature.

We also collected additional sociodemographic data from the American Community Survey 5-year estimates (2016–2020) from the US Census Bureau. The variables include the total population; the percentages of white, black, and Asian; male and female; Hispanic-or-Latino and non-Hispanic-or-Latino; and under 5 years old and 5–17 years old, along with mean household income.

2.4. Statistical Analysis

All the datasets were merged using ArcGIS Pro 3.2 software (ERSI, Redlands, CA, USA) based on each county's Federal Information Processing System (FIPS) code. A total of 3143 counties were included in the dataset. Before building regression models, we conducted exploratory analysis. We made histograms to show the distribution of each variable and conducted Pearson correlation analysis to obtain the preliminary relationship between these variables.

The Poisson regression model was used to examine the relationship between ASD prevalence and EQI. We chose the Poisson model because it is a well-established method for analyzing count data and rate-based outcomes, such as ASD prevalence. This model is particularly effective when the dependent variable represents the number of occurrences per unit of population. We examined the mean and variance of ASD prevalence and did not find evidence for over-dispersion of this variable. The model can be expressed as follows:

$$\log(\lambda_i) = \beta_0 + \beta_1 X_{1i} + \beta_2 X_{2i} + \cdots + \beta_n X_{ni} + \epsilon_i$$

where i is the index of a county and λ_i is the expected ASD prevalence in county i. β_0 is the intercept, $\beta_1, \beta_2, \ldots, \beta_n$ are the regression coefficients, $X_{1i}, X_{ni}, \ldots, X_{ni}$ are predictors, and ϵ_i is the error term. The link function is the natural logarithm.

Initially, each model only included one explanatory variable to obtain its unadjusted association with ASD prevalence. Then, each model included one EQI variable (overall EQI or domain-specific indices) and several covariates. The final model was adjusted for three covariates: race (the percentage of the black population), age (the percentage of the population aged 5–17 years), and population density. These three variables were included in the model for the following reasons. (1) The selection of race, age, and population density as covariates is based on in their significant potential to influence ASD prevalence and their ability to impact the relationship between environmental quality and ASD [54]. It has been shown that there are variations in ASD prevalence across different racial and ethnic groups. The adjustment for age ensures that the prevalence of ASD is not impacted due to variations in age distribution across counties. Population density can affect both the likelihood of ASD diagnosis and exposure to environmental factors. (2) They did not cause multicollinearity based on Pearson correlation analysis. (3) Finally, the model had a smaller Akaike information criterion (AIC) score compared with models with other variables. To determine the impacts of urbanicity and climate on the association between ASD prevalence and EQI, the models were stratified by each RUCC group and climate region, respectively. For all models, the EQI variables and other covariates were standardized (mean = 0, standard deviation = 1) to facilitate model interpretation. The association was indicated by risk ratio (RR) corresponding to a 1 standard deviation increase in explanatory variables. The association was assumed to be positive if RR is larger than 1, and negative if RR is less than 1. The significance level was set at 0.05. The analysis was conducted with SAS 9.4 (SAS Inc., Cary, NC, USA).

To determine if the ASD and EQI association varies by county, a geographically weighted regression (GWR) model was used. The GWR model was built on the above Poisson regression model. However, the regression coefficients for the Poisson model are fixed for all counties, while in the GWR model, regression coefficients were allowed to vary by county. The GWR model was chosen because it allows for the examination of spatial variations in the relationship between environmental factors and ASD prevalence. This model provides localized estimates of how the impact of environmental variables on ASD prevalence varies across different regions. This spatially explicit approach offers more precise insights into the environmental influences on ASD and supports specific interventions based on local conditions. A general GWR model can be written as below:

$$y_i = \beta_{0i} + \beta_{1i}X_{1i} + \beta_{2i}X_{2i} + \cdots + \beta_{ni}X_{ni} + \epsilon_i$$

where, y_i is the ASD prevalence at county i, β_{0i} is the intercept for county i, $\beta_{1i}, \beta_{2i}, \ldots, \beta_{ni}$ are the regression coefficients for county i, X_{1i}, $X_{ni}, \ldots, X_{ni}$ are predictors, and ϵ_i is the error term.

In GWR, the regression coefficients are estimated locally for each county i, reflecting how the relationship between ASD prevalence and EQI changes across space. This spatial variability is captured by weighting observed data based on their distance from the location of interest using a Gaussian kernel function. This approach allows the GWR model to account for spatial heterogeneity by giving more weight to nearby observations and less to those farther away. The GWR model was run on ArcGIS Pro 3.2 (ERSI, Redlands, CA, USA).

2.5. Sensitivity Analysis

Because the prevalence of ASD was estimated based on the sampling data, there is uncertainty in their values. To incorporate this uncertainty, we randomly simulated the ASD prevalence of each county 1000 times based on its point estimate and 95% confidence interval (95% CI), then ran the same Poisson regression model 1000 times using the simulated ASD prevalence as the response variable. Additionally, to examine whether the change in predictors affects the association between ASD prevalence and EQI, we included a gender variable (the percentage of the female population) in the Poisson regression model. Therefore, the model was adjusted for four variables.

3. Results

The descriptive statistics of ASD prevalence and related explanatory variables are shown in Table 1. The county-level average prevalence of ASD is 2.56% among children aged 5–17. The overall EQI and the five domain-specific indices had a mean of 0 and a standard deviation of 1. The correlation between ASD prevalence and those explanatory variables is shown in Table 2. ASD prevalence was positively correlated with the EQI's overall, air, and built indices, but negatively correlated with land and sociodemographic indices. Additionally, ASD prevalence had positive correlations with population density, percentages of total population, black population, Asian population, and non-Hispanic or Latino population, but had negative correlations with the percentages of white population, Hispanic or Latino population. No significant correlation was observed between ASD prevalence and the mean household income.

The unadjusted Poisson regression model showed that ASD prevalence had significant positive associations with the EQI's overall, air, and built indices, population density, and the percentages of black, Asian, and female, but had significant negative associations with the EQI's land and sociodemographic indices, and the percentages of white, male, and children under 5 as well as aged 5–17. No significant associations were found with the mean household income and the two ethnic groups (Hispanic or Latino population and non-Hispanic or Latino population) (Table S1).

Table 1. Descriptive statistics of the response variable and explanatory variables.

Variables	N	Mean	Standard Deviation	Minimum	Maximum
ASD prevalence	3143	2.56	0.9	0	24.28
Overall EQI	3143	0	1	−6.79	2.83
EQI—air	3143	0	1	−6.72	3.71
EQI—built	3143	0	1	−4.71	5.66
EQI—land	3143	0	1	−4.54	1.84
EQI—sociodemographic	3143	0	1	−5.13	2.76
EQI—water	3143	0	1	−1.46	2.05
County size (km^2)	3143	2965.11	9479.22	5.31	383,144.8
Mean household income ($)	3143	72,262	18,113	34,331	183,898
Total population	3143	103,904	332,097	117	10,040,682
Population density (person/km^2)	3143	103.14	689.59	0.01	27,528.08
White (%)	3143	0.82	0.17	0.03	1
Black (%)	3143	0.09	0.14	0	0.88
Asian (%0	3143	0.01	0.03	0	0.43
Hispanic or Latino (%)	3143	0.1	0.14	0	0.99
Non—Hispanic or Latino (%)	3143	0.9	0.14	0.01	1
Male (%)	3143	0.5	0.02	0.42	0.71
Female (%)	3143	0.5	0.02	0.29	0.58
Under 5 years (%)	3143	0.06	0.01	0	0.18
5 to 17 years (%)	3143	0.16	0.03	0	0.32

Table 2. Pearson correlation between ASD prevalence and explanatory variables.

Explanatory Variables	N	r	*p*	Explanatory Variables	N	r	*p*
Overall EQI	3143	0.114	<0.001	White	3143	−0.180	<0.001
EQI—air	3143	0.159	<0.001	Black	3143	0.247	<0.001
EQI—built	3143	0.049	0.006	Asian	3143	0.063	<0.001
EQI—land	3143	−0.067	<0.001	Hispanic or Latino	3143	−0.041	0.023
EQI—sociodemographics	3143	−0.138	<0.001	Non-Hispanic or Latino	3143	0.041	0.023
EQI—water	3143	−0.017	0.339	Male	3143	−0.088	<0.001
Population density	3143	0.164	<0.001	Female	3143	0.088	<0.001
Total population	3143	0.200	<0.001	Under 5 years	3143	−0.065	<0.001
Mean household income	3143	0.021	0.235	5 to 17 years	3143	−0.108	<0.001

After adjusting for age, race, and population density, ASD prevalence still had significant positive associations with the EQI's overall (RR = 1.03, 95% CI = 1.01–1.06), and air (RR = 1.04, 95% CI = 1.01–1.06) indices, but a negative association with the sociodemographic index (RR = 0.96, 95% CI = 0.94–0.98). There were no significant associations with the built, land, and water indices. The results from the multivariate models with all five domain-specific indices closely align with those obtained from the analyses with individual indices (Table 3).

Figure 2 illustrates the associations from adjusted Poisson regression models stratified by RUCC. Significant associations were only observed in the RUCC1 group, metropolitan urbanized areas, where ASD prevalence was positively associated with the air index (RR = 1.04, 95% CI: 1.00–1.09) but negatively associated with the sociodemographic index (RR = 0.96, 95% CI: 0.94–1.00). No significant associations were observed for the other indices in other areas.

Table 3. Association between ASD prevalence and EQI from Poisson regression models adjusted for race, age and population density.

Model ID	Explanatory Variables	RR (95% CI)
1	Overall EQI	1.03 (1.01–1.06)
	Black (%)	1.07 (1.05–1.10)
	5 to 17 years (%)	0.97 (0.94–0.99)
	Population density	1.03 (1.01–1.04)
2	EQI—air	1.04 (1.01–1.06)
	Black (%)	1.07 (1.05–1.09)
	5 to 17 years (%)	0.97 (0.95–0.99)
	Population density	1.03 (1.01–1.04)
3	EQI—built	1.01 (0.99–1.03)
	Black (%)	1.08 (1.06–1.10)
	5 to 17 years (%)	0.97 (0.95–0.99)
	Population density	1.03 (1.01–1.04)
4	EQI—land	0.99 (0.97–1.01)
	Black (%)	1.08 (1.06–1.10)
	5 to 17 years (%)	0.97 (0.95–0.99)
	Population density	1.03 (1.01–1.04)
5	EQI—sociodemographic	0.96 (0.94–0.98)
	Black (%)	1.08 (1.06–1.11)
	5 to 17 years (%)	0.97 (0.95–0.99)
	Population density	1.02 (1.00–1.04)
6	EQI—water	1.02 (0.99–1.04)
	Black (%)	1.08 (1.06–1.10)
	5 to 17 years (%)	0.97 (0.95–0.99)
	Population density	1.03 (1.02–1.04)
	EQI—air	1.03 (1.01–1.06)
	EQI—built	1.00 (0.98–1.02)
7	EQI—land	0.99 (0.96–1.01)
	EQI—sociodemographic	0.96 (0.94–0.98)
	EQI—water	1.01 (0.99–1.03)
	Black (%)	1.08 (1.06–1.10)
	5 to 17 years (%)	0.98 (0.95–1.00)
	Population density	1.02 (1.00–1.03)

Figure 3 shows the associations stratified by climate regions. For the overall EQI, the associations were significant in the humid subtropical (RR = 1.04, 95% CI = 1.00–1.09) and warm summer continental (RR = 1.06, 95% CI = 1.00–1.12) regions. For domain-specific indices, the air index had positive associations with ASD prevalence in the humid subtropical (RR = 1.04, 95% CI = 1.00–1.09), warm summer continental (RR = 1.08, 95% CI = 1.02–1.14), and dry (RR = 1.21, 95% CI = 1.01–1.46) regions. The land index was negatively associated with ASD prevalence in warm summer continental (RR = 0.92, 95% CI = 0.86–0.96) regions. The sociodemographic index had a negative association in humid subtropical (RR = 0.96, 95% CI = 0.92–1.00). No significant associations were found with the built and water indices in any climate regions.

Figure 4 illustrates the county-specific association between ASD prevalence and overall EQI, demonstrating how the association varied across the US. Several counties in Arizona, Texas, Illinois, and Michigan had a relatively higher positive association. For domain-specific indices, the spatial pattern of the air index association resembled that for the overall EQI (Figure S1). For the built index, a higher positive association was observed in Texas, southern California, and Wisconsin (Figure S2). The spatial patterns of the associations are similar for the land and sociodemographic indices, of which a higher positive association was found in the central region of the United States, e.g., some counties in Kansas, Missouri, and Indiana (Figures S3 and S4). For the water index, a higher positive association was concentrated in Florida and adjacent counties in Alabama and Georgia (Figure S5).

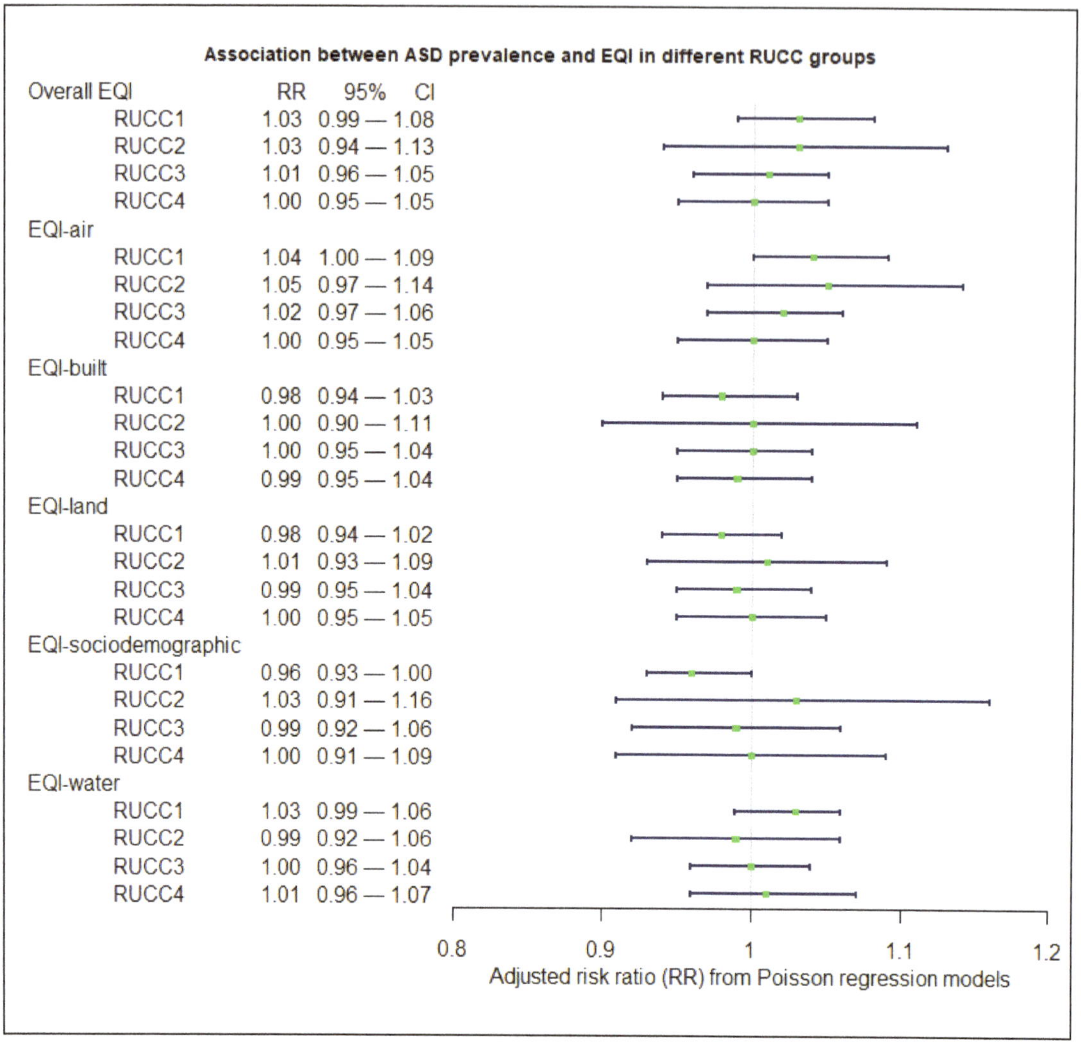

Figure 2. Association between ASD prevalence and EQI in different RUCC groups from Poisson regression models adjusted for race, age, and population density.

Sensitivity analysis showed that the association between ASD and EQI remained consistent with the simulated ASD prevalence, or when adjusted for the percentage of female. Figure 5 shows the distribution of risk ratio obtained from the model with simulated ASD prevalence. The overall EQI and air index were positively associated with ASD prevalence; the risk ratios were above 1.00 and the mean of the risk ratios were 1.03 and 1.04, respectively. The sociodemographic index was negatively associated with ASD prevalence; all the risk ratios were below 1.00 and the mean of the risk ratios was 0.96. The additional adjustment for the percentage of female had a marginal impact on the results (Table S2).

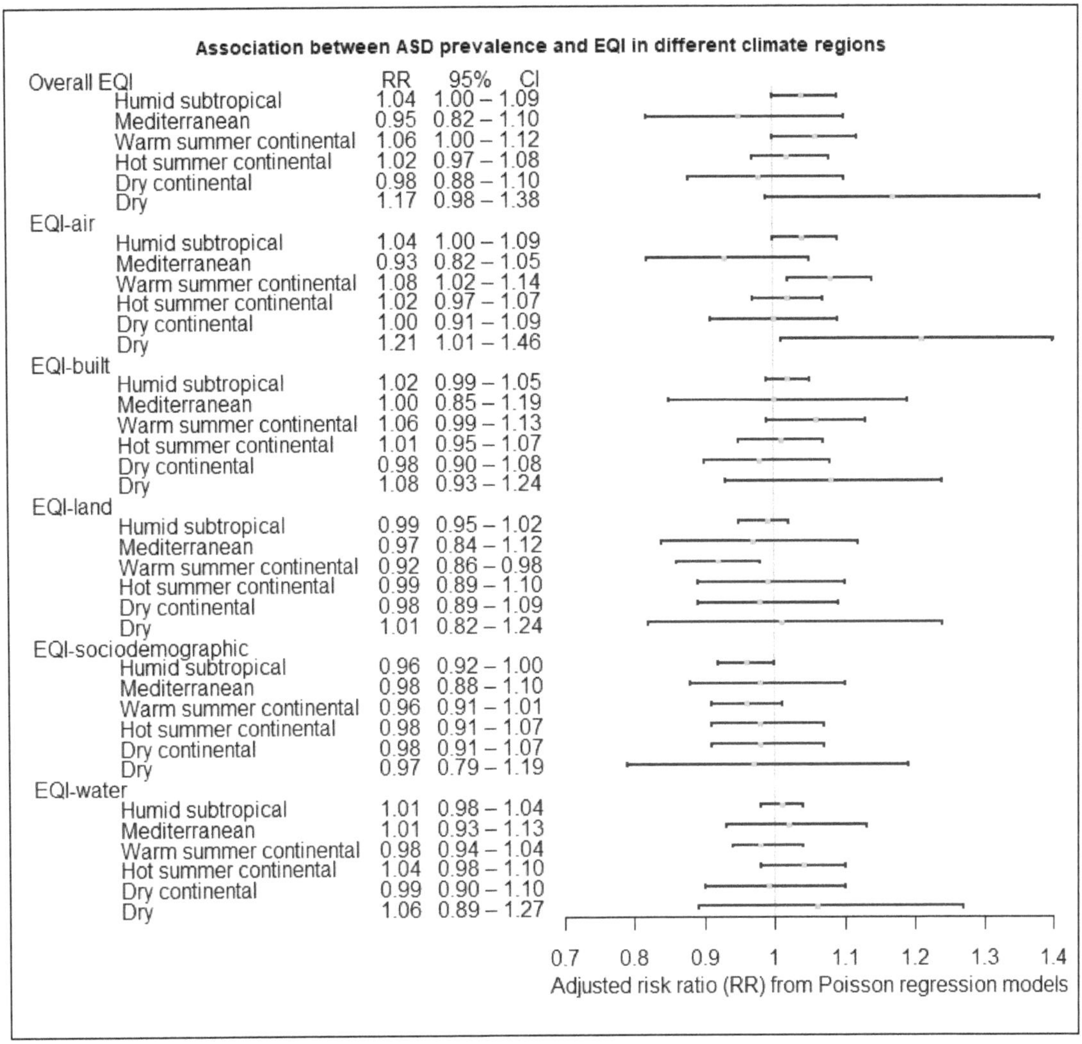

Figure 3. Association between ASD prevalence and EQI in different climate regions from Poisson regression models adjusted for race, age, and population density.

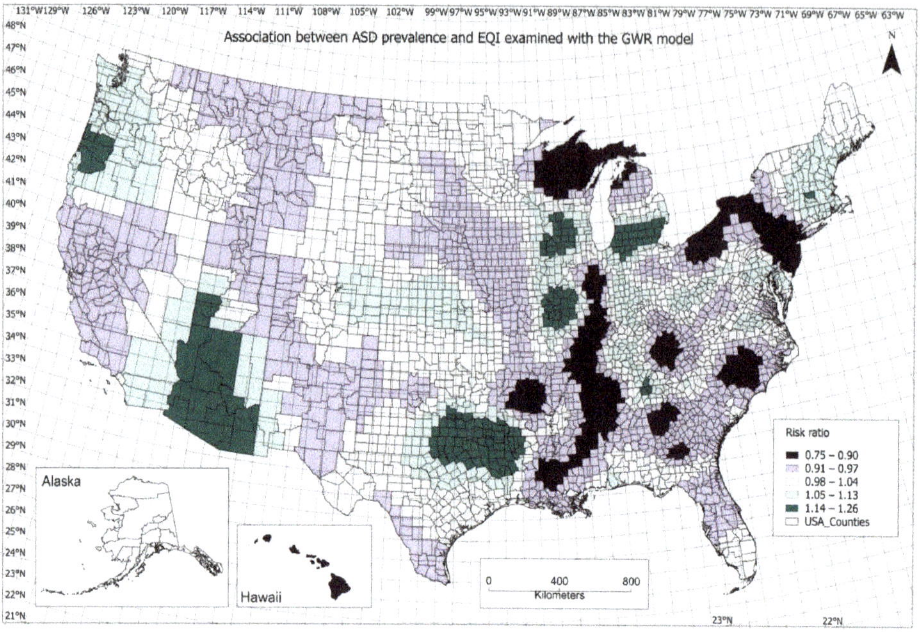

Figure 4. Association between ASD prevalence and the overall EQI from the geographically weighted regression model.

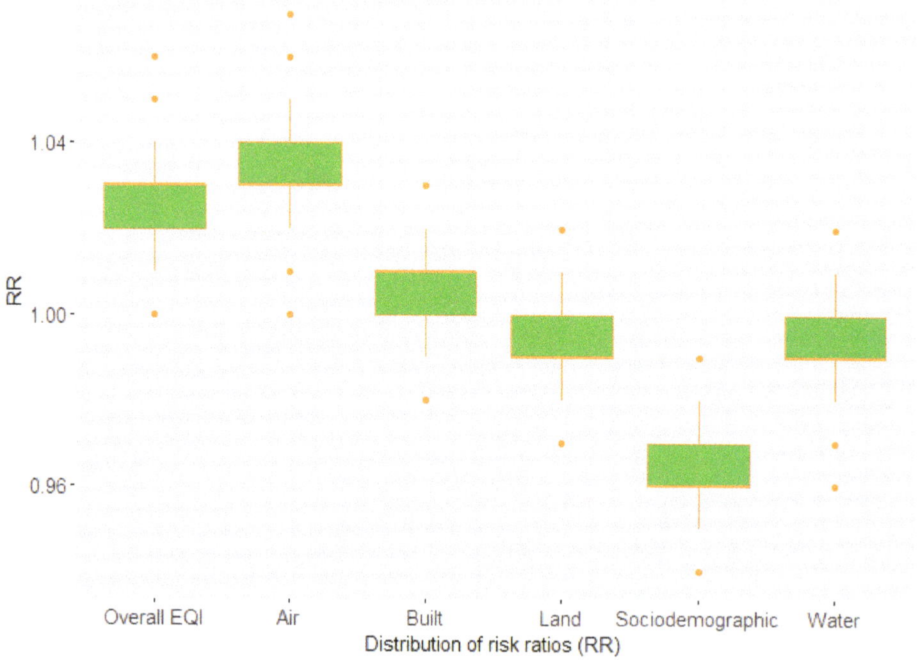

Figure 5. Distribution of risk ratios (RR) obtained from Poisson regression models with simulated ASD prevalence.

4. Discussion

We found that ASD prevalence had significant positive associations with the overall EQI and the air index, of which the risk ratios were 1.03 and 1.04, respectively, indicating the autism prevalence might increase by 3% and 4% per 1 standard deviation increase in the overall EQI and the air index, respectively. Meanwhile, a significant negative association was observed for the sociodemographic index with the risk ratio of 0.94, indicating the autism prevalence might decrease by 6% per 1-standard deviation increase in sociodemographic index. In addition, there were regional and local variations in these associations. The sensitivity analysis indicated that the results were robust. To date, the environmental contribution to the cause of ASD is still unclear; we are not aware of any studies that examined the cumulative and combined effects of environmental factors. Therefore, the study provided new insights into the relationship between ASD prevalence and environmental factors.

In this study, the results suggested that poor air quality was associated with increased ASD prevalence in metropolitan urbanized areas, which is consistent with previous reports on the associations between autism risk and individual air pollutants [15–17,21,23,24,26–28,55–57]. In metropolitan areas, traffic-related air pollution is a major source of air pollutants, particularly fine particulate matter ($PM_{2.5}$). Among many types of air pollutants, more evidence supports the conclusion that there are significant associations between $PM_{2.5}$ and ASD [21,55]. The evidence for the association between ASD risk and other air pollutants such as ozone, SO_2, and NO_2 is relatively limited. Exposure to air pollutants, such as particulate matter, may lead to inflammation and oxidative stress in the body, which may affect the developing brain, potentially leading to changes in neural development and function, thus increasing the risk of ASD [58–60]. A positive association between ASD and the air index underscores the need for strict air quality regulations and targeted interventions to reduce exposure to pollutants, particularly in areas with high pollution levels. It also points to the necessity of further research to understand the mechanisms behind this association and the potential benefits of improving air quality on reducing ASD risk.

We observed the negative association between sociodemographic index and ASD prevalence, suggesting poor sociodemographic quality was associated with a low risk of ASD. The result seems counterintuitive because it is commonly believed that poor socioeconomic status is often associated with poor health outcomes. The counterintuitive result was also observed in the associations with other health outcomes, e.g., adult asthma [48] and mortality caused by heart diseases [50], which might be attributed to the space scale used in the model. However, in terms of ASD, the negative association might not be a surprise since previous studies have linked a higher socioeconomic quality to a higher prevalence of ASD in the US [61,62]. The results also highlight the complexities in the relationship between environmental exposures and the prevalence of ASD.

The association between ASD prevalence and environmental quality was affected by climate regions. There were more significant associations in the humid subtropical and warm summer continental regions. According to the Köppen climate classification [63], a humid subtropical climate is characterized by relatively high temperatures, high humidity levels, and distinct seasons. A warm summer continental climate is characterized by distinct seasons, with warm to hot summers and cold winters. The results suggest that extreme weather events might promote the effects of environmental factors on ASD. However, the potential mechanisms need to be further investigated.

With the GWR model, we illustrated the associations in individual counties. Compared with traditional non-spatial models used in many epidemiological studies, the GWR model has several advantages. It addresses spatial autocorrelation issues in the data, thus improving model accuracy. More importantly, it captures the local effects of environmental exposure on health outcomes, thus helping policymakers and planners make more informed decisions by considering specific risk factors in local areas. For example, the results from the GWR model showed the air index had a positive association with ASD prevalence in Maricopa County, Arizona, which informs us that air pollution may cause multiple adverse effects on human health in this area, where air pollutants were associated with higher risk of mortality previously [64]. In addition, no significant association was found for the water index from the Poisson regression model. However, positive associations were found in most counties in Florida and adjacent counties in other states. Since water bodies in Florida are often affected by cyanobacterial blooms [65,66], whether cyanobacterial blooms are linked to ASD is an interesting research topic and needs further investigation.

This finding of study highlights several key Sustainable Development Goals (SDGs). First, it underscores the importance of SDG 3 (Good Health and Well-Being), as improved environmental quality can significantly promote child health and neurodevelopment. It also aligns with SDG 11 (Sustainable Cities and Communities) by advocating for better urban planning and environmental management to reduce pollution. By examining disparities in environmental quality across different sociodemographic groups, the study relates to SDG 10 (Reduced Inequalities). Overall, the findings support integrating environmental health into public policy to advance these SDGs and ensure a healthier future for all.

Most previous studies focused on single or individual environmental exposures on the risk of ASD. Since the environmental effect in the development of ASD is very complicated, it is necessary to investigate the cumulative or simultaneous effects of multiple environmental exposures. In contrast, our study examined the cumulative effects of combined air pollutants rather than focusing on individual pollutants. This study is the first to capture the multifactorial effects of environmental factors on ASD prevalence. The study is also the first to examine the associations between ASD and environmental factors at the national scale and the impact of urbanicity and climate. The large-scale study allows us to explore the spatial patterns in the associations across the US.

The study has a few limitations. First, the ecological nature of this study showed the effects of environmental factors on ASD at the population level, but not at the individual level. The associations do not suggest a cause–effect relationship. Second, because of the difficulties in collecting data on such a large scale, the environmental exposure data were collected over multiple years. There are likely temporal variations in these data. Therefore, we are unable to build temporal relationship between environmental exposure and the development of autism. Since the environmental exposure data were collected a few years earlier than the estimate of ASD prevalence, the association reflects the effects of early exposure to these environmental factors among children.

5. Conclusions

This study reveals significant associations between ASD prevalence and poor environmental quality, particularly air pollution. Our analysis shows that EQI higher values and elevated air index levels are linked to increased ASD risk, underscoring the critical impact of environmental factors on neurodevelopment. Notably, these associations are more pronounced in metropolitan urban areas and regions with humid subtropical and warm summer continental climates, suggesting that both urbanicity and climate play significant roles in amplifying the effects of environmental pollutants.

As the first comprehensive examination of the cumulative effects of environmental factors on ASD prevalence, this study provides crucial insights into how environmental quality, especially air quality, contributes to ASD risk. The findings advocate for targeted public health interventions and urban planning strategies to address environmental risks, particularly in vulnerable regions and populations. Future research will build on these results by exploring specific environmental influences on ASD within diverse locations, aiming to refine strategies for mitigating environmental impacts on neurodevelopment.

Supplementary Materials: The following supporting information can be downloaded at: https://www.mdpi.com/article/10.3390/ijgi13090308/s1, Table S1. The unadjusted association between ASD prevalence and explanatory variables from univariate Poisson regression models; Table S2. Association between ASD prevalence and environmental quality adjusted for rage, gender, age and population density; Figure S1. Association between ASD prevalence and the air index from the geographically weighted regression model; Figure S2. Association between ASD prevalence and the built index from the geographically weighted regression model; Figure S3. Association between ASD prevalence and the land index from the geographically weighted regression model; Figure S4. Association between ASD prevalence and the sociodemographic index from the geographically weighted regression model; Figure S5. Association between ASD prevalence and the water index from the geographically weighted regression model.

Author Contributions: Jianyong Wu conceived and designed the study, conducted data analysis and drafted the manuscript. Data acquisition: Jianyong Wu and Alexander C. McLain. Review & editing: Jianyong Wu, Alexander C. McLain, Paul Rosile and Darryl B. Hood. All authors have read and agreed to the published version of the manuscript.

Funding: J.W. is supported by the startup fund from the College of Public Health, The Ohio State University.

Data Availability Statement: The data of this study are available from the corresponding author upon reasonable request.

Acknowledgments: We would like to thank Yanni Cao for her assistance with GIS mapping.

Conflicts of Interest: The authors declare no conflicts of interest.

References

1. American Psychiatric Association. *Diagnostic and Statistical Manual of Mental Disorders (DSM-5®)*; American Psychiatric Pub: Washington, DC, USA, 2013.
2. Kang, L.; Liu, J.; Liu, Y.; Liang, W.; Yang, F.; Liu, M. Global, regional, and national disease burden of autism spectrum disorder among children under 5 years from 1990 to 2019: An analysis for the Global Burden of Disease 2019 Study. *Asian J. Psychiatry* **2023**, *79*, 103359. [CrossRef] [PubMed]
3. Maenner, M.J.; Warren, Z.; Williams, A.R.; Amoakohene, E.; Bakian, A.V.; Bilder, D.A.; Durkin, M.S.; Fitzgerald, R.T.; Furnier, S.M.; Hughes, M.M. Prevalence and characteristics of autism spectrum disorder among children aged 8 years—Autism and Developmental Disabilities Monitoring Network, 11 sites, United States, 2020. *MMWR Surveill. Summ.* **2023**, *72*, 1. [CrossRef] [PubMed]
4. Dietz, P.M.; Rose, C.E.; McArthur, D.; Maenner, M. National and state estimates of adults with autism spectrum disorder. *J. Autism Dev. Disord.* **2020**, *50*, 4258–4266. [CrossRef]
5. Buescher, A.V.S.; Cidav, Z.; Knapp, M.; Mandell, D.S. Costs of Autism Spectrum Disorders in the United Kingdom and the United States. *JAMA Pediatr.* **2014**, *168*, 721–728. [CrossRef] [PubMed]
6. Leigh, J.P.; Du, J. Brief Report: Forecasting the Economic Burden of Autism in 2015 and 2025 in the United States. *J. Autism Dev. Disord.* **2015**, *45*, 4135–4139. [CrossRef]
7. Newschaffer, C.J.; Croen, L.A.; Daniels, J.; Giarelli, E.; Grether, J.K.; Levy, S.E.; Mandell, D.S.; Miller, L.A.; Pinto-Martin, J.; Reaven, J.; et al. The epidemiology of autism spectrum disorders. *Annu. Rev. Publ. Health* **2007**, *28*, 235–258. [CrossRef]
8. Chaste, P.; Leboyer, M. Autism risk factors: Genes, environment, and gene-environment interactions. *Dialogues Clin. Neurosci.* **2012**, *14*, 281–292. [CrossRef]
9. Pugsley, K.; Scherer, S.W.; Bellgrove, M.A.; Hawi, Z. Environmental exposures associated with elevated risk for autism spectrum disorder may augment the burden of deleterious de novo mutations among probands. *Mol. Psychiatry* **2022**, *27*, 710–730. [CrossRef]
10. Imamura, A.; Morimoto, Y.; Ono, S.; Kurotaki, N.; Kanegae, S.; Yamamoto, N.; Kinoshita, H.; Tsujita, T.; Okazaki, Y.; Ozawa, H. Genetic and environmental factors of schizophrenia and autism spectrum disorder: Insights from twin studies. *J. Neural Transm.* **2020**, *127*, 1501–1515. [CrossRef]
11. Hansen, S.N.; Schendel, D.E.; Francis, R.W.; Windham, G.C.; Bresnahan, M.; Levine, S.Z.; Reichenberg, A.; Gissler, M.; Kodesh, A.; Bai, D. Recurrence risk of autism in siblings and cousins: A multinational, population-based study. *J. Am. Acad. Child. Adolesc. Psychiatry* **2019**, *58*, 866–875. [CrossRef]
12. Sandin, S.; Lichtenstein, P.; Kuja-Halkola, R.; Larsson, H.; Hultman, C.M.; Reichenberg, A. The familial risk of autism. *JAMA* **2014**, *311*, 1770–1777. [CrossRef] [PubMed]
13. Castelbaum, L.; Sylvester, C.M.; Zhang, Y.; Yu, Q.; Constantino, J.N. On the nature of monozygotic twin concordance and discordance for autistic trait severity: A quantitative analysis. *Behav. Genet.* **2020**, *50*, 263–272. [CrossRef] [PubMed]
14. Tick, B.; Bolton, P.; Happé, F.; Rutter, M.; Rijsdijk, F. Heritability of autism spectrum disorders: A meta-analysis of twin studies. *J. Child. Psychol. Psychiatry* **2016**, *57*, 585–595. [CrossRef]
15. Weisskopf, M.G.; Kioumourtzoglou, M.-A.; Roberts, A.L. Air pollution and autism spectrum disorders: Causal or confounded? *Curr. Environ. Health Rep.* **2015**, *2*, 430–439. [CrossRef]
16. Kalkbrenner, A.E.; Daniels, J.L.; Chen, J.C.; Poole, C.; Emch, M.; Morrissey, J. Perinatal exposure to hazardous air pollutants and autism spectrum disorders at age 8. *Epidemiology* **2010**, *21*, 631–641. [CrossRef]

17. Raz, R.; Roberts, A.L.; Lyall, K.; Hart, J.E.; Just, A.C.; Laden, F.; Weisskopf, M.G. Autism Spectrum Disorder and Particulate Matter Air Pollution before, during, and after Pregnancy: A Nested Case-Control Analysis within the Nurses' Health Study II Cohort. *Environ. Health Perspect.* **2015**, *123*, 264–270. [CrossRef] [PubMed]
18. Roberts, E.M.; English, P.B.; Grether, J.K.; Windharn, G.C.; Somberg, L.; Wolff, C. Maternal residence near agricultural pesticide applications and autism spectrum disorders among children in the California Central Valley. *Environ. Health Perspect.* **2007**, *115*, 1482–1489. [CrossRef] [PubMed]
19. Volk, H.E.; Lurmann, F.; Penfold, B.; Hertz-Picciotto, I.; McConnell, R. Traffic-Related Air Pollution, Particulate Matter, and Autism. *JAMA Psychiatry* **2013**, *70*, 71–77. [CrossRef]
20. Modabbernia, A.; Velthorst, E.; Reichenberg, A. Environmental risk factors for autism: An evidence-based review of systematic reviews and meta-analyses. *Mol. Autism* **2017**, *8*, 1–16. [CrossRef]
21. Talbott, E.O.; Arena, V.C.; Rager, J.R.; Clougherty, J.E.; Michanowicz, D.R.; Sharma, R.K.; Stacy, S.L. Fine particulate matter and the risk of autism spectrum disorder. *Environ. Res.* **2015**, *140*, 414–420. [CrossRef]
22. Li, Y.; Xie, T.; Melo, R.D.C.; de Vries, M.; Lakerveld, J.; Zijlema, W.; Hartman, C.A. Longitudinal effects of environmental noise and air pollution exposure on autism spectrum disorder and attention-deficit/hyperactivity disorder during adolescence and early adulthood: The TRAILS study. *Environ. Res.* **2023**, *227*, 115704. [CrossRef] [PubMed]
23. Pagalan, L.; Bickford, C.; Weikum, W.; Lanphear, B.; Brauer, M.; Lanphear, N.; Hanley, G.E.; Oberlander, T.F.; Winters, M. Association of prenatal exposure to air pollution with autism spectrum disorder. *JAMA Pediatr.* **2019**, *173*, 86–92. [CrossRef]
24. McGuinn, L.A.; Windham, G.C.; Kalkbrenner, A.E.; Bradley, C.; Di, Q.; Croen, L.A.; Fallin, M.D.; Hoffman, K.; Ladd-Acosta, C.; Schwartz, J. Early life exposure to air pollution and autism spectrum disorder: Findings from a multisite case–control study. *Epidemiol. Camb. Mass.* **2020**, *31*, 103. [CrossRef] [PubMed]
25. Carter, S.A.; Rahman, M.M.; Lin, J.C.; Shu, Y.-H.; Chow, T.; Yu, X.; Martinez, M.P.; Eckel, S.P.; Chen, J.-C.; Chen, Z. In utero exposure to near-roadway air pollution and autism spectrum disorder in children. *Environ. Int.* **2022**, *158*, 106898. [CrossRef]
26. Yu, X.; Rahman, M.M.; Carter, S.A.; Lin, J.C.; Zhuang, Z.; Chow, T.; Lurmann, F.W.; Kleeman, M.J.; Martinez, M.P.; van Donkelaar, A. Prenatal air pollution, maternal immune activation, and autism spectrum disorder. *Environ. Int.* **2023**, *179*, 108148. [CrossRef]
27. Oudin, A.; Frondelius, K.; Haglund, N.; Källén, K.; Forsberg, B.; Gustafsson, P.; Malmqvist, E. Prenatal exposure to air pollution as a potential risk factor for autism and ADHD. *Environ. Int.* **2019**, *133*, 105149. [CrossRef] [PubMed]
28. Rahman, M.M.; Shu, Y.-H.; Chow, T.; Lurmann, F.W.; Yu, X.; Martinez, M.P.; Carter, S.A.; Eckel, S.P.; Chen, J.-C.; Chen, Z. Prenatal exposure to air pollution and autism spectrum disorder: Sensitive windows of exposure and sex differences. *Environ. Health Perspect.* **2022**, *130*, 017008. [CrossRef]
29. Carter, C.J.; Blizard, R. Autism genes are selectively targeted by environmental pollutants including pesticides, heavy metals, bisphenol A, phthalates and many others in food, cosmetics or household products. *Neurochem. Int.* **2016**, *101*, 83–109. [CrossRef]
30. Hertz-Picciotto, I.; Schmidt, R.J.; Krakowiak, P. Understanding environmental contributions to autism: Causal concepts and the state of science. *Autism Res.* **2018**, *11*, 554–586. [CrossRef]
31. Ye, B.S.; Leung, A.O.W.; Wong, M.H. The association of environmental toxicants and autism spectrum disorders in children. *Environ. Pollut.* **2017**, *227*, 234–242. [CrossRef]
32. Becerra, T.A.; Wilhelm, M.; Olsen, J.; Cockburn, M.; Ritz, B. Ambient air pollution and autism in Los Angeles county, California. *Env. Health Perspect.* **2013**, *121*, 380–386. [CrossRef]
33. Liew, Z.; Meng, Q.; Yan, Q.; Schullehner, J.; Hansen, B.; Kristiansen, S.M.; Voutchkova, D.D.; Olsen, J.; Ersbøll, A.K.; Ketzel, M. Association between estimated geocoded residential maternal exposure to lithium in drinking water and risk for autism spectrum disorder in offspring in Denmark. *JAMA Pediatr.* **2023**, *177*, 617–624. [CrossRef] [PubMed]
34. Awadh, S.M.; Yaseen, Z.M.; Al-Suwaiyan, M.S. The role of environmental trace element toxicants on autism: A medical biogeochemistry perspective. *Ecotoxicol. Environ. Saf.* **2023**, *251*, 114561. [CrossRef] [PubMed]
35. Dou, J.F.; Schmidt, R.J.; Volk, H.E.; Nitta, M.M.; Feinberg, J.I.; Newschaffer, C.J.; Croen, L.A.; Hertz-Picciotto, I.; Fallin, M.D.; Bakulski, K.M. Exposure to heavy metals in utero and autism spectrum disorder at age 3: A meta-analysis of two longitudinal cohorts of siblings of children with autism. *Environ. Health* **2024**, *23*, 62. [CrossRef] [PubMed]
36. Kang, N.; Sargsyan, S.; Chough, I.; Petrick, L.; Liao, J.; Chen, W.; Pavlovic, N.; Lurmann, F.W.; Martinez, M.P.; McConnell, R. Dysregulated Metabolic Pathways Associated with Air Pollution Exposure and the Risk of Autism: Evidence from Epidemiological Studies. *Environ. Pollut.* **2024**, *361*, 124729. [CrossRef] [PubMed]
37. Moschetti, A.; Giangreco, M.; Ronfani, L.; Cervellera, S.; Ruffilli, M.P.; Nume, C.; Barbi, E.; Servidio, A.G. An ecological study shows increased prevalence of autism spectrum disorder in children living in a heavily polluted area. *Sci. Rep.* **2024**, *14*, 17159. [CrossRef]
38. O'Sharkey, K.; Meng, Q.; Mitra, S.; Paik, S.-a.; Liu, J.; Shen, J.; Thompson, L.K.; Chow, T.; Su, J.; Cockburn, M. Associations between brake and tire wear-related PM2. 5 metal components, particulate oxidative stress potential, and autism spectrum disorder in Southern California. *Environ. Int.* **2024**, *185*, 108573. [CrossRef]
39. Román, P.; Ruiz-González, C.; Rueda-Ruzafa, L.; Cardona, D.; Requena, M.; Alarcón, R. Exposure to Environmental Pesticides and the Risk of Autism Spectrum Disorders: A Population-Based Case-Control Study. *Medicina* **2024**, *60*, 479. [CrossRef]
40. Dietert, R.R.; Dietert, J.M.; DeWitt, J.C. Environmental risk factors for autism. *Emerg. Health Threat. J.* **2011**, *4*, 7111. [CrossRef]

41. Wu, J.; Jackson, L. Inverse relationship between urban green space and childhood autism in California elementary school districts. *Environ. Int.* **2017**, *107*, 140–146. [CrossRef]
42. Pagalan, L.; Oberlander, T.F.; Hanley, G.E.; Rosella, L.C.; Bickford, C.; Weikum, W.; Lanphear, N.; Lanphear, B.; Brauer, M.; van den Bosch, M. The association between prenatal greenspace exposure and *Autism spectrum* disorder, and the potentially mediating role of air pollution reduction: A population-based birth cohort study. *Environ. Int.* **2022**, *167*, 107445. [CrossRef] [PubMed]
43. Chen, Y.; Chen, G.; Liu, Y.; Dong, G.-H.; Yang, B.-Y.; Li, S.; Huang, H.; Jin, Z.; Guo, Y. Exposure to greenness during pregnancy and the first three years after birth and autism spectrum disorder: A matched case-control study in shanghai, China. *Environ. Pollut.* **2024**, *340*, 122677. [CrossRef] [PubMed]
44. Lavigne, É.; Abdulaziz, K.E.; Murphy, M.S.; Stanescu, C.; Dingwall-Harvey, A.L.; Stieb, D.M.; Walker, M.C.; Wen, S.W.; Shin, H.H. Associations of neighborhood greenspace, and active living environments with autism spectrum disorders: A matched case-control study in Ontario, Canada. *Environ. Res.* **2024**, *252*, 118828. [CrossRef]
45. Lobdell, D.T.; Jagai, J.S.; Rappazzo, K.; Messer, L.C. Data sources for an environmental quality index: Availability, quality, and utility. *Am. J. Public. Health* **2011**, *101*, S277–S285. [CrossRef]
46. Messer, L.C.; Jagai, J.S.; Rappazzo, K.M.; Lobdell, D.T. Construction of an environmental quality index for public health re-search. *Environ. Health* **2014**, *13*, 39. [CrossRef]
47. USEPA. *Environmental Quality Index—Technical Report, 2006–2010*; U.S. Environmental Protection Agency: Washington, DC, USA, 2020; EPA/600/R-20/367.
48. Gray, C.L.; Lobdell, D.T.; Rappazzo, K.M.; Jian, Y.; Jagai, J.S.; Messer, L.C.; Patel, A.P.; DeFlorio-Barker, S.A.; Lyttle, C.; Solway, J. Associations between environmental quality and adult asthma prevalence in medical claims data. *Environ. Res.* **2018**, *166*, 529–536. [CrossRef] [PubMed]
49. Jagai, J.S.; Krajewski, A.K.; Shaikh, S.; Lobdell, D.T.; Sargis, R.M. Association between environmental quality and diabetes in the USA. *J. Diabetes Investig.* **2020**, *11*, 315–324. [CrossRef]
50. Jian, Y.; Messer, L.C.; Jagai, J.S.; Rappazzo, K.M.; Gray, C.L.; Grabich, S.C.; Lobdell, D.T. Associations between environmental quality and mortality in the contiguous United States, 2000–2005. *Environ. Health Perspect.* **2017**, *125*, 355–362. [CrossRef]
51. Krajewski, A.K.; Rappazzo, K.M.; Langlois, P.H.; Messer, L.C.; Lobdell, D.T. Associations between cumulative environmental quality and ten selected birth defects in Texas. *Birth Defects Res.* **2021**, *113*, 161–172. [CrossRef]
52. Jagai, J.S.; Messer, L.C.; Rappazzo, K.M.; Gray, C.L.; Grabich, S.C.; Lobdell, D.T. County-level cumulative environmental quality associated with cancer incidence. *Cancer* **2017**, *123*, 2901–2908. [CrossRef]
53. Roman-Urrestarazu, A.; Yang, J.C.; van Kessel, R.; Warrier, V.; Dumas, G.; Jongsma, H.; Gatica-Bahamonde, G.; Allison, C.; Matthews, F.E.; Baron-Cohen, S. Autism incidence and spatial analysis in more than 7 million pupils in English schools: A retrospective, longitudinal, school registry study. *Lancet Child. Adolesc. Health* **2022**, *6*, 857–868. [CrossRef] [PubMed]
54. Bradshaw, J.; Eberth, J.M.; Zgodic, A.; Federico, A.; Flory, K.; McLain, A.C. County-Level Prevalence Estimates of Autism Spectrum Disorder in Children in the United States. *J. Autism Dev. Disord.* **2023**, *54*, 2710–2718. [CrossRef] [PubMed]
55. Dutheil, F.; Comptour, A.; Morlon, R.; Mermillod, M.; Pereira, B.; Baker, J.S.; Charkhabi, M.; Clinchamps, M.; Bourdel, N. Autism spectrum disorder and air pollution: A systematic review and meta-analysis. *Environ. Pollut.* **2021**, *278*, 116856. [CrossRef] [PubMed]
56. Lam, J.; Sutton, P.; Kalkbrenner, A.; Windham, G.; Halladay, A.; Koustas, E.; Lawler, C.; Davidson, L.; Daniels, N.; Newschaffer, C.; et al. A Systematic Review and Meta-Analysis of Multiple Airborne Pollutants and Autism Spectrum Disorder. *PLoS ONE* **2016**, *11*, e0161851. [CrossRef]
57. Volk, H.E.; Hertz-Picciotto, I.; Delwiche, L.; Lurmann, F.; McConnell, R. Residential Proximity to Freeways and Autism in the CHARGE Study. *Environ. Health Perspect.* **2011**, *119*, 873–877. [CrossRef]
58. Chauhan, A.; Chauhan, V. Oxidative stress in autism. *Pathophysiology* **2006**, *13*, 171–181. [CrossRef]
59. Frye, R.E.; Cakir, J.; Rose, S.; Palmer, R.F.; Austin, C.; Curtin, P. Physiological mediators of prenatal environmental influences in autism spectrum disorder. *Bioessays* **2021**, *43*, 2000307. [CrossRef]
60. Rossignol, D.A.; Frye, R.E. Evidence linking oxidative stress, mitochondrial dysfunction, and inflammation in the brain of individuals with autism. *Front. Physiol.* **2014**, *5*, 150. [CrossRef]
61. Durkin, M.S.; Maenner, M.J.; Meaney, F.J.; Levy, S.E.; DiGuiseppi, C.; Nicholas, J.S.; Kirby, R.S.; Pinto-Martin, J.A.; Schieve, L.A. Socioeconomic inequality in the prevalence of autism spectrum disorder: Evidence from a U.S. cross-sectional study. *PLoS ONE* **2010**, *5*, e11551. [CrossRef]
62. Thomas, P.; Zahorodny, W.; Peng, B.; Kim, S.; Jani, N.; Halperin, W.; Brimacombe, M. The association of autism diagnosis with socioeconomic status. *Autism* **2012**, *16*, 201–213. [CrossRef]
63. Kottek, M.; Grieser, J.; Beck, C.; Rudolf, B.; Rubel, F. World map of the Koppen-Geiger climate classification updated. *Meteorol. Z.* **2006**, *15*, 259–263. [CrossRef] [PubMed]
64. Moolgavkar, S.H. Air pollution and daily mortality in three US counties. *Environ. Health Perspect.* **2000**, *108*, 777–784. [CrossRef] [PubMed]

65. Burns, J. Toxic cyanobacteria in Florida waters. In *Cyanobacterial Harmful Algal Blooms: State of the Science and Research Needs*; Springer: Berlin/Heidelberg, Germany, 2008; pp. 127–137.
66. Glibert, P.M.; Heil, C.A.; Rudnick, D.T.; Madden, C.J.; Boyer, J.N.; Kelly, S.P. Florida Bay: Water quality status and trends, historic and emerging algal bloom problems. *Contrib. Mar. Sci.* **2009**, *38*, 5–17.

International Journal of
Geo-Information

MDPI

Article

Isochrone-Based Accessibility Analysis of Pre-Hospital Emergency Medical Facilities: A Case Study of Central Districts of Beijing

Yuan Zhao and Ying Zhou *

School of Architecture, Southeast University, Nanjing 210096, China; yuanz@seu.edu.cn
* Correspondence: zhouying@seu.edu.cn

Abstract: Pre-hospital emergency medical service (PHEMS) is critical for the treatment outcomes of life-threatening injuries and time-sensitive illnesses. Response time, influenced by traffic conditions and the site planning of pre-hospital emergency medical facilities (PHEMFs), is the main indicator for evaluating PHEMS. In 2020, the Beijing government released the "Special Plan for Spatial Layout of Pre-hospital Emergency Medical Facilities in Beijing (2020–2022)". This paper evaluates the functional efficiency and spatial equity of this plan within Beijing's central six districts using isochrone measures to assess the accessibility of the planned PHEMFs. The isochrone coverages of the area and population were calculated, and the temporal-spatial characteristics of isochrones were concluded. The analysis revealed that while the current planning meets several objectives, challenges in service availability and equity persist. Although 10-min isochrone coverage was high, 8-min coverage was insufficient, particularly during peak hours. This highlights gaps in service accessibility that necessitate additional emergency stations in underserved areas. The current planning approach leads to significant overlap at administrative boundaries, causing service oversupply and increased costs, which calls for a city-wide planning perspective that breaks administrative boundaries to optimize resource allocation. Traffic conditions significantly impact service coverage, with congestion reducing coverage in central areas and better coverage near traffic hubs. Future planning should strategically place stations based on traffic patterns and population distribution to enhance emergency medical service accessibility and equity in urban areas.

Keywords: emergency medical service; pre-hospital emergency medical facility; isochrone; accessibility analysis

1. Introduction

As an integral part of the healthcare system, pre-hospital emergency medical service (PHEMS) is the first level of healthcare response for out-of-hospital medical emergencies. It refers to a system that organizes all aspects of medical care provided to patients in pre- or out-of-hospital environments [1,2]. It is critical to the treatment outcomes of life-threatening injuries and time-sensitive illnesses, which may lead to premature mortality and serious disability. Additionally, PHEMS serves as a fundamental public resource for managing common medical conditions and is essential for effective disaster response and mass casualty management [3,4]. In particular, the administrative control policies during the COVID-19 pandemic restricted citizens' free access to emergency departments, leading to greater reliance on urban EMS under emergency conditions.

In urban settings, pre-hospital care typically starts with an emergency call to a dispatch center. Trained personnel assess the need for emergency care, and ambulances are then dispatched to provide services like triage and treatment as well as transport the patients to the proper medical facility [5]. The time between the moment an emergency call is made and the equipped ambulance's arrival at the scene is defined as the response time (RT), which is a primary metric for evaluating PHEMS performance and is crucial for the success of pre-hospital care [6]. RT is divided into three components: call time (the interval from receiving the emergency call to raising the alert), gathering time (from sending the alert to dispatching the medical team), and road time (from ambulance dispatch to arrival at the scene) [7]. Among these, road time accounts for the largest percentage and has the biggest influence on patient outcomes [8]. This is affected by both the traffic conditions and the site planning of PHEMS facilities. Reasonable site planning of EMS facilities is essential to guarantee an efficient and equitable pre-hospital emergency system, as time is crucial when dealing with a patient in an emergency.

The World Health Organization recommends that emergency medical services ambulance response time to a medical emergency is within 8 min for at least 90% of calls [6,9,10]. Nonetheless, RT differs not only between nations and regions globally but also between rural, suburban, and urban sectors all within the same region [11,12]. For instance, the median of statewide RT in Texas, US, was 7 min in 2021 [13], and the RT in Japan was 7.5 min in 2016 [6]. The average RT for life-threatening calls was 10.5 min in 2023 [14], and the RT in Greece was 28.9 min in 2016 [6]. In China, regional disparities are pronounced, with urban–suburban RT differences remaining substantial even within a single city [11]. In Beijing, the capital city of China, the RT was still 16.41 min in 2020 [11], which is far behind the 8-min standard. To address this issue, the Chinese government released new guidelines for PHEMS in 2020 [15]. Specific measures were proposed, including service area, ambulance number, and maximum dispatch time. Each municipal government still has the right to set its specified response time requirement.

To enhance PHEMS, the Beijing government released the "Special Plan for Spatial Layout of Pre-hospital Emergency Medical Facilities in Beijing (2020–2022)" (Special Plan for short) in 2020 [16]. The planning objective for this Special Plan was to achieve an average RT of less than 12 min. The plan proposed 465 pre-hospital emergency medical facility sites across the city, including 278 new sites and 187 existing sites. The planning method was based on the administrative divisions, taking Jiedao (the minimum administrative unit in urban areas of China) as the basic planning unit, establishing at least one emergency station within each Jiedao. This planning method is widely applied in Chinese urban planning, and it has the advantage of easy evaluation and assessment of the government at all levels. However, there are still several issues that need further discussion. Can this planning approach achieve the planning objectives? Is the planning outcome adequate and equitable to the population? Does a situation where emergency services are unavailable or oversupplied occur? How do traffic conditions affect planning outcomes, and how can the uncertainty caused by traffic be avoided in future planning?

To discuss the questions mentioned above, this paper takes the six central districts of Beijing as the study area and applies the isochrone measure to evaluate the accessibility of the planned pre-hospital emergency medical facilities (PHEMFs) in the Special Plan. Accessibility is a critical indicator of the functional efficiency and spatial equity of urban services; it measures the ease of reaching spatially distributed opportunities [17]. Various measures, including gravity models, cumulative opportunity measures, two-step floating-catchment area (2SFCA), and kernel density estimation (KDE), have been developed to assess urban service accessibility [17,18]. These measures are widely applied in the field of transport geography and urban planning to help urban planners and policymakers evaluate the performance of transportation and land-use systems in urban areas [19,20]. However, the measure selection still needs discussion based on the complexity and realism of the practical problem. One often-used technique for measuring accessibility without designating a destination is the isochrone approach, sometimes known as the cumulative opportunities measure within the isochrone. The isochrone defines reachable locations from a fixed starting point within the given cut-off time by a specified mode of transport. Given that response time is critical for emergency medical systems, assessing PHEMF accessibility through isochrones with stringent time thresholds provides valuable insights into functional efficiency and spatial equity. This paper aims to evaluate the functional efficiency and spatial equity of the pre-hospital emergency medical facilities (PHEMF) planning in the six central districts of Beijing by applying the isochrone measure to assess accessibility, analyze the isochrone coverage results, examine the temporal–spatial characteristics, and discuss the traffic sensitivity and equality assessment of the study area.

The remainder of this paper is structured as follows. Section 2 reviews the existing literature. Section 3 introduces the methodology and data used in this paper, including basic information about the study area, the data collection and processing methods, and the analysis method used in this study. Section 4 analyzes the results obtained by applying the methods introduced in Section 3. Section 5 discusses and concludes the accessibility assessment results from both the demand side and the supply side and proposes future planning suggestions based on the analysis results. Section 6 concludes the study.

2. Literature Review

Accessibility is a deep-seated and widely used concept in the field of transport geography and urban planning, emphasized by numerous studies for its importance in the healthcare domain [18,21,22]. Archiving adequate and equitable accessibility has become a critical objective of policy making, urban planning, and public health planning. Accessibility was also applied to various urban services, such as job opportunities [23–25], urban parks [26,27], food outlets [28,29], and so on. Despite its wide-ranging applications, the literature suggests that accessibility consists of three major components: transportation component, human activity component, and land use component [18].

Determining each component is the first step in calculating accessibility. The transportation component deals with the ease of traveling; it refers to the specific transportation network within the study area, such as the subway network or the urban road network. The human activity component focuses on the preferences of service consumers, including service facility choice preferences and transportation options preferences [18]. Both the transportation network and consumer transportation choice determine travel time. The land use component refers to the spatial distribution of service facilities, determining the traveling destination of service consumers.

This study evaluated the service accessibility of the planned PHEMFs in the Special Plan. The planned PHEMF site locations were used as the facility spatial distribution, and the driving mode in the urban road network was applied to calculate the travel time. As usual, the nearest ambulance was dispatched to the patient's location and chose the fastest route; thus, the facility preference of patients was neglected in emergency conditions.

Various formulations for measuring accessibility have been proposed in the literature and can be divided into two categories based on the calculation outcomes. One group of metrics has a result with absolute units, such as distance and travel time to the nearest service facility, population-to-provider ratios, and cumulative opportunity measure (COM). COM assesses accessibility by counting the number of opportunities reachable within a specified travel time or distance from a given location. A simple form of COM is:

$$A_i = \sum_j f E_j \tag{1}$$

where A_i is the total opportunities available of location i, E_j is the number of opportunities in location j, f is 1 for locations within a given threshold, and 0 otherwise [20]. It has the advantage of being simple in calculation, direct in interpretation, and comparable across regions, but the trade-off is low accuracy and realism [20,30].

To address these limitations, another group of methods, such as gravity models, the two-step floating catchment area (2SFCA) method, and kernel density estimation (KDE), were proposed to obtain a more accurate evaluation of accessibility through more complex computations [18]. The results are expressed in relative terms by normalizing the values over a particular range [31], and their interpretation is limited to comparisons with other outcomes. These methods are commonly used to evaluate urban service equity [19,20,32], uncover social disparities [33], and assess the unequal allocation of resources [34]. For example, 2SFCA calculates the supply-to-population ratio within a defined catchment area for each facility, considering travel time or distance. It then sums these ratios for each population point, accounting for accessible facilities within their catchment areas [18]. While 2SFCA offers a comprehensive and context-sensitive analysis, it requires more detailed data and computational effort, and its results are expressed in relative terms, which may be less intuitive than COM.

Choosing the appropriate measure depends on the practical problem and requires balancing between accuracy and simplicity. Most healthcare accessibility research focuses on primary care [35], hospital care [32,36,37], and EMS [38,39]. Methods relative units, such as 2SFCA, are more appropriate for equity discussion for primary care and hospital care because the research is focused on the physical separation and resource competition that result in uneven service distribution. For emergency care, response time is the critical metric, represented in absolute units (minutes). Since response time is paramount, service coverage is defined by the total area or population within the cut-off travel time, making the cumulative opportunity measure with response time constraints (isochrone) suitable for this study.

Recently, several platforms, such as Mapbox [40], iso4app [41], and TravelTime [42], have introduced online isochrone services that are convenient to acquire, fast in calculation, and accurate in results. However, these services have limitations. Most APIs do not account for departure times, which hinders their ability to conduct temporal analyses—studies that examine variations in accessibility at different times of the day. Additionally, some APIs have region restrictions, which results in poor service rates and accuracy for mainland Chinese cities. To address these issues and construct an accurate isochrone that reflects temporal variations, this study employs a methodology that connects sample points based on equal travel times from a starting location at various times throughout the day. By integrating these temporal characteristics, we ensure that the isochrones accurately represent how accessibility changes during peak hours, midnight hours, and normal hours of the day, providing a more reliable analysis of accessibility patterns.

The sample points are specific locations within the study area where accessibility is measured. They help in assessing the spatial accessibility of the PHEMFs by providing a reference for evaluating how far the ambulance can reach within the required time under different traffic conditions. Three techniques are often used to choose sample points: using administrative divisions' centroids [43], the centroid of grid-based raster [28,37], and radial rays. The third approach draws rays that split the circumference into equiangular slices radially spread from the origin and take identical steps along the ray as the sample points. The latter two methods are most frequently used to obtain travel data through open map APIs. Although smaller spatial units can yield more accurate findings by offering higher spatial analysis precision, they also cause a large increase in API request time, which slows down the computation speed. The radial-ray-based approach can significantly reduce the quantity of API requests while maintaining sample density. In this study, parameters were chosen to balance calculation efficiency and accuracy with a radial angle of 10 degrees and a step size of 100 m.

When calculating the equity of accessibility, both the supply and demand sides must be considered. In the healthcare system, supply-side accessibility and service coverage can be evaluated using PHEMF isochrones. On the demand side, competition exists among the patients, i.e., the medical service resources are limited. More competitors reduce the available opportunities that the patient can reach in the real world than in the ideal situation, especially in special cases like mass casualty incidents (MCIs). The actual accessibility of an opportunity depends not only on it being reachable but also on the number of other competitors that can reach it [20,44]. Therefore, it is necessary to consider competition when calculating the demand-side accessibility of emergency services. Researchers have advocated the importance of considering the competition in accessibility measures and have also pointed out that accessibility should be related to changes in demand [20,25,45,46]. Nevertheless, with the improvement in calculation accuracy, the accessibility measures that account for the competition tend to be complex in calculation and difficult to interpret. Researchers have also noted that because the COM only accounts for a single cut-off trip cost and ignores spatial distribution variance, it has the drawback of failing to take opportunity competition into account [30]. Kelobonye (2020) introduced a competition component to COM to improve its accuracy and showed its applicability and improvement in order to increase the measure's accuracy while maintaining its simplicity and broad application [20]. This study applies the cumulative opportunity measure, considering competition from the demand side, to assess the equity of emergency service accessibility.

3. Methods and Data Description

3.1. Data Description

The datasets utilized in this paper included the pre-hospital emergency medical facilities (PHEMF) data, population data, and travel time data within the study area. The sources and processing methods for these datasets are outlined below.

3.1.1. Study Area

Beijing, the capital of China, is one of the most populous metropolitan cities, with a population of 21.88 million and an area of 16.41 thousand square kilometers as of 2022 [47]. As shown in Figure 1, this study focused on the six core districts of Beijing: Dongcheng, Xicheng, Chaoyang, Haidian, Fengtai, and Shijingshan. These districts are considered the central urban regions of the city.

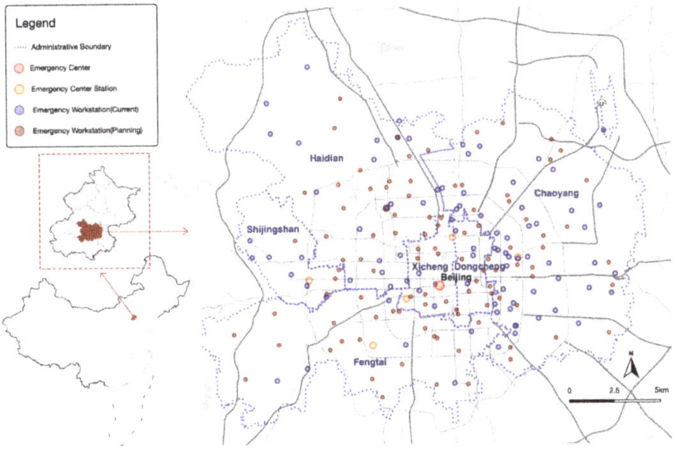

Figure 1. Spatial distribution of PHEMFs in the six central districts of Beijing.

3.1.2. Pre-Hospital Emergency Medical Facility Data

The emergency medical service system in Beijing includes three types of PHEMFs: emergency medical centers (EMCs), emergency central stations (ECSs), and emergency stations (ESs). The primary distinction is seen in the range of services offered and the size of the facilities built. EMCs are large, well-equipped facilities responsible for citywide dispatch commands. ECSs are medium-sized facilities, generally over 800 square meters, that manage, command, and provide training within designated areas. ESs are smaller, support first aid within their immediate areas, and are categorized into grade A and grade B based on the number of ambulances they can accommodate; grade A stations have six ambulance parking spots, while grade B stations have three [16].

To enhance EMS services, Beijing launched an upgrade plan in 2020, known as the Special Plan for Spatial Layout of Pre-hospital Emergency Medical Facilities in Beijing (2020–2022) [16]. It planned 456 emergency facility site locations for the entire city, including 278 new locations. Within our study area, there were 95 existing and 101 newly planned locations, as summarized in Table 1. The facility distribution included one EMC and six

ECSs (one per district), with the newly planned ECS located in Xicheng. The remaining facilities were ESs, totaling 189 stations, with 89 existing and 100 planned. The spatial distribution of the facility locations is shown in Figure 1.

Table 1. PHEMFs in the six central districts.

	Total	EMC	ECS	ES			
				Existing	Planned	Grade A	Grade B
Dongcheng	12	0	1	4	7	1	10
Xicheng	18	1	1	4	12	4	12
Chaoyang	81	0	1	48	32	10	70
Haidian	45	0	1	20	24	6	38
Fengtai	29	0	1	6	22	6	22
Shijingshan	11	0	1	7	3	3	7
Total	196	1	6	89	100	30	159

3.1.3. Population Data

The population data were obtained from WorldPop [48]. The data were aggregated and constrained with buildings from the 2020 population, with a grid of 100 m × 100 m [49]. There were 172,968 grids with population data within the study area. This dataset showed its advantage in the high accuracy of the area with satellite-based settlement images, especially in highly developed urban areas [50], which is consistent with the study area of this paper.

3.1.4. Travel Time Data

Two main trip time collection methods are commonly used: GIS-based methods and open map-based approaches. GIS-based methods, using embedded spatial analysis tools [37,51–54], provide fast calculations but often ignore actual traffic conditions. In contrast, open map-based methods use real-time and historical speed data to calculate more accurate travel times [23,55]. A large number of studies using online map data in the field of traffic analysis and transport accessibility have emerged [23,36,55], demonstrating that the open map service can provide objective and accurate travel data.

The isochrones in this study were constructed using real-time travel data from the Amap platform [56], a major location-based service provider in China. Amap offers route planning based on real-time traffic conditions and user data to estimate vehicle speeds and predict road conditions. The location of each PHEMF was used as the route origin, the surrounding sample points of each facility were used as the route destinations, and the shortest travel time strategy was applied to the route requests.

The real-time travel time data could reflect real traffic congestion during the day. To make a comparison between different traffic hours, the data acquisition hours were further divided into three time periods due to the time-varying characteristics of urban traffic: midnight period (22:00–05:00 the next day), peak period (07:00–09:00 and 17:00–20:00), and normal period (other hours). The temporal analysis in the following sections is based on the three time periods. Each origin–destination pair's travel time was measured three times within the same period, and the average was used to ensure data reliability.

3.2. Analysis Method Design for Accessibility Evaluation

3.2.1. Isochrone Construction Method

An isochrone is defined as the reachable location from a fixed starting point within the given cut-off time by a specified mode of transport. In this study, the service area of each PHEMF was evaluated by applying isochrone in three defined periods. The radial-ray-based approach was used to construct the isochrones. This method involved drawing radial rays from the origin, which divided the surrounding area into equiangular segments. Sample points were then selected along these rays at regular intervals. The travel time from the origin to each sample point was computed using an open map platform with the travel mode set to driving (i.e., by ambulance). Then, the isochrone was constructed by connecting the farthest points from the origin with identical cut-off travel time.

Figure 2 illustrates the detailed steps of constructing an isochrone with a time threshold of T. (1) Determine the coordinates of starting point O. (2) Take the starting point as the center of the circle, distance D as the radius, and set the circle as the picking range of endpoints (where D exceeds the optimal straight-line distance within time T in an urban area). (3) Select N radial rays with an identical angle that are centered at point O ($\theta = 360^{\circ}/N$). (4) Along each radial ray, take the farthest point A as the first destination to calculate the travel time from point O to point A, t_{OA}. (5) If $t_{OA} > T$, take one step toward point O, calculate the coordinates of point B ($D_{OB} = D_{OA}$-d), and calculate t_{OB}. Repeat this process until the travel time is less than or equal to T ($t_{OB} \leq T$), then point B is the farthest reachable point on this ray. (6). Repeat steps 4 and 5 for each ray to obtain the collection of the farthest reachable points in N lines. (7). Construct the isochrons of time T by connecting the farthest reachable points in all directions.

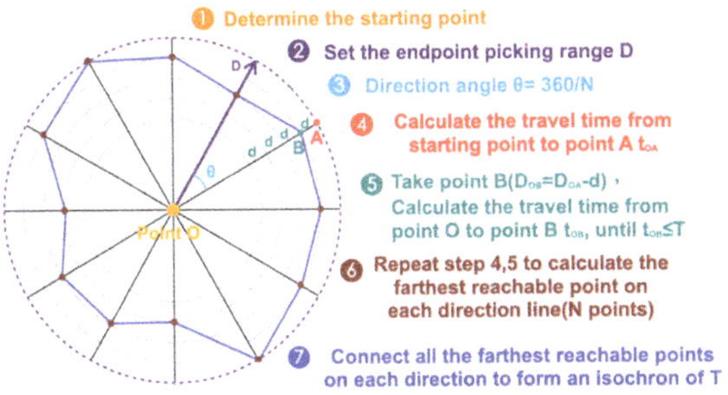

Figure 2. Steps of constructing isochrone of threshold time T.

The parameters in the isochrone construction steps affected both the result accuracy and calculation efficiency. A larger value for N (number of radial rays) and a smaller value for d (step size) improved the precision of the isochrone but also increased the number of API requests, thereby reducing computational efficiency. To find a balance between accuracy and efficiency, we conducted experiments with different parameter combinations. First, step size d was set to 100 m, which is smaller than the typical city block size in Beijing's central districts. Then, with the maximum driving speed within the urban street of 60 km/h and the largest time threshold being 10 min in this study, the farthest driving distance was 10 km. Therefore, the picking range D should be less than 10 km. We randomly selected 10 facility points from the PHEMF set as test points and calculated the farthest distance reachable in all directions. The results indicated that 6 km was the smallest integer value for D. Regarding the direction angle between radial rays, $\theta = 5, 10, 20$ (corresponding to N = 72, 36, 18), was tested on the randomly selected test points. The number of API requests ranged from 1100 to 1500 per PHEMF when $\theta = 10$, and it was halved when $\theta = 20$ and doubled when $\theta = 5$. Additionally, the isochrone results were more starlike when $\theta = 5$, while $\theta = 20$ produced less detail. Thus, $\theta = 10$ (N = 36) was selected as the optimal parameter to ensure accurate isochrone representation while maintaining manageable computational demands.

3.2.2. Accessibility of PHEMF

The cumulative opportunity measure (COM) was applied to measure the accessibility of PHEMF. It counts the number of populations that the ambulance can reach, starting from each PHEMF within travel time T. The isochrone of time T in the period h ($h \in \{midnight, peak, normal\}$) obtained for a PHEMF i was treated as its service area within time T; its covered area was expressed as $AR_i^{T,h}$. The population within the service area $P_i^{T,h}$ was calculated as

$$P_i^{T,h} = \sum_j f\left(c_{ij}^h, T\right) Pop_j \quad (2)$$

$$f\left(c_{ij}^{h}, T\right) = \begin{cases} 1 \; if \; c_{ij}^{h} \leq T \\ 0 \; if \; c_{ij}^{h} > T \end{cases} \quad (3)$$

where $f(c_{ij}^{h}, T)$ is the impedance function, it denotes the isochrone of time T in the period h of location i. c_{ij}^{h} denotes the travel time from i to j in the period h, Pop_j is the number of populations in grid j, and j is the population grid within the isochrone-covered area.

3.2.3. PHEMF Accessibility Sensitivity to Traffic

Traffic congestion significantly impacts ambulance travel times, thereby influencing the critical time available for first aid. During midnight hours, when traffic is minimal, travel times are shortest, resulting in the largest coverage area for isochrones. Conversely, during peak hours, especially in densely developed metropolitan areas, traffic congestion leads to extended travel times, which reduces the coverage area of isochrones. This variation in coverage area between the peak and midnight periods is influenced by traffic patterns, which affect response times and, consequently, the effective service area of each facility. Thus, it can serve as an indicator of how sensitive each PHEMF is to traffic conditions. To quantify this sensitivity, we introduced the accessibility sensitivity to traffic ($S_i{}^T$) as an indicator to identify the most traffic-sensitive facilities. $S_i{}^T$ was calculated using the following formula:

$$S_i^T = \frac{A_i^{T,midnight} - A_i^{T,peak}}{A_i^{T,midnight}} \quad (4)$$

where $A_i{}^{T,midnight}$ is the T isochrone coverage area of PHEMF i during the midnight period, $A_i{}^{T,peak}$ is the T isochrone coverage area of PHEMF i during the peak hours.

This metric allowed us to evaluate how traffic congestion impacted the accessibility of PHEMFs, providing insights into the variability of service coverage and identifying the facilities that were most impacted by traffic congestion. It also implies the importance of considering traffic conditions in future planning.

3.2.4. Equity Assessment

In Section 3.2.2, the accessibility of each PHEMF was calculated by measuring the area and population that a single facility served within a given time T from the supply side. It was also necessary to measure accessibility from the demand side. The demand side accessibility was used to assess the equity among the population.

In the traditional cumulative opportunities approach, the value was calculated by setting the demand point as the origin and summing up the number of reachable supply facilities within the threshold time. This method is simple but with its limitation of lack of accuracy, especially under the condition of limited resources. The value of reachable opportunities decreased when the competition for them increased, and the traditional cumulative opportunity method overestimated the actual accessible opportunities. In the case of an emergency, one may not expect an ambulance when all ambulances are on missions, even if the emergency station is quite near. To reflect the degree of competition for limited opportunities, a competition component was incorporated into the traditional cumulative opportunity method to assess the effective accessibility of population grids.

The method used the supply–demand ratio; it first estimated the share of opportunities proportional to the size of service demand for every supply location, then summed up the proportional opportunities in locations that were covered in each population grid. In the context of emergency medical services, opportunity refers to the likelihood of an ambulance reaching a location in time. The calculation was expressed as follows,

$$A_i^{T,h} = \sum\nolimits_j \frac{g\left(c_{ij}^{h}, T\right) E_j}{P_j^{T,h}} \quad (5)$$

$$g\left(c_{ij}^{h}, T\right) = \begin{cases} 1 \ if \ c_{ij}^{h} \leq T \\ 0 \ if \ c_{ij}^{h} > T \end{cases} \tag{6}$$

where $A_i^{T,h}$ is the effective accessibility at time T in the time period h of location i (ambulance available to an individual person in grid i). $g(c_{ij}^{h}, T)$ is similar to Equation (3), denotes the isochrone of PHEMF j of time T in the time period h could cover the grid i. E_j is the number of ambulances of PHEMF j. $P_j^{T,h}$ is the total population within the service area of PHEMF j of time T in the time period h, expressed by Equation (2). This method is simple in calculation and retains its practical significance. The result was expressed in opportunities (ambulances) per person.

4. Results Analysis

Emergency response time can be divided into three periods: call time, gathering time, and road time. According to the statistics of the Beijing EMS, the median response time was 16.5 min in 2005 [57], 19.18 min in 2008, and 22.26 min in 2017 [58]. The average response time was around 15 min in 2021 [59], 16.04 min in 2022 [60], and 12.20 min in 2023 [61]. The first two phases, which take place inside emergency stations and centers, are influenced by the qualifications and proficiency of the response team. The longest and most challenging to control is road time—the duration for an ambulance to arrive at the incident site. The median time from the emergency call to ambulance departure is around 4 min [58]. The median ambulance driving time in Beijing was 10.6 min in 2005 [57], 14.75 min in 2008, and 17.35 min in 2017 [58].

To meet the target of "average response time less than 12 min" in the Special Plan, the time from emergency call to ambulance departure should be controlled to 2 to 4 min; thus, the road travel time of ambulances should be less than 10 to 8 min. Based on these time ranges, this paper calculates the multiple time threshold isochrone coverages of PHEMFs during three time periods (midnight period (22:00–05:00 the next day), peak period (07:00–09:00 and 17:00–20:00), and normal period (other hours). The results are as follows.

4.1. Isochrone Coverage Results

Table 2 shows the total area and population coverage results of isochrones with different travel time thresholds in the three time periods. Figure 3 visualizes the isochrone results for 10-min and 8-min travel times, using color to distinguish between peak and midnight periods. The coverage result for 9-min travel time fell between the results for 10 and 8 min, and the normal period coverage fell between the peak and midnight periods. Therefore, only the isochrone coverage results for 10 and 8 min during the midnight and peak periods were visualized to better illustrate the disparities in the data.

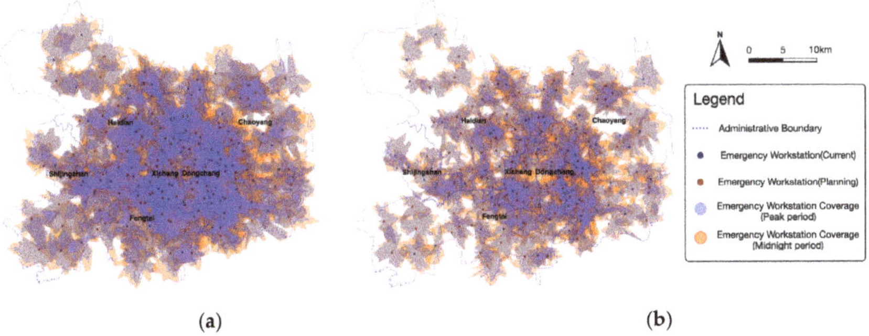

Figure 3. Isochrone results for different travel time thresholds: (**a**) 10 min, (**b**) 8 min.

Table 2. Area and population coverage of isochrones in different periods.

Periods	Coverage	Travel Time Threshold		
		10 min	**9 min**	**8 min**
Peak	Area (km^2)	1105.55	1018.95	837.62
	Area Proportion	80.39%	74.09%	60.91%
	Population (Million)	15.91	15.14	12.95
	Population Proportion	93.83%	89.31%	76.41%
Normal	Area (km^2)	1127.79	1043.0	879.9
	Area Proportion	82.01%	75.84%	63.98%
	Population (Million)	16.04	15.36	13.41
	Population Proportion	94.65%	90.64%	79.08%
Midnight	Area (km^2)	1202.22	1144.00	1035.49
	Area Proportion	87.42%	83.19%	75.30%
	Population (Million)	16.58	16.25	15.41
	Population Proportion	97.81%	95.90%	90.91%

Note: Coverage area/population refers to the coverage area/population of all isochrones within the six central districts. The coverage proportion refers to the ratio of the coverage area/population within the central six districts to the total area/population of the central six districts.

It could be seen from the results that, within a 10-min travel time, PHEMFs covered the vast majority of the urban area, with 87.42% coverage at midnight and 80.39% area coverage during peak hours. The population coverage performed even better, reaching 93.83% during peak hours and 97.81% in the midnight period. However, the coverage significantly decreased within an 8-min travel time, accounting for 75.30% of the area at midnight, and only 60.91% of the urban area and 76.41% of the population during peak hours, presenting more uncovered areas and populations.

In addition, Figure 3a illustrates a high rate of overlap in the coverage of isochrones within the central urban area for the 10-min threshold (the darker the color, the more overlapping the layers). The areas with the highest rate of overlap were found around district borders, including the border between Dongcheng and Chaoyang District, the northern border of Fengtai District, and the southeast border of Haidian District. Conversely, the coverage overlap rate for 8-min isochrone was significantly lower, with primary coverage overlap areas in the southwest of Xicheng District, the vicinity of the Dongcheng District and Chaoyang District borders, and the eastern portion of Shijingshan District.

4.2. *Temporal–Spatial Characteristics of Isochrones*

The statistics of the isochrone coverage results of 196 PHEMFs in different periods are shown in Figure 4. As illustrated in Figure 4a,b, the area coverage distribution of the isochrones varied across different periods. The midnight period (blue) displayed a relatively normal distribution with a tight relationship between the median and mean values. The distribution was right-skewed for normal and peak periods (orange and green), with a significantly reduced number of facilities with large area coverage. In the comparison of the area coverage during the peak and midnight periods, the mean values of 10-min and 8-min travel time thresholds decreased by 43.57% and 46.47%, respectively. The population coverage was similar, as shown in Figure 4c,d, with right-skewed distributions during peak and normal periods and a flatter distribution during the midnight period. This result reflects the fact that many emergency facilities have large area coverage but small population coverage, and their area coverage results are majorly affected by the travel time threshold.

By comparing population coverage during the peak and midnight periods, the mean values of 10-min and 8-min travel time thresholds decreased by 44.9% and 50%, respectively. Since 10-min isochrones covered almost twice the area and population of 8-min isochrones in all periods, increasing the travel time threshold significantly expanded the population coverage results of PHEMFs.

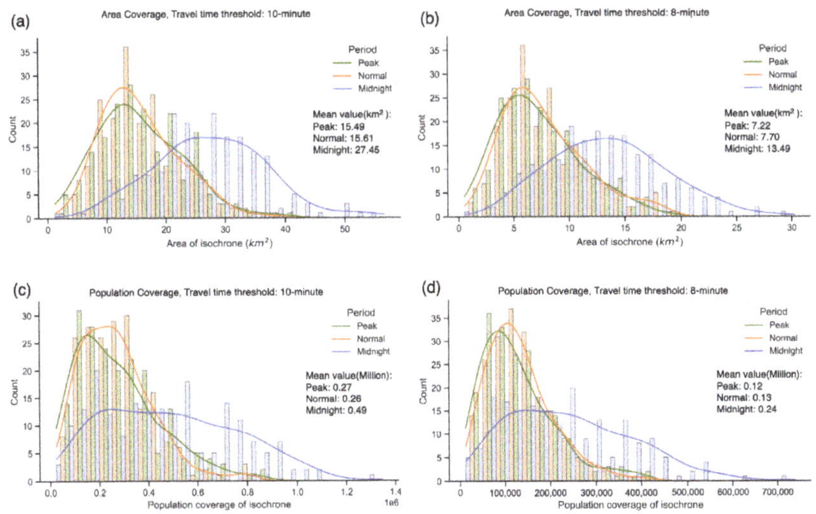

Figure 4. Isochrone distribution: (**a**) area coverage of 10 min, (**b**) area coverage of 8 min, (**c**) population coverage of 10 min, (**d**) population coverage of 8 min.

This result also showed that traffic conditions had a major influence on the isochrone coverage results, with little variation between the peak and normal periods, indicating congested traffic during non-midnight hours, making it challenging for ambulances to arrive quickly. Meanwhile, extending ambulance travel time effectively increased PHEMF service areas.

Figure 5 shows the geographical distribution of the isochrone coverage results. Table 3 categorizes these results into four groups based on their coverage characteristics. Type 1 facilities had a large area and large population coverage; they were mainly located in the area around traffic hubs, particularly in the northeastern region between the Third and Fourth Ring Roads. Type 2 facilities were located primarily in the outer areas of the central six districts, including the northeast of Chaoyang District, the south of Fengtai District, and the northwest of Haidian District, etc. These areas typically had a lower population density and lower emergency facility density. Facilities with high population coverage, including Type 1 and Type 3, were generally found near the borders of the six districts, particularly at the boundaries of Dongcheng and Xicheng Districts, as well as the southern boundary of Haidian District. Type 4 facilities, which had a small area and population coverage, were mainly located in the central areas of each district.

This distribution was significantly influenced by the underlying traffic patterns and population distribution within the city. Type 1 facilities were located near major traffic hubs, where road networks were denser and more efficient, facilitating quicker response times despite high traffic volumes. Type 2 facilities, on the other hand, were positioned in the outer regions of the central districts, where population density was lower, and traffic congestion was less intense. This allowed these facilities to cover larger geographic areas with fewer people, compensating for the longer travel distances required to reach emergency incidents. Type 3 facilities were typically found near district borders where population density was high, but traffic congestion limited extensive coverage. Finally, Type 4 facilities, characterized by their limited area and population coverage, were situated in central urban areas, where the population density was highest and road networks were most congested. The extremely heavy traffic in these areas restricted isochrone coverage within central district regions. To meet the high demand in these areas, additional emergency facilities are necessary. The distribution of these isochrones highlighted the crucial role of traffic conditions and population density in shaping the accessibility and efficiency of emergency medical services.

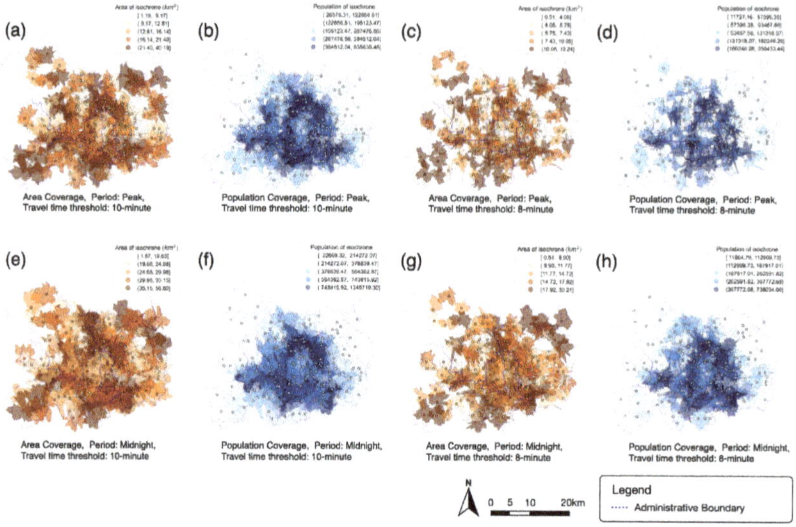

Figure 5. Spatial distribution of isochrones: (**a**) area coverage of 10-min isochrones in the peak period, (**b**) population coverage of 10-min isochrones in the peak period, (**c**) area coverage of 8-min isochrones in the peak period, (**d**) population coverage of 8-min isochrones in the peak period, (**e**) area coverage of 10-min isochrones in the midnight period, (**f**) population coverage of 10-min isochrones in the midnight period, (**g**) area coverage of 8-min isochrones in the midnight period, (**h**) population coverage of 8-min isochrones in the midnight period.

Table 3. Area and population coverage characteristics.

Type	Area Coverage	Population Coverage	Major Locations
1	Large	Large	Around traffic hubs (Near the Third Ring and Fourth Ring Roads)
2	Large	Small	Edge area of central six districts
3	Small	Large	Around borders between six districts
4	Small	Small	Middle area of each district

As shown in Figure 5, isochrone coverage overlapped significantly in the central urban area. Particularly around the border area of Dongcheng District and Xicheng District, which exhibited low area coverage but high population coverage. A comparison of the spatial distributions across different periods revealed that Type 1 locations remain relatively stable, maintaining high coverage throughout all periods due to their advantageous traffic locations. This further demonstrated the significance of the traffic to PHEMF's coverage. Conversely, some type 4 facilities had a limited area and population coverage across all periods. Their isochrones had poor coverage capacity and overlap with other facilities' isochrones. It could be integrated with the nearby facilities, which would lower operational costs without compromising service quality.

4.3. Traffic Sensitivity Analysis

Further calculating the accessibility sensitivity to the traffic of each PHEMF according to Equation (4), the results are presented in Figure 6. Accessibility sensitivity measures the proportion of area change rate between the peak and midnight periods. A higher value indicates larger area shrinkage during the peak period, demonstrating high sensitivity to traffic conditions, and vice versa.

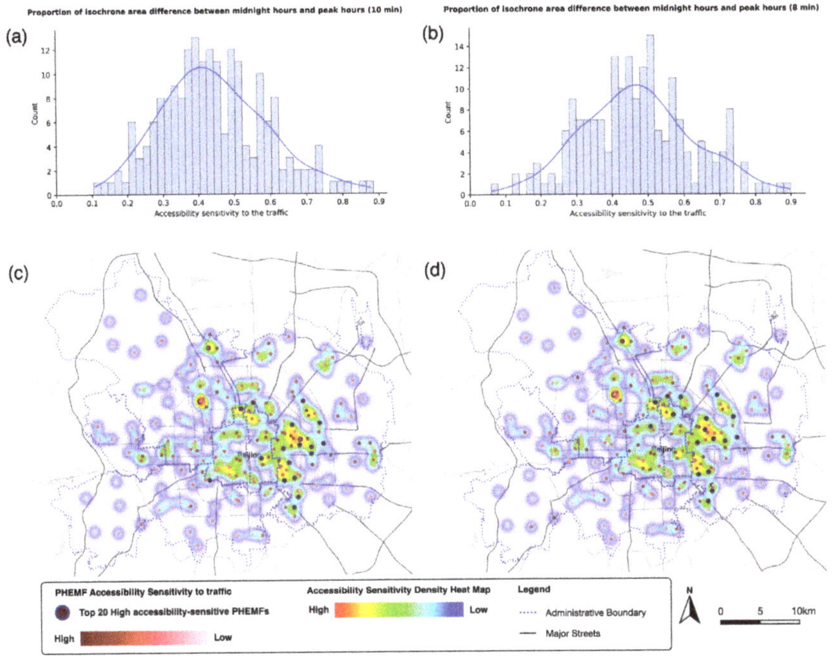

Figure 6. Distribution of PHEMF accessibility sensitivity to traffic: (**a**) 10-min travel time threshold, (**b**) 8-min travel time threshold, (**c**) accessibility sensitivity density heatmap with a 10-min travel time threshold, (**d**) accessibility sensitivity density heatmap with an 8-min travel time threshold.

The statistical results presented normal distribution patterns, with mean accessibility sensitivity around 40% and 50% for 10-min and 8-min travel time thresholds, respectively. This finding suggests that during peak times, the area coverage of the majority of PHEMFs shrank by about 50%. Additionally, the sensitivity to traffic decreased as travel time increased.

PHEMFs with accessibility sensitivity larger than 70% were identified as highly accessibility-sensitive facilities. There were 11 and 19 high accessibility-sensitive PHEMFs with a 10-min and 8-min threshold, respectively, mainly located in Chaoyang District, including the boundary region with Dongcheng District, the area between the East Third Ring Road and the Fourth Ring Road, and the northeast area between the Fourth and Fifth Ring Roads, as shown in Figure 6c,d. Furthermore, a hotspot appeared in Haidian District, located at the traffic hub between the Third and Fourth Ring Roads.

4.4. Equity Assessment Results

From the demand perspective, patients who can reach more PHEMFs within a certain time threshold have a higher chance of receiving critical medical care during emergencies. The available emergency services of each PHEMF can be represented as the available number of ambulances, the number of emergency personnel, the number of medical equipment, and so on. Each PHEMF is built and equipped according to a grade-based standard, with the fixed ambulance space representing the maximum service capacity. There are four grades of PHEMFs in Beijing: the EMC and ECSs are equipped with 30 fixed ambulance spaces, the Grade-A ESs have 6 f, and Grade-B ESs have 3. The available ambulances for each population grid (100 m × 100 m) was calculated using the method described in Section 3.2.4, with results presented in Figure 7.

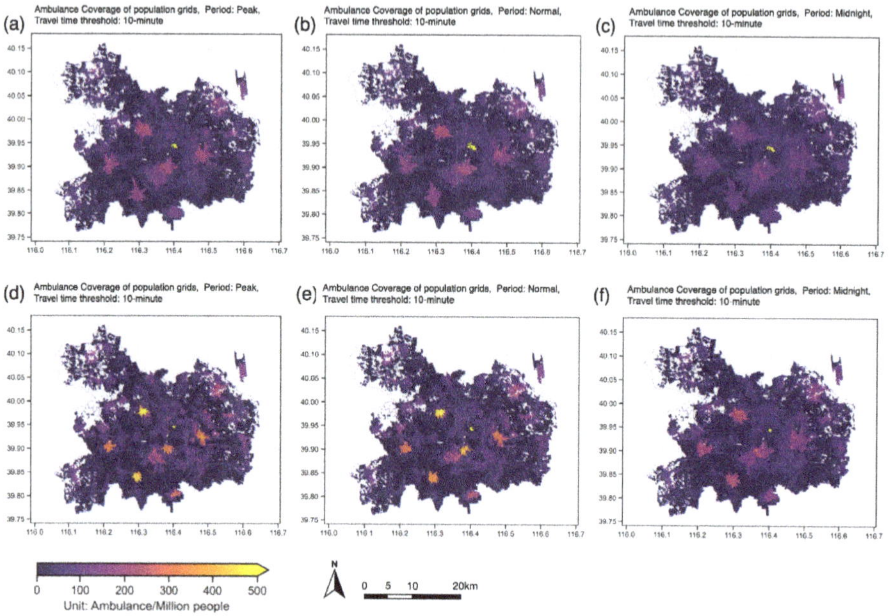

Figure 7. Accessibility of population grids with different travel time thresholds in different periods: (**a**) 10-min isochrones in the peak period, (**b**) 10-min isochrones in the normal period, (**c**) 10-min isochrones in the midnight period, (**d**) 8-min isochrones in the peak period, (**e**) 8-min isochrones in the normal period, (**f**) 8-min isochrones in the midnight period.

As shown in Figure 7, all subgraphs used a uniform color scale for easier comparison. In general, the central area of the study area had more emergency service opportunities than the outer regions. The 8-min travel time threshold showed more disparities in emergency service opportunities compared to the 10-min travel time threshold. In the peak period, as shown in Figure 7a,d, several extremely high-value regions (colored in bright yellow) existed, resulting from the reduction in coverage area during peak times. It was the calculation result of a large number of fixed ambulance spaces (EMC and ECS) but a small isochrone area coverage and small population coverage. For example, DC-001, an EMC with 30 ambulance slots, served only 36,720 population grids during peak hours, resulting in an extreme value of 816.9 ambulances per population grid.

The uneven value distribution, indicating inequality in accessibility, was more noticeable at peak and regular periods. In addition, as shown in Figure 3, there were more isochrone overlaps during the midnight hour; however, there was no obvious rise in the accessibility value of population grids compared to the peak hour. The reason lies in the high population density in the urban area, resulting in a small number of ambulances per population value and, thus, a small increment in the isochrone overlap regions. This phenomenon indicates that PHEMFs with large service area coverage and population coverage do not have an accessibility advantage in the context of resource competition. At the same time, traffic circumstances had a major impact on the service coverage of these facilities, particularly during peak hours. This results in high accessibility in local neighborhoods but an uneven distribution throughout the entire city.

Equal access to emergency services is vital for EMS planning. This analysis result provided evidence for future EMS planning and PHEMF site selection strategies. Therefore, setting more small-scale PHEMFs equipped with fewer ambulance spaces can offer better and more equitable emergency services than fewer large-scale PHEMFs equipped with more ambulances in urban areas.

5. Discussion

As a time-sensitive service, the location of pre-hospital emergency medical facilities (PHEMF) and traffic conditions directly influence service coverage and rescue efficiency. This study evaluated the accessibility of PHEMFs within Beijing's six central districts under the Special Plan by applying isochrone measures. The radial-ray-based approach and open map platform travel data used in this study showed the advantage of reflecting temporal characteristics during peak hours, midnight hours, and normal hours of the day, providing a more reliable analysis of accessibility patterns. The conducted multi-period isochrone analyses examined both the demand and supply aspects of emergency medical services, providing insights and suggestions for future planning.

Regarding the overall isochrone coverage, the coverage area for 10 min of driving was quite high, covering over 80.39% of the region at all times. In contrast, the coverage area for 8 min of driving was rather low, covering just 60.91% of the area during peak hours. This discrepancy highlights the presence of areas with low emergency service accessibility, particularly on the periphery of the study area. To address this, planning additional emergency stations in these underserved areas could improve overall coverage.

Moreover, there was a substantial overlap in isochrone coverage, with dense coverage overlap areas mostly concentrated at the intersection of different administrative districts. This resulted in an oversupply of services in certain areas, increasing operational costs, and leading to inefficient resource allocation. This phenomenon was primarily due to the current planning approach, which is based on administrative divisions. Each administrative district tends to place its facilities near its regional boundaries to meet service coverage rate requirements, resulting in overlapping coverage at these administrative boundaries. Therefore, the urban medical emergency facilities network should be designed holistically, with service coverage calculated from a city-wide perspective. Breaking the restriction of administrative boundaries is more conducive to the effective allocation of resources and efficiency optimization.

Traffic conditions significantly impacted isochrone coverage, with smooth traffic substantially increasing the coverage area. Nonetheless, the traffic in the central urban area of Beijing is relatively congested during non-night hours, with little difference observed between peak and normal periods. Facilities with larger isochrone area coverage were generally located on the periphery of the central urban area and near rapid transit nodes, while facilities in the urban core area tended to have smaller isochrone coverage areas. Therefore, future planning should adopt different strategies for various urban areas. To leverage traffic convenience, future medical emergency stations could be established near traffic hubs in less densely populated regions. In contrast, in densely populated regions, which are mostly located in the central areas of the city, the planning strategy should be adjusted to reduce the scale of a single facility but increase the local facility density and reserve isochrones overlapping. This approach aims to minimize the long service response time caused by traffic congestion.

The accessibility sensitivity to the traffic of each PHEMF was identified by calculating the change rate of the coverage area at midnight and peak periods. The higher the accessibility sensitivity to traffic, the more obvious the reduction in service area during peak hours. The calculation showed that the shorter the travel time, the more the number of facilities is sensitive to traffic. Extending the travel time can not only effectively expand the service coverage of ambulances but also reduce the number of highly traffic-sensitive facilities. Therefore, it is recommended to minimize the medical emergency system's acceptance, information transmission, and departure times to maximize ambulance driving time and broaden the range of services that PHEMFs can provide. Therefore, minimizing system acceptance, information transmission, and departure times is crucial to maximizing ambulance driving time and service range.

One possible planning approach for PHEMFs with high traffic sensitivity involves meeting coverage requirements with numerous small area coverage stations and adding more station sites surrounding the current stations. Additionally, increasing mobile vehicles as temporary emergency stations during peak hours in traffic-sensitive areas can also expedite service response times. There are two types of PHEMFs with low accessibility sensitivity to traffic: one is the facility with a larger isochrone coverage area at all times, and the other is the facility with a smaller isochrone coverage area at all times. For the former, expanding their construction scale can help meet demand within their service areas and support nearby facilities. For the latter, integrating these facilities with nearby ones can reduce operational costs without compromising overall service coverage. Furthermore, newly planned PHEMF sites are better suited to areas with less traffic.

Accessibility and demand competition significantly impact the availability of emergency medical supplies from an equity standpoint. This is especially crucial during disasters like earthquakes or the COVID-19 pandemic, where high demand for EMS poses a barrier to the equitable distribution of medical resources. PHEMFs with large area and population coverage have less competitive advantage but are more susceptible to traffic, which is consistent with the traffic sensitivity analysis results. Thus, increasing the number of small-scale stations in areas with high population density may be advantageous for both population equality and overall coverage rates. Traffic conditions significantly influence planning outcomes, necessitating future strategies to address uncertainties and improve accessibility and efficiency.

6. Conclusions

This study used isochrone measures to evaluate the accessibility of PHEMFs within Beijing's six central districts under the Special Plan. The analysis results revealed several key findings and areas for potential improvement.

The findings indicate that while the 10-min isochrone coverage was high, the 8-min coverage was insufficient, particularly during peak hours, highlighting gaps in service accessibility in the current plan. This disparity underscores the need for additional emergency stations in underserved areas to enhance overall coverage.

The current planning approach resulted in significant isochrone coverage overlap at administrative district intersections, leading to service oversupply and increased costs. Addressing this requires a city-wide planning perspective, breaking administrative boundaries to optimize resource allocation.

Traffic conditions were a critical factor affecting service coverage. Congestion reduced coverage in central areas, while facilities near traffic hubs in less populated regions showed better coverage. Future planning should strategically place emergency stations considering traffic patterns, with more stations near traffic hubs in less dense areas and increased facility density in urban cores to mitigate congestion impacts.

The sensitivity analysis highlights the importance of extending travel times to expand coverage and reduce traffic sensitivity. Minimizing system acceptance, information transmission, and departure times is crucial to maximizing ambulance driving time and service range.

In conclusion, while the current planning approach meets several objectives, challenges remain in service availability and equity. Addressing these issues requires integrated and flexible planning strategies that account for traffic conditions and population distribution. Future research should focus on refining these strategies and exploring innovative solutions to enhance the accessibility and equity of emergency medical services in urban areas.

Author Contributions: Conceptualization, Yuan Zhao; methodology, Yuan Zhao; software, Yuan Zhao; validation, Yuan Zhao; formal analysis, Yuan Zhao; investigation, Yuan Zhao; resources, Yuan Zhao; data curation, Yuan Zhao; writing—original draft preparation, Yuan Zhao; writing—review & editing, Yuan Zhao; visualization, Yuan Zhao; supervision, Ying Zhou; project administration, Ying

Zhou; funding acquisition, Ying Zhou. All authors have read and agreed to the published version of the manuscript.

Funding: This research was supported by the National Natural Science Foundation of China (Grant No. 51978143).

Data Availability Statement: The data of this work can be shared with the readers depending on the request.

Conflicts of Interest: The authors declare no conflicts of interest.

References

1. Tintinalli, J.E.; Cameron, P.; Holliman, J. *EMS: A Practical Global Guidebook*; PMPH-USA: Shelton, CT, USA, 2010; ISBN 1-60795-043-X.
2. Mehmood, A.; Rowther, A.A.; Kobusingye, O.; Hyder, A.A. Assessment of Pre-Hospital Emergency Medical Services in Low-Income Settings Using a Health Systems Approach. *Int. J. Emerg. Med.* **2018**, *11*, 53. [CrossRef] [PubMed]
3. Turner, C.D.; Lockey, D.J.; Rehn, M. Pre-Hospital Management of Mass Casualty Civilian Shootings: A Systematic Literature Review. *Crit. Care* **2016**, *20*, 362. [CrossRef]
4. Waseem, H.; Naseer, R.; Razzak, J.A. Establishing a Successful Pre-Hospital Emergency Service in a Developing Country: Experience from Rescue 1122 Service in Pakistan. *Emerg. Med. J.* **2011**, *28*, 513–515. [CrossRef]
5. Gostin, L.O.; Viswanathan, K.; Altevogt, B.M.; Hanfling, D. *Crisis Standards of Care: A Systems Framework for Catastrophic Disaster Response*; National Academies Press: Washington, DC, USA, 2012; Volume 3, ISBN 0-309-25346-2.
6. Cabral, E.L.D.S.; Castro, W.R.S.; Florentino, D.R.M.; Viana, D.A.; Costa Junior, J.F.D.; Souza, R.P.; Rêgo, A.C.M.; Araújo-Filho, I.; Medeiros, A.C. Response Time in the Emergency Services. Systematic Review. *Acta Cir. Bras.* **2018**, *33*, 1110–1121. [CrossRef] [PubMed]
7. Cai, M.; Liu, E.; Tao, H.; Qian, Z.; Lin, X.; Cheng, Z. Does Level of Hospital Matter? A Study of Mortality of Acute Myocardial Infarction Patients in Shanxi, China. *Am. J. Med. Qual.* **2018**, *33*, 185–192. [CrossRef]
8. Swan, D.; Baumstark, L. Does Every Minute Really Count? Road Time as an Indicator for the Economic Value of Emergency Medical Services. *Value Health* **2022**, *25*, 400–408. [CrossRef]
9. Pons, P.T.; Markovchick, V.J. Eight Minutes or Less: Does the Ambulance Response Time Guideline Impact Trauma Patient Outcome? *J. Emerg. Med.* **2002**, *23*, 43–48. [CrossRef]
10. Rhodes, H.; Rourke, B.; Pepe, A. Ambulance Response in Eight Minutes or Less: Are Comorbidities a Factor. *Am. Surg.* **2023**, *89*, 3478–3481. [CrossRef]
11. Jin, Y.; Chen, H.; Ge, H.; Li, S.; Zhang, J.; Ma, Q. Urban–Suburb Disparities in Pre-Hospital Emergency Medical Resources and Response Time among Patients with out-of-Hospital Cardiac Arrest: A Mixed-Method Cross-Sectional Study. *Front. Public Health* **2023**, *11*, 1121779. [CrossRef]
12. Mell, H.K.; Mumma, S.N.; Hiestand, B.; Carr, B.G.; Holland, T.; Stopyra, J. Emergency Medical Services Response Times in Rural, Suburban, and Urban Areas. *JAMA Surg.* **2017**, *152*, 983–984. [CrossRef]
13. Texas Department of State Health Services, Texas Health Data. Emergency Medical Service (EMS) 911 Run Times. Available online: https://healthdata.dshs.texas.gov/dashboard/injuries/ems-911-run-times (accessed on 10 January 2024).
14. NHS England Ambulance Quality Indicators Data 2023–2024. Available online: https://www.england.nhs.uk/statistics/statistical-work-areas/ambulance-quality-indicators/ambulance-quality-indicators-data-2023-24/ (accessed on 10 January 2024).
15. Central People's Government of the People's Republic of China Guiding Opinions on Further Improving Pre-Hospital Medical Emergency Services 2020. Available online: https://www.gov.cn/gongbao/content/2021/content_5581081.htm (accessed on 10 January 2024).
16. Beijing Municipal Health Commission Special Plan for Spatial Layout of Pre-Hospital Medical Emergency Facilities in Beijing (2020–2022). 2020. Available online: https://wjw.beijing.gov.cn/zwgk_20040/wsyj/202007/t20200728_1963964.html (accessed on 10 January 2024).
17. Páez, A.; Scott, D.M.; Morency, C. Measuring Accessibility: Positive and Normative Implementations of Various Accessibility Indicators. *J. Transp. Geogr.* **2012**, *25*, 141–153. [CrossRef]
18. Neutens, T. Accessibility, Equity and Health Care: Review and Research Directions for Transport Geographers. *J. Transp. Geogr.* **2015**, *43*, 14–27. [CrossRef]
19. Sharma, G.; Patil, G.R. Public Transit Accessibility Approach to Understand the Equity for Public Healthcare Services: A Case Study of Greater Mumbai. *J. Transp. Geogr.* **2021**, *94*, 103123. [CrossRef]
20. Kelobonye, K.; Zhou, H.; McCarney, G.; Xia, J.C. Measuring the Accessibility and Spatial Equity of Urban Services under Competition Using the Cumulative Opportunities Measure. *J. Transp. Geogr.* **2020**, *85*, 102706. [CrossRef]
21. Guagliardo, M.F. Spatial Accessibility of Primary Care: Concepts, Methods and Challenges. *Int. J. Health Geogr.* **2004**, *3*, 3. [CrossRef]
22. Wang, F. Measurement, Optimization, and Impact of Health Care Accessibility: A Methodological Review. *Ann. Assoc. Am. Geogr.* **2012**, *102*, 1104–1112. [CrossRef]

23. Xiao, W.; Wei, Y.D.; Wan, N. Modeling Job Accessibility Using Online Map Data: An Extended Two-Step Floating Catchment Area Method with Multiple Travel Modes. *J. Transp. Geogr.* **2021**, *93*, 103065. [CrossRef]
24. Pan, Q.; Jin, Z.; Liu, X. Measuring the Effects of Job Competition and Matching on Employment Accessibility. *Transp. Res. Part Transp. Environ.* **2020**, *87*, 102535. [CrossRef]
25. Cheng, J.; Bertolini, L. Measuring Urban Job Accessibility with Distance Decay, Competition and Diversity. *J. Transp. Geogr.* **2013**, *30*, 100–109. [CrossRef]
26. Park, K. Psychological Park Accessibility: A Systematic Literature Review of Perceptual Components Affecting Park Use. *Landsc. Res.* **2017**, *42*, 508–520. [CrossRef]
27. Rigolon, A. A Complex Landscape of Inequity in Access to Urban Parks: A Literature Review. *Landsc. Urban Plan.* **2016**, *153*, 160–169. [CrossRef]
28. Järv, O.; Tenkanen, H.; Salonen, M.; Ahas, R.; Toivonen, T. Dynamic Cities: Location-Based Accessibility Modelling as a Function of Time. *Appl. Geogr.* **2018**, *95*, 101–110. [CrossRef]
29. Smith, D.M.; Cummins, S.; Taylor, M.; Dawson, J.; Marshall, D.; Sparks, L.; Anderson, A.S. Neighbourhood Food Environ-ment and Area Deprivation: Spatial Accessibility to Grocery Stores Selling Fresh Fruit and Vegetables in Urban and Rural Settings. *Int. J. Epidemiol.* **2010**, *39*, 277–284. [CrossRef]
30. Kelobonye, K.; McCarney, G.; Xia, J.C.; Swapan, M.S.H.; Mao, F.; Zhou, H. Relative Accessibility Analysis for Key Land Uses: A Spatial Equity Perspective. *J. Transp. Geogr.* **2019**, *75*, 82–93. [CrossRef]
31. Batty, M. Accessibility: In Search of a Unified Theory. *Environ. Plan. B Plan. Des.* **2009**, *36*, 191–194. [CrossRef]
32. Zhao, P.; Li, S.; Liu, D. Unequable Spatial Accessibility to Hospitals in Developing Megacities: New Evidence from Beijing. *Health Place* **2020**, *65*, 102406. [CrossRef]
33. Liu, L.; Kar, A.; Tokey, A.I.; Le, H.T.; Miller, H.J. Disparities in Public Transit Accessibility and Usage by People with Mobil-ity Disabilities: An Evaluation Using High-Resolution Transit Data. *J. Transp. Geogr.* **2023**, *109*, 103589. [CrossRef]
34. Li, C.; Wang, J. A Hierarchical Two-Step Floating Catchment Area Analysis for High-Tier Hospital Accessibility in an Urban Agglomeration Region. *J. Transp. Geogr.* **2022**, *102*, 103369. [CrossRef]
35. McGrail, M.R.; Humphreys, J.S. Measuring Spatial Accessibility to Primary Health Care Services: Utilising Dynamic Catch-ment Sizes. *Appl. Geogr.* **2014**, *54*, 182–188. [CrossRef]
36. Mayaud, J.R.; Tran, M.; Nuttall, R. An Urban Data Framework for Assessing Equity in Cities: Comparing Accessibility to Healthcare Facilities in Cascadia. *Comput. Environ. Urban Syst.* **2019**, *78*, 101401. [CrossRef]
37. Wang, J.; Du, F.; Huang, J.; Liu, Y. Access to Hospitals: Potential vs. Observed. *Cities* **2020**, *100*, 102671. [CrossRef]
38. Xia, T.; Song, X.; Zhang, H.; Song, X.; Kanasugi, H.; Shibasaki, R. Measuring Spatio-Temporal Accessibility to Emergency Medical Services through Big GPS Data. *Health Place* **2019**, *56*, 53–62. [CrossRef]
39. Shang, Q.; Guo, X.; Li, J.; Wang, T. Post-Earthquake Health Care Service Accessibility Assessment Framework and Its Appli-cation in a Medium-Sized City. *Reliab. Eng. Syst. Saf.* **2022**, *228*, 108782. [CrossRef]
40. Mapbox Isochrone API | API Docs | Mapbox. Available online: https://docs.mapbox.com/api/navigation/isochrone/ (accessed on 10 January 2024).
41. ISO4APP API Isochrones Map (Travel Time Map). Available online: https://www.iso4app.net/ (accessed on 10 January 2024).
42. TravelTime Isochrones Map. Available online: https://traveltime.com/apis/isochrones (accessed on 10 January 2024).
43. Hu, S.; Song, W.; Li, C.; Lu, J. A Multi-Mode Gaussian-Based Two-Step Floating Catchment Area Method for Measuring Ac-cessibility of Urban Parks. *Cities* **2020**, *105*, 102815. [CrossRef]
44. Bunel, M.; Tovar, E. Key Issues in Local Job Accessibility Measurement: Different Models Mean Different Results. *Urban Stud.* **2014**, *51*, 1322–1338. [CrossRef]
45. Geurs, K.T.; Van Wee, B. Accessibility Evaluation of Land-Use and Transport Strategies: Review and Research Directions. *J. Transp. Geogr.* **2004**, *12*, 127–140. [CrossRef]
46. Merlin, L.A.; Hu, L. Does Competition Matter in Measures of Job Accessibility? Explaining Employment in Los Angeles. *J. Transp. Geogr.* **2017**, *64*, 77–88. [CrossRef]
47. The People's Government of Beijing Municipality Overview of Beijing. Available online: https://www.beijing.gov.cn/renwen/bjgk/ (accessed on 10 January 2024).
48. WorldPop WorldPop. Available online: https://hub.worldpop.org/ (accessed on 10 January 2024).
49. Bondarenko, M.; Kerr, D.; Sorichetta, A.; Tatem, A. Census/Projection-Disaggregated Gridded Population Datasets, Adjusted to Match the Corresponding UNPD 2020 Estimates, for 51 Countries across Sub-Saharan Africa Using Building Footprints. University of Southampton: Southampton, UK, 2020. [CrossRef]
50. WorldPop Top-Down Estimation Modelling: Constrained vs. Unconstrained. Available online: https://www.worldpop.org/methods/top_down_constrained_vs_unconstrained/ (accessed on 10 January 2024).
51. Esri An Overview of the Network Analyst Toolbox. Available online: https://pro.arcgis.com/en/pro-app/latest/tool-reference/network-analyst/an-overview-of-the-network-analyst-toolbox.htm (accessed on 10 January 2024).
52. Xi, Y.; Miller, E.J.; Saxe, S. Exploring the Impact of Different Cut-off Times on Isochrone Measurements of Accessibility. *Transp. Res. Rec.* **2018**, *2672*, 113–124. [CrossRef]
53. Esri Service Area Analysis. Esri an Overview of the Network Analyst Toolbox. Available online: https://desktop.arcgis.com/en/arcmap/latest/extensions/network-analyst/service-area.htm (accessed on 10 January 2024).

54. TravelTime TravelTime ArcGIS Plugin. Esri an Overview of the Network Analyst Toolbox. Available online: https://docs.traveltime.com/arcgis/about/overview (accessed on 10 January 2024).
55. Wang, F.; Xu, Y. Estimating O–D Travel Time Matrix by Google Maps API: Implementation, Advantages, and Implications. *Ann. GIS* **2011**, *17*, 199–209. [CrossRef]
56. Amap Amap Web API. Available online: https://lbs.amap.com/api/webservice/summary (accessed on 10 January 2024).
57. Zhang, J.; Wang, L.; Li, H.; Zhao, Y. Response Time of the Beijing 120 Emergency Medical Service. *Emerg. Med. J.* **2010**, *27*, 784–785. [CrossRef]
58. Huang, W.; Wang, T.-B.; He, Y.-D.; Zhang, H.; Zhou, X.-H.; Liu, H.; Zhang, J.-J.; Tian, Z.-B.; Jiang, B.-G. Trends and Character-istics in Pre-Hospital Emergency Care in Beijing from 2008 to 2017. *Chin. Med. J.* **2020**, *133*, 1268–1275. [CrossRef] [PubMed]
59. Beijing Emergency Medical Center the Transformation of Pre-Hospital Emergency Care in the Capital in Ten Years: 120 Vehicles Increased by More Than 130%. Available online: https://www.beijing120.com/content/9393?channelId=200 (accessed on 27 July 2024).
60. The Standing Committee of Beijing Municipal People's Congress Research on the Status Quo, Problems and Countermeasures of Pre-Hospital Medical Emergency Services in Beijing. Available online: http://www.bjrd.gov.cn/rdzl/rdcwhgb/ssljrdcwhgb202305/202312/t20231212_3498429.html (accessed on 27 July 2024).
61. Beijing Municipal Health Commission 2023 Beijing Health and Medical Statistics Report. Available online: https://wjw.beijing.gov.cn/sjfb/bjstjgb/bjstjgb2023/ (accessed on 27 July 2024).

isprs International Journal of *Geo-Information*

MDPI

Article

City Transmission Networks: Unraveling Disease Spread Dynamics

Hend Alrasheed [1,*], Norah Alballa [2], Isra Al-Turaiki [2], Fahad Almutlaq [3] and Reham Alabduljabbar [1]

1 Department of Information Technology, College of Computer and Information Sciences, King Saud University, Riyadh 11421, Saudi Arabia; rabduljabbar@ksu.edu.sa
2 Department of Computer Science, College of Computer and Information Sciences, King Saud University, Riyadh 11421, Saudi Arabia; nalballa@ksu.edu.sa (N.A.); ialturaiki@ksu.edu.sa (I.A.-T.)
3 Department of Geography, College of Humanities and Social Sciences, King Saud University, Riyadh 11451, Saudi Arabia; falmutlaq@ksu.edu.sa
* Correspondence: halrasheed@ksu.edu.sa

Abstract: In the midst of global efforts to curb the spread of infectious diseases, researchers worldwide are striving to unravel the intricate spatial and temporal patterns of disease transmission dynamics. Mathematical models are indispensable tools for understanding the dissemination of emerging pathogens and elucidating the evolution of epidemics. This paper introduces a novel approach by investigating city transmission networks as a framework for analyzing disease spread. In this network, major cities are depicted as nodes interconnected by edges representing disease transmission pathways. Subsequent network analysis employs various epidemiological and structural metrics to delineate the distinct roles played by cities in disease transmission. The primary objective is to identify superspreader cities. Illustratively, we apply this methodology to study COVID-19 transmission in Saudi Arabian cities, shedding light on the specific dynamics within this context. These insights offer valuable guidance for decision-making processes and the formulation of effective intervention strategies, carrying significant implications for managing public health crises.

Keywords: transmission network; epidemiological measures; structural measures; superspreader cities; COVID-19; GIS

1. Introduction

The transmission dynamics of infectious diseases are multifaceted, influenced by myriad factors such as demographic characteristics, population movements, host behaviors and immune responses, healthcare infrastructure, and environmental conditions [1,2]. Recent studies underscore that a minority of infected individuals, often termed superspreaders, can drive the majority of disease cases in an outbreak [3]. Furthermore, studies suggest that imported cases play a substantial role in seeding local transmission in various epidemic contexts, often accounting for a considerable proportion of total infections in many countries [4,5]. Interestingly, some cities exhibit characteristics that significantly influence the spread of diseases, similar to the role of individual superspreaders in an outbreak, prompting the adoption of the concept of superspreader cities[6]. Effective control strategies necessitate comprehensive measures, including both *within city* lockdowns and *between city* movement restrictions, to mitigate disease transmission rates [7].

Mathematically modeling disease transmission is a crucial step toward effective disease management, enabling better resource allocation in healthcare, the evaluation of control measures' effectiveness, and the prediction of transmission patterns. Epidemic modeling provides a potent tool for predicting the trajectory of an outbreak and devising strategies to contain it. Such models prove particularly useful in scenarios where data on mobility and travel are limited or inaccurate. Various mathematical modeling approaches have been employed in epidemiological contexts, including statistical models [8], mathematical formulations [9–11], and network-based analyses [12–14]. These models contribute significantly to our understanding of disease dynamics and aid in developing evidence-based interventions for public health. However, most traditional epidemic models focus on the temporal aspect of the disease and are non-spatial [15]. While there are some studies that have successfully modeled disease spread within cities and among individuals [16–22], there remains a considerable gap in understanding and modeling between-city and cross-regional disease transmission.

In this study, we explore between-city transmission patterns utilizing a spatiotemporal network-based epidemic model. Spatiotemporal network-based epidemic models have been widely recognized and utilized in the field of epidemiology to study disease transmission dynamics, particularly in the context of infectious diseases. While there are various modeling approaches available, we choose the spatiotemporal network-based model due to its ability to capture both spatial and temporal dimensions of disease transmission patterns. It allows us to assess the role of different cities in the spread of a disease and identify potential superspreaders (cities with the highest potential to disseminate the disease). This highlights the critical importance of managing these influential nodes in disease control efforts [23,24].

Initially, we establish a city transmission network where nodes represent distinct cities and edges signify disease transmission from one city to another. Subsequently, the network is partitioned into multiple epidemic trees, each originating from a city with initial cases. These trees are then subjected to analysis using various epidemiological and structural metrics, offering quantitative insights for comparing the distinct roles cities play in disease propagation. Epidemiological measures delineate the spread of the epidemic among cities, while structural metrics scrutinize the static interconnectivity between them. Our approach emphasizes city connectivity over population size when studying disease propagation, recognizing that population size alone has limitations as a reliable predictor of disease spread [25].

We apply our framework to examine the case of COVID-19 in Saudi Arabia, leveraging authentic epidemiological data [26]. Our findings reveal that the impact of city infections is not confined to local boundaries but can extend across regional borders, affecting neighboring areas. Furthermore, we assert that the identification of superspreader cities holds greater significance than pinpointing infection sources. These results serve as valuable guidance for policymakers in setting priorities and refining quarantine strategies.

The rest of this work is organized as follows: Section 2 presents some preliminary concepts and definitions, and Section 3 presents the related work. Section 4 discusses the method, including network construction and analysis. Section 5 presents an illustrative example. Lastly, Section 6 concludes this paper.

2. Preliminaries

A crucial role in disease transmission is played by node accessibility (the local environment of the node) and reachability (the global environment of the node) within network structures [27–29]. Several network structures have been used to model disease propagation including social networks, contact networks, and disease transmission networks. In this work, we use the epidemic tree [15,30,31] structure to track disease transmission.

In graph theory, an *epidemic tree* $T_c = (V, E)$ rooted at node $c \in V$, where V is the set of nodes (infection cases) and E is the set of edges, is a directed rooted tree that allows understanding disease spread by its hidden structural properties [32]. The root of the tree c represents a primary case in the infection process.

Each tree edge represents a parent–child relationship in the disease spread process, where the parent node infects the child node. The creation of edges follows the chronological order of the infection of each pair of nodes such that a parent node is infected before its children nodes. The infection process from a parent node to a child node can be *deterministic* using node attributes such as the spatial distance to an infected parent node, or *stochastic* using probability [15,33–35].

An *epidemic forest* is a collection of epidemic trees which accrues when there are multiple primary cases. This representation assists the extraction of epidemic information at different spatial and temporal scales. It can also be used to reveal disease–environmental associations and guide disease control interventions.

The *neighborhood* of a node $u \in V$, denoted by $N(u)$, is the set of neighbors of u, i.e., $N(u) = v|u,v \in E$. The *degree* of node u is the size of its neighborhood ($d(u) = |N(u)|$). Node degrees have been shown to have a great impact on disease propagation [36,37].

A *path* in the tree connecting a pair of nodes u and v is a sequence of adjacent nodes that starts at u and ends with v. The *length* of a given path is the number of edges on the path. The *diameter* of a tree T_c, denoted by $diam\ (T_c)$, is the number of nodes on a longest path between any two nodes in the tree. The tree diameter and average path length provide indications about the possibility of infection throughout the epidemic tree. For instance, the shorter the average path length between nodes, the higher the possibility of infection [28].

A *Breadth First Search* (BFS) starting at a given node u traverses the entire tree, level by level, by increasing distances from node u. That is, it starts traversing all nodes one hop away from u (u's neighbors). Then, it visits all nodes at two hops away from u, and so on. This systematic exploration helps in visualizing the spread and reach of potential infections across the network.

Node centrality measures rank nodes with respect to their importance by assigning a numerical value to each node according to its location in the network, which influences the overall dynamics of the network interactions. *Degree centrality* considers the central nodes to be those with the highest number of connections, highlighting potential hubs of activity or transmission. *Closeness centrality* identifies the center of the network as the subset of nodes with the shortest average distance to all other nodes, thereby highlighting those that can most efficiently spread or gather information, or, in the context of epidemics, transmit infections. In tree-structured networks, closeness centrality offers profound insights; the center, often referred to as the median and typically consisting of one or two nodes, is deemed the pivotal point of the network. This designation underscores its importance in strategic interventions and control measures. The application of closeness centrality is crucial for identifying key nodes, which are prioritized for thorough analysis and targeted in preventive strategies within epidemiological studies. This approach ensures that efforts are concentrated where they can be most effective in mitigating the spread of disease.

3. Related Work

Understanding how infections spread is crucial for controlling disease transmission. Epidemiology can greatly benefit from studying contact networks, as they provide valuable insights into disease propagation between individuals [12–14].

Recent studies have focused on utilizing advanced tools and methodologies to analyze city transmission networks and uncover hidden patterns of disease spread within cities. For instance, the study by John [38] investigated the impact of high connectivity and human movement on infectious disease transmission within city networks. The results indicated that travel time was the most crucial factor influencing disease transmission, followed by human movement. The study by Guo et al. [39] focused on a dynamic model of respiratory disease transmission by population mobility based on city networks, highlighting the importance of considering population mobility and disease transmission dynamics in urban settings. Leung et al. [40] conducted a systematic review on simulating contact networks for livestock disease epidemiology. The research altered the resulting network by randomly rewiring edges connecting node types that were not connected in the empirical network while preserving the clustering coefficient and mean degree of the Barabasi–Albert model simulation. This approach aimed to enhance the understanding of livestock disease transmission dynamics.

Luo et al. [29] studied COVID-19 transmission in the Chinese cities of Tianjin and Chengdu using visualization techniques, finding that transmission characteristics varied among cities. Büttner and Krieter [41] demonstrated various disease transmission routes within animal trade networks, emphasizing the integration of different transmission pathways into simulation models. Xie et al. [42] investigated the impact of asymmetric activity on interactions between networks, highlighting the role of network structures. In a related study, Hearst et al. [43] identified potential superspreaders and disease transmission hotspots using white-tailed deer scraping networks. Krbylvik et al. [19] conducted network analysis of the detained and staff member movements in the Cook County Jail in Chicago, Illinois. The study, based on the movement of 5884 persons from 1 March to 30 April 2020, identified fewer COVID-19 links than expected among detained persons, implying that interventions and medical isolation policies were effective. In the networks of staff members, there were more links than predicted, indicating possible areas of concentration for further transmission.

Recent studies have also focused on the spatiotemporal dynamics of disease transmission. For instance, Shaw et al. [44] focused on modeling contacts and the spread of COVID-19 in the context of the return to work, demonstrating that limiting social contact through strategies such as reducing the number of people or time spent in the workplace are effective measures. Silva et al. [45] quantitatively analyzed the effectiveness of public health measures on COVID-19 transmission, emphasizing the importance of social isolation policies. Gayawan et al. [46] looked at the spatiotemporal dynamics of COVID-19 in 47 African countries. The study focused on the first 62 days of the disease's appearance in Africa, revealing that neighboring countries pose a major importation risk to each other. Chan and Wen [47] examined the impact of changes in intercity passenger rail travel on COVID-19 early spatial transmission in mainland China, investigating the association between structural changes in the railway origin-destination network and the prevalence of COVID-19 cases using Bayesian multivariate regression. Dlamini et al. [48] integrated various variables to spatially model COVID-19 transmission risk in Eswatini, analyzing case data for the period under strict lockdown. Pribadi et al. [49] studied the policy of Large-Scale Social Restriction (LSSR) in Jakarta, Indonesia, using hotspot analysis and space–time scan statistics to examine infection and transmission risk. The results suggest that spatial transmission continues despite a decrease in the overall pandemic curve during LSSR adoption.

In the context of Saudi Arabia, which serves as the case study for this work, the majority of COVID-19 research primarily focuses on statistical and mathematical models [50–56]. However, there is an opportunity to explore network-based approaches to better understand city-to-city disease transmission. While existing studies have utilized network-based SIR models [13], they often overlook the spatiotemporal aspect of the infection. Consequently, in this work, we propose a spatiotemporal network-based model to shed light on the dynamics of city-to-city disease transmission in Saudi Arabia.

4. Methods

We investigate between-city disease transmission patterns by analyzing city transmission networks. To achieve this goal, we initially build a city transmission network using data on infection and disease importation history. Subsequently, we conduct a quantitative analysis of the network's global, epidemiological, and structural characteristics.

4.1. Transmission Network Construction

To understand the dynamics of disease transmission across cities, we establish a city transmission network characterized by three fundamental components: central nodes denoting cities with initial imported cases (patient zero), nodes representing the remaining cities, and edges indicating the direction of transmission from one city to another. All central nodes are considered infected because they host at least one individual who contracted the disease while traveling. The remaining cities become infected when a person in that city is confirmed to have the disease. Each of these cities is linked to another city from which they contract the disease and to another city to which they transmit the infection. The resulting city transmission network is denoted by $G = (V, C, E)$ where V is the set of nodes, $C \subset V$ is the set of central nodes, and E indicates the set of edges.

This construction results in a network with a tree-like structure. Each node is attributed with an infection date. The ensemble of epidemic trees rooted at each central node constitutes an epidemic forest. The resulting network is undirected; however, we use directed edges to emphasize the chronological flow of disease transmission. See Figure 1 for an example of a transmission network.

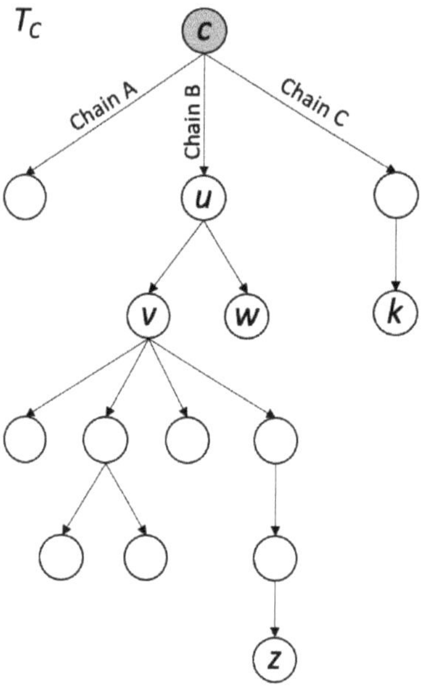

Epidemiological propoerties

Measure	Value		
Total Number of Chains	3		
Average Chain Size	4.7		
	Chain		
	A	B	C
Chain Size	1	11	2
Maximum Length of Chain	0	4	1
Chain Diameter	0	5	1

Structural propoerties

Measure	Value
Size	14
Diameter	7
Height	5
Median	Nodes *u* and *v*
Degree Center	Node *u*

Figure 1. An example of a transmission network. Tables list the epidemiological and structural properties of the epidemic tree rooted at node c with three transmission chains.

4.2. Transmission Network Analysis

Our goal is to use the topological properties of the transmission network to understand the role of cities and their connectivity in the disease propagation patterns. To do so, we analyze the developed network global properties such as node degree distribution and pair of node distances. Then, we analyze the epidemic tree rooted at each central node using two sets of measures: epidemiological and structural. Epidemiological measures are used to assess the evolving epidemiology of a disease. These metrics are crucial for understanding how infections propagate between nodes within the network, highlighting key transmission paths and the overall reach of the disease. Structural measures focus on the overall topology and connectivity of the epidemic network. These metrics are important for understanding the static properties of the network that might impact disease propagation. They provide insights into the network's connectivity and the hierarchical organization of infected nodes. Figure 1 shows an example of all properties.

In an epidemic tree, the root (source node) represents a source of infection. A transmission chain shows generations of infected nodes generated as a result of direct or indirect contact with the source node. Let T_c be the epidemic tree rooted at central node c, and $T_c = \{V, E\}$ be the set of epidemiological measures which include the following.

- **Total Number of Chains:** The Total Number of Chains indicates the number of chains starting at a central node [29]. The Total Number of Chains of a given central node c equals the number of node c's direct neighbors. It can be used to rank central nodes according to their role in direct disease spread. For example, in Figure 1, the Total Number of Chains of the shown epidemic tree is 3. This metric indicates the number of direct transmission paths originating from a central node, reflecting the node's direct impact on disease spread.
- **Chain Size:** The Chain Size indicates the number of nodes in each transmission chain excluding the central node [29]. The Chain Size of a given node v, where $v \in N(c)$ and c is a central node, equals the number of nodes in the Breadth First Search (BFS) tree rooted at v. It can be used to measure the influence of non-central nodes in spreading the disease. For example, the Chain Size of Chain B in Figure 1 is 11 since node u spreads the disease to 10 other nodes.
- **Maximum Length of Chains:** The Maximum Length of Chains shows the maximum number of directional edges in each chain [29]. The Maximum Length of Chains of a node v, where $v \in N(c)$ and c is a central node is equal to the height of the Breadth First Search (BFS) tree rooted at v. This metric captures the furthest extent a disease can travel within a chain. The Maximum Length of Chains of Chain B in Figure 1 is 4, showing the number of generations the disease traveled.
- **Average Chain Size:** The Average Chain Size represents the average number of cases resulting from an infection started at given central node [29]. It is computed by dividing the summation of Chain Sizes starting with same central node by the number of chains starting at a central node, providing an average measure of transmission spread. For example, the Average Chain Size of the epidemic tree in Figure 1 is 4.7 $((1 + 11 + 2)/3)$.
- **Chain Diameter:** The Chain Diameter measures the longest distance between any two nodes in a chain (excluding the central node), indicating the maximal spread within a chain. It can be obtained by computing the diameter of the undirected BFS tree rooted at node v, where $v \in N(c)$ and c is a central node. In Figure 1, the diameter of Chain B is five since the maximum distance connecting two nodes is five (path between nodes w and z).

The set of structural measures compares the hierarchical structures of each epidemic tree rooted at a central node. This set of measures includes:

- **Size:** The size of T_c indicates the total number of nodes that are infected as a result of a direct or indirect relationship with c, reflecting the infection's reach. It is computed as $|T_c| - 1$. The size measure provides a quantification of the infection ability of each central node. The size of the epidemic tree T_c in Figure 1 is 14.
- **Diameter:** The diameter of T_u represents the maximum path length between any two nodes in T_u. It is computed as $\max_{w,z \in V}\{d(w,z)\}$. The Diameter provides an estimation of the disease transmission distances. Note that the diameter does not take edge directions into account. In Figure 1, the diameter of T_c equals $d(k,z)$, which is seven.
- **Height:** The height of T_c shows the maximum number of directional edges in a path connecting c to a leaf node. It is computed as $\max_{v \in V}\{d(c,v)\}$. This measure is similar to the Maximum Length of Chains, except that it selects the maximum over all chains. In Figure 1, the height of the epidemic tree is five since $d(c,z) = 5$.
- **Median:** The median of T_c represents the vertex (or two connected vertices) closest to every other vertex in T_c (edge directions are not considered). It identifies disease spreader nodes with respect to node closeness to other nodes in the tree. The two nodes that represent the median of the epidemic tree in Figure 1 are nodes u and v.
- **Degree Center:** The Degree Center decides which node (or nodes) are most central with respect to their number of connections in an epidemic tree. It identifies disease spreader nodes with respect to node degrees. The central node according to degree in Figure 1 is node u.

- **Temporal Information:** A given epidemic tree can be temporally characterized by starting and ending dates [29]. The starting date of an epidemic tree T_c is equal to the infection date of its root node c, and its ending date is the last date on which a leaf node $v \in V$ was infected. The two dates define the disease spreading period [15].
- **Spatial Information:** A given epidemic tree can be spatially characterized by its geographic coverage [29], which describes the geographic area coverage by the tree [15].

5. Illustrative Example

We study the role and impact of city connectivity on COVID-19 disease spread in Saudi Arabia to demonstrate the proposed method.

5.1. Data

We utilize a COVID-19 dataset. The dataset is procured from the Saudi Ministry of Health [26], covering the period from 2 March 2020, to 25 April 2020, and consisting of 198,018 records. Each record within the dataset contains personal details, including age, gender, race, and city of residence. Additionally, the dataset encompasses information related to COVID-19 testing, such as the date of the test, the hospital where it was conducted, the test outcome, and the date the results were received. It also includes travel history, specifically noting whether individuals had visited any countries where the virus was endemic.

Two main data cleaning steps are applied to the dataset. First, we exclude any records that indicated a negative or not confirmed COVID-19 outcome, ensuring that our dataset focuses exclusively on confirmed cases. Second, records of individuals who tested positive for COVID-19 but had no travel history are excluded. This step ensures that the analysis concentrates on cities with initial imported cases. After applying these cleaning steps, the dataset is reduced to 1366 records.

After that, information from the individual records is extracted to build the COVID-19 city infection history file which includes the following sections (see Table A1 in Appendix A): city name, city region, date of first reported case (confirmation as a positive case), and date of first imported tested case (taking the swap). We include 119 main cities in Saudi Arabia. Not all cities appear in the obtained file. The reported dates for those cities are obtained from the daily dates provided by the online COVID-19 Dashboard: Saudi Arabia [57]. Table A1 shows that the date of the first imported tested case is much earlier compared to the date of the first reported case in 27 cities such as Arriad, Addammam, and Abha. This indicates that positive imported COVID-19 cases are actively spreading the disease for a period of time. This set of cities is considered to have a central role in disease transmission. The generated COVID-19 city infection history file and the constructed transmission network dataset are all available at https://github.com/halrashe/Covid19-Transmission-Network (accessed on 1 August 2024).

We assume that the potential infectious range of a city to cover the entire country since Saudi Arabia has well-developed road networks and transportation systems, and thus travel between any two cities is possible.

Our city transmission network, denoted by $G = (V, C, E)$ where V is the set of nodes, $C \subset V$ is the set of central nodes, and E is the set of edges, has a total of 119 nodes, 20 central nodes, and 118 edges (see Figure 2). The first positive COVID-19 case in Saudi Arabia was confirmed on 2 March 2020 in the city of Alqatif. Therefore, Alqatif city is selected to be the first infected node in the network. The remaining cities are added based on their first reported date (breaking ties arbitrarily). Let $I \subseteq V$ be a set of infected nodes, $S \subseteq V$ be a set of susceptible nodes, and $w \in I$ and $z \in S$ be two nodes (cities). A directed edge e_{wz} connects node w to node z if w is the closest in distance to node z than every other node $v \in I$. Because we focus on between-city analysis, nodes with an imported tested case after the date of 21 March 2020 (the date when all domestic transportation was suspended) are not considered central.

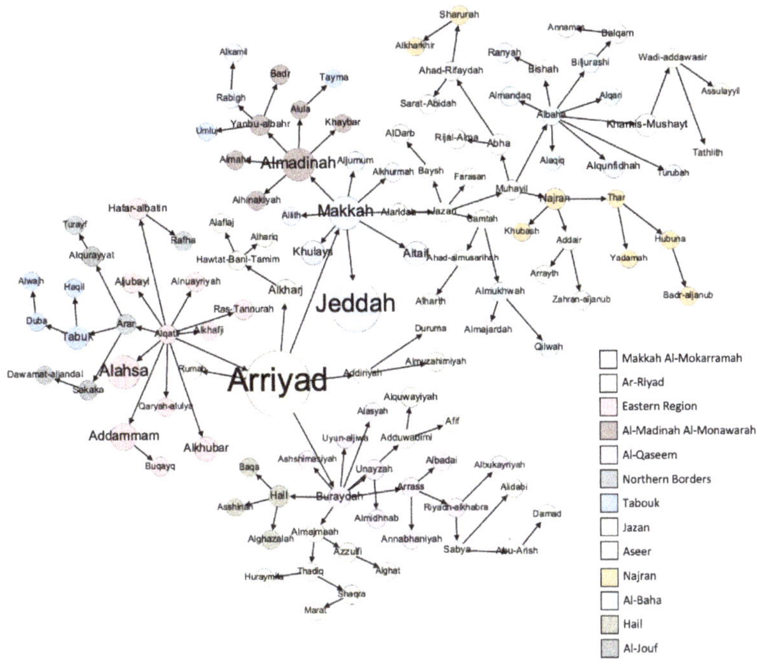

Figure 2. COVID-19 city transmission network between in Saudi Arabia. Nodes are partitioned according to their administrative regions. Node sizes are proportional to their populations.

5.2. Experimental Setup

Network construction and analyses were all conducted using the Python-based Networkx library [58]. Network visualizations were implemented using Gephi [59]. All experiments were run using a MacBook Pro, with the macOS Catalina operating system, version 10.15.4, and a 2 GHz Quad-Core Intel Core i5 with 16 GB RAM.

5.3. Results

Several cases test positive for COVID-19 after visiting infected countries in 27 Saudi cities, 20 of which occur before or on 21 March 2020 (the date when all domestic transportation was suspended). We consider all 20 cities as central nodes in the transmission network. Then, we measure several global, epidemiological, and structural properties of the transmission network and its chains. Tables 1 and 2 list several quantitative epidemiological and structural properties of COVID-19 transmission in Saudi Arabia.

5.3.1. Global Properties of Transmission Network

The network (epidemic forest) has 119 nodes and 118 edges (single connected component). The epidemic forest consists of 20 epidemic trees, each rooted at a central node. In total, 71% of edges connect cities that belong to the same administrative region. The maximum, minimum, and average outdegrees over all nodes are 11, 0, and 1, respectively. Figure 3 shows the degree distribution of all nodes. The degree distribution depicted in Figure 3 highlights a skewed pattern, with most nodes having a low outdegree and a few nodes exhibiting higher connectivity. This heterogeneity indicates that certain cities play disproportionately influential roles in disease transmission, acting as hubs in the network. Irrespective of edge directions, the average path length between nodes is three, and the network diameter is eight.

Table 1. Epidemiological properties of the transmission network chains for COVID-19 in Saudi Arabia.

	Central Node	Total Num of Chains	Avg Chain Size	Chain Size	Num of Chains	Max Length of Chains	Chain Diam
1	Alqatif	11	10.7	1 2 9 98	7 2 1 1	1 2 4 8	0 1 5 13
2	Makkah almukarramah	8	7.4	1 11 42	6 1 1	1 4 6	0 5 8
3	Arriyad	5	19.4	1 3 4 29 60	1 1 1 1 1	1 2 3 6 7	0 2 2 9 10
4	Jazan	5	8.2	1 2 6 31	2 1 1 1	1 2 3 5	0 1 4 8
5	Almadinah almunawwarah	5	2	1 2 5	3 1 1	1 2 4	0 1 4
6	Muhayil	3	10	6 9 15	1 1 1	4 4 4	4 5 6
7	Najran	3	2.7	1 3 4	1 1 1	1 2 3	0 2 3
8	Abha	2	2.5	1 4	1 1	1 3	0 3
9	Adduwadimi	2	1	1	2	1	0
10	Alkharj	1	3	3	1	2	2
11	Addammam	1	1	1	1	1	0
12	Duba	1	1	1	1	1	0
13	Hafar-albatin	1	1	1	1	1	0
14	Aljubayl	0	0	0	0	0	0
15	Jeddah	0	0	0	0	0	0
16	Annamas	0	0	0	0	0	0
17	Alahsa	0	0	0	0	0	0
18	Altaif	0	0	0	0	0	0
19	Alkhubar	0	0	0	0	0	0
20	Alqunfidhah	0	0	0	0	0	0

5.3.2. Epidemiological Properties of Transmission Networks

Different epidemiological characteristics were captured by the quantitative measures of the transmission network: Total Number of Chains, Chain Size, Maximum Length of Chains, Average Chain Size, and Chain Diameter. The Total Number of Chains, Chain Size, and Average Chain Size describe the scope of COVID-19 transmission through one source of infection (one central node). The Maximum Length of Chains and Chain Diameter describe the scale of COVID-19 transmission through one source of infection.

Table 2. Quantitative structural properties of transmission chains for COVID-19 in Saudi Arabia.

	Central Node	Size	Diameter	Height	Median	Degree Center
1	Alqatif	118	13	8	Arriyad Makkah	Alqatif
2	Makkah	59	10	6	Jazan	Albaha
3	Arriyad	97	13	7	Arriyad Makkah	Albaha Makkah Buraydah
4	Jazan	41	8	5	Muhayil	Albaha
5	Almadinah	10	5	3	Almadinah Yanbu-albahr	Almadinah
6	Muhayil	30	8	4	Muhayil	Albaha
7	Najran	8	5	3	Najran Thar	Najran Thar Addair
8	Abha	5	4	3	Ahad-rifaydah	Ahad-rifaydah
9	Adduwadimi	2	2	1	Adduwadimi	Adduwadimi
10	Alkharj	3	2	2	Hawtat-bani-tamim	Hawtat-bani-tamim
11	Addammam	1	1	1	Addammam Buqayq	Addammam Buqayq
12	Duba	1	1	1	Duba Duba	Alwajh Alwajh
13	Hafar-albatin	1	1	1	Hafar-albatin Hafar-albatin	Rafha Rafha
14	Aljubayl	0	0	0	Aljubayl	Aljubayl
15	Jeddah	0	0	0	Jeddah	Jeddah
16	Annamas	0	0	0	Annamas	Annamas
17	Alahsa	0	0	0	Alahsa	Alahsa
18	Altaif	0	0	0	Altaif	Altaif
19	Alkhubar	0	0	0	Alkhubar	Alkhubar
20	Alqunfidhah	0	0	0	Alqunfidhah	Alqunfidhah

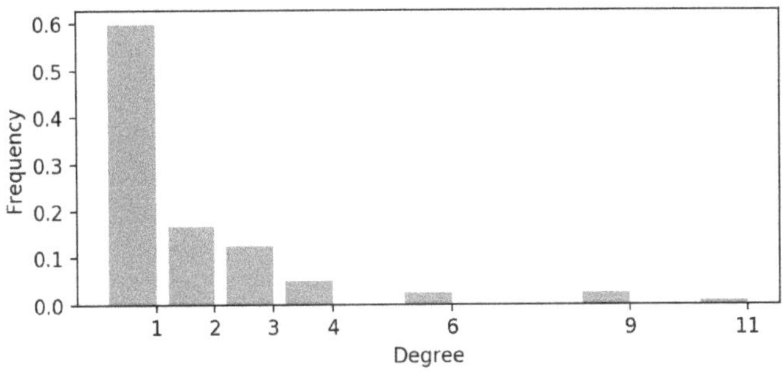

Figure 3. Degree distribution of the transmission network nodes.

According to Table 1, Alqatif city appears to have a bigger role in the spread of COVID-19 (Total Number of Chains is 11). This can be due to the fact that Alqatif was the first city to host a positive COVID-19 case in Saudi Arabia. This can also be due to Alqatif's geographic location (or a combination of both). The Maximum Length of a Transmission

Chain in Alqatif reaches 8, which suggests that the spread of COVID-19 in Saudi Arabia was highly affected by in-between city transmission. The Average Chain Size is 10.7 (the smallest Chain Size is one and the largest is 98). This suggests that COVID-19 may have traveled to 10 cities (depth-wise) before it was controlled.

Table 1 also shows that Makkah, the holiest city, was a vital source of the disease's transmission. A total of eight transmission chains originated from Makkah with a Maximum Length of 6 and a Chain Size of 42. Each of Arriyad, Jazan, and Almadinah generated a total of five transmission chains with average sizes of 19.4, 8.2, and 2, respectively. The Maximum Length of Chains is 7 in Arriyad, 5 in Jazan, and 4 in Almadinah.

Several central cities generated fewer transmission chains including Muhayil, Najran, Abha, and Adduwadimi (Total Number of Chains is between two and three). Interestingly, the produced transmission chains are not necessarily shorter (compared with the Average Chain Size of central cities that produced more chains). For example, Muhayil's Average Chain Size is larger than Makkah's Average Chain Size, although Makkah produced eight chains and Muhayil produced three chains.

Some cities appear to have more negligible transmission effects during the disease transmission period. For example, Addamam, Duba, and Hafar-albatin caused a transmission to only a single city. Aljubayl, Jeddah, Annamas, Alahsa, Altaif, Alkhubar, and Alqunfidhah did not produce any disease transmissions across the network.

Figure 4 show two epidemic trees rooted at central nodes Jazan (T_{Jazan}) and Almadinah ($T_{Almadinah}$), respectively. The different nodes are colored according to the administrative regions they belong to. The figure shows that both central nodes have caused disease transmission within and outside of their administrative regions (Jazan spread the disease to five other regions and Almadinah to two other regions). Both trees have the same Total Number of Chains. However, the Average Chain Size of T_{Jazan} is larger than that of $T_{Almadinah}$.

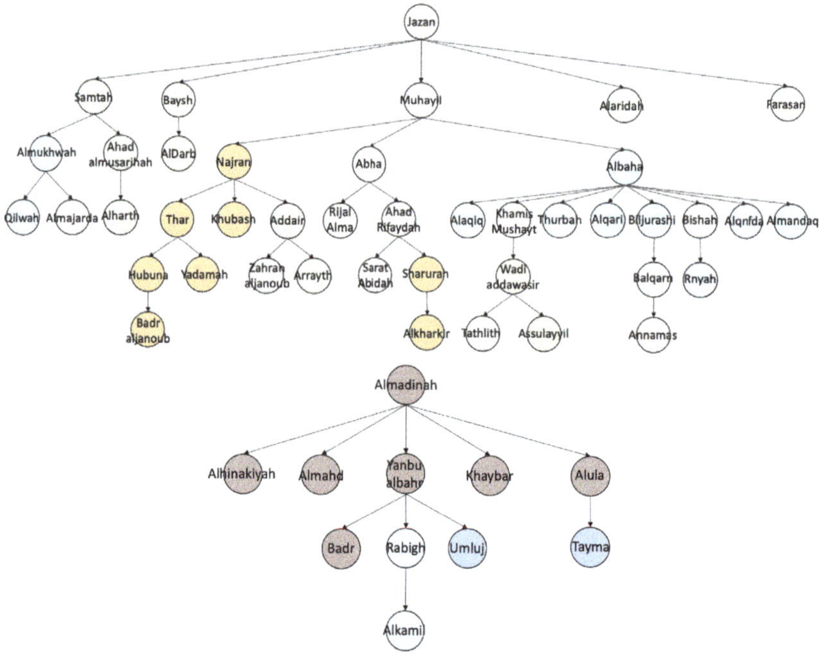

Figure 4. The epidemic trees rooted at two central nodes: Jazan (**top**) and Almadinah (**bottom**).

5.3.3. Structural Properties of Transmission Networks

The second set of measures examines the structural properties of the epidemic trees rooted at each central node. Those measures provide insights about the between-city transmission events. Seven measures were considered for each epidemic tree: Size, Diameter, Height, Median, Degree Center, and Temporal and Spatial Information. The Size property indicates the total number of infections arising from each infected central node. Table 2 shows that the epidemic trees rooted at Alqatif, Arriyad, and Makkah resulted in larger infection sizes compared to the other epidemic trees. The three trees also have the largest diameters and heights, indicating their significant role in the disease spread. The Diameters of each of $T_{Alqatif}$, T_{Makkah}, and $T_{Arriyad}$ are 13, 10, and 13, respectively. The Heights of $T_{Alqatif}$, T_{Makkah}, and $T_{Arriyad}$ are 8, 6, and 7, respectively.

Additionally, Jazan generated a total of 41 infections with a Diameter of eight and a Height of five. Muhayil produced a total of 30 infections. The Diameter and Height of $T_{Muhayil}$ are 8 and 4, respectively. Almadinah and Najran (with sizes of 10 and 8, respectively) both have a Diameter of 5 and Height of 3. Abha, Alkharj, and Adduwadimi generated 5, 3, and 2 total infections. The Diameters are 4, 2, and 2, and the Heights are 3, 2, and 1, respectively.

Node centrality measures identify superspreader nodes in each tree. We use two centrality measures: Median (node or nodes closest to every other node with respect to distance) and Degree Center (node or nodes with the largest number of connections). Interestingly, the central node and the median are represented by different nodes in most epidemic trees. For example, the Median in $T_{Alqatif}$ is represented by two nodes: Arriyad and Makkah. The Median in T_{Makkah} is represented by one node: Jazan. Similarly, in most epidemic trees, the central node and the Degree Center are not necessarily equal. For example, the Degree Center in both T_{Makkah} and T_{Jazan} is Albaha (see Figure 4. In fact, Albaha appears to represent the Degree Center in several epidemic trees including T_{Makkah}, $T_{Arriyad}$, and $T_{Muhayil}$.

Figure 5 and Table 3 show the temporal and spatial information of several epidemic trees. Multiple epidemic trees have overlapping temporal information and geographic coverages. For example, $T_{Muhayil}$ is a subset of T_{Jazan}.

Table 3. Temporal and spatial information of 13 epidemic trees.

	Central Node	Starting Date	Ending Date	Coverage (km^2)
1	Alqatif	2 March 2020	23 June 2020	1,862,582
2	Arriyad	9 March 2020	23 June 2020	1,066,118
3	Makkah	10 March 2020	22 June 2020	642,964
4	Jazan	16 March 2020	22 June 2020	351,874
5	Muhayil	19 March 2020	22 June 2020	339,969
6	Almadinah	20 March 2020	23 June 2020	206,758
7	Najran	23 March 2020	11 June 2020	65,481
8	Abha	24 March 2020	22 June 2020	88,921
9	Adduwadmi	30 March 2020	26 April 2020	79,475
10	Alkharj	9 April 2020	23 May 2020	81,057
11	Addammam	15 March 2020	24 April 2020	7778
12	Duba	3 April 2020	6 April 2020	23,046
13	Hafar-albatin	20 March 2020	24 April 2020	87,496

5.3.4. Validation

Our goal is to validate our city transmission network generation. Our proposed network generation model uses geographic distance between cities as the single factor that affect the infection process (the infection always progresses to a susceptible city from the closest infected one). To validate the generated network, we need to decide the factor or factors that most affect disease transmission between cities, for example, mobility and population.

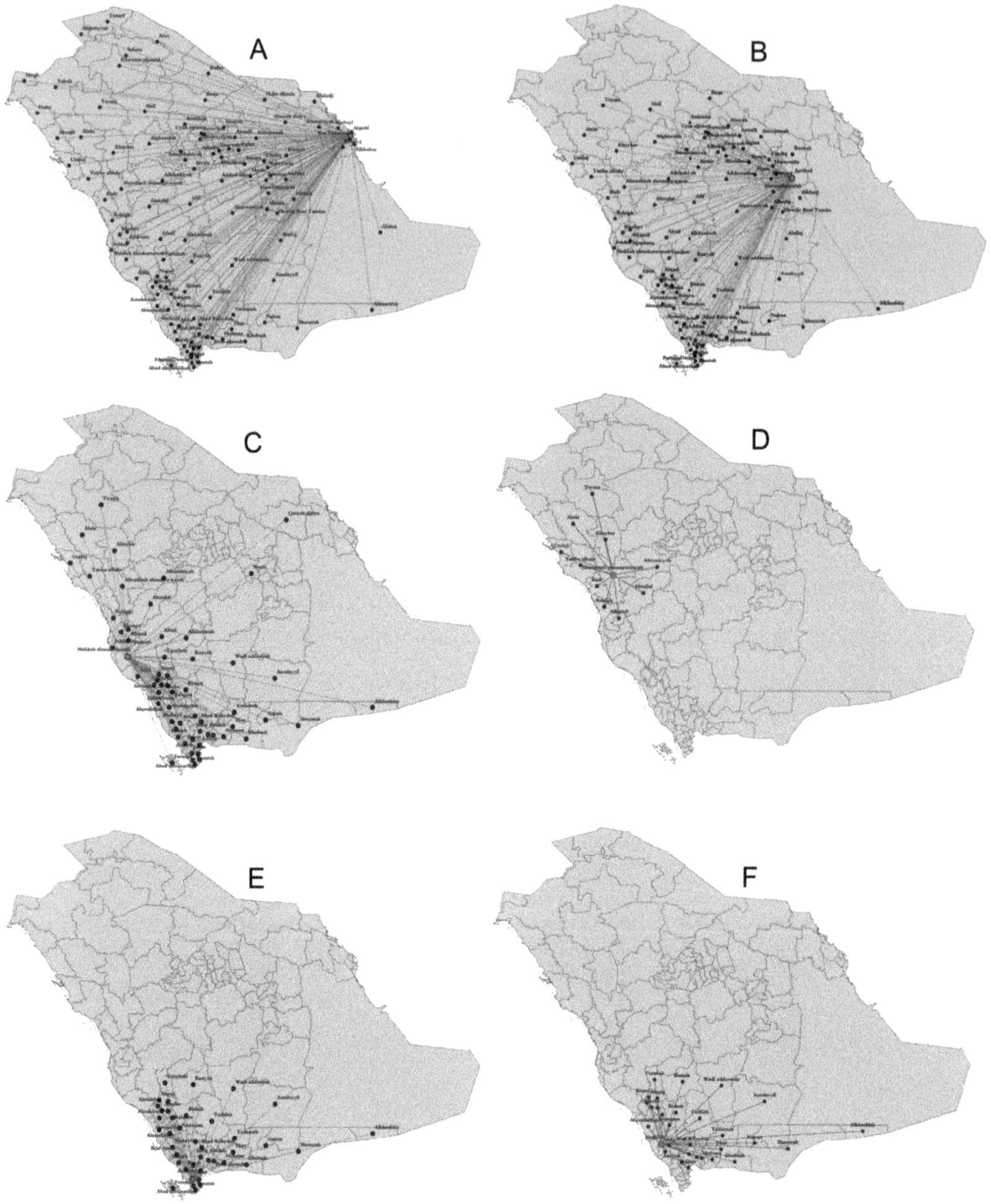

Figure 5. Geographic coverages of six epidemic trees: (**A**) $T_{Alqatif}$, (**B**) $T_{Arriyad}$, (**C**) T_{Makkah}, (**D**) $T_{Almadinah}$, (**E**) T_{Jazan}, and (**F**) $T_{Muhayil}$. The red dots indicate the root cities of the respective epidemic trees.

We analyze the relationship between city populations and the order by which each city was infected. We use Pearson's product–moment correlation to find the correlation between the population and the order (see Figure 6). The analysis indicates a moderate negative relationship ($r = -0.39$), suggesting that nodes with higher populations are more likely to become infected earlier than lower population nodes.

Based on this result, we create another transmission model that takes destination city population into account. Given an infected node u and a non-infected node v, the spread of infection from u to v occurs with a probability p_{uv} proportional to the population of node v (resembling city mobility) as follows $p_{uv} = \alpha * (population_u / population_{sum})$, where α is a constant and $population_{sum}$ is the population sum over all cities.

We use this model to create several transmission network ensembles, each of which simulates a disease transmission incident. The first infected node is set to Alqatif, and α is set to 0.1. For each network, we count the Size (number of infected nodes in the tree rooted at a central node) of each central node and compare them with the tree sizes of the original transmission network. Figure 7 compares the epidemic tree sizes of the original network and the average of 100 simulated networks using the model described above. The Pearson correlation coefficient between the two curves is 0.78, indicating a positive relationship. This implies that no matter what the infection order is, a city population plays a big role in its infectivity.

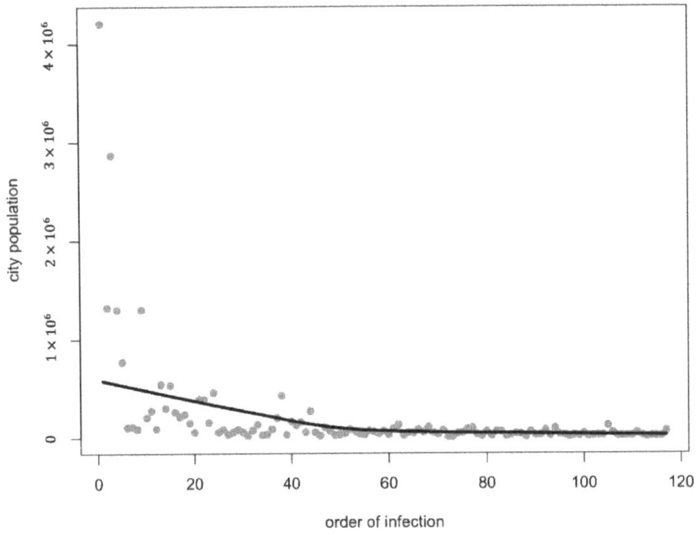

Figure 6. The correlation between city populations and the order in which cities were infected.

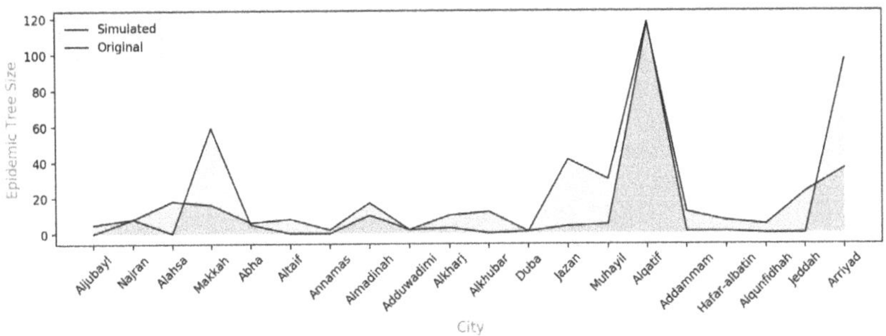

Figure 7. Comparing tree sizes of original and simulated transmission networks.

5.4. Discussion

Understanding the behavior and the spread patterns of a disease helps to effectively and cost-efficiently contain it. Tracing the transmission chains across the cities is one of the crucial tools for managing the pandemic. It can assist authorities in tailoring their efforts and setting the appropriate control measures, focusing on superspreader cities instead of overall lockdowns, to alleviate the otherwise devastating effects on economies.

Considering the importance of between-city movement in disease transmission, we propose constructing a city transmission network that models the spread of a disease. Network-based approaches provide additional insights into disease spread dynamics that are not captured by alternative methods. Unlike traditional models, network-based approaches can incorporate more information and handle complex interactions between geographical locations. This level of information richness offers a better representation of disease transmission through specific pathways and superspreader cities. The network-based method improves epidemic forecasting accuracy while also providing actionable information for more effective disease control and prevention strategies.

Our network is built based on epidemiological data about the disease and geographic distances between cities. Then, quantitative analysis is used to compare the impact of different cities on the disease transmission process. We focus on epidemiological and structural effects of each source of infection, including tracing the infection and discovering superspreader cities.

Identifying the source (or sources) of an infection is important; however, deciding superspreader cities (with the highest potential to spread an infection) is vital for disease prevention. In our example, Alqatif was the first city with a positive COVID-19 case in Saudi Arabia. However, tracing the transmission chains in the city transmission network revealed that the median (center) of this tree was Arriyad and Makkah. This indicates that the role played by Arriyad and Makkah cities during disease transmission was bigger compared to that of Alqatif. Consequently, authorities should prioritize enforcing lockdowns in these cities to effectively mitigate the spread of disease. By focusing the preventative measures and resources in Arriyad and Makkah, where the transmission dynamics have demonstrated a central role in the network, targeted interventions can be more strategically implemented. This approach not only curtails the further spread of the virus from these hubs but also allows for a more efficient allocation of healthcare resources and public health responses, potentially leading to a quicker containment of outbreaks.

Our analysis also shows that a city infection impact is not always local. In most cases, the impact crosses the regional borders of a city to other cities in different regions. For example, Makkah city spread the disease to other cities within its region (Altaif, Alqunfidhah, and Khulays) and others in Almadinah, Jazan, and Albaha regions. This type of analysis can help decision makers with disease prevention and control strategies, for example, determining priorities and narrowing the scope of quarantine.

Because the model relies on the daily number of confirmed cases, it enables the real-time identification of critical locations for early intervention with a certain degree of precision. It uses epidemiological metrics, such as the Total Number of Chains at each central node, to decide the role of these nodes in disease spread, even before the pandemic ends and without complete time series data. This capability for early detection could have allowed authorities to implement targeted quarantine measures to effectively mitigate the impact of an outbreak. Furthermore, our model facilitates the efficient allocation and management of healthcare resources, thereby reducing the pressures on national healthcare systems. It empowers authorities to more effectively distribute medical supplies and other essential items to strategically important cities. By preparing essential nodes in the virus propagation network ahead of time, we can ensure better readiness for potential outbreaks.

6. Conclusions

In order to better control a running disease, it is important to understand how it propagates. Individuals and the disease transmission between them or (groups of them) can be represented as a network. Such a network can be constructed to provide important information on the epidemiological dynamics. Looking into the network structure and possible disease transmission paths may help with disease management and control. Here, we proposed building a city transmission network to simulate the spread of a disease. The constructed network supports comparing the impact of cities on disease transmission using quantitative methods.

For each source of infection, we investigated the epidemiological and structural impacts, as well as superspreaders. Our analysis suggests that identifying superspreader cities is crucial in the early stages of an epidemic, more so than community-level disease transmission. This is because the effects of infections in these cities are not confined to local boundaries but can extend across regional borders, impacting neighboring areas. We show the example of COVID-19 in Saudi Arabia. In this example, there is evidence that Arriyad and Makkah played a larger influence in the spread of disease than the city of Alqatif.

The proposed method for investigating superspreading events and disease transmission dynamics can be applied in different regions by considering region-specific factors, human mobility patterns, and transmission dynamics. The methodology's adaptability and effectiveness in estimating superspreading environments make it a valuable tool for studying disease transmission dynamics across various geographical settings. Moreover, the model can be applied in real time to offer insights into the role of cities in disease transmission.

The proposed method has a few challenges and limitations. First, the available epidemiological data of each infected individual usually lack complete contact history. The exact exposure history (including domestic travel history) of each individual is important for accurate network construction. Second, while it is often straightforward to identify individuals' international travel history, tracking their domestic travel can be more challenging. Third, the between-city distance was the only criterion used to decide disease transmission from one city to another. A probabilistic model that considers other criteria (human mobility, city population, etc.) would have provided more realistic results.

Author Contributions: Conceptualization, Hend Alrasheed; methodology, Hend Alrasheed and Reham Alabduljabbar; software, Hend Alrasheed; validation, Hend Alrasheed, Isra Al-Turaiki and Norah Alballa; formal analysis, Hend Alrasheed and Fahad Almutlaq; investigation, Hend Alrasheed and Reham Alabduljabbar; resources, Fahad Almutlaq; data curation, Fahad Almutlaq; writing—original draft preparation, Hend Alrasheed, Isra Al-Turaiki, Norah Alballa, Fahad Almutlaq and Reham Alabduljabbar; writing—review and editing, Isra Al-Turaiki and Reham Alabduljabbar; visualization, Hend Alrasheed and Norah Alballa; supervision, Hend Alrasheed; project administration, Hend Alrasheed All authors have read and agreed to the published version of the manuscript.

Funding: This research project was supported by Researchers Supporting Project number (RSPD2024R905), King Saud University, Riyadh, Saudi Arabia.

Data Availability Statement: The history file and the constructed transmission network dataset and analysis code are all available at https://github.com/halrashe/Covid19-Transmission-Network (accessed on 1 August 2024).

Conflicts of Interest: The authors declare no conflicts of interest.

Appendix A

Table A1. COVID-19 city infection history file with the following sections: cities, their regions, date and frequency of first reported case, and first tested case in each city, respectively.

	City	Region	Reported Date	Freq	Tested Date	Freq
1	Alahsa	Eastern Region	14 March 2020	1	11 March 2020	2
2	Alaflaj	Ar-Riyad	6 May 2020	1		
3	Alasyah	Al-Qaseem	23 May 2020	1		
4	Albaha	Al-Baha	20 March 2020	1	20 March 2020	1
5	Albadai	Al-Qaseem	31 March 2020	1		
6	Albukayriyah	Al-Qaseem	18 April 2020	1		
7	Alhariq	Ar-Riyad	23 May 2020	1		
8	Addiriyah	Ar-Riyad	4 April 2020	1		
9	Addammam	Eastern Region	15 March 2020	1	3 March 2020	1
10	Adduwadimi	Ar-Riyad	30 March 2020	1	28 March 2020	1
11	Alaridah	Jazan	26 April 2020	14		
12	Alaqiq	Al-Baha	23 April 2020	1		
13	Alghat	Ar-Riyad	22 June 2020	2		
14	Alghazalah	Hail	6 May 2020	1		
15	Abha	Aseer	24 March 2020	6	19 March 2020	2
16	Abu Arish	Jazan	26 April 2020	10		
17	Ahad almusarihah	Jazan	26 May 2020	1		
18	Ahad Rifaydah	Aseer	2 April 2020	1		
19	Afif	Ar-Riyad	26 April 2020	2		
20	Addair	Jazan	7 May 2020	1		
21	Alharth	Jazan	1 June 2020	1		
22	Alhinakiyah	Al-Madinah Al-Monawarah	1 April 2020	1		
23	Alidabi	Jazan	4 May 2020	1		
24	Aljubayl	Eastern Region	25 March 2020	1	21 March 2020	1
25	Aljumum	Makkah Al-Mokarramah	21 May 2020	3		
26	Alkamil	Makkah Al-Mokarramah	6 May 2020	1		
27	Alkhafji	Eastern Region	26 March 2020	1		
28	Alkharj	Ar-Riyad	9 April 2020	2	6 April 2020	1
29	Alkharkhir	Najran	22 June 2020	4		
30	Alkhubar	Eastern Region	22 March 2020	4	11 March 2020	1
31	Alkhurmah	Makkah Al-Mokarramah	23 April 2020	1		
32	Allith	Makkah Al-Mokarramah	16 April 2020	2		

Table A1. *Cont.*

	City	Region	Reported Date	Freq	Tested Date	Freq
33	Almadinah almunawwarah	Al-Madinah Al-Monawarah	20 March 2020	1	19 March 2020	2
34	Almahd	Al-Madinah Al-Monawarah	24 April 2020	3		
35	Almajardah	Aseer	26 April 2020	1		
36	Almajmaah	Ar-Riyad	4 April 2020	1		
37	Almandaq	Al-Baha	23 April 2020	1		
38	Almidhnab	Al-Qaseem	22 April 2020	1		
39	Almukhwah	Al-Baha	21 April 2020	3		
40	Almuzahimiyah	Ar-Riyad	24 April 2020	1		
41	Alnuayriyah	Eastern Region	21 March 2020	1		
42	Alqari	Al-Baha	21 May 2020	1		
43	Alqatif	Eastern Region	2 March 2020	1	19 March 2020	1
44	AlDarb	Jazan	2 May 2020	1		
45	Alqunfidhah	Makkah Al-Mokarramah	23 March 2020	1	20 March 2020	1
46	Alqurayyat	Al-Jouf	16 April 2020	2		
47	Alquwayiyah	Ar-Riyad	10 April 2020	2		
48	Altaif	Makkah Al-Mokarramah	23 March 2020	6	19 March 2020	1
49	Alula	Al-Madinah Al-Monawarah	7 April 2020	1		
50	Alwajh	Tabouk	6 April 2020	1		
51	Annabhaniyah	Al-Qaseem	11 June 2020	1		
52	Annamas	Aseer	22 May 2020	1	19 March 2020	2
53	Arar	Northern Borders	25 March 2020	2	22 March 2020	2
54	Arrass	Al-Qaseem	30 March 2020	1	26 March 2020	1
55	Arrayth	Jazan	10 June 2020	1		
56	Arriyad	Ar-Riyad	9 March 2020	1	7 March 2020	1
57	Ashshimasiyah	Al-Qaseem	22 June 2020	11		
58	Asshinan	Hail	20 June 2020	1		
59	Assulayyil	Ar-Riyad	13 May 2020	1		
60	Azzulfi	Ar-Riyad	15 April 2020	1		
61	Badr	Al-Madinah Al-Monawarah	23 June 2020	1		
62	Badr aljanub	Najran	11 June 2020	1		
63	Balqarn	Aseer	17 May 2020	7		
64	Baqa	Hail	22 May 2020	1		
65	Baysh	Jazan	19 April 2020	1		
66	Biljurashi	Al-Baha	24 April 2020	1		

Table A1. *Cont.*

	City	Region	Reported Date	Freq	Tested Date	Freq
67	Bishah	Aseer	20 March 2020	1		
68	Buqayq	Eastern Region	24 April 2020	3		
69	Buraydah	Al-Qaseem	26 March 2020	1	22 March 2020	1
70	Damad	Jazan	27 May 2020	1		
71	Dawamat aljandal	Al-Jouf	27 April 2020	1		
72	Duba	Tabouk	3 April 2020	1	18 March 2020	1
73	Duruma	Ar-Riyad	4 May 2020	1		
74	Farasan	Jazan	10 June 2020	2		
75	Hafar albatin	Eastern Region	20 March 2020	1	18 March 2020	1
76	Hail	Hail	14 April 2020	1	12 April 2020	1
77	Haqil	Tabouk	16 May 2020	1		
78	Hawtat Bani Tamim	Ar-Riyad	4 May 2020	1		
79	Hubuna	Najran	3 June 2020	1		
80	Huraymila	Ar-Riyad	12 May 2020	1		
81	Jazan	Jazan	16 March 2020	1	14 March 2020	1
82	Jeddah	Makkah Al-Mokarramah	11 March 2020	1	8 March 2020	2
83	Khamis Mushayt	Aseer	28 March 2020	3		
84	Khaybar	Al-Madinah Al-Monawarah	4 May 2020	1		
85	Khubash	Najran	22 May 2020	1		
86	Khulays	Makkah Al-Mokarramah	10 April 2020	1		
87	Makkah almukarramah	Makkah Al-Mokarramah	10 March 2020	1	9 March 2020	4
88	Marat	Ar-Riyad	15 May 2020	1		
89	Muhayil	Aseer	19 March 2020	1	17 March 2020	1
90	Najran	Najran	23 March 2020	1	18 March 2020	1
91	Qaryah alulya	Eastern Region	20 May 2020	1		
92	Qilwah	Al-Baha	11 May 2020	1		
93	Rabigh	Makkah Al-Mokarramah	19 April 2020	2		
94	Rafha	Northern Borders	24 April 2020	1		
95	Ranyah	Makkah Al-Mokarramah	28 May 2020	1		
96	Ras Tannurah	Eastern Region	29 March 2020	1		
97	Rijal Alma	Aseer	16 April 2020	3		
98	Riyadh alkhabra	Al-Qaseem	9 April 2020	1	6 April 2020	1
99	Rumah	Ar-Riyad	16 May 2020	1		

Table A1. *Cont.*

	City	Region	Reported Date	Freq	Tested Date	Freq
100	Sabya	Jazan	12 April 2020	2		
101	Sakaka	Al-Jouf	24 April 2020	5		
102	Samtah	Jazan	30 March 2020	1		
103	Sarat Abidah	Aseer	9 May 2020	1		
104	Shaqra	Ar-Riyad	12 May 2020	1		
105	Sharurah	Najran	7 April 2020	4		
106	Tabuk	Tabouk	29 March 2020	1	1 April 2020	2
107	Tathlith	Aseer	8 May 2020	1		
108	Tayma	Tabouk	15 May 2020	1		
109	Thadiq	Ar-Riyad	8 May 2020	1		
110	Thar	Najran	25 May 2020	6		
111	Turayf	Northern Borders	12 May 2020	18		
112	Turubah	Makkah Al-Mokarramah	25 April 2020	1		
113	Umluj	Tabouk	30 April 2020	1		
114	Unayzah	Al-Qaseem	9 April 2020	2		
115	Uyun aljiwa	Al-Qaseem	21 May 2020	5		
116	Wadi addawasir	Ar-Riyad	26 April 2020	2		
117	Yadamah	Najran	1 June 2020	1		
118	Yanbu albahr	Al-Madinah Al-Monawarah	8 April 2020	1		
119	Zahran aljanub	Aseer	21 May 2020	2		

References

1. Eames, K.T.D.; Read, J.M. Networks in Epidemiology. In Proceedings of the Bio-Inspired Computing and Communication, Berlin/Heidelberg, Germany, 2–5 April 2008; Lecture Notes in Computer Science; pp. 79–90.
2. Sun, K.; Wang, W.; Gao, L.; Wang, Y.; Luo, K.; Ren, L.; Zhan, Z.; Chen, X.; Zhao, S.; Huang, Y.; et al. Transmission heterogeneities, kinetics, and controllability of SARS-CoV-2. *Science* **2021**, *371*, eabe2424. [CrossRef]
3. Van Gunten, T. Visualizing the Network Structure of COVID-19 in Singapore. *Socius* **2021**, *7*, 23780231211000171. [CrossRef] [PubMed]
4. Russell, T.W.; Wu, J.T.; Clifford, S.; Edmunds, W.J.; Kucharski, A.J.; Jit, M. Effect of internationally imported cases on internal spread of COVID-19: A mathematical modelling study. *Lancet Public Health* **2021**, *6*, e12–e20. [CrossRef] [PubMed]
5. Godin, A.; Xia, Y.; Buckeridge, D.L.; Mishra, S.; Douwes-Schultz, D.; Shen, Y.; Lavigne, M.; Drolet, M.; Schmidt, A.M.; Brisson, M.; et al. The role of case importation in explaining differences in early SARS-CoV-2 transmission dynamics in Canada—A mathematical modeling study of surveillance data. *Int. J. Infect. Dis.* **2021**, *102*. [CrossRef] [PubMed]
6. Lewis, D. Superspreading drives the COVID pandemic–and could help to tame it. *Nature* **2021**, *590*, 544–547. [CrossRef] [PubMed]
7. Oka, T.; Wei, W.; Zhu, D. The effect of human mobility restrictions on the COVID-19 transmission network in China. *PLoS ONE* **2021**, *16*, e0254403. [CrossRef]
8. Benvenuto, D.; Giovanetti, M.; Vassallo, L.; Angeletti, S.; Ciccozzi, M. Application of the ARIMA model on the COVID-2019 epidemic dataset. *Data Brief* **2020**, *29*, 105340. [CrossRef]
9. Biala, T.A.; Afolabi, Y.O.; Khaliq, A.Q.M. How efficient is contact tracing in mitigating the spread of COVID-19? A mathematical modeling approach. *Appl. Math. Model.* **2022**, *103*, 714–730. [CrossRef]
10. Yang, Z.; Zeng, Z.; Wang, K.; Wong, S.S.; Liang, W.; Zanin, M.; Liu, P.; Cao, X.; Gao, Z.; Mai, Z.; et al. Modified SEIR and AI prediction of the epidemics trend of COVID-19 in China under public health interventions. *J. Thorac. Dis.* **2020**, *12*, 165. [CrossRef]

11. Lin, Q.; Zhao, S.; Gao, D.; Lou, Y.; Yang, S.; Musa, S.S.; Wang, M.H.; Cai, Y.; Wang, W.; Yang, L.; et al. A conceptual model for the coronavirus disease 2019 (COVID-19) outbreak in Wuhan, China with individual reaction and governmental action. *Int. J. Infect. Dis.* **2020**, *93*, 211–216. [CrossRef]
12. Liu, F.; Li, X.; Zhu, G. Using the contact network model and Metropolis-Hastings sampling to reconstruct the COVID-19 spread on the "Diamond Princess". *Sci. Bull.* **2020**, *65*, 1297–1305. [CrossRef] [PubMed]
13. Alrasheed, H.; Althnian, A.; Kurdi, H.; Al-Mgren, H.; Alharbi, S. COVID-19 Spread in Saudi Arabia: Modeling, Simulation and Analysis. *Int. J. Environ. Res. Public Health* **2020**, *17*, 7744. [CrossRef] [PubMed]
14. Peirlinck, M.; Linka, K.; Costabal, F.S.; Kuhl, E. Outbreak dynamics of COVID-19 in China and the United States. *Biomech. Model. Mechanobiol.* **2020**, *19*, 2179–2193. [CrossRef] [PubMed]
15. Li, M.; Shi, X.; Li, X.; Ma, W.; He, J.; Liu, T. Epidemic forest: A spatiotemporal model for communicable diseases. *Ann. Am. Assoc. Geogr.* **2019**, *109*, 812–836. [CrossRef]
16. Gürsakal, N.; Batmaz, B.; Aktuna, G. Drawing transmission graphs for COVID-19 in the perspective of network science. *Epidemiol. Infect.* **2020**, *148*, e269. [CrossRef] [PubMed]
17. Hâncean, M.G.; Perc, M.; Lerner, J. Early spread of COVID-19 in Romania: Imported cases from Italy and human-to-human transmission networks. *R. Soc. Open Sci.* **2020**, *7*, 200780. [CrossRef] [PubMed]
18. Wong, N.S.; Lee, S.S.; Kwan, T.H.; Yeoh, E.K. Settings of virus exposure and their implications in the propagation of transmission networks in a COVID-19 outbreak. *Lancet Reg. Health West. Pac.* **2020**, *4*, 100052. [CrossRef] [PubMed]
19. Kırbıyık, U. Network Characteristics and Visualization of COVID-19 Outbreak in a Large Detention Facility in the United States—Cook County, Illinois, 2020. *MMWR Morb. Mortal. Wkly. Rep.* **2020**, *69*, 1625–1630 .
20. Changruenngam, S.; Bicout, D.J.; Modchang, C. How the individual human mobility spatio-temporally shapes the disease transmission dynamics. *Sci. Rep.* **2020**, *10*, 11325. [CrossRef]
21. Maheshwari, P.; Albert, R. Network model and analysis of the spread of COVID-19 with social distancing. *Appl. Netw. Sci.* **2020**, *5*, 100. [CrossRef]
22. Klise, K.; Beyeler, W.; Finley, P.; Makvandi, M. Analysis of mobility data to build contact networks for COVID-19. *PLoS ONE* **2021**, *16*, e0249726. [CrossRef] [PubMed]
23. Loeffler-Wirth, H.; Schmidt, M.; Binder, H. Covid-19 transmission trajectories–monitoring the pandemic in the worldwide context. *Viruses* **2020**, *12*, 777. [CrossRef] [PubMed]
24. Cardoso, B.H.F.; Gonçalves, S. Universal scaling law for human-to-human transmission diseases. *Europhys. Lett.* **2021**, *133*, 58001. [CrossRef]
25. Hu, H.; Nigmatulina, K.; Eckhoff, P. The scaling of contact rates with population density for the infectious disease models. *Math. Biosci.* **2013**, *244*, 125–134. [CrossRef] [PubMed]
26. Ministry of Health Saudi Arabia. Ministry of Health Saudi Arabia. 2022. Available online: https://www.moh.gov.sa/en/Pages/Default.aspx (accessed on 1 August 2024).
27. Newman, M.E.; Strogatz, S.H.; Watts, D.J. Random graphs with arbitrary degree distributions and their applications. *Phys. Rev. E* **2001**, *64*, 026118. [CrossRef] [PubMed]
28. Kiss, I.Z.; Green, D.M.; Kao, R.R. The network of sheep movements within Great Britain: Network properties and their implications for infectious disease spread. *J. R. Soc. Interface* **2006**, *3*, 669–677. [CrossRef] [PubMed]
29. Luo, C.; Ma, Y.; Jiang, P.; Zhang, T.; Yin, F. The construction and visualization of the transmission networks for COVID-19: A potential solution for contact tracing and assessments of epidemics. *Sci. Rep.* **2021**, *11*, 8605. [CrossRef] [PubMed]
30. Williamson, S.G. *Combinatorics for Computer Science*; Courier Corporation: North Chelmsford, MA, USA, 2002.
31. Mesbahi, M.; Egerstedt, M. *Graph Theoretic Methods in Multiagent Networks*; Princeton University Press: Princeton, NJ, USA, 2010.
32. Kansky, K.; Danscoine, P. Measures of network structure. *FLUX Cah. Sci. Int. RÉSeaux Territ.* **1989**, *5*, 89–121. [CrossRef]
33. Haydon, D.T.; Chase-Topping, M.; Shaw, D.; Matthews, L.; Friar, J.; Wilesmith, J.; Woolhouse, M. The construction and analysis of epidemic trees with reference to the 2001 UK foot–and–mouth outbreak. *Proc. R. Soc. Lond. Ser. Biol. Sci.* **2003**, *270*, 121–127. [CrossRef]
34. Napp, S.; Allepuz, A.; Purse, B.; Casal, J.; García-Bocanegra, I.; Burgin, L.; Searle, K. Understanding spatio-temporal variability in the reproduction ratio of the bluetongue (BTV-1) epidemic in Southern Spain (Andalusia) in 2007 using epidemic trees. *PLoS ONE* **2016**, *11*, e0151151. [CrossRef]
35. Lau, M.S.; Dalziel, B.D.; Funk, S.; McClelland, A.; Tiffany, A.; Riley, S.; Metcalf, C.J.E.; Grenfell, B.T. Spatial and temporal dynamics of superspreading events in the 2014–2015 West Africa Ebola epidemic. *Proc. Natl. Acad. Sci. USA* **2017**, *114*, 2337–2342. [CrossRef] [PubMed]
36. Diekmann, O.; Heesterbeek, J.A.P. *Mathematical Epidemiology of Infectious Diseases: Model Building, Analysis and Interpretation*; John Wiley & Sons: Hoboken, NJ, USA, 2000; Volume 5.
37. Kao, R.R.; Danon, L.; Green, D.M.; Kiss, I.Z. Demographic structure and pathogen dynamics on the network of livestock movements in Great Britain. *Proc. R. Soc. Biol. Sci.* **2006**, *273*, 1999–2007. [CrossRef] [PubMed]
38. John, R.S.; Miller, J.C.; Muylaert, R.L.; Hayman, D.T. High connectivity and human movement limits the impact of travel time on infectious disease transmission. *J. R. Soc. Interface* **2024**, *21*, 20230425. [CrossRef] [PubMed]
39. Guo, Z.; Li, J.; Xiao, G.; Gong, L.; Wang, Y. Dynamic model of respiratory infectious disease transmission by population mobility based on city network. *R. Soc. Open Sci.* **2022**, *9*, 221232. [CrossRef] [PubMed]

40. Leung, W.T.; Rudge, J.W.; Fournié, G. Simulating contact networks for livestock disease epidemiology: A systematic review. *J. R. Soc. Interface* **2023**, *20*, 20220890. [CrossRef] [PubMed]
41. Büttner, K.; Krieter, J. Illustration of different disease transmission routes in a pig trade network by monopartite and bipartite representation. *Animals* **2020**, *10*, 1071. [CrossRef] [PubMed]
42. Xie, X.; Zhao, L.; Qian, Y. Impact of asymmetric activity on interactions between information diffusion and disease transmission in multiplex networks. *Commun. Theor. Phys.* **2023**, *75*, 075001. [CrossRef]
43. Hearst, S.; Huang, M.; Johnson, B.; Rummells, E. Identifying potential super-spreaders and disease transmission hotspots using white-tailed deer scraping networks. *Animals* **2023**, *13*, 1171. [CrossRef] [PubMed]
44. Shaw, A.K.; White, L.A.; Michalska-Smith, M.; Borer, E.T.; Craft, M.E.; Seabloom, E.W.; Snell-Rood, E.C.; Travisano, M. Lessons from movement ecology for the return to work: Modeling contacts and the spread of COVID-19. *PLoS ONE* **2021**, *16*, e0242955. [CrossRef]
45. Silva, T.C.; Anghinoni, L.; Zhao, L. Quantitative Analysis of the Effectiveness of Public Health Measures on COVID-19 Transmission. *medRxiv* **2020**. Available online: https://www.medrxiv.org/content/10.1101/2020.05.15.20102988v1.full.pdf+html (accessed on 1 August 2024).
46. Gayawan, E.; Awe, O.O.; Oseni, B.M.; Uzochukwu, I.C.; Adekunle, A.; Samuel, G.; Eisen, D.P.; Adegboye, O.A. The spatio-temporal epidemic dynamics of COVID-19 outbreak in Africa. *Epidemiol. Infect.* **2020**, *148*, e212. [CrossRef]
47. Chan, C.H.; Wen, T.H. Revisiting the Effects of High-Speed Railway Transfers in the Early COVID-19 Cross-Province Transmission in Mainland China. *Int. J. Environ. Res. Public Health* **2021**, *18*, 6394. [CrossRef] [PubMed]
48. Dlamini, W.M.D.; Simelane, S.P.; Nhlabatsi, N.M. Bayesian network-based spatial predictive modelling reveals COVID-19 transmission dynamics in Eswatini. *Spat. Inf. Res.* **2021**, *30*, 183–194. [CrossRef]
49. Pribadi, D.O.; Saifullah, K.; Putra, A.S.; Nurdin, M.; Iman, L.O.S.; Rustiadi, E. Spatial analysis of COVID-19 outbreak to assess the effectiveness of social restriction policy in dealing with the pandemic in Jakarta. *Spat. -Spatio-Temporal Epidemiol.* **2021**, *39*, 100454. [CrossRef] [PubMed]
50. Abuhasel, K.A.; Khadr, M.; Alquraish, M.M. Analyzing and forecasting COVID-19 pandemic in the Kingdom of Saudi Arabia using ARIMA and SIR models. *Comput. Intell.* **2020**, *38*, 770–783. [CrossRef] [PubMed]
51. Alboaneen, D.; Pranggono, B.; Alshammari, D.; Alqahtani, N.; Alyaffer, R. Predicting the epidemiological outbreak of the coronavirus disease 2019 (COVID-19) in Saudi Arabia. *Int. J. Environ. Res. Public Health* **2020**, *17*, 4568. [CrossRef] [PubMed]
52. Elhassan, T.; Gaafar, A. Mathematical Modeling of the COVID-19 Prevalence in Saudi Arabia. *medRxiv* **2020**. Available online: https://www.medrxiv.org/content/10.1101/2020.06.25.20138602v1 (accessed on 1 August 2024).
53. Komies, S.; Aldhahir, A.M.; Almehmadi, M.; Alghamdi, S.M.; Alqarni, A.; Oyelade, T.; Alqahtani, J.S. COVID-19 Outcomes in Saudi Arabia and the UK: A Tale of Two Kingdoms. *medRxiv* **2020**. Available online: https://www.medrxiv.org/content/10.1101/2020.04.25.20079640v1 (accessed on 1 August 2024).
54. Khoj, H.; Mujallad, A.F. Epidemic Situation and Forecasting if COVID-19 in Saudi Arabia Using SIR Model. Technical Report. 2020. Available online: https://www.medrxiv.org/content/10.1101/2020.05.05.20091520v1 (accessed on 1 August 2024).
55. Awwad, F.A.; Mohamoud, M.A.; Abonazel, M.R. Estimating COVID-19 cases in Makkah region of Saudi Arabia: Space-time ARIMA modeling. *PLoS ONE* **2021**, *16*, e0250149. [CrossRef]
56. Al-Turaiki, I.; Almutlaq, F.; Alrasheed, H.; Alballa, N. Empirical Evaluation of Alternative Time-Series Models for COVID-19 Forecasting in Saudi Arabia. *Int. J. Environ. Res. Public Health* **2021**, *18*, 8660. [CrossRef]
57. Ministry of Health Saudi Arabia. COVID-19 Dashboard: Saudi Arabia. 2022. Available online: https://covid19.moh.gov.sa/ (accessed on 1 November 2021).
58. Networkx Network Analysis in Python. Networkx Documentation. 2021. Available online: https://networkx.github.io (accessed on 1 August 2024).
59. Gephi. Gephi—The Open Graph Viz Platform. 2021. Available online: https://gephi.org (accessed on 1 August 2024).

International Journal of
Geo-Information

MDPI

Article

Sensing the Environmental Inequality of $PM_{2.5}$ Exposure Using Fine-Scale Measurements of Social Strata and Citizenship Identity

Li He [1,†], Lingfeng He [1,*,†], Zezheng Lin [2], Yao Lu [3], Chen Chen [4], Zhongmin Wang [5], Ping An [6], Min Liu [6], Jie Xu [7] and Shurui Gao [1]

1 Institute for Empirical Social Science Research, School of Humanities and Social Science, Xi'an Jiaotong University, Xi'an 710049, China; lihegeo@xjtu.edu.cn (L.H.); gaoshurui@stu.xjtu.edu.cn (S.G.)
2 Steering Committee of ESG & Carbon Neutral Investment, United Nations Industrial Development Organization, Beijing 100060, China; jasonlinzezheng@gmail.com
3 Rackham Graduate School, University of Michigan, Ann Arbor, MI 48109, USA
4 Xi'an Jiaotong University Press, Xi'an 710049, China
5 Xi'an Public Security Bureau, Xi'an 710002, China
6 School of Management, Xi'an Jiaotong University, Xi'an 710049, China; anping@stu.xjtu.edu.cn (P.A.); liumin0@stu.xjtu.edu.cn (M.L.)
7 School of Economics and Finance, Xi'an Jiaotong University, Xi'an 710049, China
* Correspondence: helingfeng@stu.xjtu.edu.cn
† These authors contributed equally to this work.

Abstract: Exposure to $PM_{2.5}$ pollution poses substantial health risks, with the precise quantification of exposure being fundamental to understanding the environmental inequalities therein. However, the absence of high-resolution spatiotemporal ambient population data, coupled with an insufficiency of attribute data, impedes a comprehension of the environmental inequality of exposure risks at a fine scale. Within the purview of a conceptual framework that interlinks social strata and citizenship identity with environmental inequality, this study examines the environmental inequality of $PM_{2.5}$ exposure with a focus on the city of Xi'an. Quantitative metrics of the social strata and citizenship identities of the ambient population are derived from housing price data and mobile phone big data. The fine-scale estimation of $PM_{2.5}$ concentrations is predicated on the kriging interpolation method and refined by leveraging an advanced dataset. Employing geographically weighted regression models, we examine the environmental inequality pattern at a fine spatial scale. The key findings are threefold: (1) the manifestation of environmental inequality in $PM_{2.5}$ exposure is pronounced among individuals of varying social strata and citizenship identities within our study area, Xi'an; (2) nonlocal residents situated in the northwestern precincts of Xi'an are subject to the most pronounced $PM_{2.5}$ exposure; and (3) an elevated socioeconomic status is identified as an attenuating factor, capable of averting the deleterious impacts of $PM_{2.5}$ exposure among nonlocal residents. These findings proffer substantial practical implications for the orchestration of air pollution mitigation strategies and urban planning initiatives. They suggest that addressing the wellbeing of the marginalized underprivileged cohorts, who are environmentally and politically segregated under the extant urban planning policies in China, is of critical importance.

Keywords: $PM_{2.5}$ exposure; environmental inequality; social stratum; citizenship identity; spatial analysis

1. Introduction

Air pollution exposure is recognized as a complex and multifaceted challenge that intersects the disciplines of geography, public health, environmental science, and the social sciences. The exposure to air pollutants, both short-term and long-term, whether acute or chronic, has been consistently associated with an array of adverse health outcomes, including an elevated risk of cardiopulmonary and respiratory diseases [1–4], as well as increased mortality rates [1,5,6]. Moreover, emerging evidence suggests that air pollution may induce cognitive decline [7] and depressive disorder [8]. A substantial body of research has demonstrated that the health risks associated with air pollution are not evenly distributed across the population, with disparities often linked to socioeconomic status and ethnicity, a phenomenon that reflects the spatial distribution of pollution and is encapsulated by the concept of environmental inequality [9,10].

Environmental inequality has risen as a critical issue in air pollution exposure research [10]. A substantial body of research has furnished compelling evidence highlighting the disproportionate impact on vulnerable populations characterized by low socioeconomic status, including limited education, low occupational status, unemployment, and poverty [11,12]. Additionally, the lack of housing ownership [13,14] and racial or ethnic-based social exclusion, particularly affecting Black, Latinx, and Indigenous communities [15–17], have been identified as significant factors contributing to disparities in air pollution exposure and the ensuing health consequences. These patterns of disparity have been extensively studied from the 1970s to the present, transcending geographical boundaries and manifesting in both urban and rural settings [12,14,16,18], across developing and developed nations [12,16,19,20], and even in societies considered to be more egalitarian [21].

In recent years, fruitful advancements have been made in understanding environmental inequality in air pollution exposure in China [10,22]. However, the reliance on static population data sourced from censuses and yearbooks at the administrative division level presents limitations, as it does not account for the dynamic nature of human activities and the daily spatial distribution of the ambient population [23–25]. It is important to recognize two key limitations when working with static data such as census records. First, residents' daily activities are not confined by the boundaries of blocks, census tracts, or administrative districts. Analyzing spatial patterns using a regular grid as the unit of assessment, instead of administrative divisions, mitigates the issue of arbitrarily assigning demographic and socioeconomic indicators based on artificial boundaries, further ensuring the validity of pollution exposure assessments. Second, static data such as census population data fail to account for residents' characteristics of travel activities, making it unconducive to accurately depicting the daily average spatial distribution of the population.

To address these limitations, there has been a shift towards utilizing high-resolution global population data represented through regular grids, such as footfall data [26], LandScan [27,28], and WorldPop [29]. These data offer enhanced spatial resolution, but are limited by the absence of attribute data that characterize the ambient population (i.e., spatiotemporally dynamic population) [30]. This ongoing gap constrains scholars' capacity to fully comprehend the risks associated with pollution exposure and environmental equality at the fine scale.

Advancements in data collection technology present an opportune avenue for overcoming the aforementioned challenges [31,32]. In this regard, spatially referenced mobile phone data have emerged as a promising data source because of their extensive coverage, high penetration rate, and remarkable spatial–temporal continuity [33,34]. They adeptly capture the spatial distribution, mobility patterns, and social activities of the ambient population. Furthermore, mobile phone data have proven to be particularly efficacious in quantifying multifaceted attributes of the ambient population at finer spatiotemporal resolutions [32,35]. Although early research focused predominantly on estimating the number of ambient populations, recent methodological developments have broadened the scope of analysis to include multidimensional attributes of the ambient population, while ensuring the preservation of anonymity and desensitizing sensitive information to protect privacy [36]. In the domain of spatial equity evaluation, the identification of high-resolution proxies for socioeconomic status is paramount. To this end, a diverse array of data sources have been harnessed, including remote sensing [37], social media [38,39], and street view data [40]. The most recent research has leveraged machine learning methods to predict spatial variations in socioeconomic status at the neighborhood level, predicated on online housing advertising text [41]. These endeavors demonstrate the feasibility of employing housing-related information as a metric for estimating the spatial distribution of socioeconomic status.

The primary objective of this study is to investigate the environmental inequality of $PM_{2.5}$ pollution exposure among residents. Our goal is to delineate the spatial distribution patterns of $PM_{2.5}$ concentrations and their association with the social strata and citizenship identities at a fine-scale level (1 km × 1 km). Xi'an, a representative industrial city in northern China, was selected as our study area. The technical route of this study is shown in Figure 1. Leveraging the kriging method, we generated the spatiotemporal distribution of $PM_{2.5}$ concentration from daily air pollution monitoring data over a one-year period, from 1 January 2021 to 31 December 2021. Subsequently, we conducted an analysis of the spatiotemporal patterns of the environmental inequality of $PM_{2.5}$ exposure, integrating data on the distribution of citizenship identities derived from mobile phone data with the distribution of social strata estimated though secondhand housing prices. The empirical findings highlight significant environmental inequality in $PM_{2.5}$ exposure in Xi'an, with pronounced disparities observed among individuals of different social strata and citizenship identities.

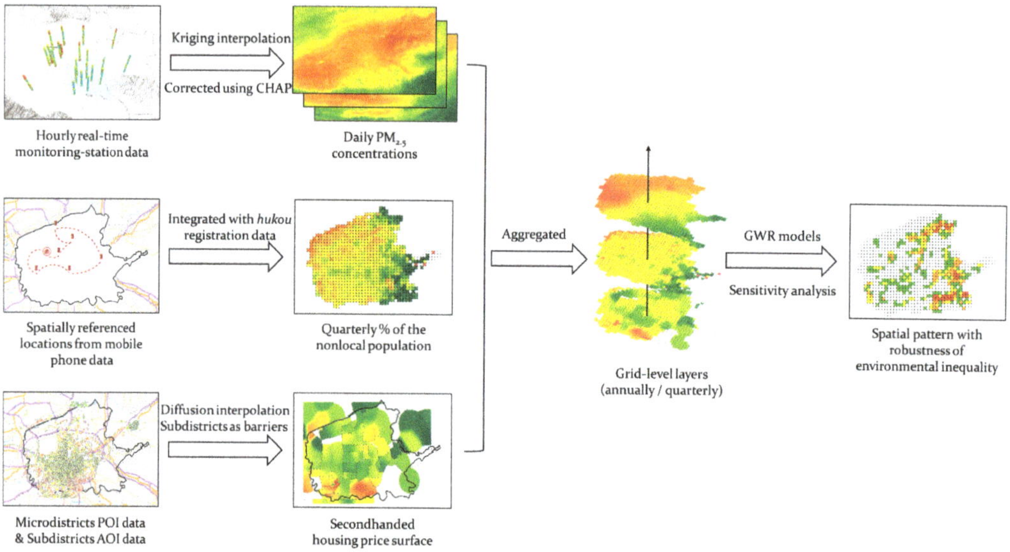

Figure 1. The flowchart of the study.

2. Materials and Methods

2.1. Study Area

The study area is the main urban area of Xi'an, situated within the Shaanxi Province of China. The region is located in the central Shaanxi Plain, nestled in the middle Yellow River Basin. As a quintessential industrial city, Xi'an boasts a diverse economic landscape, featuring key sectors such as infrastructure development, energy and chemical industries, and equipment manufacturing. Figure 2 shows the location of the study area in China.

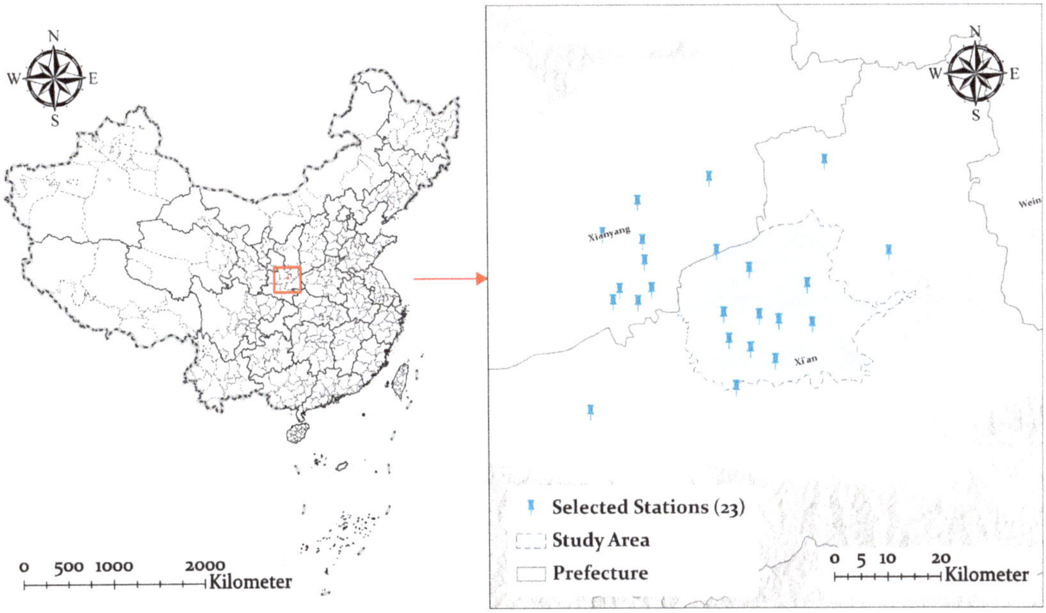

Figure 2. The location of the study area and selected air pollution monitoring stations.

2.2. Data

2.2.1. Air Pollution Data

In this investigation, we acknowledge the diurnal and seasonal fluctuations in human activities; accordingly, we employ a geostatistical method that leverages hourly real-time monitoring station data. To mitigate the constraints inherent in geostatistical analyses, we integrate a refined daily gapless 1 km × 1 km global ground-level $PM_{2.5}$ dataset to enhance the accuracy of our estimates [42].

The air quality data were procured from the National Urban Air Quality Real-Time Release Platform of China (www.cnemc.cn) [43]. This dataset compiles hourly $PM_{2.5}$ concentrations, reading from an extensive network of 2024 monitoring stations in China. Considering proximity and topographical factors (as depicted in Figure 2), this study selected a subset of 23 monitoring stations situated within the study area and their immediate environs. Considering the significant perturbations in human behavior and atmospheric quality induced by the COVID-19 outbreak and consequent lockdown protocols in 2020 [44–46], our analysis is focused on the timeframe from 1 January 2021 to 31 December 2021.

The process of calculating the $PM_{2.5}$ dataset in this study is delineated as follows:

1. The hourly station data were aggregated, and the daily $PM_{2.5}$ concentrations during the entire day, daytime (9 a.m. to 6 p.m.), and nighttime (12 a.m. to 6 a.m.) were calculated for each station.
2. The kriging method was used to generate daily $PM_{2.5}$ concentrations throughout the entire day, daytime (9 a.m. to 6 p.m.), and nighttime (12 a.m. to 6 a.m.).
3. The estimated daytime and nighttime surfaces were corrected with the daily gapless 1 km × 1 km global ground-level $PM_{2.5}$ dataset. For each cell:

$$CPM_{i,d,t} = UPM_{i,d,t} \times \frac{GHPM_{i,d}}{UPME_{i,d}} \quad (1)$$

where $CPM_{i,d,t}$ is the corrected $PM_{2.5}$ concentration for cell i during time t (daytime or nighttime) on day d, $UPM_{i,d,t}$ is the uncorrected $PM_{2.5}$ concentration for cell i during time t (daytime or nighttime) on day d, $GHPM_{i,d}$ is the daily $PM_{2.5}$ concentration for cell i on day d according to the daily gapless 1 km global ground-level $PM_{2.5}$ dataset, and $UPME_{i,d}$ is the uncorrected entire day $PM_{2.5}$ concentration for cell i during day d.

2.2.2. Spatially Referenced Mobile Phone Data

In the sociopolitical fabric of China, the possession of a local *hukou* serves as a determinant of urban citizenship, fundamentally influencing an individual's eligibility for municipal public services [47]. Consequently, the hukou system is venerated as a pivotal metric for delineating citizenship identities. To attain precise measurements of *hukou* at a fine scale, this study employs spatially referenced mobile phone data, amalgamated with demographic and social activity data extracted from an anonymized cohort of users. This data consortium is procured through a collaborative endeavor with the Xi'an Public Security Bureau, which manages the data of all mobile phone users in Xi'an. Subjected to a stringent protocol of anonymization and aggregation, the data are distilled into a matrix of 1 km × 1 km grid cells for analysis. The dataset encompasses key variables, including the percentage of nonlocal residents within the municipal confines of Xi'an, which is calculated as follows:

1. The historical locations during the daytime (i.e., 9 a.m. to 6 p.m.) were spatially mapped onto the grid cells, and the population within each grid was computed.
2. The historical locations during the nighttime (i.e., 12 a.m. to 6 a.m.) were spatially mapped onto the grid cells, and the population within each grid was computed.
3. The daytime population and nighttime population within each grid were combined and integrated with *hukou* registration data. The percentage of nonlocal residents within each grid is then determined as the percentage of residents with *hukou* registered in cities other than Xi'an relative to the total population within that grid.

Given the onerous computational demands of processing an entire annum of mobile phone data, a judicious balance was struck between computational complexity and analytical precision. To this end, we opted to focus on eight discrete and specific dates from the year 2021, selected to capture a spectrum of seasonal variations and weekly intervals. The chosen dates include 17 March (Wednesday), 20 March (Saturday), 16 June (Wednesday), 19 June (Saturday), 15 September (Wednesday), 18 September (Saturday), 24 November (Wednesday), and 27 November (Saturday). The selection of these dates is predicated on their representation of both weekdays and weekends, unencumbered by traditional Chinese festivals, which are known to induce aberrations in the typical spatial mobility patterns of individuals.

2.2.3. House Price Data

Relative residential property value, or housing price, is regarded as a socioeconomic status (SES) measure in geographical research [48]. Hence, this study uses the secondhand housing price per unit area as an indicator of neighborhood SES. The data were acquired from KE Holdings Inc., Beijing, China (also known as *Beike*), China's leading online and offline real estate brokerage and portal company, accessible via www.ke.com. Acknowledging the dynamic nature of real estate data subject to real-time market oscillations, this study meticulously selected housing price data that reflect the prevailing market conditions as of the 11th day of March in the year 2023, thereby ensuring the temporal relevance and accuracy of the SES indicators utilized in the analysis.

The house price data are stratified across two spatial hierarchical dimensions: (1) subdistricts, represented as polygon geometries; and (2) microdistricts, denoted as points. The term "subdistricts" refers to designated areas under the jurisdiction of local suburban governments. The term "microdistricts" alludes to enclosed areas with essential services provided within these gated communities and has been employed as a mechanism for smaller-scale administration by the Chinese government, as elucidated by Tomba [49]. These dual classifications provide critical stratigraphic signifiers for the spatially variable socioeconomic status and the segmentation of social collectives along the spectrum of social strata. Employing geostatistical interpolation techniques, this study harnesses subdistrict boundaries as natural barriers and microdistricts as anchor points for the spatial modeling process. Consequently, the resultant house price surface is collapsed into a homogenized grid system, with each cell measuring 1 km × 1 km, thereby rendering the data amenable to subsequent analytical endeavors. This aggregation not only streamlines the dataset for tractable analysis but also preserves the nuanced spatial dynamics that are intrinsic to the socioeconomic landscape under investigation.

2.3. *Dependent Variable and Independent Variables*

In geographically weighted regression analysis (see Section 2.4.3), the dependent variable at the grid level is determined as follows:

- $PM_{2.5}$ exposure is empirically quantified through the calculation of the mean $PM_{2.5}$ concentration during both daytime and nighttime.

The independent variables include:

- Citizenship identity is measured by the percentage of the nonlocal population residing in a given grid.
- Social stratum is operationalized as socioeconomic status and measured by the mean price of secondhand houses within a particular grid.

2.4. *Analytical Methods*

2.4.1. Interpolation Techniques

The daily $PM_{2.5}$ concentrations, in their unadjusted form, were estimated using the general kriging method. The kriging operations were executed within the ArcGIS Pro® 3.2 environment, with default parameter settings.

To establish the secondhand housing price surface, a diffusion interpolation with barriers was employed, wherein the boundaries of subdistricts function as barriers to the interpolation process. This computational procedure was also performed using ArcGIS Pro® 3.2.

2.4.2. Global and Local Spatial Autocorrelation

The Global Moran's I index is used as a diagnostic tool to assess the presence and strength of spatial autocorrelation. This metric quantifies the linear correlation between the values of a given variable within a specific geographic unit and the spatially weighted mean values of the same variable across neighboring geographic units. In our analysis, Global Moran's I was applied to quantify the degree of spatial autocorrelation observed in several important variables, including the percentage of nonlocal residents and housing prices. Furthermore, it was employed in the measurement of spatial autocorrelation within the residuals of the GWR (geographically weighted regression) model. To gain deeper insight into pinpointing clusters with high or low values, as well as identifying spatial outliers, we further employed Anselin Local Moran's I, also known as cluster and outlier analysis. The global Moran's I and Anselin Local Moran's I were calculated using ArcGIS Pro® 3.2.

2.4.3. Geographically Weighted Regression

The primary aim of this paper is to uncover spatial inequities in $PM_{2.5}$ exposure, with a particular focus on identifying areas where there exists a positive correlation between the percentage of the nonlocal residents (a proxy for citizenship identity) and $PM_{2.5}$ concentration levels, and, conversely, areas where there is a negative correlation between the average housing price (a proxy for social stratum) and $PM_{2.5}$ concentration. To achieve this, it is imperative to employ an algorithm capable of detecting localized patterns among these variables.

Geographically weighted regression (GWR) facilitates the exploration of varying relationships between independent and dependent variables across locales [50,51]. In this study, we employed GWR to elucidate the spatially varying relationships between $PM_{2.5}$

exposure and two key independent variables: the percentage of the nonlocal population and the average housing price. The GWR model computes localized estimates of β_p at each location i by utilizing the centroids associated with the grid data. The construction of three models are as follows.

Model 1: The mathematical representation of the model regarding daytime $PM_{2.5}$ concentrations and the nonlocal population is as follows:

$$y_i = \beta_{i0} + \beta_{i1}X_{i1} + \varepsilon_i \quad (2)$$

where y_i denotes the daytime $PM_{2.5}$ concentration at grid i in 2021, X_{i1} denotes the percentage of the nonlocal population at grid i in 2021, β_{i0} denotes the localized realization of the constant at grid i, β_{i1} denotes the localized realization of the coefficient of the percentage of the nonlocal population at grid i, and ε_i denotes the localized realization of the error item at grid i.

Model 2: The mathematical representation of the model regarding nighttime $PM_{2.5}$ concentrations and the nonlocal population is the same as Equation (2), but y_i denotes the nighttime $PM_{2.5}$ concentrations at grid i in 2021.

Model 3: The mathematical representation of the model for nighttime $PM_{2.5}$ concentrations and the housing price follows Equation (2), where y_i denotes the nighttime $PM_{2.5}$ concentration at grid i in 2021, and X_{i1} denotes the average housing price at grid i in 2021.

Given that the urban population typically gravitates towards the city center for employment and leisure activities during daytime hours, giving rise to an inconsistency between the population and their residences, the model regarding daytime $PM_{2.5}$ concentrations and the housing price is not applicable and will not be fitted.

To estimate the models, we leveraged the package "spgwr" in the R programming environment (version 4.1.3), as detailed by Bivand [52]. The "gwr.sel" function from the "spgwr" package is invoked to ascertain the optimal bandwidth selection for the GWR models.

2.4.4. Sensitivity Analysis

Given that the estimation of the nonlocal residents at each grid for the year 2021 is predicated on a mere eight-day sample, it is important to apply a sensitivity analysis to determine whether the choice of which days to select has an impact on the results. Hence, we fit the following quarter-specific models:

Model 4: The mathematical representation of the quarter-specific relationship between daytime $PM_{2.5}$ concentrations and the nonlocal population is as follows:

$$y_{i,q} = \beta_{i0,q} + \beta_{i1,q}X_{i1,q} + \varepsilon_{i,q} \quad (3)$$

where $y_{i,q}$ denotes the daytime $PM_{2.5}$ concentration at grid i in quarter q, $X_{i1,q}$ denotes the percentage of the nonlocal population at grid i in quarter q, $\beta_{i0,q}$ denotes the localized realization of the constant at grid i in quarter q, $\beta_{i1,q}$ denotes the localized realization of the coefficient of the percentage of the nonlocal population at grid i in quarter q, and $\varepsilon_{i,q}$ denotes the localized realization of the error item at grid i in quarter q.

Model 5: The mathematical representation of the quarter-specific relationship between nighttime $PM_{2.5}$ concentrations and the nonlocal population is formed in the same way as Equation (3), but where $y_{i,q}$ denotes the nighttime $PM_{2.5}$ concentrations at grid i in quarter q; the others remain the same as in Model 4.

Finally, we construct a pattern robustness indicator to describe the robustness of the detected inequality pattern regarding the citizenship identities in each grid, given as

$$R_{t,i} = \sum_{q=1}^{4} Sig_{t,q,i} \quad (4)$$

where $R_{t,i}$ refers to the pattern robustness of grid i for timespan t (daytime or nighttime), and $Sig_{t,q,i}$ is defined as

$$Sig_{t,q,i} = \begin{cases} 1, \; b_{t,q,i} > 0 \; and \; is \; significant \\ 0, \; otherwise \end{cases} \tag{5}$$

where $b_{t,q,i}$ refers to the localized realization of the coefficient of the percentage of the nonlocal population at grid i in quarter q for timespan t (i.e., daytime or nighttime, coming from Model 4 and Model 5, respectively). The level of significance was set to 0.05.

The sensitivity analysis was also performed in the R programming environment (version 4.1.3), with the "spgwr" package.

3. Results

3.1. The Spatiotemporal Patterns of the $PM_{2.5}$ Concentration

As illustrated in Figure A1, by 2021, the prevailing conditions in Xi'an had largely returned to prepandemic norms. Hence, it is reasonable to examine the $PM_{2.5}$ concentration in 2021 in this study.

Figure 3 presents the daily estimated $PM_{2.5}$ concentration in Xi'an throughout 2021, subdivided into three panels representing the entire day, daytime, and nighttime. Notably, Friday exhibits the peak $PM_{2.5}$ concentration levels, whereas Monday exhibits the lowest concentration (excluding during the daytime) over the course of the week. Figure 3 further signifies a progressive increase in concentrations from Monday to Friday, followed by a subsequent decrease from Friday to the ensuing Monday.

In terms of seasonal fluctuations, $PM_{2.5}$ concentrations typically increase from late fall through early spring, encompassing a five-month period from November to March. During this interval, the recorded concentrations predominantly align with the Interim Target 2, with values ranging from 37.5 to 50 $\mu g/m^3$ and even more severe concentrations. These values are juxtaposed against the "recommended long- and short-term AQG levels and interim targets" as stipulated by the World Health Organization [53]. Conversely, from mid-May to mid-October, concentrations tend to be relatively lower, primarily falling within the range of the AQG level (0 to 15 $\mu g/m^3$) and Interim Target 3 (25 to 37.5 $\mu g/m^3$). Figure A2 presents the corresponding results according to the ambient air quality standards issued by the Ministry of Ecology and Environment of the People's Republic of China [54].

Figure 4 shows the spatial distribution of the $PM_{2.5}$ concentration in Xi'an for the year 2021. It visualizes both annual data and quarterly variations. With respect to the annual tendencies, heightened $PM_{2.5}$ concentrations are noted in the northwestern sectors of the city, whereas comparatively diminished levels are observed in the southeastern reaches. During the nighttime, $PM_{2.5}$ concentrations are higher in the northwest and lower in the southeast of the city, while $PM_{2.5}$ concentrations are higher in the center of the city in the daytime. In the southeast, the daytime and nighttime concentrations are relatively similar. Conversely, the daytime concentrations are significantly lower than the nighttime concentrations in the northwest.

Quarterly fluctuations in the spatial distribution patterns of the $PM_{2.5}$ concentration are observed. In the first quarter, the distribution pattern shows higher concentrations in the west and lower concentrations in the east. In the second and third quarters, a southward dip in concentrations is observed, with concentrations radiating outward to the surrounding areas. In the fourth quarter, the distribution pattern aligns with the annual trend, exhibiting lower concentrations in the southeast and higher concentrations in the northwest. According to the analysis of diurnal variations, significant differences existed between daytime and nighttime concentrations in the first and fourth quarters. In the second and third quarters, the daytime and nighttime concentrations exhibit less pronounced differences; however, the nighttime concentrations in the southern part of the city are surprisingly lower than the daytime concentrations, which is contrary to the observed annual pattern. Furthermore, the daytime $PM_{2.5}$ concentrations are greater than the nighttime $PM_{2.5}$ concentrations in the third quarter, which is also contrary to the observed annual pattern.

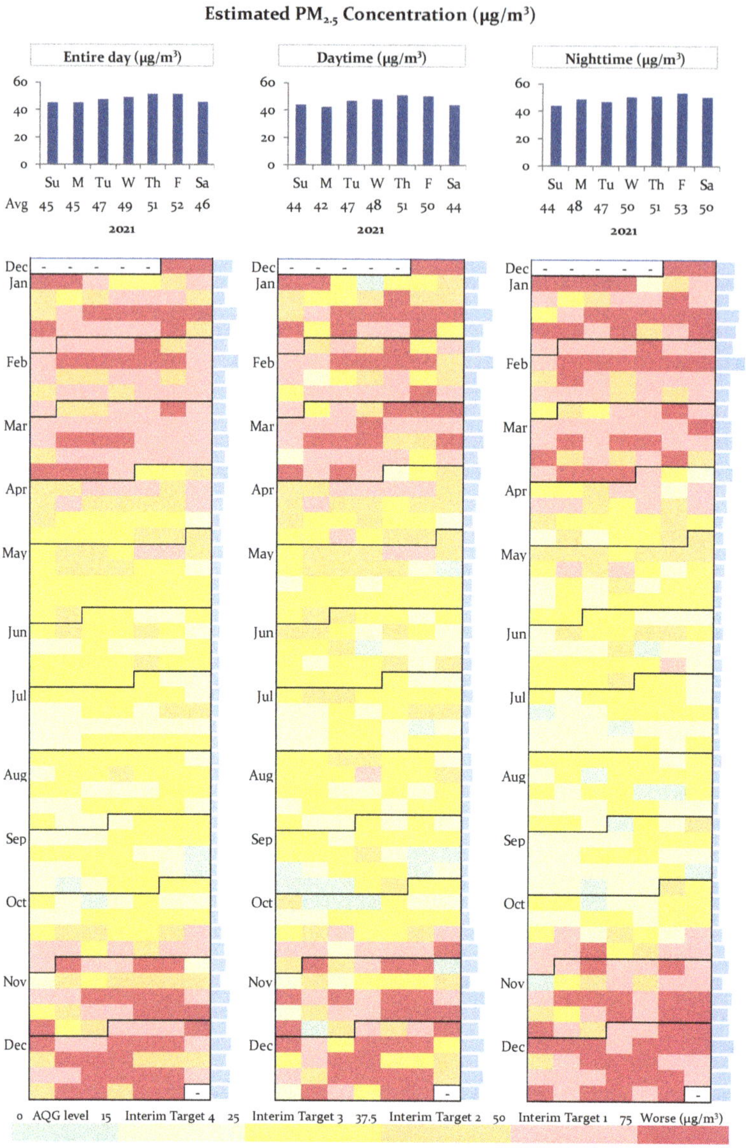

Figure 3. Temporal distribution of the $PM_{2.5}$ concentration across 2021, depicting the daily, weekly, and weekly mean variations in the $PM_{2.5}$ concentration. The breaks and labels of $PM_{2.5}$ concentration adhere to the guidelines established by the World Health Organization [53]. The "entire day" corresponds to 00:00 to 23:59; "daytime" spans from 9 a.m. to 6 p.m.; and "nighttime" encompasses the hours from 12 a.m. to 6 a.m. The definitions of daytime and nighttime align with those used for mobile phone data. This chart was created using the Calendar Chart Template from Vertex42.com [55].

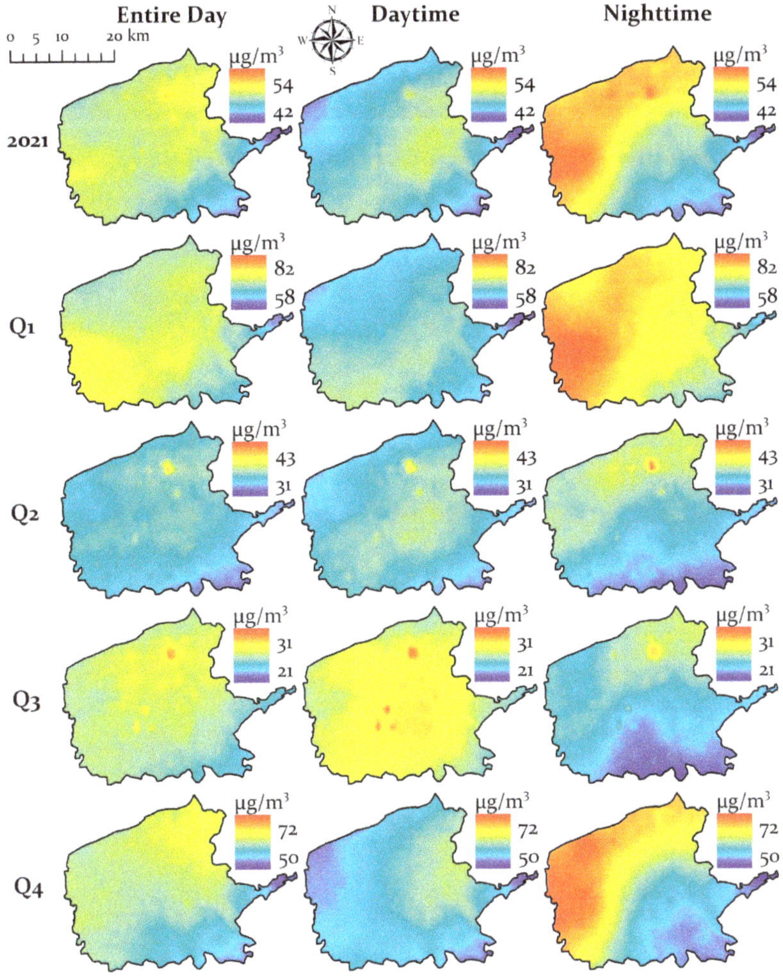

Figure 4. Spatial distribution of the $PM_{2.5}$ concentration in Xi'an in 2021. To account for the significant differences among quarters, the color bar ranges are consistent within each quarter (or for annual subplots). Q1 to Q4 refer to quarters 1 to 4, respectively. The "entire day" corresponds to 00:00 to 23:59; "daytime" spans from 9 a.m. to 6 p.m.; and "nighttime" encompasses the hours from 12 a.m. to 6 a.m. The definitions of daytime and nighttime align with those used for mobile phone data.

3.2. Environmental Inequality in Terms of $PM_{2.5}$ Exposure

Figure 5 illustrates the spatial distribution of the percentage of nonlocal residents in the four quarters of 2021 and housing price (CNY/m^2) for the same year. The spatial distribution of the percentage of nonlocal residents reveals a distinct pattern, with elevated values in the northwestern sector and diminished values in the southeastern sector. Housing prices display a characteristic centralized distribution pattern. Notably, three clusters with low values are observed in the northwestern, northern, and eastern sections of the urban area, while the southern and northeastern parts of the city exhibit three clusters with high-value concentrations.

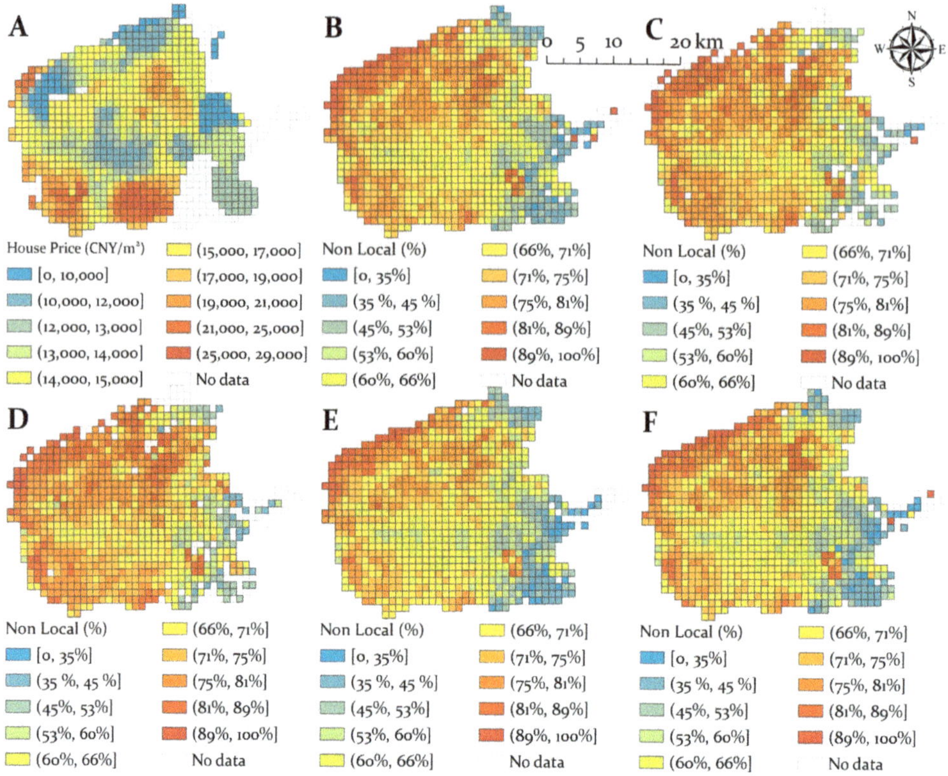

Figure 5. Spatial distributions of the independent variables. (**A**) The estimated housing price in 2021 (using data from 11 March 2023); (**B**) the percentage of nonlocal residents in 2021; (**C**) the percentage of nonlocal residents in 2021 quarter 1; (**D**) the percentage of nonlocal residents in 2021 quarter 2; (**E**) the percentage of nonlocal residents in 2021 quarter 3; (**F**) the percentage of nonlocal residents in 2021 quarter 4.

As indicated in Table 1 and Figure 6, the percentage of nonlocal residents and the housing price both exhibit significant global and local spatial autocorrelation, suggesting the reasonableness of using GWR models. Figure A3 displays the bivariate relationship between independent and dependent variables, suggesting the potential for both linear and polynomial relationships. In response to this, an exhaustive enumeration of parameter combinations was conducted, encompassing variable relationships (linear, quadratic, or cubic) and bandwidth parameters (including bandwidth adaptivity, optimization method, and geographical weighting function). A comparative assessment of their goodness of fit was executed, with the findings presented in Table S1. The results reveal that the incorporation of polynomial relationships does not confer a superior fit for the models. Consequently, linear models, specifically Models 1, 2, and 3, as per Equation (2), were selected for their optimal balance of fit and interpretability. The parameters of these chosen models are presented in Table S2.

Table 1. Global Moran's I of independent variables.

Variable	Moran's I	Z Score	p Value
Estimated housing price in 2021	0.751	62.665	0.000
Percentage of nonlocal residents in year 2021	0.652	58.688	0.000
Percentage of nonlocal residents in 2021 quarter 1	0.600	50.443	0.000
Percentage of nonlocal residents in 2021 quarter 2	0.628	52.484	0.000
Percentage of nonlocal residents in 2021 quarter 3	0.730	65.472	0.000
Percentage of nonlocal residents in 2021 quarter 4	0.650	58.252	0.000

Parameters used in ArcGIS Pro tool Spatial Autocorrelation (Global Moran's I) (Spatial Statistics Tools): Conceptualization of Spatial Relationships: FIXED_DISTANCE_BAND; Distance Method: EUCLIDEAN_DISTANCE; Standardization: ROW; Distance Band or Threshold Distance: 2341.

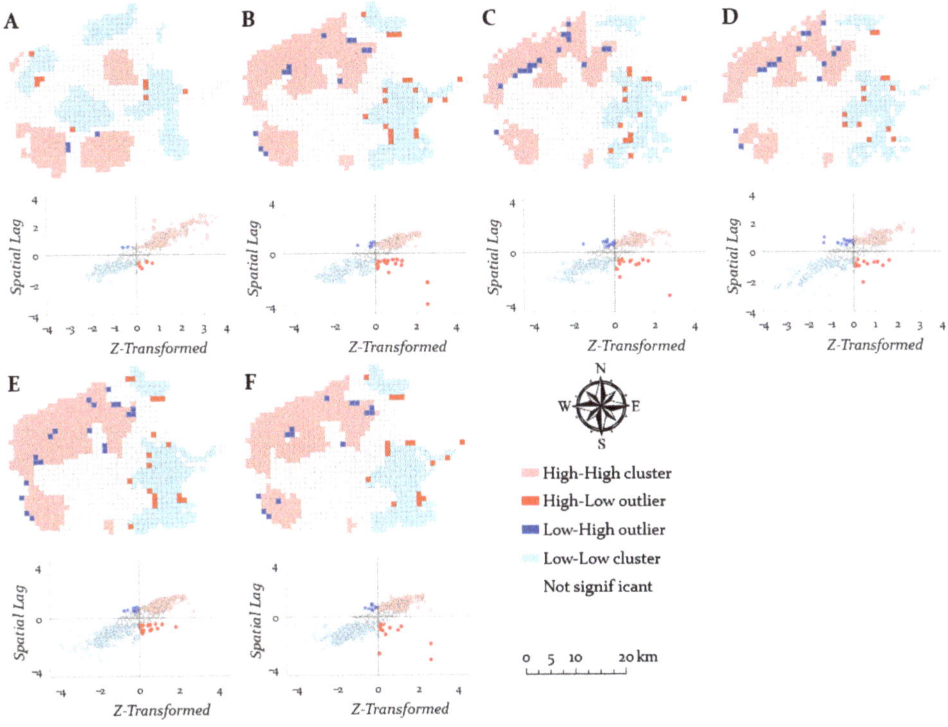

Figure 6. Moran's scatterplots and Anselin Local Moran's I for the independent variables. (**A**) The estimated housing price in 2021 (using data from 11 March 2023); (**B**) the percentage of nonlocal residents in 2021; (**C**) the percentage of nonlocal residents in 2021 quarter 1; (**D**) the percentage of nonlocal residents in 2021 quarter 2; (**E**) the percentage of nonlocal residents in 2021 quarter 3; (**F**) the percentage of nonlocal residents in 2021 quarter 4.

Figure 7A–C present the results of GWR models investigating spatiotemporal patterns of inequality in $PM_{2.5}$ exposure, regarding the percentage of nonlocal residents and housing prices, across the city. Positive significance indicates greater $PM_{2.5}$ exposure in areas with a greater percentage of nonlocal residents, as shown in Figure 7A,B. Conversely, negative significance denotes areas with reduced housing prices correlating with increased $PM_{2.5}$

exposure, as shown in Figure 7C. The inequality related to the percentage of nonlocal residents is particularly pronounced in the northwestern and southern sectors of the city, which are characterized by lower housing prices, as identified in Figure 5. The inequality related to housing prices is observed in various urban regions, indicating a more complex spatial dynamic. Figure 7D,E graphically represent the robustness of the inequality pattern (i.e., significant outcomes observed in quarterly regressions), particularly focusing on the daytime and nighttime percentages of nonlocal residents exposed to $PM_{2.5}$, respectively. The consistency of spatial distributions of daytime and nighttime $PM_{2.5}$ exposure inequality patterns across different quarters suggests the robustness of the observed trends. Notably, nighttime patterns display more enhanced robustness than daytime patterns. Hence, Figure 7D,E illustrate that the choice of which days to select has a slight impact on the results presented in Figure 7A,B.

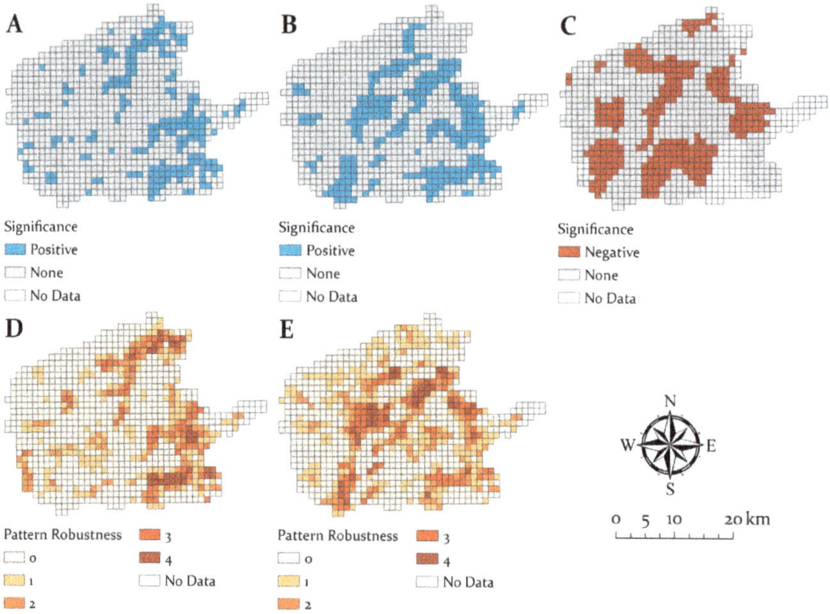

Figure 7. Localized $PM_{2.5}$ exposure inequality pattern and sensitivity analysis. (**A**) Results of Model 1, regarding daytime $PM_{2.5}$ concentration and the percentage of nonlocal population. (**B**) Results of Model 2, regarding nighttime $PM_{2.5}$ concentration and the percentage of nonlocal population. (**C**) Results of Model 3, regarding nighttime $PM_{2.5}$ concentration and the secondhand housing price. (**D**) Sensitivity analysis based on Model 4, regarding daytime $PM_{2.5}$ concentration and the percentage of nonlocal population in quarterly data. (**E**) Sensitivity analysis based on Model 5, regarding nighttime $PM_{2.5}$ concentration and the percentage of nonlocal population in quarterly data.

4. Discussion

4.1. Principal Findings

This study conducted a microscale analysis of $PM_{2.5}$ exposure variability within Xi'an city, leveraging housing price and mobile phone data to explore the correlation between $PM_{2.5}$ concentrations and pivotal social determinants: citizenship identity and socioeconomic status. The findings indicate that residents lacking local registration exhibit increased exposure to $PM_{2.5}$. Additionally, the research uncovers a mitigating effect of elevated socioeconomic status, which may afford individuals the agency to select residences in areas with reduced $PM_{2.5}$ concentrations. This suggests a social gradient in air pollution exposure, with implications for environmental justice and urban planning.

4.2. Comparison with Previous Work

This research augments the burgeoning literature on environmental inequality in the context of air pollution exposure. A number of recent studies have endeavored to elucidate the environmental inequality in air pollution exposure in China [10,22–25,30]. At the macroscale (e.g., national scale), existing studies have predominantly discovered correlations between spatial distribution of $PM_{2.5}$ concentration and regional population density and land cover types, among several others [28,56].

At the urban scale, research (e.g., studies focused on Beijing, Nanjing and Wuhan) has found the association between $PM_{2.5}$ concentration and walkability of streets, land uses, and found that air pollution exposure risks for children and the elderly are uneven [10,23,57]. Studies in China found that the risk of $PM_{2.5}$ exposure varies with age, income, gender, etc. [22,57]. Notably, the elderly, who experience higher risk of air pollution exposure, are mainly located in the central and peripheral urban zones [10]. J. Chen et al. [58] found that risk of environmental pollution exposure of residents varies with migration status, and migrants from rural places have higher risk of environmental pollution exposure. However, the study was aimed at the national scale, and there is a lack of understanding of the microscale variation within the city.

Our study bridges this gap by dissecting the environmental inequality in $PM_{2.5}$ exposure at grid scale. We have unveiled the spatial distribution of $PM_{2.5}$ concentration and their associations with social strata and citizenship identity of the ambient population at a grid scale. This microscale analysis complements the national-level studies by extending the discourse to include the intricate relationship between an individual's socioeconomic status and citizenship, and their exposure to air pollution risks. This approach provides a more nuanced understanding of environmental inequality, transitioning from a macroscopic perspective to a more localized scale.

4.3. Practical Implications

Our findings suggest that the observed environmental inequality in $PM_{2.5}$ exposure in Xi'an can be partly attributed to historical and ongoing disparities in urban planning. While the specific reasons behind these disparities require further investigation, our analysis of the city's general master plan (2008–2035) reveals a persistent neglect of the northwestern sector, characterized by an absence of environmental amenities, such as green belts, and a dearth of access to vital public services [59,60]. This neglect has rendered the area's residents susceptible to the adverse effects of air pollution, reflecting a broader pattern of environmental injustice where marginalized communities are disproportionately affected by environmental hazards.

The spatial distribution of $PM_{2.5}$ exposure may also be influenced by social dynamics, with nonlocal residents potentially forming residential clusters due to weaker social ties or cultural integration with the local community [61,62]. The concentration of nonlocal residents in the northwestern district, exacerbated by limited policy focus and economic development, further contributes to the environmental inequality.

To address these intertwined issues, a comprehensive and multifaceted strategy is warranted:

Housing affordability issue in less polluted areas. Introduce financial assistance programs and subsidies aimed at making housing in less polluted areas accessible to low-income nonlocal residents. Additionally, invest in affordable housing development in less polluted areas to alleviate the concentration of vulnerable populations near pollution sources.

Mitigating pollution sources in the northwestern district. Implement stricter environmental regulations for industries in the northwestern district to curtail $PM_{2.5}$ emissions. Promote sustainable development through investment in clean technologies and alternative energy sources, and consider the strategic relocation of polluting industries to less populated industrial zones.

Enhancing public services in less developed areas. Direct investment towards infrastructure improvements in underdeveloped areas, with an emphasis on public transportation, healthcare facilities, and educational opportunities. The development of green spaces and parks can simultaneously enhance air quality and offer residents access to recreational spaces.

Promoting social integration and reducing discrimination. Enact antidiscrimination policies to protect nonlocal residents from biased housing practices, and ensuring equitable access to opportunities regardless of their citizenship status. Encourage social integration programs to build a cohesive community with a collective commitment to environmental health.

Utilizing environmental justice frameworks in urban planning. Embed principles of environmental justice into urban planning frameworks to ensure a just distribution of environmental resources and to mitigate the disparate impacts of environmental hazards across different socioeconomic and citizenship groups. Mandate comprehensive environmental impact assessments for new developments to evaluate and balance air quality implications and environmental benefits equitably.

These policy recommendations, grounded in the study's findings, necessitate a nuanced understanding of local contexts, collaborative efforts among diverse stakeholders, and vigilant monitoring to ensure their efficacy in redressing environmental inequalities.

4.4. Strengths and Limitations

This study presents a useful attempt to quantitatively evaluate the fine-scale disparities in air pollution exposure predicated on social strata and citizenship identity. Our empirical study affirms the viability of examining the spatial variation of air pollution exposure at grid scale. Two important measures, citizenship identity and social stratum, can be quantified using mobile phone big data. To be specific, the citizenship identity can be quantified using the percentage of nonlocal population residing in a grid, and social stratum can be operationalized as socioeconomic status and measured by the average price of secondhand houses within in a grid.

Despite the study's contributions, it is circumscribed by limitations that set the stage for future research. The findings are limited to the grid scale, which warrants exploration of more discrete geographical entities such as subdistricts and microdistricts to attain a heightened level of granularity. Additionally, the research's scope did not encompass occupational-based inequalities due to an absence of professional data on residents, underscoring the need for multifaceted data sources in subsequent studies.

The utilization of housing prices as an index of socioeconomic status is not without its challenges, particularly given the constraints in procuring data for the year 2021. The COVID-19 pandemic's variegated effects on housing prices further complicate the use of 2023 data as a proxy for the preceding year. While the robust correlation coefficient of 0.7449 between the average housing prices of 2021 and March 2023 at the subdistrict level substantiates the study's data strategy (as detailed in Appendix B), the acquisition of historical data remains an imperative for future research endeavors.

Furthermore, the calculation of the nonlocal resident ratio is currently anchored in data from a mere eight days, casting uncertainty over the established weekday–weekend pattern. Although sensitivity analysis indicates minimal impact from the specific days selected, a more expansive temporal framework is advisable for future research to solidify this metric. Lastly, the potential influence of unaccounted confounding factors on $PM_{2.5}$ exposure cannot be discounted, necessitating the integration of a wider array of variables in forthcoming studies to deepen our comprehension of this intricate phenomenon.

5. Conclusions

This study elucidates the environmental inequality pertaining to $PM_{2.5}$ exposure in Xi'an, with a particular focus on the inordinate burden shouldered by nonlocal residents in the city's northwestern quadrant. A stark contrast is observed in the $PM_{2.5}$ concentrations experienced by these residents as opposed to those inhabiting the southern regions, who are generally characterized by higher socioeconomic status and are favored with improved air quality. Our paper identifies citizenship identity and social strata as key factors contributing to the observed inequality. Furthermore, we explored potential underlying causes related to historical and ongoing disparities in urban planning and the *hukou* system, which can limit access to opportunities and resources based on residency status. This research contributes to a growing body of knowledge on environmental justice, highlighting the complex interplay between social and spatial factors in shaping environmental exposure risks.

In sum, this research provides a spatial lens through which to view the social inequalities engendered by identity, power, and economic factors, as reflected in $PM_{2.5}$ exposure levels in Xi'an. By acknowledging the limitations and identifying areas for future research, this study sets the stage for the advancement of efficacious strategies aimed at redressing environmental inequalities and promoting a more just and equitable urban milieu that is sensitive to the environmental rights and wellbeing of all its inhabitants.

Supplementary Materials: The following supporting information can be downloaded at: https://www.mdpi.com/article/10.3390/ijgi13070257/s1, Figure S1: Bivariate relationship between $PM_{2.5}$ concentration and the percentage of nonlocal population; Table S1: Parameter and goodness of fit of all models; Table S2: Parameter and goodness of fit of selected models.

Author Contributions: Conceptualization, Li He; methodology, Li He and Lingfeng He; software, Lingfeng He; validation, Li He and Lingfeng He; formal analysis, Li He and Lingfeng He; investigation, Li He, Lingfeng He, Zhongmin Wang, Ping An, and Min Liu; resources: Li He and Lingfeng He; data curation, Lingfeng He, Zhongmin Wang, Ping An, and Min Liu; writing—original draft preparation, Li He, Lingfeng He, Zezheng Lin, Yao Lu, and Shurui Gao; writing—review and editing, Li He, Lingfeng He, Zezheng Lin, Chen Chen, and Jie Xu; visualization, Li He and Lingfeng He; supervision, Li He; project administration, Li He; funding acquisition, Li He. Li He and Lingfeng He contributed equally to this work. All authors have read and agreed to the published version of the manuscript.

Funding: This research was funded by the Ministry of Education, Humanities and Social Sciences Research Youth Foundation, China (No. 20YJC840014), the National Natural Science Foundation of China (No. 42001164), and Research Project on Forging a Sense of Community for the Chinese Nation in Shaanxi Province (No. 2024MZW001). The APC was funded by the Ministry of Education, Humanities and Social Sciences Research Youth Foundation, China (No. 20YJC840014) and the National Natural Science Foundation of China (No. 42001164).

Data Availability Statement: Mobile phones are not available due to the information security requirements. House price data and code used in data collection, data processing, and data analysis are available via https://github.com/CenterForSocialComputing/ijgi-spatial-inequality-of-PM2.5-exposure.

Conflicts of Interest: The authors declare no conflicts of interest.

Appendix A. Explanation of Variables Selection

For residents in China's big cities, whether they hold a household registration system is an important factor in whether they can buy a home and in which geographical area they can buy a home. The hukou system pointed out in this paper as a phenomenon of social strata division in China's big cities has been proved by many existing studies (e.g., [63–65]). The impact on the purchase of housing is mainly reflected in the following aspects:

Whether residents have local hukou directly affects the eligibility of residents to buy a house. Since the 2010s, all major cities have had limited home purchase policies. Most big cities have restrictions on who can buy a home, and one of the most important restrictions is household registration. Nonresidents usually need to meet certain conditions to buy a home, such as paying local social security or personal income taxes for a certain number of years. The vast majority of mainstream cities only allow qualified nonresident residents to settle down and, thus, qualify for a house purchase.

In addition, even for some urban residential areas which can allow nonregistered people to buy homes, they still bear higher loan rates and down payments than registered residents. For example, *Notice of the People's Bank of China on Adjusting the Policy on Personal Housing Loans* [66] stipulates that the down payment ratio of nonregistered residents to buy a first home shall not be less than 35%, and the loan interest rate shall not be less than 1.1 times the benchmark interest rate. Another example is *Notice on Adjusting and Optimizing the Standards for Ordinary Housing and Personal Housing Loan Policies in Beijing* [67], which stipulates that nonhousehold resident families must pay social security or personal income tax for five consecutive years when purchasing a house in Beijing.

Another example is that in the same city, different residents enjoy completely different public services. Registered residents can enjoy more public services, such as children's education and medical security. For example, *the Compulsory Education Law of the People's Republic of China* stipulates that school-age children and adolescents at the stage of compulsory education shall only receive education in schools where their "hukou registration is located". In addition, in many mainstream cities, many benefits, including pension insurance and unemployment insurance, are also highly tied to household registration.

Finally, the segregation of economic and social status caused by the household registration system causes the different economic status of different groups, and also affects the economic ability of more nonlocal residents to buy property in areas with better public services. The first is the barrier to migration: the household registration system restricts the freedom of migrant workers. Many are unable to move to higher-paying areas and attain better-paying formal jobs. Forced to perform more manual labor in big cities, they are confined to the primary labor market, known as "migrant workers", and are destined to struggle to buy better-served property. The existing high housing prices may cause the labor force to be unable to find long-term stable employment in the place of employment, and further aggravate the differentiation of social strata.

Appendix B. Explanation of Using House Price Data in 2023

Currently there are two methods to obtain the house price data: (1) online map services (e.g., API of Ke.com), and (2) the list of house sales (e.g., Web Pages of Anjuke.com). The advantage of Method 1 is that the collected data contain spatially referenced information that can be spatially matched with other spatial data used in this analysis, whereas the disadvantage is that we can only obtain real-time house prices; the historical house price data are not available. Method 2, on the contrary, is characterized by its capacity to yield historical data. However, this method is encumbered by the limitation that the data procured lack spatial referencing, a critical component for spatial analysis. Moreover, despite the inclusion of geographic textual descriptors within the dataset obtained through Method 2, the nonstandardized structure of this textual information poses significant challenges. The alignment of such data with that derived from Method 1 is rendered infeasible owing to these structural discrepancies. Additionally, the prevalent challenges associated with geocoding in the context of Chinese-based geospatial data are widely acknowledged within both industrial and academic spheres. Consequently, after a thorough evaluation of the methodological constraints and data integrity considerations, the utilization of data sourced via Method 2 was deliberately eschewed in favor of alternative datasets that better align with the spatial analysis requirements of our research.

As supplementary support for adopting Method 1, we conducted a correlation analysis on the historical data obtained through Method 2. These are subdistrict-level data, and after removing missing values, a total of $N = 118$ subdistricts located in the study area were taken into analysis. In the correlation analysis, X is the housing price of the subdistrict in March 2023, and Y is the average housing price of the subdistrict in 2021. We find that the correlation between X and Y is 0.7449. The high degree of linear correlation ensures the validity of the direction and significance of the GWR coefficients, as we only focus on the relative size of the coefficients rather than absolute size. This can serve as proof of the rationality of our data collection method.

Appendix C. Figures

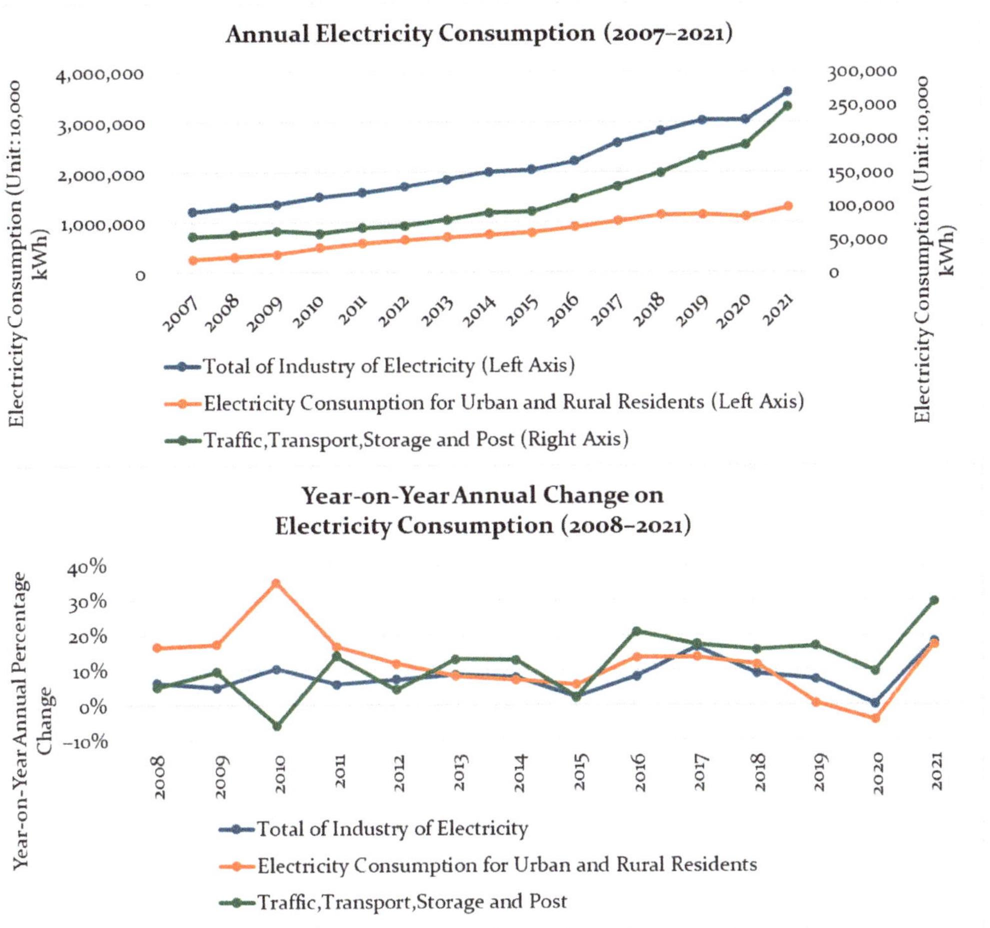

Figure A1. The annual electricity consumption and its year-on-year annual change from 2007 to 2021.

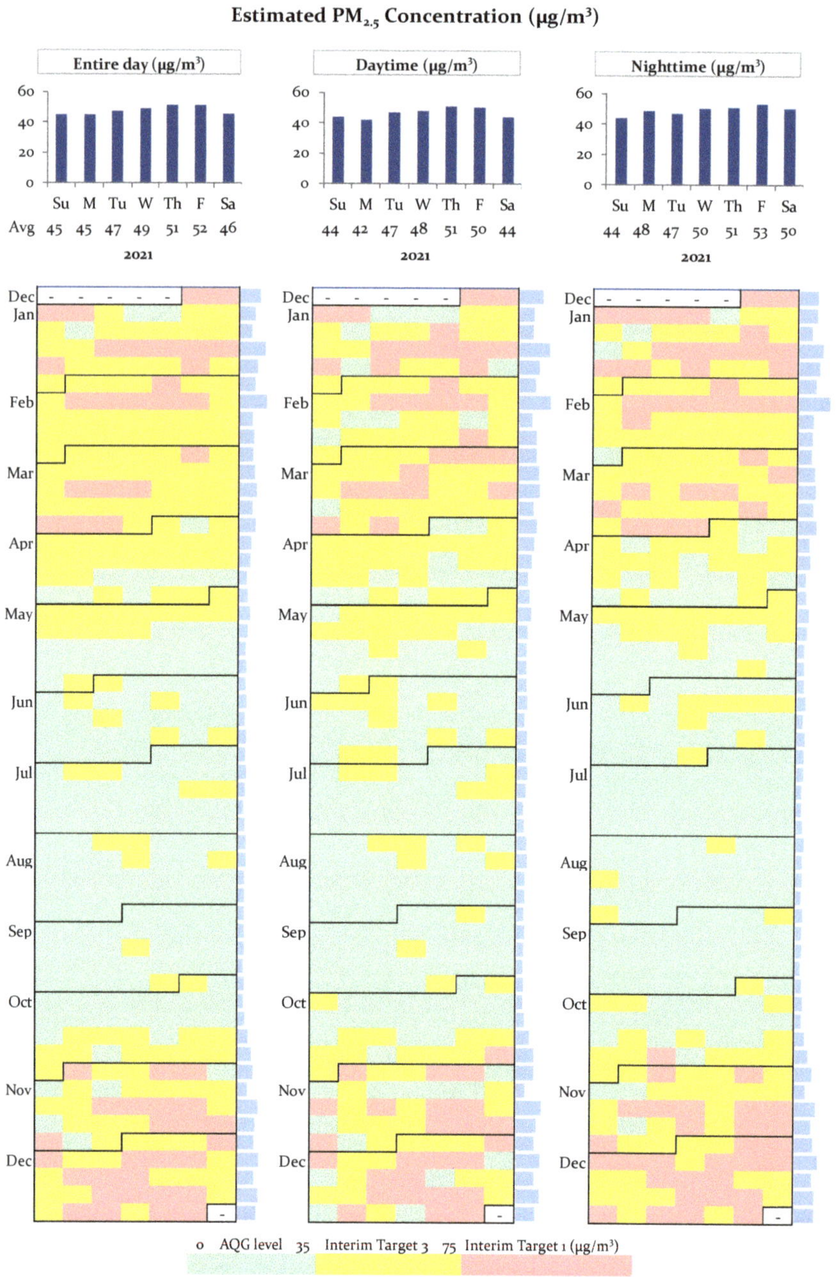

Figure A2. Temporal distribution of the $PM_{2.5}$ concentration across 2021, depicting the daily, weekly, and weekly mean variations in the $PM_{2.5}$ concentration. The breaks and labels of $PM_{2.5}$ concentration adhere to the guidelines established by the Ministry of Ecology and Environment of the People's Republic of China [54]. The "entire day" corresponds to 00:00 to 23:59; "daytime" spans from 9 a.m. to 6 p.m.; and "nighttime" encompasses the hours from 12 a.m. to 6 a.m. The definitions of daytime and nighttime align with those used for mobile phone data. This chart was created using the Calendar Chart Template from Vertex42.com [55].

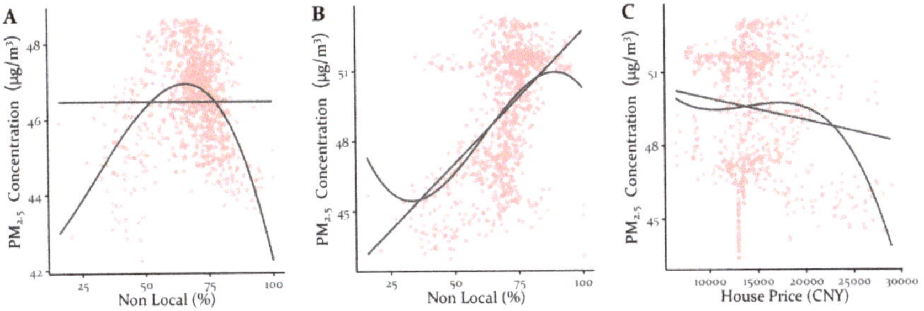

Figure A3. Bivariate relationship between $PM_{2.5}$ concentration and the percentage of nonlocal population and house price. (**A**) The daytime $PM_{2.5}$ concentration~the percentage of nonlocal. (**B**) The nighttime $PM_{2.5}$ concentration~the percentage of nonlocal population. (**C**) The daytime $PM_{2.5}$ concentration~housing price. Smooth lines are fitted using linear regression and polynomial regression, respectively. The "daytime" spans from 9 a.m. to 6 p.m.; and the "nighttime" encompasses the hours from 12 a.m. to 6 a.m.

References

1. Fiordelisi, A.; Piscitelli, P.; Trimarco, B.; Coscioni, E.; Iaccarino, G.; Sorriento, D. The Mechanisms of Air Pollution and Particulate Matter in Cardiovascular Diseases. *Heart Fail. Rev.* **2017**, *22*, 337–347. [CrossRef]
2. Hamra, G.B.; Guha, N.; Cohen, A.; Laden, F.; Raaschou-Nielsen, O.; Samet, J.M.; Vineis, P.; Forastiere, F.; Saldiva, P.; Yorifuji, T.; et al. Outdoor Particulate Matter Exposure and Lung Cancer: A Systematic Review and Meta-Analysis. *Environ. Health Perspect.* **2014**, *122*, 906–911. [CrossRef] [PubMed]
3. Liu, C.; Chen, R.; Sera, F.; Vicedo-Cabrera, A.M.; Guo, Y.; Tong, S.; Coelho, M.S.Z.S.; Saldiva, P.H.N.; Lavigne, E.; Matus, P.; et al. Ambient Particulate Air Pollution and Daily Mortality in 652 Cities. *N. Engl. J. Med.* **2019**, *381*, 705–715. [CrossRef] [PubMed]
4. Pui, D.Y.H.; Chen, S.-C.; Zuo, Z. PM2.5 in China: Measurements, Sources, Visibility and Health Effects, and Mitigation. *Particuology* **2014**, *13*, 1–26. [CrossRef]
5. Cao, J.; Xu, H.; Xu, Q.; Chen, B.; Kan, H. Fine Particulate Matter Constituents and Cardiopulmonary Mortality in a Heavily Polluted Chinese City. *Environ. Health Perspect.* **2012**, *120*, 373–378. [CrossRef]
6. Crouse, D.L.; Peters, P.A.; van Donkelaar, A.; Goldberg, M.S.; Villeneuve, P.J.; Brion, O.; Khan, S.; Atari, D.O.; Jerrett, M.; Pope, C.A.; et al. Risk of Non Accidental and Cardiovascular Mortality in Relation to Long-Term Exposure to Low Concentrations of Fine Particulate Matter: A Canadian National-Level Cohort Study. *Environ. Health Perspect.* **2012**, *120*, 708–714. [CrossRef]
7. Weuve, J.; Puett, R.C.; Schwartz, J.; Yanosky, J.D.; Laden, F.; Grodstein, F. Exposure to Particulate Air Pollution and Cognitive Decline in Older Women. *Arch. Intern. Med.* **2012**, *172*, 219–227. [CrossRef] [PubMed]
8. Braithwaite, I.; Zhang, S.; Kirkbride, J.B.; Osborn, D.P.J.; Hayes, J.F. Air Pollution (Particulate Matter) Exposure and Associations with Depression, Anxiety, Bipolar, Psychosis and Suicide Risk: A Systematic Review and Meta-Analysis. *Environ. Health Perspect.* **2019**, *127*, 126002. [CrossRef]
9. Asch, P.; Seneca, J.J. Some Evidence on the Distribution of Air Quality. *Land Econ.* **1978**, *54*, 278–297. [CrossRef]
10. Shan, Z.; Li, H.; Pan, H.; Yuan, M.; Xu, S. Spatial Equity of PM2.5 Pollution Exposures in High-Density Metropolitan Areas Based on Remote Sensing, LBS and GIS Data: A Case Study in Wuhan, China. *Int. J. Environ. Res. Public Health* **2022**, *19*, 12671. [CrossRef]
11. Gouveia, N.; Slovic, A.D.; Kanai, C.M.; Soriano, L. Air Pollution and Environmental Justice in Latin America: Where Are We and How Can We Move Forward? *Curr. Environ. Health Rep.* **2022**, *9*, 152–164. [CrossRef] [PubMed]
12. Jerrett, M.; Burnett, R.T.; Kanaroglou, P.; Eyles, J.; Finkelstein, N.; Giovis, C.; Brook, J.R. A GIS—Environmental Justice Analysis of Particulate Air Pollution in Hamilton, Canada. *Environ. Plan. A* **2001**, *33*, 955–973. [CrossRef]
13. Chakraborty, J. Cancer Risk from Exposure to Hazardous Air Pollutants: Spatial and Social Inequities in Tampa Bay, Florida. *Int. J. Environ. Health Res.* **2012**, *22*, 165–183. [CrossRef] [PubMed]
14. Zhou, Q.; Zhang, X.; Chen, J.; Zhang, Y. Do Double-Edged Swords Cut Both Ways? Housing Inequality and Haze Pollution in Chinese Cities. *Sci. Total Environ.* **2020**, *719*, 137404. [CrossRef] [PubMed]
15. Abel, T.D.; White, J. Skewed Riskscapes and Gentrified Inequities: Environmental Exposure Disparities in Seattle, Washington. *Am. J. Public Health* **2011**, *101*, S246–S254. [CrossRef] [PubMed]
16. Jiang, Y.; Yang, Y. Environmental Justice in Greater Los Angeles: Impacts of Spatial and Ethnic Factors on Residents' Socioeconomic and Health Status. *Int. J. Environ. Res. Public Health* **2022**, *19*, 5311. [CrossRef] [PubMed]
17. Maantay, J. Asthma and Air Pollution in the Bronx: Methodological and Data Considerations in Using GIS for Environmental Justice and Health Research. *Health Place* **2007**, *13*, 32–56. [CrossRef]

18. Stuart, A.L.; Mudhasakul, S.; Sriwatanapongse, W. The Social Distribution of Neighborhood-Scale Air Pollution and Monitoring Protection. *J. Air Waste Manag. Assoc.* **2009**, *59*, 591–602. [CrossRef] [PubMed]
19. Chakraborty, J.; Green, D. Australia's First National Level Quantitative Environmental Justice Assessment of Industrial Air Pollution. *Environ. Res. Lett.* **2014**, *9*, 044010. [CrossRef]
20. Ghorbani, S.; Salehi, E.; Faryadi, S.; Jafari, H.R. Geospatial Analysis of the Distribution of Air Pollutant Emissions in Tehran with a Focus on Environmental Justice. *Int. J. Ecosyst. Ecol. Sci.* **2020**, *10*, 235–248. [CrossRef]
21. Chaix, B.; Gustafsson, S.; Jerrett, M.; Kristersson, H.; Lithman, T.; Boalt, A.; Merlo, J. Children's Exposure to Nitrogen Dioxide in Sweden: Investigating Environmental Injustice in an Egalitarian Country. *J. Epidemiol. Community Health* **2006**, *60*, 234–241. [CrossRef] [PubMed]
22. Gu, L.; Rosenberg, M.; Zeng, J. The impacts of socioeconomic and environmental factors on self-rated health status among different income groups in China. *Geogr. Res.* **2017**, *36*, 1257–1270. [CrossRef]
23. Chen, X.; Feng, J. Health effects of built environment based on a comparison of walkability and air pollution:A case study of Nanjing City. *Prog. Geogr.* **2019**, *38*, 296–304. [CrossRef]
24. Fotheringham, A.S.; Yue, H.; Li, Z. Examining the Influences of Air Quality in China's Cities Using Multi-scale Geographically Weighted Regression. *Trans. GIS* **2019**, *23*, 1444–1464. [CrossRef]
25. Long, Y.; Wang, J.; Wu, K.; Zhang, J. Population Exposure to Ambient PM2.5 at the Subdistrict Level in China. *Int. J. Environ. Res. Public Health* **2018**, *15*, 2683. [CrossRef] [PubMed]
26. Crols, T.; Malleson, N. Quantifying the Ambient Population Using Hourly Population Footfall Data and an Agent-Based Model of Daily Mobility. *Geoinformatica* **2019**, *23*, 201–220. [CrossRef] [PubMed]
27. Liu, H.; Liu, J.; Li, M.; Gou, P.; Cheng, Y. Assessing the Evolution of PM2.5 and Related Health Impacts Resulting from Air Quality Policies in China. *Environ. Impact Assess. Rev.* **2022**, *93*, 106727. [CrossRef]
28. Zhang, Z.; Wang, J.; Hart, J.E.; Laden, F.; Zhao, C.; Li, T.; Zheng, P.; Li, D.; Ye, Z.; Chen, K. National Scale Spatiotemporal Land-Use Regression Model for PM2.5, PM10 and NO2 Concentration in China. *Atmos. Environ.* **2018**, *192*, 48–54. [CrossRef]
29. Xu, Y.; Wei, M.; Zou, B.; Guo, Z.; Li, S. Spatial-Temporal Variation and Spatial Differentiation Geographic Detection of PM2.5 Concentration in Shandong Province Based on Spatial Scale Effect. *Environ. Sci.* **2023**. *Online First*. [CrossRef]
30. Chen, B.; Song, Y.; Jiang, T.; Chen, Z.; Huang, B.; Xu, B. Real-Time Estimation of Population Exposure to PM2.5 Using Mobile- and Station-Based Big Data. *Int. J. Environ. Res. Public Health* **2018**, *15*, 573. [CrossRef]
31. He, L.; Páez, A.; Liu, D. Built Environment and Violent Crime: An Environmental Audit Approach Using Google Street View. *Comput. Environ. Urban Syst.* **2017**, *66*, 83–95. [CrossRef]
32. He, L.; Páez, A.; Jiao, J.; An, P.; Lu, C.; Mao, W.; Long, D. Ambient Population and Larceny-Theft: A Spatial Analysis Using Mobile Phone Data. *ISPRS Int. J. Geo-Inf.* **2020**, *9*, 342. [CrossRef]
33. Lai, S.; Bogoch, I.I.; Ruktanonchai, N.W.; Watts, A.; Lu, X.; Yang, W.; Yu, H.; Khan, K.; Tatem, A.J. Assessing Spread Risk of COVID-19 in Early 2020. *Data Sci. Manag.* **2022**, *5*, 212–218. [CrossRef]
34. Panigutti, C.; Tizzoni, M.; Bajardi, P.; Smoreda, Z.; Colizza, V. Assessing the Use of Mobile Phone Data to Describe Recurrent Mobility Patterns in Spatial Epidemic Models. *R. Soc. Open Sci.* **2017**, *4*, 160950. [CrossRef] [PubMed]
35. Reades, J.; Calabrese, F.; Ratti, C. Eigenplaces: Analysing Cities Using the Space—Time Structure of the Mobile Phone Network. *Environ. Plann. B* **2009**, *36*, 824–836. [CrossRef]
36. Sun, L.; Zhang, H.; Fang, C. Data Security Governance in the Era of Big Data: Status, Challenges, and Prospects. *Data Sci. Manag.* **2021**, *2*, 41–44. [CrossRef]
37. Abitbol, J.L.; Karsai, M. Interpretable Socioeconomic Status Inference from Aerial Imagery through Urban Patterns. *Nat. Mach. Intell.* **2020**, *2*, 684–692. [CrossRef]
38. Guo, S.; Fang, F.; Zhou, T.; Zhang, W.; Guo, Q.; Zeng, R.; Chen, X.; Liu, J.; Lu, X. Improving Google Flu Trends for COVID-19 Estimates Using Weibo Posts. *Data Sci. Manag.* **2021**, *3*, 13–21. [CrossRef]
39. Llorente, A.; Garcia-Herranz, M.; Cebrian, M.; Moro, E. Social Media Fingerprints of Unemployment. *PLoS ONE* **2015**, *10*, e0128692. [CrossRef] [PubMed]
40. Suel, E.; Bhatt, S.; Brauer, M.; Flaxman, S.; Ezzati, M. Multimodal Deep Learning from Satellite and Street-Level Imagery for Measuring Income, Overcrowding, and Environmental Deprivation in Urban Areas. *Remote Sens. Environ.* **2021**, *257*, 112339. [CrossRef]
41. Wang, L.; He, S.; Su, S.; Li, Y.; Hu, L.; Li, G. Urban Neighborhood Socioeconomic Status (SES) Inference: A Machine Learning Approach Based on Semantic and Sentimental Analysis of Online Housing Advertisements. *Habitat Int.* **2022**, *124*, 102572. [CrossRef]
42. Wei, J.; Li, Z.; Lyapustin, A.; Wang, J.; Dubovik, O.; Schwartz, J.; Sun, L.; Li, C.; Liu, S.; Zhu, T. First Close Insight into Global Daily Gapless 1 Km PM2.5 Pollution, Variability, and Health Impact. *Nat. Commun.* **2023**, *14*, 8349. [CrossRef] [PubMed]
43. Wang, X. Historical Data of Air Quality in China. Available online: https://quotsoft.net/air/ (accessed on 7 June 2022).
44. He, G.; Pan, Y.; Tanaka, T. The Short-Term Impacts of COVID-19 Lockdown on Urban Air Pollution in China. *Nat. Sustain.* **2020**, *3*, 1005–1011. [CrossRef]
45. Kumari, P.; Toshniwal, D. Impact of Lockdown on Air Quality over Major Cities across the Globe during COVID-19 Pandemic. *Urban Clim.* **2020**, *34*, 100719. [CrossRef] [PubMed]

46. Romanillos, G.; García-Palomares, J.C.; Moya-Gómez, B.; Gutiérrez, J.; Torres, J.; López, M.; Cantú-Ros, O.G.; Herranz, R. The City Turned off: Urban Dynamics during the COVID-19 Pandemic Based on Mobile Phone Data. *Appl. Geogr.* **2021**, *134*, 102524. [CrossRef] [PubMed]
47. Chan, K.W.; Zhang, L. The *Hukou* System and Rural-Urban Migration in China: Processes and Changes. *China Q.* **1999**, *160*, 818–855. [CrossRef] [PubMed]
48. Coffee, N.T.; Lockwood, T.; Hugo, G.; Paquet, C.; Howard, N.J.; Daniel, M. Relative Residential Property Value as a Socio-Economic Status Indicator for Health Research. *Int. J. Health Geogr.* **2013**, *12*, 22. [CrossRef] [PubMed]
49. Tomba, L. *The Government Next Door: Neighborhood Politics in Urban China*; Cornell University Press: Ithaca, NY, USA, 2014.
50. Páez, A.; Farber, S.; Wheeler, D. A Simulation-Based Study of Geographically Weighted Regression as a Method for Investigating Spatially Varying Relationships. *Environ. Plan. A* **2011**, *43*, 2992–3010. [CrossRef]
51. Lu, B.; Hu, Y.; Yang, D.; Liu, Y.; Liao, L.; Yin, Z.; Xia, T.; Dong, Z.; Harris, P.; Brunsdon, C.; et al. GWmodelS: A Software for Geographically Weighted Models. *SoftwareX* **2023**, *21*, 101291. [CrossRef]
52. Bivand, R.; Yu, D.; Nakaya, T.; Garcia-Lopez, M.-A. Spgwr: Geographically Weighted Regression. Available online: https://CRAN.R-project.org/package=spgwr (accessed on 25 March 2023).
53. World Health Organization. *WHO Global Air Quality Guidelines: Particulate Matter (PM2.5 and PM10), Ozone, Nitrogen Dioxide, Sulfur Dioxide and Carbon Monoxide*; World Health Organization: Geneva, Switzerland, 2021; ISBN 978-92-4-003422-8.
54. Ministry of Ecology and Environment of the People's Republic of China. Ambient Air Quality Standards. Available online: https://www.mee.gov.cn/ywgz/fgbz/bz/bzwb/dqhjbh/dqhjzlbz/201203/t20120302_224165.shtml (accessed on 22 June 2024).
55. Wittwer, J. Calendar Heat Map Template. Available online: https://www.vertex42.com/ExcelTemplates/calendar-chart.html (accessed on 12 April 2022).
56. Lu, D.; Xu, J.; Yue, W.; Mao, W.; Yang, D.; Wang, J. Response of PM2.5 Pollution to Land Use in China. *J. Clean. Prod.* **2020**, *244*, 118741. [CrossRef]
57. Ma, J.; Liu, B.; Mitchell, G.; Dong, G. A Spatial Analysis of Air Pollution and Environmental Inequality in Beijing, 2000–2010. *J. Environ. Plan. Manag.* **2019**, *62*, 2437–2458. [CrossRef]
58. Chen, J.; Chen, S.; Landry, P.F. Migration, Environmental Hazards, and Health Outcomes in China. *Soc. Sci. Med.* **2013**, *80*, 85–95. [CrossRef] [PubMed]
59. Xi'an Municipal People's Government Xi An Cheng Shi Zong Ti Gui Hua 2008–2020. Available online: http://zygh.xa.gov.cn/ywpd/cxghgsgb/ghgsgb/62876060f8fd1c0bdc995ed3.html (accessed on 26 October 2023).
60. Xi'an Natural Resources and Planning Bureau Xi An Shi Guo Tu Kong Jian Gui Hua 2021–2035 Cao An Gong Shi. Available online: http://www.xa.gov.cn/index/tttp/636a2fa2f8fd1c4c21276937.html (accessed on 3 March 2023).
61. Solinger, D.J. *Contesting Citizenship in Urban China: Peasant Migrants, the State, and the Logic of the Market*; University of California Press: Berkeley, CA, USA, 1999.
62. Somers, M.R.; Gibson, G.D. Reclaiming the Epistemological "Other": Narrative and the Social Constitution of Identity. In *Social Theory and the Politics of Identity*; Craig, C., Ed.; Blackwell: Oxford, UK; Cambridge, MA, USA, 1994; pp. 37–99.
63. Li, Y.; Zhu, D.; Zhao, J.; Zheng, X.; Zhang, L. Effect of the Housing Purchase Restriction Policy on the Real Estate Market: Evidence from a Typical Suburb of Beijing, China. *Land Use Policy* **2020**, *94*, 104528. [CrossRef]
64. Liu, Y. Introduction to Land Use and Rural Sustainability in China. *Land Use Policy* **2018**, *74*, 1–4. [CrossRef]
65. Yu, Q.; Hui, E.C.-M.; Shen, J. Do Local Governments Capitalise on the Spillover Effect in the Housing Market? Quasi-Experimental Evidence from House Purchase Restrictions in China. *Land Use Policy* **2023**, *133*, 106851. [CrossRef]
66. The People's Bank of China. Notice of the People's Bank of China on Adjusting the Policy on Personal Housing Loans. Available online: http://www.pbc.gov.cn/goutongjiaoliu/113456/113469/3014377/index.html (accessed on 28 February 2024).
67. The People's Government of Beijing. Municipality Notice on Adjusting and Optimizing the Standards for Ordinary Housing and Personal Housing Loan Policies in Beijing. Available online: https://www.beijing.gov.cn/zhengce/zhengcefagui/202312/t20231214_3500672.html (accessed on 28 February 2024).

isprs International Journal of *Geo-Information*

MDPI

Article

A Novel Flexible Geographically Weighted Neural Network for High-Precision PM2.5 Mapping across the Contiguous United States

Dongchao Wang [1], Jianfei Cao [1], Baolei Zhang [1,*], Ye Zhang [2] and Lei Xie [2]

[1] College of Geography and Environment, Shandong Normal University, Jinan 250358, China
[2] Shandong Provincial Territorial Spatial Ecological Restoration Center, Jinan 250014, China
* Correspondence: 110118@sdnu.edu.cn

Abstract: Air quality degradation has triggered a large-scale public health crisis globally. Existing machine learning techniques have been used to attempt the remote sensing estimates of PM2.5. However, many machine learning models ignore the spatial non-stationarity of predictive variables. To address this issue, this study introduces a Flexible Geographically Weighted Neural Network (FGWNN) to estimate PM2.5 based on multi-source remote sensing data. FGWNN incorporates the Flexible Geographical Neuron (FGN) and Geographical Activation Function (GWAF) within the framework of Artificial Neural Network (ANN) to capture the intricate spatial non-stationary relationships among predictive variables. A robust air quality remote sensing estimation model was constructed using remote sensing data of Aerosol Optical Depth (AOD), Normalized Difference Vegetation Index (NDVI), Temperature (TMP), Specific Humidity (SPFH), Wind Speed (WIND), and Terrain Elevation (HGT) as inputs, and Ground-Based PM2.5 as the observation. The results indicated that FGWNN successfully generates PM2.5 remote sensing data with a 2.5 km spatial resolution for the contiguous United States (CONUS) in 2022. It exhibits higher regression accuracy compared to traditional ANN and Geographically Weighted Regression (GWR) models. FGWNN holds the potential for applications in high-precision and high-resolution remote sensing scenarios.

Keywords: FGWNN; spatial non-stationary; high-precision PM2.5 inversion; multi-source remote sensing

1. Introduction

Atmospheric pollution is primarily composed of PM2.5 particles, which can persist in the atmosphere and exert widespread and profound impacts on human health and the environment [1]. Environmental remote sensing provides a means for globally, continuously, and in real-time retrieving PM2.5 concentrations [2]. The PM2.5 data from the United States (U.S.) Environmental Protection Agency (EPA), as a product of the U.S. ground-based air quality monitoring network, have undergone rigorous quality validation [3], and are widely utilized in environmental science [4], atmospheric science [5], public health [6], disaster management [7], and other fields. This dataset furnishes researchers and policymakers with crucial data support, aiding in our better understanding and addressing of atmospheric pollution issues [8]. Nevertheless, existing remote sensing-derived PM2.5 products commonly suffer from low spatial resolution, failing to delineate local details [9]. To overcome this limitation, acquiring high-resolution PM2.5 spatial distribution data is of paramount importance for the dynamic monitoring and control of atmospheric PM2.5 pollution [10–12].

In the task of retrieving PM2.5 concentrations, the selection of predictive factors is a critical step. The choice of predictors should be based on atmospheric physical and chemical processes, ecological environment quality, meteorological factors, and geographic information. Common parameters include Aerosol Optical Depth (AOD), Normalized Difference Vegetation Index (NDVI), meteorological conditions, and topographic features [13]. AOD provides global atmospheric optical information and is a significant indicator of the atmospheric physical and chemical evolution of air pollutants [14]. Numerous studies have demonstrated a significant correlation between AOD and surface PM2.5 concentration, making AOD one of the most reliable explanatory factors in PM2.5 prediction [15–17]. NDVI reflects vegetation health, land use changes, and ecosystem productivity, serving as an essential measure of ecological environment quality. Studies have shown that NDVI significantly impacts PM2.5 concentrations by reducing dust, adsorbing particles, improving microclimate conditions, reducing pollution sources, and enhancing ecosystem purification functions [18]. Meteorological conditions actively influence the dispersion, dilution, and deposition of pollutants, significantly affecting the spatiotemporal distribution of PM2.5 concentrations [19]. Topographic features alter atmospheric morphology by adjusting air flow, forming the temperature inversion layers, influencing meteorological conditions, and creating urban heat island effects, indirectly affecting the spatial distribution of PM2.5 concentrations [20].

The estimation of PM2.5 through remote sensing involves methods such as AOD inversion [21], atmospheric chemical transport models [22], spatiotemporal interpolation [23], data assimilation [24], among others. The most widely used parameter is the satellite-monitored AOD. To estimate ground-level PM2.5 from AOD, a typical strategy is to establish the statistical relationship between AOD and PM2.5 [25]. The accuracy of these methods is constrained by the number of monitoring stations, remote sensing data resolution, and model quality [26], and a comprehensive approach incorporating multiple data sources and methods is often necessary to enhance inversion accuracy. However, the reality is that traditional spatial statistical tools tend to focus on detecting spatial relationships in sample data [27], and when the spatial density and uniformity of sampling points are insufficient, the estimation accuracy and confidence significantly decrease [28]. The air quality products derived from ground-based stations can solve these problems.

In recent years, new research has emerged in which geostatistical tools and machine learning methods are used for PM2.5 inversion. Scholars have designed geographically weighted regression (GWR) models [29,30] and mixed-effects models [31] for detecting geographical relationships between PM2.5 and data such as AOD, meteorological parameters, and land use information. The novel convolutional neural network (CNN) model can utilize the spatial correlation between predictor variables to increase the ground-level PM2.5 estimation accuracy to some extent [32]. Combining AOD and big data, the PM2.5 regression model using the random forest algorithm can assess the risk of air pollution exposure in the Yangtze River Delta urban agglomeration region during COVID-19 [33]. These inverse models are not perfectly compatible with nonlinear fitting and spatial relationship detection. Traditional geostatistical models cannot fit complex nonlinear relationships, while machine learning methods cannot express spatial non-stationarity.

As studies on PM2.5 spatial patterns increase, various machine learning-related methods (e.g., CNN, Artificial Neural Network (ANN) and Generalized Regression Neural Network (GRNN)) have gradually been introduced. To more accurately calculate geographically weighted kernels, the Geographically Neural Network Weighted Regression (GNNWR) innovatively combines Ordinary Least Squares (OLS) and neural networks to successfully estimate complex geographical processes [34]. In addition to spatial relationships, temporal series are also important research objects in the field of GWR. The Geographically and Temporally Weighted Neural Network (GTWNN) accounts for both spatial and temporal non-stationarity and has been applied in high-precision crop yield prediction modeling [35]. To address nonlinearity and spatiotemporal heterogeneity, researchers have proposed another GTWNN using GRNN, which shows a superior performance in exploring the spatiotemporal relationship between AOD and PM2.5 [36]. However, these GWR-ANN methods mainly focus on improving the accuracy of regression relationships without considering the impact of training samples on the accuracy of spatial dependence, resulting in a certain degree of discount in predictive performance.

Many studies have used GWR or neural networks for PM2.5 inversion, with their data processing methods being essentially similar. When faced with imperfect training samples, the common approach is to first train the optimal regression model [37]. If the prediction samples are also not ideal, one can choose to enhance the density of prediction samples using interpolation techniques, effectively filling the entire target resolution space, or proceed without any further adjustments [38]. Finally, the prediction samples are input into the regression model to obtain the prediction results. If non-ideal prediction samples are left unprocessed, interpolation methods are used to complete the prediction data [39]. This posteriori method results in predictions with high specificity, greatly limiting the model's generalization capability [40]. In contrast, constructing a uniform and dense spatial network would lead to a more comprehensive and accurate understanding of spatial non-stationarity.

This study endeavors to incorporate spatial non-stationary into a machine learning model for the high-precision estimation of PM2.5 via remote sensing data. The proposed Flexible Geographically Weighted Neural Network (FGWNN) model is designed with the Flexible Geographical Neuron (FGN) and Geographically Weighted Activation Function (GWAF) to mitigate the negative impacts of uniform and sparse samples on regression accuracy. It enables the simultaneous learning of spatial non-stationarity and global non-linear relationships within the neural network. The 2.5 km spatial resolution PM2.5 data over the contiguous U.S. (CONUS) can be predicted by FGWNN with conventional satellite remote sensing product data. The organization of this paper is as follows. Section 2 elaborates on the study region and data materials associated with this study. Section 3 provides a detailed description of the FGWNN model design and evaluation. Section 4 demonstrates the FGWNN's performance and spatiotemporal patterns of PM2.5. Recommendations and further discussions based on this research will be presented in Section 5. Finally, we conclude in Section 6.

2. Study Region and Material

2.1. Study Area

The CONUS (Figure 1), excluding Alaska and Hawaii, comprises 48 states and the District of Columbia, with a total area of approximately 7.6 million square kilometers, representing over 80% of the nation's land area. The terrain generally exhibits a west-to-east elevation gradient, featuring high mountains and plateaus such as the Rocky Mountains, the Cascade Range, and the Colorado Plateau in the west, and low mountains and plains including the Appalachian Mountains, the Great Plains, and coastal plains in the east. The population of the CONUS is predominantly concentrated in the eastern and western coastal regions, as well as some inland states in the south and west. California, Texas, Florida, and New York are the four most populous states in the CONUS [41].

The influence factors of air quality exhibit regional variations in the CONUS (Figure 2). These variations are attributed to factors such as meteorological conditions, terrain features, and the distribution of emission sources [42]. Extreme events, such as forest fires, dust storms, and volcanic eruptions, can also impact air quality in the CONUS. In recent years, large-scale forest fires in Canada have led to a surge in PM2.5 concentrations, affecting millions of people in the CONUS [43].

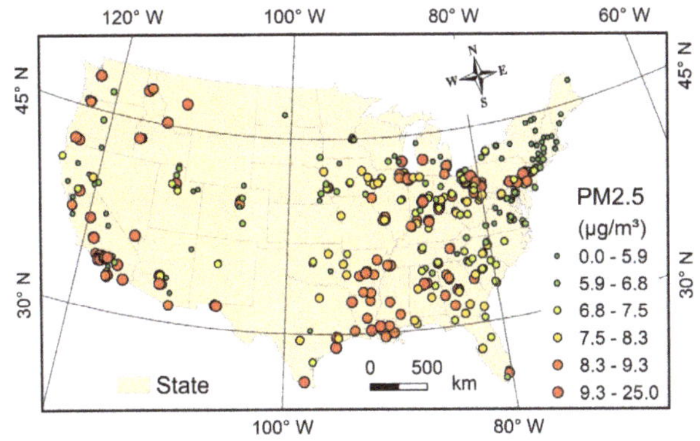

Figure 1. The spatial distribution of PM2.5 concentration monitored by ground-based stations over the CONUS in 2022.

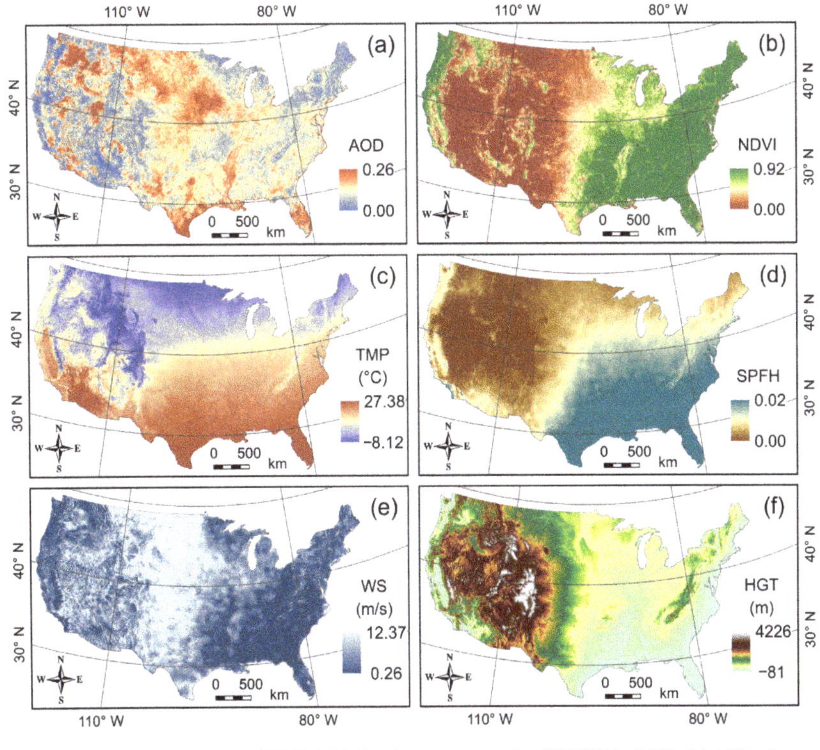

Figure 2. Mean distribution of PM2.5 driving factors across the CONUS in 2022. (**a**) AOD: Aerosol Optical Depth; (**b**) NDVI: Normalized Difference Vegetation Index; (**c**) TMP: temperature; (**d**) SPFH: specific humidity; (**e**) WIND: wind speed; (**f**) HGT: terrain elevation.

2.2. Data Sources

In the field of air pollution research, obtaining large-scale and long-term remote sensing data is crucial for understanding the spatiotemporal patterns of air pollutants. Remote sensing datasets from MODIS, Landsat, Sentinel, and others, combined with ground-level air quality monitoring data, have greatly facilitated collaboration and research in the field of air pollution [44]. However, existing air quality data sources exhibit significant differences in spatial resolution, with low-resolution data diminishing the utility and quality of high-resolution data.

2.2.1. EPA PM2.5

Ground-level PM2.5 monitoring data for the CONUS are derived from the EPA's Outdoor Air Quality Data (https://aqs.epa.gov/aqsweb/airdata/download_files.html, accessed on 21 March 2024) [45]. We selected data records from 20 March 2022, to 21 March 2023 as the initial dataset for our study. The annual and seasonal averages of pollutant concentrations were calculated based on 24 h average PM2.5 values (pollutant standard: PM25 24 h 2012). Furthermore, sites included in the average calculation were required to have monitoring data for more than 100 days. A total of 473 valid PM2.5 ground-level monitoring sites were obtained within the study area. The average PM2.5 concentrations for all sites are depicted in Figure 1, reflecting the overall spatial distribution of PM2.5 in the CONUS in 2022.

2.2.2. MODIS AOD

The MCD19A2 V6.1 data product is a Level-2 gridded product of land-based AOD from the MODIS Terra and Aqua instruments, generated daily at a pixel resolution of 1 km (https://lpdaac.usgs.gov/products/mcd19a2v061/, accessed on 21 March 2024) [46]. The product includes relevant AOD layers, such as 0.47 μm blue band AOD, 0.55 μm green band AOD, and AOD uncertainty. In this study, the 0.47 μm blue band AOD is selected as the research data.

2.2.3. MODIS NDVI

The MODIS Vegetation Index (MYD13Q1) V6.1 data are generated every 16 days (https://lpdaac.usgs.gov/products/myd13q1v061/, accessed on 21 March 2024) [47] with a spatial resolution of 250 m for Level-3 products. MODIS NDVI products are calculated from atmospherically corrected bi-directional surface reflectance and are processed to mask water, clouds, heavy aerosols, and cloud shadows.

2.2.4. NOAA RTMA

The Real-Time Mesoscale Analysis (RTMA) is part of the NOAA Analysis and Observation (AoR) project (https://www.nco.ncep.noaa.gov/pmb/products/rtma/, accessed on 21 March 2024) [48]. It is a high spatiotemporal resolution near-surface weather analysis approach. The product provides hourly analysis data at 2.5 km resolution for CONUS grid cells. The analysis product includes surface-observable weather elements and accounts for terrain effects. It also provides analysis for total cloud cover and visibility. In this study, RTMA is responsible for providing accurate weather conditions (temperature, specific humidity, wind speed) and model terrain elevation data (model terrain elevation) for PM2.5 inversion.

2.3. Data Preprocessing and Integration

Before modeling, it is necessary to preprocess and integrate the acquired remote sensing and ground-level datasets to ensure the data quality and consistency. Firstly, the spatial projection system of the remote sensing datasets was integrated and reprojected to the Albers Equal Area Conic projection (ESRI:102003). Secondly, the meteorological and topographic datasets were processed using the nearest neighbor method, sampling aerosol and meteorological variables based on the coordinates of the PM2.5 monitoring points. Then, a square buffer with a 2.5 km spatial resolution was created for each PM2.5 monitoring station, and the mean values of AOD and NDVI within the buffer were resampled onto the corresponding PM2.5 monitoring point. The preprocessing and integration steps are crucial for generating reliable and robust input data for subsequent modeling work.

2.4. AOD-PM2.5 Model Structure

In this study, PM2.5 is used as the dependent variable, and AOD, NDVI, TMP, SPFH, WIND, and HGT are used as independent variables to construct the PM2.5 inversion model as follows:

$$PM2.5 \sim AOD + NDVI + TMP + SPFH + WIND + HGT \quad (1)$$

We used the average data of 2022 to conduct multicollinearity diagnosis (Table 1). The analysis results indicate that the variance inflation factor (VIF) for all independent variables are less than 10, suggesting no significant collinearity among the variables. After standardization of the regression coefficients (Beta), TMP, NDVI, and AOD have the most significant positive impacts on PM2.5.

Table 1. Multicollinearity diagnosis result.

	Unstandardized Coefficients		Standardized Coefficients	t	Sig.	Collinearity Statistics	
	Beta	Std. Error	Beta			Tolerance	VIF
(Constant)	−12.468	1.016		−12.268	0.000		
AOD	70.799	2.727	0.589	25.958	0.000	0.510	1.960
NDVI	18.214	0.888	0.845	20.509	0.000	0.154	6.476
TMP	0.878	0.029	1.256	30.649	0.000	0.156	6.399
SPFH	−1656.648	69.137	−1.167	−23.962	0.000	0.111	9.039
WIND	0.192	0.095	0.051	2.014	0.044	0.408	2.452
HGT	0.000	0.000	0.095	3.554	0.000	0.364	2.746

3. FGWNN Model for PM2.5 Estimation

3.1. Model Development

To overcome the influence on modeling from the spatial distribution and density of training data, this study designed a specific network structure for FGWNN (Figure 3). The input layer with n represents the number of training samples, while it stands for the number of prediction data when the model is used for prediction. It's important to note that the number m in the hidden layer always represents the number of FGN and does not change with the working mode. The new network architecture brings two significant advantages, namely significant savings in computer storage space and computation time.

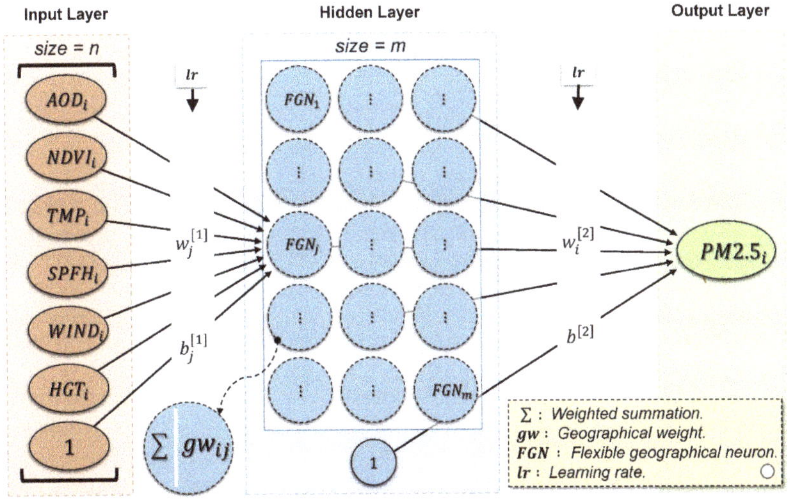

Figure 3. The FGWNN network architecture for PM2.5 inversion.

The input layer is responsible for assembling the independent variables (AOD, NDVI, TMP, SPFH, WIND, and HGT) as inputs. The hidden layer stores FGNs, and the GWAF is synchronously set above the corresponding FGNs. The output layer contains only one neuron corresponding to the dependent variable (PM2.5) output. The network weights ($w_j^{[1]}$) and biases ($b_j^{[1]}$) in the input layer are consistent with ANN.

$$X_i = \begin{bmatrix} 1 & x_{i1} & \cdots & x_{ip} \end{bmatrix} \tag{2}$$

$$W^{[1]} = \begin{bmatrix} b_1^{[1]} & \cdots & b_n^{[1]} \\ w_{11}^{[1]} & \cdots & w_{1n}^{[1]} \\ \vdots & \ddots & \vdots \\ w_{p1}^{[1]} & \cdots & w_{pn}^{[1]} \end{bmatrix} \tag{3}$$

$$W_{origin}^{[2]} = \begin{bmatrix} w_1^{[2]} \\ \vdots \\ w_m^{[2]} \end{bmatrix} \tag{4}$$

Existing neural network activation functions primarily focus on global function transformations of input signals without considering the influence of spatial location on output signals. The GWAF can utilize spatial weighting to establish spatial connections between neurons on the same layer, where different input samples activate the neurons differently. It is a local activation function, and it controls the activation level of neurons through geographical weighting. The specific formula is as follows:

$$\varnothing^{GW}(net_{ij}) = net_{ij} \times gw_{ij} \tag{5}$$

The GWAF utilizes spatial weighting to measure spatial correlations, and the activation level of neurons depends on the spatial distance between the neuron and the target sample. This achieves feature transformation of input signals and spatial smoothing. The GWAF couples neurons with spatial positions, transforming ordinary neurons into FGNs. The contribution of the output signal to the result depends on the height of spatial weights. In other words, the GWAF reflects the spatial non-stationarity characteristics of samples.

The regression process of FGWNN can be represented by a matrix equation as follows:

$$y_i = X_i W^{[1]} \left(GW_i^T \otimes W_{origin}^{[2]} \right) + b^{[2]} \tag{6}$$

In equation, the logical multiplication symbol $\otimes$ represents the element-wise multiplication of the corresponding sub-elements of the matrices on both sides. This operation results in a new matrix with the original dimension.

3.2. Model Hyperparameters Setting

The FGWNN model has various hyperparameters required for neural network learning, and including the spatial bandwidth (bw) among them would increase the computational cost of model training. Considering that the new model inherits the characteristics of GWR, we can use GWR for bandwidth selection, which can save a significant amount of computational resources and time.

In GWR, spatial weighting is a tool used to measure geographical proximity. It defines the strength of the relationship between each geographical location and its surrounding neighboring locations, reflecting the spatial correlation of geographical data in the study area. The commonly used Fixed-Gaussian spatial weight calculation formula is as follows:

$$gw_{ij} = exp\left(-\left(\frac{dist_{ij}}{bw} \right)^2 \right) \tag{7}$$

The choice of the optimal *bw* directly determines the estimation accuracy of the GWR model, and different diagnostic indicators yield different optimal bandwidths. In the GWR field, the *AICc* criterion is typically used for bandwidth selection [49], and the mathematical formula is as follows:

$$AICc = 2nln\left(\hat{\sigma}^2\right) + nln(2\pi) + n\left[\frac{n + tr(S)}{n - 2 - tr(S)}\right] \quad (8)$$

Different information feature recognition results at different spatial scales exhibit some differences, where a smaller spatial resolution provides more details but consumes more computational resources. When conducting geographical observations, the observation scale needs to match the spatial scale of the geographical phenomenon. The setting of the FGN number in FGWNN should depend on the real situation. To construct the ideal state of the geographical neural network, the FGN's positions need to be homogeneous (uniformly distributed) and compact (moderate density) in the study area.

FGWNN uses a single-neuron output layer with an L2 norm loss function. In the field of gradient descent, many new algorithms have been developed, and in practice, there is no strict categorization of algorithms. Multiple algorithms can be used together. The SGD algorithm (Mini-Batch SGD) [50] is widely used for distributing the training set. The NAdam algorithm [51] has stronger constraints on the learning rate and more direct impact on gradient updates. The learning rate can control the step size of hyperparameter iteration in neural networks. A high value can lead to non-convergence, while a low value can increase the learning cost. In the FGWNN model, the learning rate between network layers is used to fine-tune the overall learning rate of the neural network.

3.3. Model Evaluation

The error function compares the predicted output with the expected output, calculating the difference between them. Commonly used error functions include Residual Sum of Squares (RSS), Mean Squared Error (MSE), and Cross-Entropy Error. When employing an ANN to handle regression problems, the model's loss function typically uses the RSS. Dividing by 2 in the formula make it easier to calculate the derivative. The specific formula is as follows:

$$LOSS = \frac{1}{2}\sum_{i=1}^{n}(target_i - output_i)^2 \quad (9)$$

where *LOSS* denotes the amount of loss, target denotes the amount of goal, and output denotes the amount of output.

Common evaluation metrics for machine learning regression problems include Root Mean Squared Error (RMSE), LOSS, R^2, and adjusted R^2 (R^2_{adj}). These evaluation metrics are suitable for different scenarios in regression problems, and the choice of the appropriate metric depends on the nature of the problem and the specific requirements for model performance. Given FGWNN's ability to detect spatial non-stationarity, considering introducing local R^2 and local RMSE to jointly evaluate the model.

This study uses K-Fold cross-validation [52] to evaluate the model's performance. In this process, the dataset is divided into K subsets, and the model undergoes K rounds of training and validation. K-Fold cross-validation can reduce the risk of overfitting, improve model robustness, and provide reliable performance estimates. During each round of K-Fold training, FGWNN employs the early-stopping strategy [53]. It stops the model's training when the performance on the validation set no longer improves, helping to avoid local optima and overfitting traps. The combination of K-Fold cross-validation and Early-Stopping strategy significantly enhances the model's performance and stability. It ensures that the model not only learns effective features on the training data but also generalizes well to new data.

4. Results

4.1. Model Parameter Optimization

4.1.1. Uniformization Strategy Performance

The FGWNN model can operate in two modes: nonuniform mode and uniform mode. Before activating the uniformization strategy, the geographic neurons (GNs) in the neural network are aligned with the positions of ground monitoring stations (473 in total). Their spatial distribution is uneven, with dense coverage along coastal areas and sparse coverage in inland regions (Figure 4a). After uniformization, GNs are uniformly distributed across the CONUS (Figure 4b). Comparing the learning curves under the two modes (Figure 4c,d), it is observed that the convergence period for non-uniformization is later than that for uniformization, and the fluctuation in learning is higher for non-uniformization. The optimal global R^2 for the uniformization mode is slightly higher than that for the non-uniformization mode. To quantify the fitting performance of the FGWNN model under different strategies, we introduce the local R^2 metric in Figure 4e,f. The results show that, under the non-uniformization mode, the local R^2 values are higher in densely sampled areas but significantly lower in sparsely sampled areas. After activating the uniformization strategy, the difference in local R^2 is notably reduced, with a decrease in local R^2 in dense areas and an increase in local R^2 in sparse areas. In other words, the uniformization strategy transforms GNs into FGWs, effectively eliminating regression disparities caused by uneven samples.

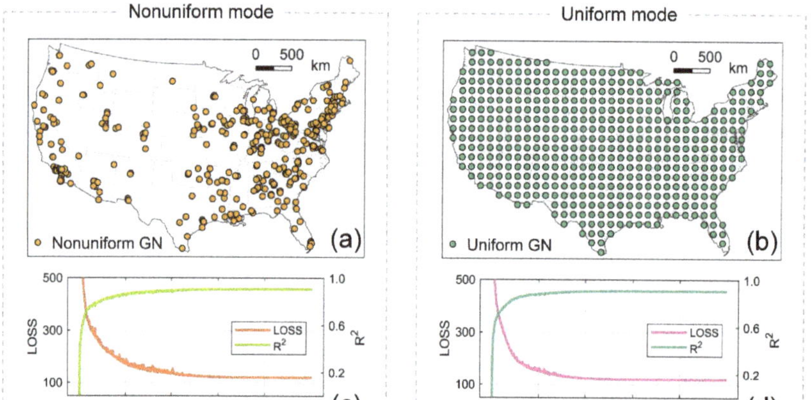

Figure 4. Comparison of the effects before and after implementing the uniformization strategy. (**a**) Non-uniformization GN; (**b**) Uniformization GN; (**c**) Learning curve under non-uniformization mode; (**d**) Learning curve under uniformization mode; (**e**) Estimated local R^2 for non-uniformization mode; (**f**) Estimated local R^2 for uniformization mode.

4.1.2. FGN Number Optimization

Figure 5 illustrates the diagnostic results of the training effectiveness of the FGWNN model under different numbers of FGNs after activating the uniformization strategy. The upper part of the figure illustrates the change patterns of LOSS and R^2. As the number of FGNs increases, LOSS initially decreases rapidly, reaching a turning point (5000), and then gradually converges. In contrast, R^2 exhibits an opposite change pattern to LOSS. To quantify the memory consumption and runtime associated with a different FGN size, this experiment focuses on the data storage of the spatial weight matrix and the learning time of the FGWNN model. The results indicate that both memory consumption and runtime follow a logarithmic growth pattern. When the number of FGNs is set to 5000, both memory consumption and runtime remain at relatively low levels. This indicates that the process of optimizing the number of FGNs needs to consider a balance between learning effectiveness and training costs, aiming to minimize the dependence on computational resources while ensuring high learning effectiveness.

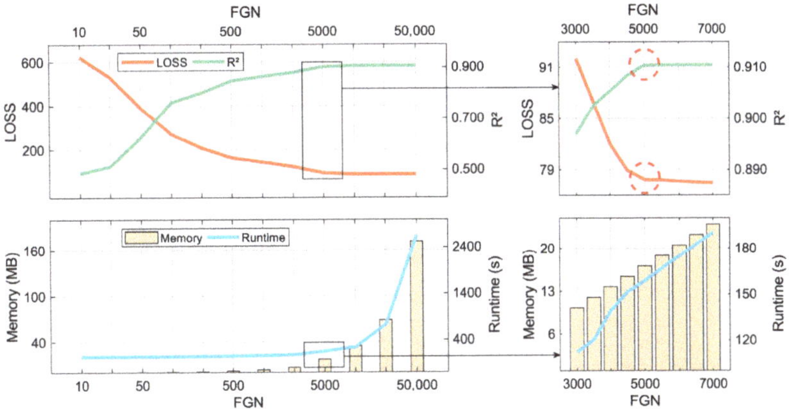

Figure 5. FGN number optimization (marked by red dotted circle) and comparison of computational cost changes.

4.2. Comparison with Other Models

4.2.1. Overall Comparison of Different Models

Table 2 presents the regression results of five models (MLR, ANN, GWR, GNNWR, and FGWNN) on the PM2.5 data cross the CONUS region in 2022. Specifically, the learning rate of all three models (ANN, GNNWR, and FGWNN) is 0.001, with 5000 neurons in the hidden layer of ANN and FGWNN, compared to 473 in GNNWR. A comparison of the computational time across different models reveals that FGWNN consumes the most time at 161 s, followed by GNNWR at 109 s, ANN at 93 s, GWR at 86 s, and MLR with the lowest consumption at 28 s. The RMSE and LOSS metrics exhibit decreasing trend, with values ranking from highest to lowest as MLR, ANN, GWR, GNNWR, and FGWNN. Conversely, R^2 and R^2_{adj} demonstrate a progressively increasing trend. Overall, the regression performance of FGWNN notably surpasses that of MLR, ANN, and GWR models, with a small improvement over GNNWR.

Table 2. Comparison of PM2.5 regression with different models over the CONUS in 2022.

Model	lr	Time	RMSE	LOSS	R^2	R^2_{adj}
MLR		28	1.794	741.982	0.168	0.158
ANN	0.001	93	1.512	527.249	0.409	0.401
GWR		86	1.061	259.493	0.709	0.705
GNNWR	0.001	109	0.604	84.085	0.906	0.905
FGWNN	0.001	161	0.581	77.887	0.913	0.912

Note: Time is in second (s), and RMSE is in μg/m^3.

Figure 6 depicts the scatter plots of PM2.5 estimated values versus observed values for the four models, along with their evaluation metric scores and linear fitting equations. Both GWR and FGWNN exhibit the ability to detect spatial non-stationarity, with significantly improved fitting accuracy compared to MLR and ANN. In comparison to the traditional GWR approach, FGWNN demonstrates an exceptional fitting capability. Its R^2_{adj} increases from less than 0.72 to nearly 0.92, with a reduction in LOSS by over 180 and RMSE decreased to within 0.60 μg/m^3. These results indicate that the FGWNN method possesses a robust generalization performance, accurately reproducing the original state of the PM2.5-AOD model. In summary, FGWNN outperforms MLR, ANN, and GWR models in the 2022 assessment.

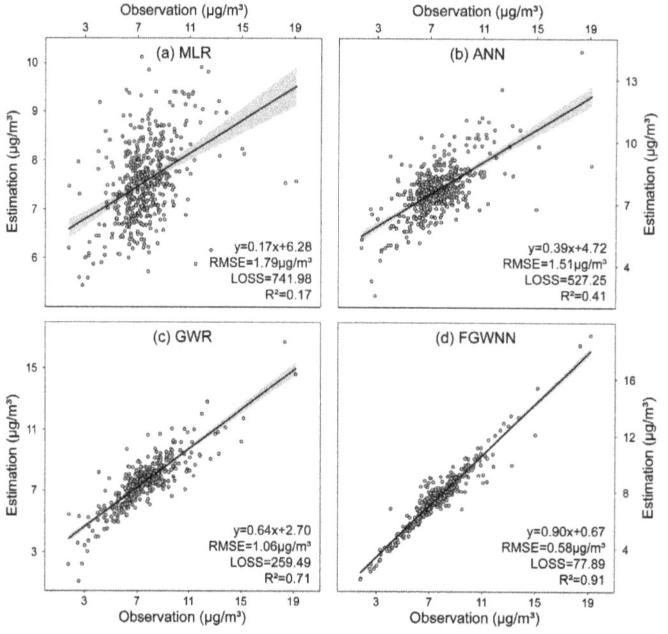

Figure 6. Scatter plots of estimated versus observed PM2.5 for the (**a**) MLR, (**b**) ANN, (**c**) GWR, and (**d**) FGWNN models.

4.2.2. Seasonal Performance Comparison for Various Models

Figure 7 presents the seasonal performance of the MLR, ANN, GWR, and FGWNN models. From the graph, it is evident that, for an equal sample dataset, the FGWNN model outperforms the other three models in all four seasons. Following FGWNN, the GWR and ANN models rank next, while the MLR model performs the poorest, with R^2 values of 0.41, 0.35, 0.46, and 0.20 for the four seasons, respectively. The seasonal performance trend of the MLR model aligns with that of the ANN model, with the highest R^2 value in autumn and the lowest in winter. Conversely, the performance of the GWR model, like the FGWNN model, initially rises, stabilizes, and then declines. Despite the results shown in the RMSE figures, which are contrary to those of the R^2 metrics, the FGWNN model maintains optimal performance.

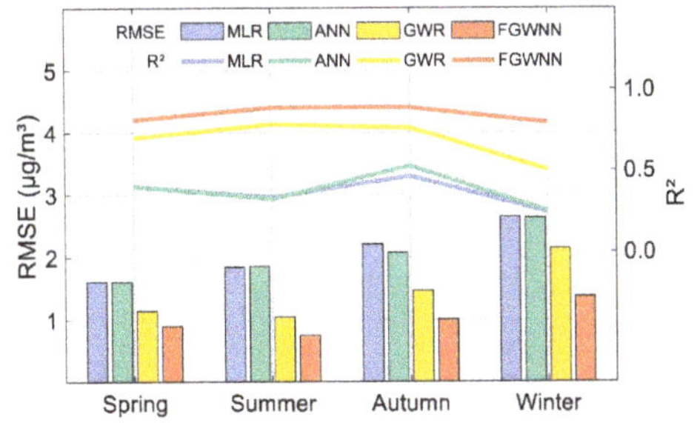

Figure 7. Trends in global regression metrics across the four seasons of 2022.

Utilizing the local R^2 and local RMSE results of each model across the four seasons, we constructed boxplots to illustrate the spatial performance of each model. Regarding the local RMSE results (Figure 8a,b,e,f), the average RMSE values for the four seasons are 0.64, 0.53, 0.68, and 0.99 for the FGWNN model. Additionally, minor spatial variability can be observed in the boxplots of the FGWNN model. By comparing the local R^2 values (Figure 8c,d,g,h), the FGWNN model once again demonstrates significant superiority, with average R^2 values of 0.89, 0.92, 0.88, and 0.81, respectively. Hence, from a statistical perspective, the FGWNN model is more suitable for satellite-based PM2.5 mapping compared to the MLR, ANN, and GWR models.

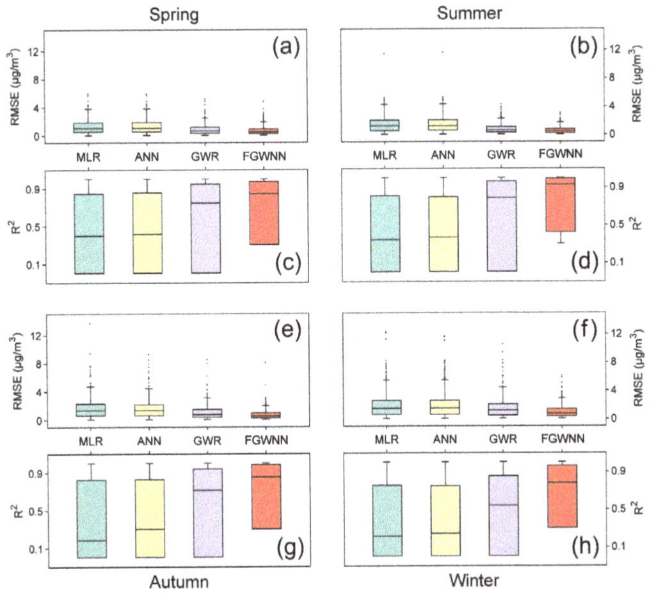

Figure 8. Boxplots of local regression metrics across the four seasons of 2022. (**a**) Local RMSE in Spring; (**b**) Local RMSE in Summer; (**c**) Local R^2 in Spring; (**d**) Local R^2 in Summer; (**e**) Local RMSE in Autumn; (**f**) Local RMSE in Winter; (**g**) Local R^2 in Autumn; (**h**) Local R^2 in Winter.

4.2.3. Annual and Seasonal Performance of FGWNN Model

To further understand the annual and seasonal performance of the FGWNN model, we evaluated its spatial performance. Table 3 presents the RMSE results for both the annual and quarterly assessments in 2022, with global RMSE values consistently below 1.0 μg/m^3 for all four seasons. From the results, the order of global RMSE magnitudes is as follows: summer < annual < spring < autumn < winter. Local RMSE values between observed and estimated PM2.5 values were calculated for each monitoring station (see Figure 9). Overall, the FGWNN model demonstrates a reliable spatial prediction capability. Indeed, the FGWNN model performs well in the central regions of station clusters but relatively poorer in the peripheral areas of these clusters. This phenomenon may be attributed to the FGWNN model's ability to smooth regression variations between station points. Despite the uneven spatial distribution of the model performance, the FGWNN model demonstrates an excellent predictive capability overall, with over 64% of sites reporting local RMSE values below 1 μg/m^3. A comparative analysis suggests that the FGWNN model proposed in this study holds significant potential for satellite-based PM2.5 mapping.

Table 3. RMSE results for year and seasons in 2022.

	Annual	Spring	Summer	Autumn	Winter
Stations	473	403	401	396	410
Global RMSE (μg/m^3)	0.581	0.644	0.534	0.684	0.989
Local RMSE < 1.0 (%)	82.7	80.1	86.0	78.5	64.6

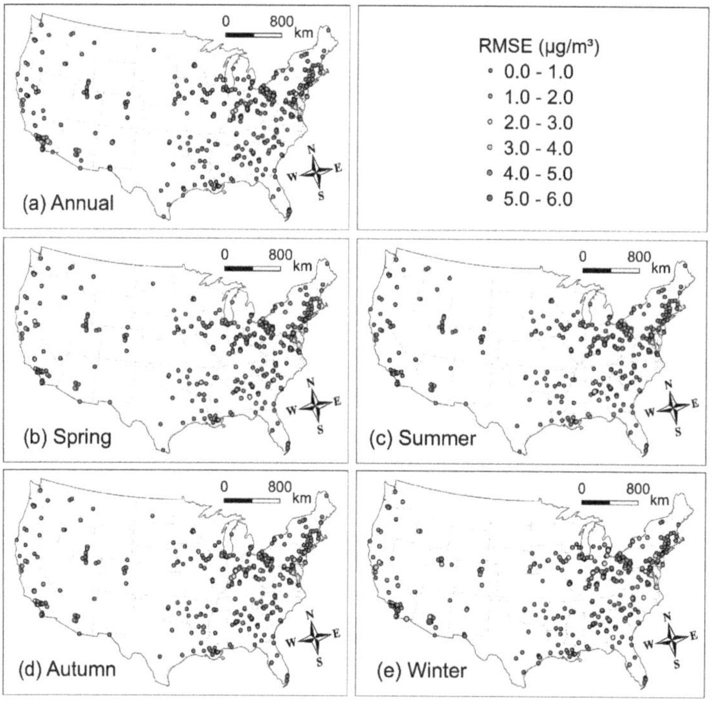

Figure 9. Local RMSE results for year and seasons in 2022 via FGWNN model.

4.3. PM2.5 Prediction over CONUS

Once the predictive capability of the FGWNN model is sufficiently validated, the continuous predictions of PM2.5 spatial concentrations in the CONUS region can be made.

Figure 10 displays the annual and seasonal distribution of ground-level PM2.5, based on the inversion of FGWNN (with 5000 FGNs). Overall, the average annual PM2.5 concentration is 7.45 μg/m^3, representing a 37.9% decrease compared to the Level 1 standard (12 μg/m^3) defined by the US-EPA in 2016. Additionally, it is predicted that approximately 43% of pixel cells in CONUS have an annual PM2.5 concentrations exceeding 12 μg/m^3. These findings suggest that CONUS still experiences mild PM2.5 pollution, and the combination of satellite remote sensing can provide a more detailed spatial distribution information of atmospheric pollutants than ground-based monitoring alone [54].

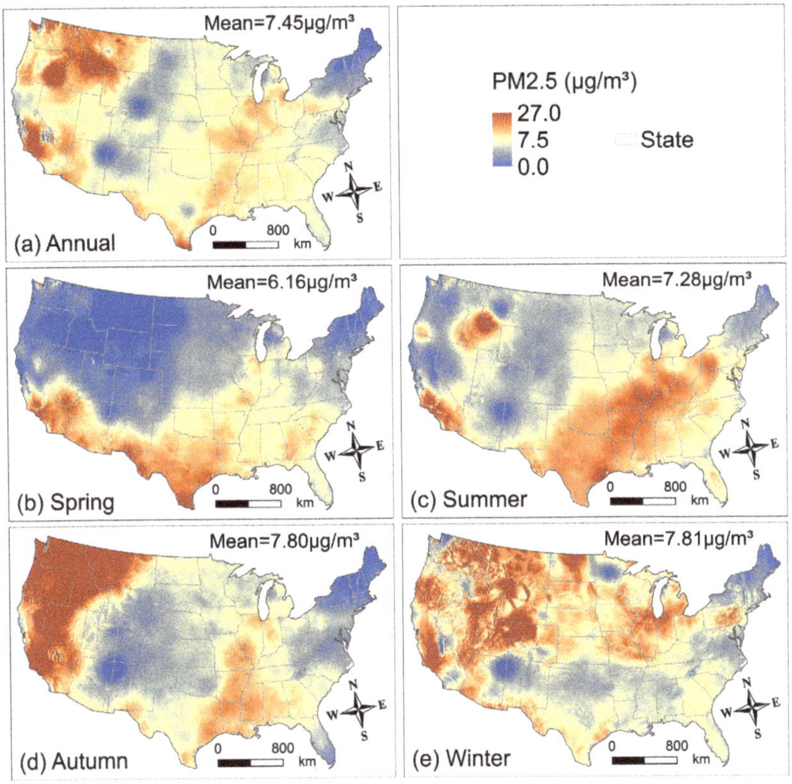

Figure 10. Satellite-derived mapping of ground-level PM2.5 concentration over CONUS in 2022.

The results from the five periods reveal a general trend of the decreasing spatial distribution of PM2.5 from coastal to inland areas, with the western and southeastern regions being more susceptible to air pollution than the central and northern regions (Figure 10). PM2.5 concentrations are generally higher in regions with a Mediterranean climate and tropical desert climate. The western, northeastern, and southern regions constitute the three major industrial zones in the United States, emitting significant amounts of particulate pollutants. Across the first three seasons, the air quality in CONUS shows a worsening trend, with PM2.5 concentrations increasing from 6.16 μg/m^3 to 7.80 μg/m^3. By winter, the air pollution peaks at 7.81 μg/m^3, covering almost the entire CONUS region. Air quality deteriorates progressively in the west as the seasons advance, while pollutants in the east shift from south to north. Additionally, Canadian forest wildfires serve as significant sources of air pollution in North America, with smoke particles transported into the CONUS airspace by atmospheric movements [55]. The northeastern and western coastal regions are major population and urban centers, yet PM2.5 accumulates continuously during this period, undoubtedly increasing health risks for local residents [56].

5. Discussion

The spatial distance between geographical objects determines the strength of their spatial relationships, referred to as spatial dependency [57]. Spatial weighting in GWR [58] describes the varying spatial dependency between individual objects and all objects. In this paper, we define the strong or weak variation in the region as the spatial dependency field (SDF). Although GWR can effectively detect spatial non-stationarity, the SDF used in the model has two limitations. First, in the sparse state (Figure 11a), training samples are homogeneously distributed in space but with low sample density. The SDF can only roughly reflect the spatial dependency pattern of the original data, overlooking the finer details. Second, when spatial density is insufficient, training samples are heterogeneously distributed in space (eccentric and uneven), which falls into the biased state (Figure 11b). This situation can cause the significant deformation of the SDF, affecting the accurate representation of the original spatial dependency pattern, and significantly diminishing the quality of the final model. In conclusion, if the ideal SDF (Figure 11c) adapted to the target spatial scale is constructed, its learned spatial non-stationarity will be more comprehensive and accurate.

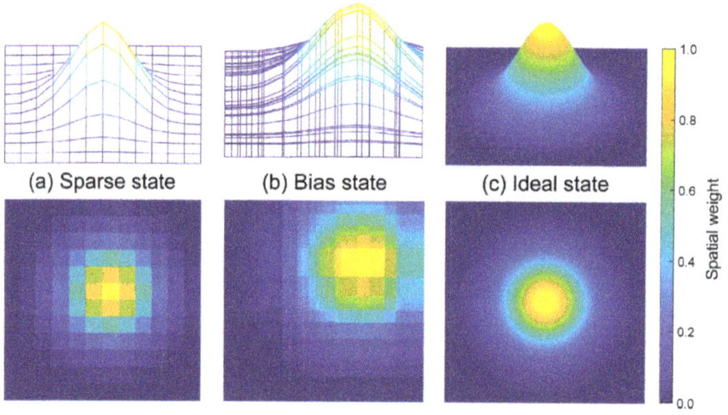

Figure 11. Three states of SDF. (**a**) Sparse state; (**b**) Biased state; (**c**) Ideal state: uniform and dense placement of FGNs.

Large-scale, low spatial resolution remote sensing images inevitably suffer from issues related to insufficient spatial details, challenging target identification, limited image quality, and application constraints [59]. The high-definition images inferred and predicted using FGWNN can facilitate the precise identification of areas with air pollution anomalies, providing strong evidence for the analysis of air pollution driving factors [60]. The quality of the SDF constructed by traditional geographical detectors depends on the density and uniformity of the spatial distribution of samples, which often suffer from sparsity and non-homogeneity in real-world data [61]. To overcome this limitation, FGWNN automatically allocates homogeneous and moderate FGNs to the hidden layer, achieving an ideal SDF state. The FGWNN method proposed in this paper realizes the effective detection of spatial relationships through the establishment of a flexible SDF, which can accurately reconstruct the real features of geographical data. Additionally, it significantly enhances the regression accuracy and spatial resolution of PM2.5 inversion, making it a reliable-efficient remote sensing mapping technique.

In exploring the spatial and temporal patterns of PM2.5 using high-precision remote sensing products from FGWNN inversion, different levels of the study area require the use of products with a compatible spatial resolution. This aims to strike a balance between inversion accuracy and computational efficiency. Figure 12 shows the study area at four administrative levels, i.e., national level (CONUS), division-level (Pacific Division), state level (California State), and county level (Los Angeles County). When the spatial resolution of the remote sensing image is not less than 20 km, PM2.5 data within the CONUS can be obtained with clear image details and no obvious jaggedness. Increasing the spatial resolution of remote sensing products to 10 km can fully demonstrate the spatial distribution characteristics of PM2.5 in the Pacific Division. In order to clearly detect the air quality distribution pattern in California State, the spatial resolution of remote sensing images is required to be higher than 5 km. Remote sensing products inverted from existing data with a maximum spatial resolution of 2.5 km can roughly reflect the general situation in Los Angeles County. Theoretically, the FGWNN model is able to complete the inversion of remote sensing products with arbitrary target resolution when the spatial resolutions of the independent variables meet the requirements.

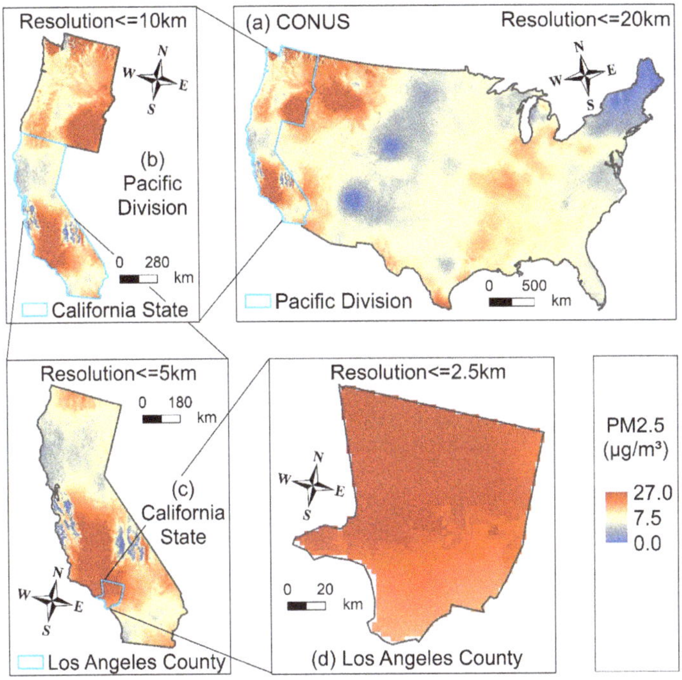

Figure 12. Spatial resolutions corresponding to the different study region levels. (**a**) CONUS; (**b**) Pacific Division; (**c**) California State; (**d**) Los Angeles County.

Although the FGWNN has made some progress, there are still some limitations. These potential issues should be further considered in subsequent research or when applying the method more widely. The choice of spatial bandwidth relies on GWR calculations [62], which may limit its practicality in spatiotemporal analysis scenarios. In high-resolution remote sensing data contexts, model training and geographical activation processes incur substantial computational costs [63]. In the future, we plan to optimize the acquisition of spatial bandwidth by embedding this process within FGWNN. Simultaneously, we aim to refine the FGWNN network structure to reduce its dependence on computer resources. It is our hope that the FGWNN model can be extended to the spatiotemporal analysis field, further advancing the development of remote sensing spatiotemporal mapping technology.

6. Conclusion

In-depth research into the spatiotemporal patterns of air pollution risk in a region can help alleviate concerns about public health crises. Building upon the foundations of GWR and ANN, this study has introduced a novel neural network structure, FGWNN. It can automatically allocate the positions and quantities of FGNs based on the characteristics of the study area, providing simultaneous analysis of the spatial non-stationarity and global nonlinear relationships within the original data. Notably, the ideal state SDF constructed by the new method can perfectly fit complex spatial non-stationary relationships. We successfully predicted PM2.5 concentrations across the CONUS in 2022, with the regression model's fitting accuracy improved to above 0.90. Despite variations in model performance across different seasons, the PM2.5 products generated at a 2.5 km resolution to maintain a high level of fidelity. The remote sensing data produced by FGWNN possess a high spatial resolution, meeting the needs of researchers for air quality assessments at different scales. In the future, it is planned to enhance the model's temporal detection capability and expand its application prospects in the spatiotemporal remote sensing domain.

Author Contributions: Conceptualization, Dongchao Wang; methodology, Dongchao Wang; validation, Dongchao Wang; resources, Dongchao Wang, Ye Zhang and Lei Xie; writing—original draft, Dongchao Wang, Jianfei Cao, Baolei Zhang, Ye Zhang and Lei Xie; visualization, Dongchao Wang and Jianfei Cao; supervision, Baolei Zhang; project administration, Baolei Zhang. All authors have read and agreed to the published version of the manuscript.

Funding: This research was funded by Shandong Province Undergraduate Teaching Reform Project (Z20220004), Jinan City-School Integration Project (JNSX2023036), National Natural Science Foundation of China (42201308), and Natural Science Foundation of Shandong Province, China (ZR2021QD127, ZR2021ME203).

Data Availability Statement: The raster dataset has been shared and accessed at https://github.com/sd19891020/FGWNN (accessed on 23 March 2024).

Conflicts of Interest: The authors declare no conflicts of interest.

References

1. Jia, N.; Li, Y.; Chen, R.; Yang, H. A Review of Global $PM_{2.5}$ Exposure Research Trends from 1992 to 2022. *Sustainability* **2023**, *15*, 10509. [CrossRef]
2. Christopher, S.; Gupta, P. Global Distribution of Column Satellite Aerosol Optical Depth to Surface $PM_{2.5}$ Relationships. *Remote Sens.* **2020**, *12*, 1985. [CrossRef]
3. Kelly, J.T.; Reff, A.; Gantt, B. A Method to Predict $PM_{2.5}$ Resulting from Compliance with National Ambient Air Quality Standards. *Atmos. Environ.* **2017**, *162*, 1–10. [CrossRef]
4. Zhang, D.; Wang, W.; Xi, Y.; Bi, J.; Hang, Y.; Zhu, Q.; Pu, Q.; Chang, H.; Liu, Y. Wildland Fires Worsened Population Exposure to $PM_{2.5}$ Pollution in the Contiguous United States. *Environ. Sci. Technol.* **2023**, *57*, 19990–19998. [CrossRef] [PubMed]
5. Lin, Y.-C.; Li, Y.-C.; Amesho, K.T.T.; Shangdiar, S.; Chou, F.-C.; Cheng, P.-C. Chemical Characterization of $PM_{2.5}$ Emissions and Atmospheric Metallic Element Concentrations in $PM_{2.5}$ Emitted from Mobile Source Gasoline-Fueled Vehicles. *Sci. Total Environ.* **2020**, *739*, 139942. [CrossRef] [PubMed]
6. Mailloux, N.A.; Abel, D.W.; Holloway, T.; Patz, J.A. Nationwide and Regional $PM_{2.5}$ -Related Air Quality Health Benefits from the Removal of Energy-Related Emissions in the United States. *GeoHealth* **2022**, *6*, e2022GH000603. [CrossRef] [PubMed]
7. Pan, S.; Gan, L.; Jung, J.; Yu, W.; Roy, A.; Diao, L.; Jeon, W.; Souri, A.H.; Gao, H.O.; Choi, Y. Quantifying the Premature Mortality and Economic Loss from Wildfire-Induced $PM_{2.5}$ in the Contiguous U.S. *Sci. Total Environ.* **2023**, *875*, 162614. [CrossRef] [PubMed]
8. Hill, A.E.; Burkhardt, J.; Bayham, J.; O'Dell, K.; Ford, B.; Fischer, E.V.; Pierce, J.R. Air Pollution, Weather, and Agricultural Worker Productivity. *Am. J. Agric. Econ.* **2023**, *Early View*, 1–25. [CrossRef]
9. Bai, K.; Li, K.; Guo, J.; Chang, N.-B. Multiscale and Multisource Data Fusion for Full-Coverage $PM_{2.5}$ Concentration Mapping: Can Spatial Pattern Recognition Come with Modeling Accuracy? *ISPRS J. Photogramm. Remote Sens.* **2022**, *184*, 31–44. [CrossRef]
10. Ghasempour, F.; Sekertekin, A.; Kutoglu, S.H. Google Earth Engine Based Spatio-Temporal Analysis of Air Pollutants before and during the First Wave COVID-19 Outbreak over Turkey via Remote Sensing. *J. Clean. Prod.* **2021**, *319*, 128599. [CrossRef]
11. Shen, L.; Hu, W.; Zhao, T.; Bai, Y.; Wang, H.; Kong, S.; Zhu, Y. Changes in the Distribution Pattern of $PM_{2.5}$ Pollution over Central China. *Remote Sens.* **2021**, *13*, 4855. [CrossRef]
12. Deng, C.; Qin, C.; Li, Z.; Li, K. Spatiotemporal Variations of $PM_{2.5}$ Pollution and Its Dynamic Relationships with Meteorological Conditions in Beijing-Tianjin-Hebei Region. *Chemosphere* **2022**, *301*, 134640. [CrossRef] [PubMed]

13. Aguilera, R.; Luo, N.; Basu, R.; Wu, J.; Clemesha, R.; Gershunov, A.; Benmarhnia, T. A Novel Ensemble-Based Statistical Approach to Estimate Daily Wildfire-Specific $PM_{2.5}$ in California (2006–2020). *Environ. Int.* **2023**, *171*, 107719. [CrossRef] [PubMed]
14. Gui, K.; Che, H.; Wang, Y.; Xia, X.; Holben, B.N.; Goloub, P.; Cuevas-Agulló, E.; Yao, W.; Zheng, Y.; Zhao, H.; et al. A Global-Scale Analysis of the MISR Level-3 Aerosol Optical Depth (AOD) Product: Comparison with Multi-Platform AOD Data Sources. *Atmos. Pollut. Res.* **2021**, *12*, 101238. [CrossRef]
15. Karimian, H.; Li, Y.; Chen, Y.; Wang, Z. Evaluation of Different Machine Learning Approaches and Aerosol Optical Depth in $PM_{2.5}$ Prediction. *Environ. Res.* **2023**, *216*, 114465. [CrossRef] [PubMed]
16. Jing, Y.; Pan, L.; Sun, Y. Estimating $PM_{2.5}$ Concentrations in a Central Region of China Using a Three-Stage Model. *Int. J. Digit. Earth* **2023**, *16*, 578–592. [CrossRef]
17. He, Q.; Ye, T.; Wang, W.; Luo, M.; Song, Y.; Zhang, M. Spatiotemporally Continuous Estimates of Daily 1-Km $PM_{2.5}$ Concentrations and Their Long-Term Exposure in China from 2000 to 2020. *J. Environ. Manag.* **2023**, *342*, 118145. [CrossRef] [PubMed]
18. Jin, H.; Chen, X.; Zhong, R.; Liu, M. Influence and Prediction of $PM_{2.5}$ through Multiple Environmental Variables in China. *Sci. Total Environ.* **2022**, *849*, 157910. [CrossRef] [PubMed]
19. Zhang, W.; Wang, H.; Zhang, X.; Peng, Y.; Zhong, J.; Wang, Y.; Zhao, Y. Evaluating the Contributions of Changed Meteorological Conditions and Emission to Substantial Reductions of $PM_{2.5}$ Concentration from Winter 2016 to 2017 in Central and Eastern China. *Sci. Total Environ.* **2020**, *716*, 136892. [CrossRef]
20. Shu, Z.; Zhao, T.; Liu, Y.; Zhang, L.; Ma, X.; Kuang, X.; Li, Y.; Huo, Z.; Ding, Q.; Sun, X.; et al. Impact of Deep Basin Terrain on $PM_{2.5}$ Distribution and Its Seasonality over the Sichuan Basin, Southwest China. *Environ. Pollut.* **2022**, *300*, 118944. [CrossRef]
21. Hua, Z.; Sun, W.; Yang, G.; Du, Q. A Full-Coverage Daily Average $PM_{2.5}$ Retrieval Method with Two-Stage IVW Fused MODIS C6 AOD and Two-Stage GAM Model. *Remote Sens.* **2019**, *11*, 1558. [CrossRef]
22. Li, S.; Chen, L.; Huang, G.; Lin, J.; Yan, Y.; Ni, R.; Huo, Y.; Wang, J.; Liu, M.; Weng, H.; et al. Retrieval of Surface $PM_{2.5}$ Mass Concentrations over North China Using Visibility Measurements and GEOS-Chem Simulations. *Atmos. Environ.* **2020**, *222*, 117121. [CrossRef]
23. Ma, J.; Ding, Y.; Cheng, J.C.P.; Jiang, F.; Wan, Z. A Temporal-Spatial Interpolation and Extrapolation Method Based on Geographic Long Short-Term Memory Neural Network for $PM_{2.5}$. *J. Clean. Prod.* **2019**, *237*, 117729. [CrossRef]
24. Wang, Y.; Yuan, Q.; Li, T.; Tan, S.; Zhang, L. Full-Coverage Spatiotemporal Mapping of Ambient $PM_{2.5}$ and PM10 over China from Sentinel-5P and Assimilated Datasets: Considering the Precursors and Chemical Compositions. *Sci. Total Environ.* **2021**, *793*, 148535. [CrossRef]
25. Xu, X.; Zhang, C.; Liang, Y. Review of Satellite-Driven Statistical Models $PM_{2.5}$ Concentration Estimation with Comprehensive Information. *Atmos. Environ.* **2021**, *256*, 118302. [CrossRef]
26. Feng, Y.; Fan, S.; Xia, K.; Wang, L. Estimation of Regional Ground-Level $PM_{2.5}$ Concentrations Directly from Satellite Top-of-Atmosphere Reflectance Using A Hybrid Learning Model. *Remote Sens.* **2022**, *14*, 2714. [CrossRef]
27. Tang, Y.; Xie, S.; Huang, L.; Liu, L.; Wei, P.; Zhang, Y.; Meng, C. Spatial Estimation of Regional $PM_{2.5}$ Concentrations with GWR Models Using PCA and RBF Interpolation Optimization. *Remote Sens.* **2022**, *14*, 5626. [CrossRef]
28. Wu, S.; Wang, Z.; Du, Z.; Huang, B.; Zhang, F.; Liu, R. Geographically and Temporally Neural Network Weighted Regression for Modeling Spatiotemporal Non-Stationary Relationships. *Int. J. Geogr. Inf. Sci.* **2021**, *35*, 582–608. [CrossRef]
29. Hu, X.; Waller, L.A.; Al-Hamdan, M.Z.; Crosson, W.L.; Estes, M.G.; Estes, S.M.; Quattrochi, D.A.; Sarnat, J.A.; Liu, Y. Estimating Ground-Level $PM_{2.5}$ Concentrations in the Southeastern U.S. Using Geographically Weighted Regression. *Environ. Res.* **2013**, *121*, 1–10. [CrossRef] [PubMed]
30. Van Donkelaar, A.; Martin, R.V.; Spurr, R.J.D.; Burnett, R.T. High-Resolution Satellite-Derived $PM_{2.5}$ from Optimal Estimation and Geographically Weighted Regression over North America. *Environ. Sci. Technol.* **2015**, *49*, 10482–10491. [CrossRef]
31. Zhang, X.; Chu, Y.; Wang, Y.; Zhang, K. Predicting Daily $PM_{2.5}$ Concentrations in Texas Using High-Resolution Satellite Aerosol Optical Depth. *Sci. Total Environ.* **2018**, *631–632*, 904–911. [CrossRef] [PubMed]
32. Park, Y.; Kwon, B.; Heo, J.; Hu, X.; Liu, Y.; Moon, T. Estimating $PM_{2.5}$ Concentration of the Conterminous United States via Interpretable Convolutional Neural Networks. *Environ. Pollut.* **2020**, *256*, 113395. [CrossRef] [PubMed]
33. Lu, D.; Mao, W.; Zheng, L.; Xiao, W.; Zhang, L.; Wei, J. Ambient $PM_{2.5}$ Estimates and Variations during COVID-19 Pandemic in the Yangtze River Delta Using Machine Learning and Big Data. *Remote Sens.* **2021**, *13*, 1423. [CrossRef]
34. Du, Z.; Wang, Z.; Wu, S.; Zhang, F.; Liu, R. Geographically Neural Network Weighted Regression for the Accurate Estimation of Spatial Non-Stationarity. *Int. J. Geogr. Inf. Sci.* **2020**, *34*, 1353–1377. [CrossRef]
35. Feng, L.; Wang, Y.; Zhang, Z.; Du, Q. Geographically and Temporally Weighted Neural Network for Winter Wheat Yield Prediction. *Remote Sens. Environ.* **2021**, *262*, 112514. [CrossRef]
36. Li, T.; Shen, H.; Yuan, Q.; Zhang, L. Geographically and Temporally Weighted Neural Networks for Satellite-Based Mapping of Ground-Level $PM_{2.5}$. *ISPRS J. Photogramm. Remote Sens.* **2020**, *167*, 178–188. [CrossRef]
37. Jin, X.; Ding, J.; Ge, X.; Liu, J.; Xie, B.; Zhao, S.; Zhao, Q. Machine Learning Driven by Environmental Covariates to Estimate High-Resolution $PM_{2.5}$ in Data-Poor Regions. *PeerJ* **2022**, *10*, e13203. [CrossRef] [PubMed]
38. Yu, X.; Xi, M.; Wu, L.; Zheng, H. Spatiotemporal Weighted for Improving the Satellite-Based High-Resolution Ground $PM_{2.5}$ Estimation Using the Light Gradient Boosting Machine. *Remote Sens.* **2023**, *15*, 4104. [CrossRef]
39. Zhang, H.; Zhan, Y.; Li, J.; Chao, C.-Y.; Liu, Q.; Wang, C.; Jia, S.; Ma, L.; Biswas, P. Using Kriging Incorporated with Wind Direction to Investigate Ground-Level $PM_{2.5}$ Concentration. *Sci. Total Environ.* **2021**, *751*, 141813. [CrossRef]

40. Jin, Y.; Yin, Z.; Zhou, W.; Shao, J. Bayesian Model Selection for Sand with Generalization Ability Evaluation. *Num. Anal. Meth. Geomech.* **2019**, *43*, 2305–2327. [CrossRef]
41. Jo, Y.; Shrestha, S.; Gomes, I.; Marks, S.; Hill, A.; Asay, G.; Dowdy, D. Model-Based Cost-Effectiveness of State-Level Latent Tuberculosis Interventions in California, Florida, New York, and Texas. *Clin. Infect. Dis.* **2021**, *73*, e3476–e3482. [CrossRef] [PubMed]
42. Li, Y.; Tong, D.; Ma, S.; Zhang, X.; Kondragunta, S.; Li, F.; Saylor, R. Dominance of Wildfires Impact on Air Quality Exceedances During the 2020 Record-Breaking Wildfire Season in the United States. *Geophys. Res. Lett.* **2021**, *48*, e2021GL094908. [CrossRef]
43. Velasco Hererra, V.M.; Soon, W.; Pérez-Moreno, C.; Velasco Herrera, G.; Martell-Dubois, R.; Rosique-de La Cruz, L.; Fedorov, V.M.; Cerdeira-Estrada, S.; Bongelli, E.; Zúñiga, E. Past and Future of Wildfires in Northern Hemisphere's Boreal Forests. *For. Ecol. Manag.* **2022**, *504*, 119859. [CrossRef]
44. Bai, K.; Li, K.; Sun, Y.; Wu, L.; Zhang, Y.; Chang, N.-B.; Li, Z. Global Synthesis of Two Decades of Research on Improving $PM_{2.5}$ Estimation Models from Remote Sensing and Data Science Perspectives. *Earth-Sci. Rev.* **2023**, *241*, 104461. [CrossRef]
45. US-EPA AirData Website File Download Page. Available online: https://aqs.epa.gov/aqsweb/airdata/download_files.html (accessed on 21 March 2024).
46. Lyapustin, A.; Wang, Y. *MODIS/Terra+Aqua Land Aerosol Optical Depth Daily L2G Global 1 km SIN Grid V061*; NASA EOSDIS Land Processes DAAC: Sioux Falls, SD, USA, 2022. [CrossRef]
47. Didan, K. *MODIS/Aqua Vegetation Indices 16-Day L3 Global 250m SIN Grid V061*; NASA EOSDIS Land Processes DAAC: Sioux Falls, SD, USA, 2021. [CrossRef]
48. NCEP Central Operations NCEP Data Products RTMA/URMA. Available online: https://www.nco.ncep.noaa.gov/pmb/products/rtma/ (accessed on 21 March 2024).
49. Brunsdon, C.; Fotheringham, A.S.; Charlton, M. Geographically Weighted Summary Statistics—A Framework for Localised Exploratory Data Analysis. *Comput. Environ. Urban Syst.* **2002**, *26*, 501–524. [CrossRef]
50. Li, M.; Zhang, T.; Chen, Y.; Smola, A.J. Efficient Mini-Batch Training for Stochastic Optimization. In Proceedings of the 20th ACM SIGKDD International Conference on Knowledge Discovery and Data Mining, New York, NY, USA, 24 August 2014; pp. 661–670. [CrossRef]
51. Dozat, T. Incorporating Nesterov Momentum into Adam. In Proceedings of the 4th International Conference on Learning Representations, Workshop Track, San Juan, Puerto Rico, 2–4 May 2016.
52. Fushiki, T. Estimation of Prediction Error by Using K-Fold Cross-Validation. *Stat. Comput.* **2011**, *21*, 137–146. [CrossRef]
53. Zhang, T.; Yu, B. Boosting with Early Stopping: Convergence and Consistency. *Ann. Statist.* **2005**, *33*, 1538–1579. [CrossRef]
54. Wei, J.; Li, Z.; Lyapustin, A.; Wang, J.; Dubovik, O.; Schwartz, J.; Sun, L.; Li, C.; Liu, S.; Zhu, T. First Close Insight into Global Daily Gapless 1 Km $PM_{2.5}$ Pollution, Variability, and Health Impact. *Nat. Commun.* **2023**, *14*, 8349. [CrossRef]
55. Wang, Z.; Wang, Z.; Zou, Z.; Chen, X.; Wu, H.; Wang, W.; Su, H.; Li, F.; Xu, W.; Liu, Z.; et al. Severe Global Environmental Issues Caused by Canada's Record-Breaking Wildfires in 2023. *Adv. Atmos. Sci.* **2024**, *41*, 565–571. [CrossRef]
56. Liu, C.; Hu, H.; Zhou, S.; Chen, X.; Hu, Y.; Hu, J. Change of Composition, Source Contribution, and Oxidative Effects of Environmental $PM_{2.5}$ in the Respiratory Tract. *Environ. Sci. Technol.* **2023**, *57*, 11605–11611. [CrossRef]
57. Legendre, P.; Fortin, M.J. Spatial Pattern and Ecological Analysis. *Vegetatio* **1989**, *80*, 107–138. [CrossRef]
58. Brunsdon, C.; Fotheringham, A.S.; Charlton, M.E. Geographically Weighted Regression: A Method for Exploring Spatial Nonstationarity. *Geogr. Anal.* **1996**, *28*, 281–298. [CrossRef]
59. Wen, D.; Huang, X.; Bovolo, F.; Li, J.; Ke, X.; Zhang, A.; Benediktsson, J.A. Change Detection from Very-High-Spatial-Resolution Optical Remote Sensing Images: Methods, Applications, and Future Directions. *IEEE Geosci. Remote Sens. Mag.* **2021**, *9*, 68–101. [CrossRef]
60. Sokhi, R.S.; Singh, V.; Querol, X.; Finardi, S.; Targino, A.C.; Andrade, M.D.F.; Pavlovic, R.; Garland, R.M.; Massagué, J.; Kong, S.; et al. A Global Observational Analysis to Understand Changes in Air Quality during Exceptionally Low Anthropogenic Emission Conditions. *Environ. Int.* **2021**, *157*, 106818. [CrossRef]
61. Tian, Z.; Wei, J.; Li, Z. How Important Is Satellite-Retrieved Aerosol Optical Depth in Deriving Surface $PM_{2.5}$ Using Machine Learning? *Remote Sens.* **2023**, *15*, 3780. [CrossRef]
62. Yang, X.; Yang, Y.; Xu, S.; Han, J.; Chai, Z.; Yang, G. A New Algorithm for Large-Scale Geographically Weighted Regression with K-Nearest Neighbors. *IJGI* **2023**, *12*, 295. [CrossRef]
63. Zhang, C.; Yue, P.; Tapete, D.; Shangguan, B.; Wang, M.; Wu, Z. A Multi-Level Context-Guided Classification Method with Object-Based Convolutional Neural Network for Land Cover Classification Using Very High Resolution Remote Sensing Images. *Int. J. Appl. Earth Obs. Geoinf.* **2020**, *88*, 102086. [CrossRef]

International Journal of
Geo-Information

MDPI

Article

Exploring the Effects of Light and Dark on Crime in London

Ezgi Erturk *, Peter Raynham and Jemima Unwin Teji

Institute of Environmental Design and Engineering, Bartlett Faculty of the Built Environment, University College London (UCL), London WC1H 0NN, UK; p.raynham@ucl.ac.uk (P.R.); jemima.unwin@ucl.ac.uk (J.U.T.)
* Correspondence: ezgi.erturk.21@ucl.ac.uk

Abstract: Safety from crime is a fundamental human need. In Maslow's hierarchy, safety is one of the foundational needs of well-being. The built environment should be safe to use at all times of the day and for all groups of people. After dark, the appearance of the outdoor environment changes dramatically, and this could impact the opportunities for crime. This study investigated the impact of daylight on the rates of different types of crime by comparing the crime rates during selected periods of daylight and darkness. The study used records of crime data from the Metropolitan Police Service. By studying crimes in the week on either side of the twice-yearly clock change, it is possible to compare periods that are dark in one week and light in the other at the same clock time. Where the time at which the crime took place was known, and using the GPS coordinates of the specific crime, the solar altitude was calculated and used to determine if it was light or dark at the time of the crime. A similar calculation was used to see if the crime would have been in the dark or light in the week on the other side of the clock change. The headline result is that there was 4.8% (OR 1.07) more crime in the dark periods than the light ones. However, this increase was not uniform across all crime types, and there were some further complications in some results due to potential changes in the behavior of some victims after dark. For the crimes of theft from a person and robbery of personal property, there was a significant increase during the dark period. The availability of light had an impact on the rate of certain crimes. Whilst this does not provide any information about the impact of street lighting on crime, it does provide some idea of by how much crime could be reduced if better lighting was provided.

Keywords: ambient lighting; crime; spatial analysis; clock changes; safety; London

1. Introduction

Safety from crime is important for well-being and mental and physical health. However, environmental conditions such as darkness can cause fear of crime [1]. Whether this fear is founded in reality and supported by real crime data has yet to be conclusively determined. The importance of safety from crime is reinforced by the United Nations in their sustainable development goal to provide a peaceful and safe built environment for all citizens [2]. Features of the physical environment can have an impact on the opportunity for crime. For example, Jacobs [3] claimed that most new residential projects could cause a rise in crime and less safe streets and parks by isolating citizens from the streets and local businesses. In the book "The Death and Life of Great American Cities" she criticizes the construction of high-density social housing projects and the design of streets for car use in the USA, which began in the 1950s, forcing people to live in more unsafe and dangerous places. Jacobs [3] also claims that the presence of other people might increase surveillance of potential criminals by providing "eyes on the street". Welsh et al. [4] support Jacob's concept of surveillance. For example, they state that removing objects which prevent the clear sight of the windows of homes and stores enhances surveillance. Clarke, R.V. [5] explained three ways that surveillance deters offenders. Firstly, formal surveillance includes security guards and CCTV cameras, which increase the chance that offenders are seen. Secondly, place managers who are in the environment due to their duties, not for security matters, such as bus drivers, city council employees, and parking lot attendants, might act as deterrents. Lastly, natural surveillance observers are citizens who use the built environment as part of their daily routines and could also help deter offenders. Newman [6] claimed that improved street lighting as part of an enhanced built environment is also part of natural surveillance. Street lighting is important because it enables pedestrians to see other people after dark.

The problem is that lighting designers need to know how to use lighting design to contribute to the safety of the environment. However, this is difficult when there is very little convincing evidence that lighting affects crime. The research presented by this paper presents evidence that some outdoor crimes are affected by ambient lighting conditions (whether it is light or dark). This means that light does matter to the incidence of crime and that the impact of electric lighting conditions on crime should be investigated in future work. If whether it is light or dark matters to crime, then it is likely that lighting design could also have an effect. It is also proposed that this be explored for future work.

2. Literature Review

There are many complex reasons that cause someone to commit a crime. These reasons are multi-faceted, and it is impossible to provide all of them in this paper. This paper focuses on the possible influence of the built environment. However, factors such as population density and seasonal or one-off events such as widespread protesting and looting can also encourage crime. For example, after Mark Duggan was killed by a police officer in London, riots between 6 and 11 August 2011 caused looting and arson in London, which later spread across England [7]. Some types of crime may also be related to seasonal differences. Andresen, M. A., and Malleson, N. [8] examined crime records in Vancouver (Canada) in 2001 based on seasonal differences. While there are exceptions, the summer season tended to see a rise in crime across several categories, including all crimes, assault, theft, theft from vehicles, and theft of vehicles. However, other crimes, such as burglary, robbery, and sexual assault, did not display a significant seasonal pattern. Another study by Shiode et al. [9] observed 12 crime types which took place in London between 2013 and 2020. While burglary and thefts from the person peak in winter, especially in November, non-property crimes such as bicycle theft and antisocial behavior peak in the summer.

The built environment, for example, the morphology of streets, also plays a key role in mitigating fear of crime. Three main aspects, prospect, escape, and concealment, affect the fear of crime and people's perceived safety in the outdoor environment [10,11]. For example, wide-open streets with escape routes reassure people more than narrow streets with limited escape routes. Zigzag paths, sharp edges on the turning points, and hedges on paths in the outdoor environment make it possible for criminals to hide [6] (p. 82). Boyce and Gutkowski [12] asserted that crime could also be related to the travel time and accessibility of locations where criminals tend to commit crimes; therefore, street lighting may not be enough to prevent crimes. For example, criminals might commit a crime in places that are easy to access, hide, and run away from, regardless of lighting conditions.

Other than the elements outlined above, the role of lighting conditions on crime and the fear of crime cannot be underestimated. Darkness could cause crime opportunities and encourage criminals to commit crimes. Using the 1992 British Crime Survey, Mayhew et al. [13] observed that most violent crimes take place in public places between 6:00 pm and midnight. According to the British Standard Institution [14], road lighting helps in tackling crime and the fear of crime. Combating crime by utilizing street lighting goes back to the date 16th Century. At the end of the 16th Century, Paris established street lighting under the control of the police administration. Police administration lighted Paris's streets from the end of October to the beginning of April after 6 pm [15]. Upgrading street lighting is assumed to be a significant environmental factor in tackling crime [16]; however, convincing evidence is rare. Welsh and Farrington [17] also state that improved lighting can reduce crime. In past studies, improved lighting was generally defined as illuminating an environment that was not lit before or increasing the level of illuminance where it was already lit. One of the earlier studies by Wright et al. [18] found that replacing light sources to provide higher illuminance can decrease crime rates in high-level crime streets. The study examined the crime rates in commercial and residential areas in Missouri and Kansas Cities between 1970 and 1973, where incandescent lamps (20–23 lumens per watt) were replaced with mercury (40–55 lumens per watt) and sodium vapor (100–130 lumens per watt) lamps. The findings showed that the incidence of violence, such as robbery and assault, decreased significantly in residential and commercial areas with upgraded street lighting.

Instead of looking at larger areas, such as Wright et al. [18], Painter [19] focused on a particular location (in Edmonton), outer London. Light sources were changed from LPS (Low-Pressure Sodium) to HPS (High-Pressure Sodium), which increased the level of illuminance from 0.6–4.5 lx to 6–25 lx on the selected streets. A survey asked about people's experiences of crime and fear of crime on the streets before and after the lighting was upgraded, with reference to the following outdoor crime types: violence against people (robbery, physical and sexual offenses, theft), vehicle offenses, and harassment. On-the-street surveys asking about pedestrians' direct experiences of street crimes were conducted immediately before and 6 weeks after the lighting installation. The question referred to a specific 6-week time period prior to the installation and a 6-week time period after the installation. They reported that 21 of 207 people had experienced crime before the lighting installation. This was in the categories of violence against the person (4), vehicle crime (12), and harassment on the street (5). After the lighting installation, only three crime incidents were reported: vehicle crime (2) and harassment on the street (1). This suggests a reduction in crime in the 6 weeks after lighting change. In addition, the installation seemed to affect perceived safety, as shown in a follow-up after the installation survey of 153 individuals: 62% responded that they felt safer, 3% of participants felt less safe, 4% of participants said "do not know", and 31% of participants said there was no change in their perceived safety. The questionnaire did not ask questions directly related to lighting to the participants (153 + 207 = 360). This is useful in contributing to avoiding bias related to socially desirable responses, in which participants could be included to say that lighting improves safety. The study asked participants' feelings about going out after dark, and also whether there were changes in their perception during the 6 weeks. Of the 360 participants in total, only 105 noticed that the lighting had been changed. Only these 105 participants who noticed the changes made to lighting were asked more questions about the lighting. For example, they were asked whether the new lighting was brighter or more attractive. When the questionnaire asked 105 participants about lighting issues, the participants might have understood that this study was related to lighting improvement. That may cause bias and affect participants' perceptions. In addition, we do not know the effect of the fact that participants lived in the same or nearby apartment blocks. Painter [19] also used the Edmonton Police records between January–March 1987 and 1988 in her study. Interestingly, police records of violence against the person increased post-lighting installation by 77% compared to the same time period the year before, whereas autocrime for the same period went down by around 6%. That result might show that reported crime could increase post-lighting installation because people could see what is happening more clearly and could, therefore, report it.

However, Nair and Ditton [20] claimed that the impact of improved lighting on crime prevention might not last in the long term. The upgrading of lighting in Bellgrove and High Blantyre indicated significant improvement in 3 months; however, this effect was not evident in interviews conducted over a year later. In addition, not all studies have found a link between lighting and crime. For example, Welsh and Farrington [17] found that despite the overall reduction in crime rates by 21% after improved street lighting, there was an increase in 3 out of 13 studies on crime rates after upgraded street lighting. Painter [21] observed the impact of upgrading the lighting in three residential high-rise buildings that are surrounded by smaller residential buildings on the West Park Estate, Ashton Under Lyne, using surveys and police records. A total of 197 households were interviewed before and after the upgrading of the lighting was completed. Of the 197 households, 65% of the residents who participated were the same people surveyed both before and after the upgrade. Although both surveys and police records demonstrate an overall decrease in the level of crime after improving the lighting, in the survey, it was reported that while the incidents of theft from vehicles increased from 5 to 15 with a 200% rise, and incidents of public physical assault increased from 9 to 19 by 89% after 12 months post-lighting installation. However, the study does not include repeated measurements beyond a year. For example, crime counts might be affected by different seasons, but this is hard to determine due to the study being confined to winter. Comparing winter and winter either side of the year is a more efficient approach than comparing autumn and winter in the same year. Additionally, if the policy for the recording of crimes by police changed during the year, the results might not be clear. For instance, the number of burglaries was 22 in 1989 before the upgrading of the lighting, and 24 in 1990 after the upgrade. However, the incident of burglaries in police records dramatically decreased to zero.

Steinbach et al. [22] observed crime records using police data in which four changes to street lighting were applied in 62 locations provided by city councils between 2010 and 2013. Firstly, the study explored crime records when street lighting was switched off; secondly, when the lighting was on for part-night only; for example, the lighting was switched off after midnight. Thirdly, when the street lighting was dimmed, and lastly, when sodium light sources were replaced with whiter light LED sources. The study found that switching off (RR 0.11; 95% CI 0.01 to 2.75)and part-night (RR 0.96; 95% CI 0.86 to 1.06) approaches did not affect the crime rates, whereas white light (RR 0.89; 95% CI 0.77 to 1.03) and dimming lighting (RR 0.84; 95% CI 0.70 to 1.02) had a small impact on reducing risk rates. Additionally, the study found that part-night lighting (RR 1.48; 95% CI 0.99 to 2.21) may increase the risk of robbery, whereas dimming (RR 0.78; 95% CI 0.60 to 1.01) may decrease the risk of violence. White lighting may decrease the risk of all types of crimes (robbery, burglary, vehicle, violence, aggregate). However, these results need to be approached cautiously as local authorities are unlikely to randomly allocate part-night lighting. The problem is that the grounds for selecting the areas to be switched off or to undergo lighting changes are unknown. It is possible that low crime rates could have played an important role in the local authorities' choices. In addition, the study did not present the changes in the locations adjacent to the case studies. Therefore, the crime might have been displaced to the adjacent streets.

Peng et al. [23] also claimed that night-time light brightness can increase criminal arrest and prosecution rates. They investigated the correlation between the brightness of night-time lighting and the crime rate in China between 2000 and 2013. By using 1 km $\times$ 1 km grids in 227 cities using the Defense Meteorological Satellite Program (DMSP), 70% of all crime records, including homicide, robbery, and theft in the China City Statistical Yearbook, were tested. Other crime types, such as rape and arson, were excluded due to a lack of information in the dataset. The study found that a 1% increase in brightness resulted in higher crime rates in bright areas; the crime rates were found to be higher in developed cities such as Shanghai, Beijing, Foshan, and Guangzhou compared to rural areas. However, the effect of the rise in crime rates was not significant.

Another approach is to compare crimes in daylight and darkness because ambient lighting conditions could help us understand whether lighting affects crime rates. Unwin et al. [24], emphasized the importance of first exploring the effects of large-scale ambient lighting conditions before honing in on optimum electric lighting conditions as if the behavior is not affected by the former, then fine-tuning the latter might be a moot point in terms of its effect on pedestrian flows. Investigating the impact of the change in ambient lighting conditions can also provide a wide perspective on the impact of lighting on crime. If ambient light does not make a difference, variations in electric lighting conditions are less likely to matter as they are more subtle than the change from daylight to dark.

Examining crime reports using ambient lighting conditions over many years of clock changes helps reduce the effects of public bias caused by media, which can have more of an influence in the short term before and after lighting installation studies. For example, the news in South Yorkshire Times [25], "Kids Make Town A 'Living Hell'" in the local newspapers, negatively affected Raynham and Mansfield's [26] study, as the headline appeared after a lighting upgrade and was likely to have affected the survey results. Two sites had 35 street lights replaced and 80 new luminaires installed. Over 3500 visitors were interviewed before and after re-lighting. Two types of surveys targeted at local businesses and pedestrians in Swinton were carried out before and after re-lighting part of the town center. After the re-lighting installation, although there was a slight increase in the town center's night visits, visitors responded that lighting alone is not enough to make streets attractive at night. They still did not feel safe because of young people, graffiti, and vandalism. Additionally, local businesses responded that there was no significant change in their perceived safety and business performance. Moreover, business owners reported that the street lighting improvements actually worsened youth nuisance by encouraging larger gangs to gather.

Ambient lighting (light/dark) depends on the time of the day. Most previous studies, such as Sullivan et al. [27], Uttley and Fotios [28], and Ferguson et al. [29], did not correctly define light, dark, or twilight conditions when they calculated daylight availability using this approach. This uncertainty might cause some miscalculations and a lack of robust analysis. For example, the twilight period was counted as dark in Fergusen et al.'s [29] work on motor vehicle crashes; however, during this period, there was a significant probability that illuminance was anywhere in the range of 10–140 lux. Muneer T. and Kambezidis H. [30] described twilight using three different levels of solar altitude. When the sun's altitude was between 0° and -6°, -6° and -12°, and -12° and -18°, it was defined as civil twilight, nautical twilight, and astronomical twilight, respectively. Raynham et al. [31] developed a method which categorized daylight to be when the sun has an altitude of greater than 0° and darkness when solar altitude is less than -6° in their study on traffic collisions. This approach removed the uncertainty associated with twilight. The method was also later applied by Fotios and Robbins, C. [32], and Fotios et al. [33] in road collision and crime studies.

Using the spring and autumn clock changes can provide a reliable approach to understanding the impact of lighting on crime because a given time may be light one week and dark in the other and can, therefore, be compared. Some studies use this method, for example, Sullivan et al. [27], Unwin et al. [24], Umbach et al. [34], Raynham et al. [31], and Tealde, E. [35]. Umbach et al. [34] investigated the effect of the mild, short-term sleep loss/gain due to Daylight Saving time on assault rates in Chicago, New York, Philadelphia, and Los Angeles between 2001 and 2014. According to a study, there was a 2.9% decrease in assaults right after Daylight Saving Time (DST) began in spring, when we lost an hour of sleep, compared to a week later. On the other hand, there was an increase of 2.8% in assaults immediately following the return to standard time in autumn, when an hour was gained, compared to a week later. The study showed that mild and short-term changes in sleep can significantly reduce/increase the rates of assault. The study implies that mild sleepiness, which is possibly associated with an hour's loss of sleep, could result in reduced assaults. Between 2004 and 2014, Tealde, E. [35] conducted a study in Montevideo, Uruguay that analyzed geolocated data on crime and public lighting. The study found that DST (Daylight Saving Time) resulted in a significant decrease of 17% in robberies. The decrease was even larger during sunset hours, up to 23%.

However, even research using specific time windows can have problems. For example, Fotios et al. [33] used the clock change method to analyze reports of crime in the U.S. from 2010 and 2019. This study found a significant rise in robbery in the dark. According to the findings, it appears that when it is dark, incidents of arson and loitering during curfew tend to rise, while cases of disorderly conduct, non-violent family offenses, and prostitution tend to decrease. The problem was that as the database used the Crime Open Database [36], which only contains dates and times that crimes were reported, rather than when they occurred, it was not possible to determine with certainty whether the crime took place in light or dark. This is because many crimes are only discovered sometime after the crime took place. Thus, it is not possible to determine if the crime took place in light or dark. In addition, all crimes cannot be limited to one specific time. For example, prostitution does not take place at a single set time. Therefore, the database might cause inaccuracy in the findings.

In summary, there are limited studies about the impact of ambient lighting conditions on crime counts, and the studies which do exist fail to measure daylight availability accurately and are unclear about the exact time window in which crime took place. In order to answer the main question, "Do ambient lighting conditions (daylight or darkness) affect crime occurrence?" this paper uses a precise calculation of the solar altitude at the time the crime took place and only uses crimes where the time was known to have taken place within a window of 5 mins or less.

The aim of the study is to examine whether there is a relationship between ambient lighting outdoors and crimes where the time is known to within 5 min. As our paper discusses, most of the approaches used before have limitations. Our research aims to find different approaches to the lighting design of external urban environments that could matter, could reduce crime, and would be worth exploring further.

To address this aim, we define four hypotheses:

1. There are seasonal differences in the effects of light and dark on crime. In autumn, we would expect a bigger difference compared to spring due to the onset of darkness.
2. Crime rates vary within the day (24 h period).
3. If light has an impact on crime, then crime at night/dark should be different from crime during the day/light.
4. Light and dark impact crime types differently. For example, outdoor crimes such as robbery and theft increase after dark, whereas other crime types do not.

This paper uses data from Metropolitan Police Services (MPS), which provides a time window in which each crime took place. By using this data, the study applied the precise clock change calculation method to assess changes in crime between light and dark.

3. Methodology

The study uses a quantitative method by using the Metropolitan Police Service (MPS) dataset of 4,790,048 crime reports that have taken place in London between 1 January 2013 and 31 August 2019. All analyses were done securely in the Jill Dando Institute Research Lab (JDIRL), which cooperates with MPS. The MPS dataset in the JDIRL [37] includes the following details (Table 1).

Table 1. Dictionary of MPS data.

Crime ID	A Unique Identifier for each Crime Record
Time Crime Recorded	The date and time the crime was verified as an actual crime.
Time Crime Reported	The date and time when the crime was first reported (usually by a member of the public) to the police.
Time Committed From	The earliest date and time at which the crime could have happened.
Time Committed To	The latest date and time at which the crime could have happened.
Location	An approximate description of where the crime happened. Of the form "On or near X Road". It is believed to be in the order of approximately 20–40 m.
Easting Coordinate	Ordinance Survey Map- British National Grid coordinate for the crime location.

Table 1. *Cont.*

Crime ID	A Unique Identifier for each Crime Record
Northing Coordinate	Ordinance Survey Map—British National Grid coordinates for the crime location.
Major Crime	Major crime classification as per the MPS rules. (Metropolitan Office, 2022).
Minor Crime	Minor crime classification as per the MPS rules. (Metropolitan Office, 2022).

The study includes 55 crime types. The major crime types in the MPS dataset are described in Table 2, according to the Metropolitan Police Office [38].

Table 2. Definition of crimes according to MPS.

Burglary	Burglary is an attempt or theft in a building where access is not allowed. It also includes damaging property.
Arson and criminal damage	Arson and criminal damage involve damaging a premises on purpose.
Drug offenses	Drug offenses consist of an attempt to sell illegal drugs, consumption, and possession of a drug.
Miscellaneous crimes against society	Miscellaneous crimes against society include all crimes against society without having a direct victim.
Possession of weapons	Possession of weapons is carrying knives and any other weapons that are illegal.
Robbery	Robbery is the theft of business or personal property by forcing or threatening someone.
Theft	Theft is stealing someone's property without the use of force.
Violence against the person	Violence against the person consists of harming the body, murder, harassment, and assault.
Vehicle offenses	Vehicle offenses include breaking traffic rules and leaving or parking a car inappropriately.
Sexual offenses	Sexual offenses involve sexual harassment and sexual interaction with an underage victim.
Public order offense	Public order offenses are defined as a crime which prevents individuals or groups of people's activities in public places.

Due to the massive amount of data and complexity of the data, this research used automated data analysis, using Python and Excel tools, and then presented the results. To reach the most reliable results in the analysis, the time accuracy of data plays a key role. Therefore, before beginning the analysis, the study cleaned up the potential errors with regard to time. 61,757 of 4,790,048 crime records were removed from the analysis where the date information contained anomalies or was void. Examples of anomalies are the crime being reported before it occurred, mistakes in data entry such as the boundaries of the time window being the wrong way around, and some crimes not being recorded fully. For example, if there was no "time committed from" data, the record was deleted from the analysis. To summarize, the below instructions were used:

Time Crime Recorded $\geq$ Time Crime Reported

If Time Committed To not void, then

Time Committed To $\geq$ Time Committed From

Else

Time Crime Reported ≥ Time Committed From

Also, Time Committed From + 365 days ≥ Time Crime Recorded.

The method of the study is described in the flow chart below, which shows the process step by step (Figure 1).

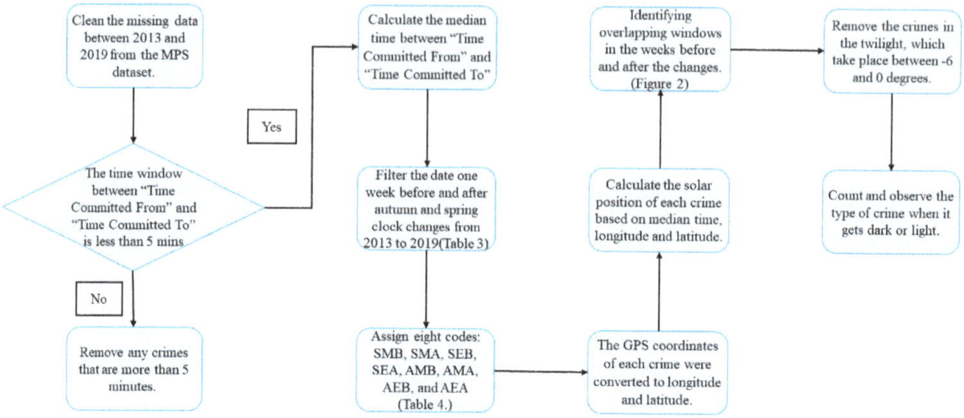

Figure 1. Flow chart of the study. Missing data refers to the lack of or incorrect information in the dataset. For example, the time committed column was empty or the type of crime was written in the time column. GPS coordinates refer to the British National Grid reference numbers.

Knowing the precise time that the crime happened is essential for accurate filtering of the data. Crimes which could have taken place in longer time periods are not useful for analysis. For example, a victim can be aware of a burglary after waking up or coming home from work, which does not provide accurate information about the time the crime occurred. For most crimes, the exact time is not known; the MPS dataset provides a window between "Time committed from" and "Time committed to" during which the crime is likely to have occurred. As this study depends on knowing if it was light or dark at the time the crime took place, only crimes where the time is known within 5 min were included. A total of 4,728,291 crimes were analyzed. To calculate solar altitude, a precise time is required. Therefore, following filtering the data by the 5 min window criteria, 2,145,398 of 4,728,921 crimes were used, which corresponds to 45.4% of the dataset. The median time of "Time Committed From" and "Time Committed To" was taken into consideration while calculating the solar position. The observing clock change time method was adopted as Unwin et al. [24] did. Therefore, the first step of the study is to define the interest of periods, which are four time periods, the week before and after spring and autumn clock changes (Table 3).

Table 3. Spring and autumn clock changes within the weeks and years of interest.

One Week before Spring Clock Change		One Week after Spring Clock Change		One Week before Autumn Clock Change		One Week after Autumn Clock Change	
Start	**End**	**Start**	**End**	**Start**	**End**	**Start**	**End**
24 March 2013	30 March 2013	31 March 2013	6 April 2013	20 October 2013	26 October 2013	27 October 2013	2 November 2013
23 March 2014	29 March 2014	30 March 2014	5 April 2014	19 October 2014	25 October 2014	26 October 2014	1 November 2014
22 March 2015	28 March 2015	29 March 2015	4 April 2015	18 October 2015	24 October 2015	25 October 2015	31 October 2015
20 March 2016	26 March 2016	27 March 2016	2 April 2016	23 October 2016	29 October 2016	30 October 2016	5 November 2016
19 March 2017	25 March 2017	26 March 2017	1 April 2017	22 October 2017	28 October 2017	29 October 2017	4 November 2017
18 March 2018	24 March 2018	25 March 2018	31 March 2018	21 October 2018	27 October 2018	28 October 2018	3 November 2018
24 March 2019	30 March 2019	31 March 2019	6 April 2019				

The second step was to assign eight periods to these weeks when there was a change between light and dark for the same time (Table 4). The process enabled us to compare the crime rates based on seasons, days and time slots in a day, and the solar position of crime based on time and location.

Table 4. Assign codes for interested weeks.

Code	Season	Time of Day	Week	Light Condition
SMB	Spring	Morning	Before	Light
SMA			After	Dark
SEB		Evening	Before	Dark
SEA			After	Light
AMB	Autumn	Morning	Before	Dark
AMA			After	Light
AEB		Evening	Before	Light
AEA			After	Dark

After filtering the data according to the time accuracy of the record (crime time known to within 5 min), the study compared crime rates in daylight and darkness. Raynham et al. [31] stated that solar altitude would provide an accurate and innovative method for understanding daylight availability. The solar altitude of crimes in the MPS dataset was calculated using the National Atmospheric Administration (NOAA) [39] method and Astral Anaconda and Geopanda Python Library [40]. The MPS dataset provides the location of each crime with an Easting and Northing coordinate used by the U.K. Ordinance Survey Mapping (British National Grid Reference). This was then converted into latitude and longitude for the calculation of solar altitude.

The twilight period can cause ambiguity in classifying dark and light conditions because the twilight period is variable, and it can still be daylight during this period. Illuminance over the twilight period was explored using a dataset consisting of over 1,600,000 records of illuminance made at 5 min intervals over 2 years in eight locations across the UK in previous research. All illuminance records were binned according to solar altitude. Analysis of illuminance percentiles revealed an illuminance of 10 lux at the 99th percentile at a solar altitude of −6 degrees and an illuminance of 50 lux at the first percentile at 0 degrees. This means that we can say with some certainty that it is dark at −6 degrees and light at 0 degrees. Local authorities tend to pick 30 lux as the threshold at which to turn street lighting on, so 50 lux is a safe estimate for conditions deemed daylit enough for street lighting not to be required. At −5 degrees, the 99th percentile value was 40 lux, and at 1 degree the first percentile value was 80 lux; these illuminance values do not provide enough certainty of darkness and daylight, which is why solar altitudes of −6 degrees and 0 degrees were used to define darkness and daylight [31]. Therefore, this study removed crimes which took place between −6 degrees and 0 degrees, which amounted to 7592 crimes in the weeks of interest. Crimes in the twilight period were added back into the dataset when the study reported crimes by the hour. Figure 2 gives an example (spring 2018) of the effect of the clock change, in this case from GMT (Greenwich Mean Time) to BST (British Summer Time), on daylight availability.

The test period refers to the time window that is dark before the clock change and light after the clock change or vice versa the following week. It is possible that the change in the number of crimes during the week of daylight saving time was not solely due to the change in daylight. Therefore, "control" periods were used so that differences between them could also be compared, as there are other factors which could affect behavior, such as changes in weather, school holidays, and events (such as Easter). The number of crimes was tallied for each control period to ensure that other major factors were not influencing the results during the clock change periods.

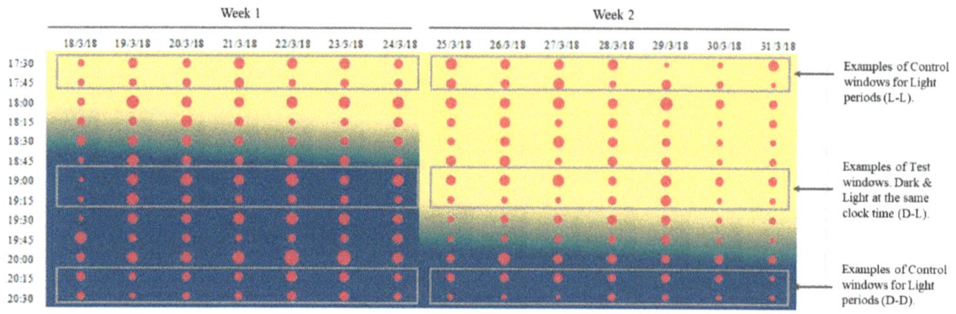

Figure 2. Chart illustrating the change in light and dark times on either side of the spring clock change in 2018. Blue indicates dark, and yellow indicates light. In between dark and light is twilight.

Lastly, to assess findings in terms of the risk of crimes in darkness, the dark/light ratio of crime in the test period and control period were compared. The odds ratio calculation that Johansson et al. [41] used in their traffic casualties paper was used, and the following formula (Equation (1)) was applied to overall crime and the breakdown of crime types:

$$OR = \frac{Crimes\ in\ test\ period\ in\ dark\ (A)/Crimes\ in\ the\ test\ period\ in\ daylight\ (B)}{Crimes\ in\ control\ period\ when\ test\ period\ is\ dark\ (C)/Crimes\ in\ control\ period\ when\ test\ period\ is\ daylight\ (D)} \quad (1)$$

When an odds ratio is greater than 1, it demonstrates higher odds of more crimes occurring in the dark; an odds ratio of less than 1 indicates lower odds of crime in the dark. The p value of each finding was calculated using the Chi-Square test. 95% confidence intervals (CI) related to the odds ratio of the findings were calculated using the following steps of Fleiss et al. [42] and Shadish et al. [43]. A, B, C, and D are the estimates of risk that are given inversely proportional to their variance in the calculation of the estimates of risk based on the odds ratio. Equation (2) provides the logarithm of the odds ratio.

$$\upsilon\mathrm{i} = \frac{1}{A} + \frac{1}{B} + \frac{1}{C} + \frac{1}{D} \quad (2)$$

wi represents the statistical weight of each estimate, incorporating both the fixed-effects and random effects models. Equation (3).

$$\mathrm{wi} = \frac{1}{\upsilon\mathrm{i}} \quad (3)$$

To find the statistically weighted mean ($\bar{y}$), the potential outcomes of different scenarios in generalized estimating (g) were calculated with Equation (4).

$$\bar{y} = \exp\left(\frac{\sum_{i=1}^{g} wiyi}{\sum_{i=1}^{g} wi}\right) \quad (4)$$

95% CI of the weighted mean was calculated, according to Equation (5).

$$95\%\ \text{confidence interval} = \exp\left[\frac{\left(\sum_{i=1}^{g} wiyi/\sum_{i=1}^{g} wi\right) \pm 1.96 \times 1}{\sqrt{\sum_{i=1}^{g} wi}}\right] \quad (5)$$

4. Results

Each crime location was recorded using GPS coordinates from the Ordnance Survey National Grid, also known as the British National Grid reference system. Figure 3 demonstrates the overall distribution and density of all reported crimes, bi-yearly, in London between 2013 and 2019.

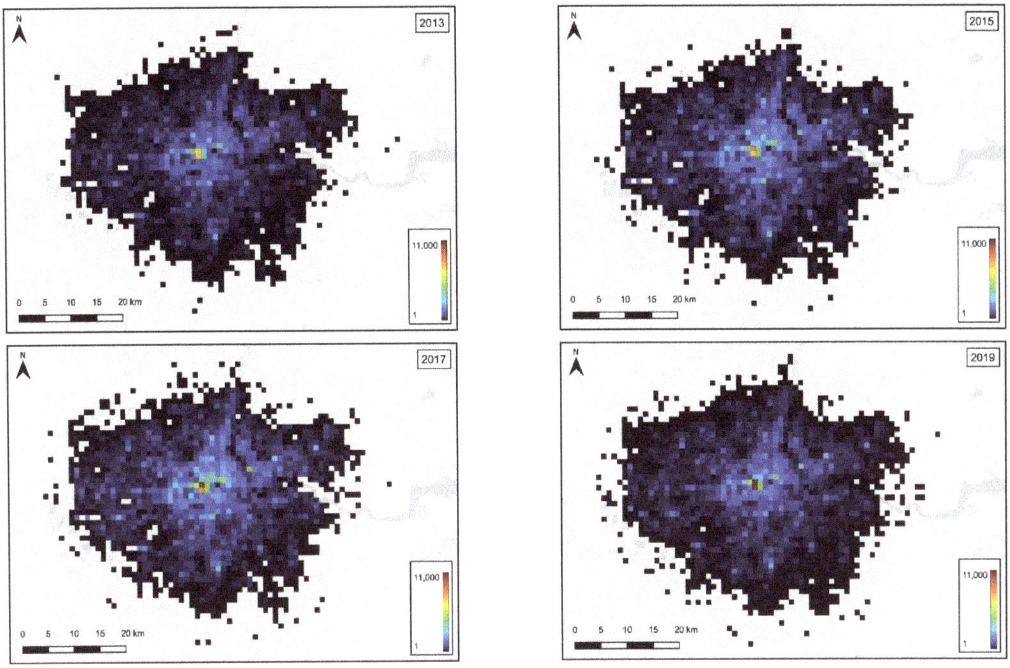

Figure 3. Map of Greater London showing total reported crime distribution and density over time, using 2013, 2015, 2017, and 2019 as example years.

After calculating the solar position, some crimes were removed because there were not enough of them for ambient lighting conditions to be shown convincingly to have an effect. Therefore, crimes with less than 20,000 records were excluded, and 20 crime types were reported. Table 5 shows the number of crimes with their definitions and the percentages of the total dataset reported to within the 5 min crime window that occurred in the controlled time periods in which the crimes occurred in the dark one week before the clock change and in the light one week after the clock change or vice versa. The results demonstrated a 4.82% (OR 1.07) rise in overall crime rates in the dark.

Table 5. The most common crimes listed with all others lumped together and the number of cases that occurred each week of interest from 2013 to 2019.

Crime Definition		Number of Crimes			Results			
Major Crime Category	Minor Crime Types	Total Crimes	Crime Known to 5 min	Percentage	Light	Dark	Light to Dark Change	Odds Ratio
Arson and Criminal Damage	**Criminal damage**	**354,720**	**143,738**	**40.5%**	**161**	**183**	**14%**	**1.07**
Burglary	Burglary—business and community	154,228	38,312	24.8%	27	52	93%	
Burglary	**Burglary—residential**	**324,535**	**71,054**	**21.9%**	**66**	**105**	**59%**	**1.59**
Drug offenses	Drug trafficking	20,166	14,039	69.6%	21	21	0%	
Drug offenses	**Possession of drugs**	**236,981**	**194,826**	**82.2%**	**262**	**217**	**−17%**	**0.80**
Public order offenses	Other offenses against the state	36,579	22,420	61.3%	24	24	0%	
Public order offenses	Public fear alarm or distress	165,928	99,080	59.7%	127	124	−2%	
Public order offenses	Racially or religiously aggravated public fear	46,983	27,567	58.7%	35	38	9%	
Robbery	**Robbery of personal property**	**149,981**	**89,897**	**59.9%**	**117**	**138**	**18%**	**1.29**
Sexual offenses	Other sexual offenses	52,057	23,869	45.9%	25	31	24%	

Table 5. *Cont.*

Crime Definition		Number of Crimes			Results			
Major Crime Category	Minor Crime Types	Total Crimes	Crime Known to 5 min	Percentage	Light	Dark	Light to Dark Change	Odds Ratio
Sexual offenses	Rape	22,352	6249	28.0%	7	4	−43%	
Theft	Bicycle theft	119,843	23,222	19.4%	44	39	−11%	
Theft	Other theft	707,220	299,821	42.4%	378	394	4%	
Theft	Shoplifting	275,729	192,439	69.8%	308	310	1%	
Theft	**Theft from person**	**254,391**	**114,593**	**45.0%**	**142**	**180**	**27%**	**1.27**
Vehicle offenses	Interfering with a motor vehicle	70,627	21,227	30.1%	17	25	47%	
Vehicle offenses	Theft from a motor vehicle	369,387	64,299	17.4%	70	60	−14%	
Vehicle offenses	Theft or taking of a motor vehicle	160,825	32,490	20.2%	28	46	64%	**1.38**
Violence against the person	Violence with injury	433,632	244,117	56.3%	284	284	0%	
Violence against the person	Violence without injury	640,149	337,734	52.8%	402	409	2%	
Other	Other	131,978	84,405	64.0%	109	98	−10%	
Total		**4,728,291**	**2,145,398**	**45.4%**	**2654**	**2782**	**4.8%**	**1.07**

The findings show that there is an overall increase in total of 4.8% (OR 1.07). Table 6 demonstrates the crime types for which the change from light to dark (or vice versa) had the most effect. Vehicle offenses (theft or taking of a motor vehicle) and burglary-residential increased dramatically by 64% (OR 1.38) and 59% (1.59), while theft from a person, robbery, and arson, and criminal damage increased by 27% (OR 1.27), 18% (OR 1.29), and 14%(1.07), respectively. In contrast, possession of drugs decreased by 17% (0R 0.80).

Table 6. Breakdown of highlighted crime types listed in Table 6 with the number of cases, odds ratio, 95% CI and *p*-values that occurred in each week of interest from 2013 to 2019.

	Number of Crimes			Analysis		
Crime Types	**Classification**	**Light**	**Dark**	**Odds Ratio**	**95% CI**	***p* Value**
Criminal damage	Test Control	158 776	177 816	1.07	0.84–1.35	0.229
Burglary-residential	Test Control	60 374	95 372	1.59	1.11–2.26	0.001
Possession of drugs	Test Control	254 1100	204 1106	0.80	0.65–0.98	0.010
Robbery of personal property	Test Control	111 554	134 519	1.29	0.95–1.70	0.066
Theft from person	Test Control	140 699	176 698	1.27	0.98–1.61	0.025
Theft or taking of a motor vehicle	Test Control	26 150	40 167	1.38	0.80–2.37	0.058
Total	Test Control	2525 11,265	2645 11,009	1.07	1.01–1.14	0.059

Table 7 shows the time of controlled periods for the evening with the results. The morning period was not analyzed because crime in the morning was much less common than crime in the afternoon; see Figure 4.

Table 7. Times of the control periods for the evening lighting conditions in spring and autumn.

Code	Condition			Time		Before	After	Percentage Change
				Start Time	End Time	Number of Crimes		
SED	Spring	Evening	Dark	20:30	21:30	2288	2495	8%
SEL	Spring	Evening	Light	17:00	18:00	3008	3253	8%
AED	Autumn	Evening	Dark	18:30	19:30	2557	2834	10%
AEL	Autumn	Evening	Light	15:30	16:30	2960	2879	−3%

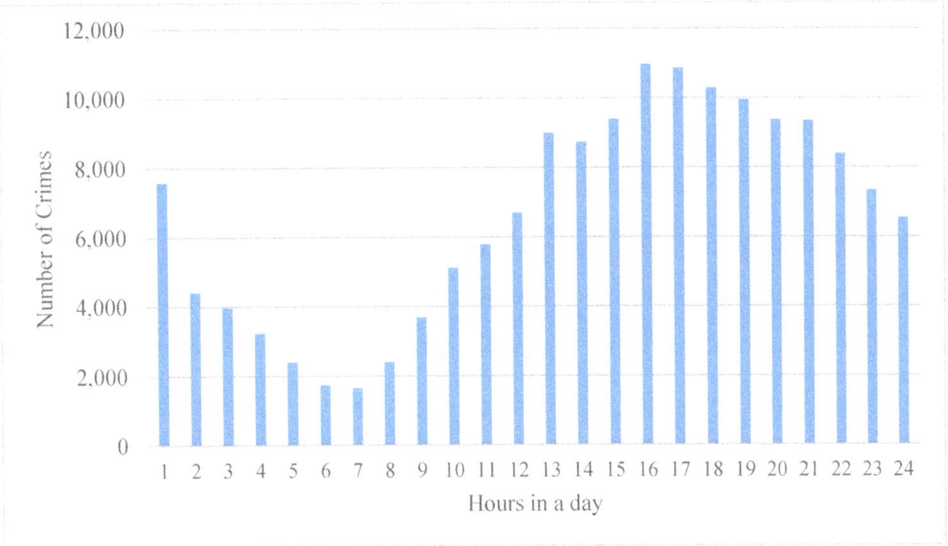

Figure 4. Total crime rates by each hour during the day.

The study also reports the distribution of crime rates in London by each hour throughout the day. Figure 4 presents 158,933 recorded crimes where the time of the crime was known to 5 min or less, within 1 week before and after autumn and spring clock changes for all years. Figure 4, therefore, only represents 45.4% of crimes reported in the week of interest. All types of crimes mentioned above are included in Figure 4. Number 1 shows the crime counts between midnight and 1 am. The results demonstrate that crime is lowest around 6 am, whereas crime rates increase significantly in the afternoon, and incidents of crime peak between 3 pm and 5 pm. A total of 30.65% of crime occurs in the morning, and 69.35% of crime occurs in the afternoon.

5. Discussion

GPS coordinates enable us to assess the crime distribution over the years. Figure 3 demonstrates crime rates were more widespread in central London than in outer London in the time period analyzed for this research. The study explored crime rates during periods in the weeks on either side of the spring and autumn clock changes where in one week at a given time, it was dark, and in the other week, it was light. The aim was to understand the impact of lighting on crime. However, this is a complex topic. There are limited past studies to which to compare the results, and it is difficult to provide predictions. For example, Tompson et al. [44] found that vehicle crimes after dark occur more where street lighting exists compared to non-lit environments; however, there is the potential for displacement of crime to adjacent streets.

In the study of Fotios et al. [33], the precise time the crime occurred is not clear. Other studies focus on crime patterns within a year instead of over the longer term [19,20]. Crime rates also might depend on other features of the built environment, such as surveillance and street morphology and criminals' purposes [6].

Nevertheless, ambient lighting conditions play a role in some crimes. The studies described previously by Doleac et al. [45], Tealde, E. [35], and Fotios et al. [33] investigated the relationship between Daylight Saving Time and crime and found that outdoor crimes such as robbery and violent attacks tend to increase due to darkness. Additionally, Doleac et al. [45] found an impact of DST on the economy, estimating that the extension of Daylight Saving in the United States in 2007 resulted in an annual cost savings to society of $59 million due to the prevention of robberies.

This study also supports these studies because we found that the fall of darkness (as opposed to daylight conditions) affects some crime types by using the DST approach. Overall, the increase in the risk of crime associated with darkness is fairly significant (5% OR 1.07). When broken down by crime type, there was a rise in theft from the person, robbery, arson and criminal damage, burglary, and vehicle offenses in the dark. Theft from a person (OR 1.27), robbery of personal property (OR 1.29), arson and criminal damage (OR 1.07), burglary (OR 1.59), and theft or taking of a motor vehicle (OR 1.38), increased after dark, while drug offenses decreased after dark. This supports the third and fourth hypotheses that "If light has an impact on crime, then crime at night/dark should be different from crime during the day/light" and "Light and dark impact crime types differently. For example, outdoor crimes such as robbery and theft increase after dark, whereas other crime types do not." When looking at drug-related (OR 0.80) crimes, there is a question about the way this type of crime is reported because the victim and the perpetrator of the crime are usually the same person. If someone has possession of drugs, they do not want to report to the police that a crime has taken place. Thus, it is suspected that the crime is normally reported when the police find the person with drugs. A total of 82% of possession of drugs crimes are known to be reported within 5 min of taking place (Table 5). This may explain the fall in the reported drug crimes after dark, as poor lighting may make it harder to find offenders.

Burglary (p-value = 0.001) and theft from the person (p-value = 0.025) show statistically significant findings ($p < 0.05$). Although the p-values of the rest of the crime types are greater than 0.05, theft or taking of a motor vehicle (p-value = 0.051), robbery of personal property (p-value = 0.066), and overall crime (p-value = 0.059) are close to 0.05, which could be described as approaching significance. Additionally, the odds ratio enables a more accurate calculation of the potential risk by considering the broader perspective by including confounding variables and creating a control period [41].

Additionally, only 22% of burglary and 17% of vehicle offenses have times known within a 5 min window, which is too low to make a convincing statement. This is because a small change in victim behavior, such as coming home soon after dark, could have a large influence on the number of crimes reported. The number of incidents (Table 5) of other crimes is too low to make any reliable claims. For example, the numbers for burglary—business and community are 27 and 52 (light, dark test period), other sexual offenses are 25 and 31, and rape are 7 and 4.

The study can convincingly report that the crimes of robbery of personal property and theft from the person seem to be typically street crimes, and the increase after dark shows a possible link with darkness, which requires further investigation. Although overall crime rates in Figure 4 in daylight are higher than after dark, crime is much more widespread in the afternoon than in the morning. It could be related to the population of the people; for example, students and adults go out to study or work. In addition, there is an increase in crime in the afternoon (PM) compared with the morning in daylight (am). Figure 4 supports the second hypothesis that "Crime rates vary within the day (24 h period)." The study helps understand whether there is a link between the occurrence of crime and external lighting conditions. The counts of all crimes increased by around 5% (OR 1.07) in the relevant daily windows using the comparison between the adjacent weeks' equivalent light-dark pairing. Table 7 shows that even though there is no significant difference between spring and autumn crime counts in the dark before and after the clock change (SED and AED), in the light periods (SEL and AEL), there is a difference. This finding affirms the hypothesis 1 that "There are seasonal differences in the effects of light and dark on crime. In autumn, we would expect a bigger difference compared to spring due to the onset of darkness". Exploration of the breakdown of each crime type, such as robbery, theft, and burglary, in spring and autumn, requires further investigation.

There were two main limitations of the study. Firstly, the Crime Lab from which the data were extracted has stringent rules. Research in crime requires vetting processes for individuals, and the crime data are preserved in a high-security room. For example, accessing data and the Lab took around 3 months due to our security vetting process. There was no internet access, and no technological devices such as laptops, mobile phones, and smartwatches were allowed in the Lab to protect the data. There were limited tools and libraries that we could use. Uploading some libraries in Python had to be done by the administrative team. Secondly, some crime data were incomplete or duplicated. For example, there were two different files for the same crime incident in 2013. While one had 600,000 records, the other had 580,000 records. We had to clean the data by comparing, matching, and interpreting each file before we began the analysis.

6. Conclusions

Analysis of total crime, using GPS coordinates to show crime distribution across greater London, demonstrated that crime did not considerably change within the year or over the years available in this dataset. However, using a reliable method, this study demonstrated that ambient light conditions impacted some crimes, in particular outdoor crimes. Robbery and theft from a person were affected by lighting conditions and increased if it was dark. This finding shows that lighting affects the behavior of criminals in the built environment, which could also contribute to the fear of becoming victimized after dark for citizens. This has wider implications for lighting design which could be used as a tool in combating crime because a better-designed lit environment could also lead to less crime. There is now a valid reason to investigate the impact of location-specific geographic features further.

The driving problem is that lighting designers need to know how to use lighting design to contribute to the safety of the environment. However, until now, there has been very little convincing evidence that lighting affects crime. Our research provides important evidence that lighting conditions impact some outdoor crimes. This finding means that different approaches to the lighting design of external urban environments matter, could reduce crime, and that the effect of local lighting conditions should be explored further.

Author Contributions: Conceptualization: Ezgi Erturk, Jemima Unwin Teji and Peter Raynham. Data Curation: Ezgi Erturk. Formal analysis: Ezgi Erturk. Funding acquisition: Ezgi Erturk, Jemima Unwin Teji and Peter Raynham. Methodology: Ezgi Erturk, Jemima Unwin Teji and Peter Raynham. Software: Ezgi Erturk and Peter Raynham. Validation: Ezgi Erturk, Peter Raynham and Jemima Unwin Teji. Supervision: Jemima Unwin Teji and Peter Raynham. Visualization: Ezgi Erturk and Peter Raynham. Writing-original draft: Ezgi Erturk, Writing-review and editing: Jemima Unwin Teji and Peter Raynham. All authors have read and agreed to the published version of the manuscript.

Funding: Access to the secure crime database of the Jill Dando Institute Research Laboratory was provided by Bartlett School of Environment Energy and Resources (BSEER-UCL). The study presented in this article is part of the PhD study of the first author, who is sponsored by the Turkish Ministry of National Education at University College London (UCL).

Data Availability Statement: The 3rd Party Data was used in this study. Restrictions apply to the availability of these data. Data were obtained from the Jill Dando Institute Research Laboratory (JDIRL Lab) at UCL and are available from https://www.ucl.ac.uk/jill-dando-institute/about-us/jdi-rl (accessed on 12 March 2024). with the permission of the JDIRL Lab at UCL. The data for the study was provided by the Jill Dando Institute Research Laboratory (JDIRL Lab) at UCL after the authors passed the vetting process, which permitted access. This is a completely secure, confidential database that is not publicly available due to the sensitivity of the data, which contains locations and times of crimes. The data were analyzed in the JDIRL Lab because data cannot be removed from the laboratory. Supplementary details are described in the methodology section. The study was also approved as a low-risk study by the Research Ethics Committee at the UCL. The study did not collect any personal data16.

Conflicts of Interest: The authors declared no potential conflicts of interest with respect to the research, authorship, and/or publication of this article.

References

1. Nasar, J.L.; Fisher, B. 'Hot spots' of fear and crime: A multi-method investigation. *J. Environ. Psychol.* **1993**, *13*, 187–206. [CrossRef]
2. United Nations. *Sustainable Development Goals*; United Nations: San Francisco, CA, USA, 2014; pp. 34–37. Available online: https://sdgs.un.org/goals/goal16 (accessed on 12 March 2024).
3. Jacobs, J. *The Death and Life of Great American Cities*; The Failure of Town Planning: New York, NY, USA, 1961.
4. Welsh, B.C.; Mudge, M.E.; Farrington, D.P. Reconceptualizing public area surveillance and crime prevention: Security guards, place managers and defensible space. *Secur. J.* **2010**, *23*, 299–319. [CrossRef]
5. Clarke, R.V. Introduction. In *Situational Crime Prevention Successful Case Studies*, 2nd ed.; Clarke, R.V., Ed.; Harrow and Heston: Guilderland, NY, USA, 1997; pp. 1–47.
6. Newman, O. *Defensible Space: Crime Prevention through Urban Design*; Collier Books: New York, NY, USA, 1973.
7. Duggan, M. Killing of Mark Duggan. 2024, pp. 1–23. Available online: https://en.wikipedia.org/wiki/Killing_of_Mark_Duggan (accessed on 13 December 2023).
8. Andresen, M.A.; Malleson, N. Crime seasonality and its variations across space. *Appl. Geogr.* **2013**, *43*, 25–35. [CrossRef]
9. Shiode, N.; Shiode, S.; Nishi, H.; Hino, K. Seasonal characteristics of crime: An empirical investigation of the temporal fluctuation of the different types of crime in London. *Comput. Urban. Sci.* **2023**, *3*, 19. [CrossRef]
10. Appleton, J. *The Experience of Landscape*; Wiley: London, UK, 1975.
11. Fisher, B.S.; Nasar, J.L. Fear of crime in relation to three exterior site features: Prospect, Refuge, and Escape. *Environ. Behav.* **1992**, *24*, 31. [CrossRef]
12. Boyce, P.; Gutkowski, J. The if, why and what of street lighting and street crime: A review. *Light. Res. Technol.* **1995**, *27*, 10. [CrossRef]
13. Mayhew, P.; Aye Maung, N.; Mirrlees-Black, C. *The 1992 British Crime Survey/by Pat Mayhew, Natalie Aye Maung and Catriona Mirrlees-Black*; HMSO: London, UK, 1993.
14. *BS 5489-1: 2020*; Design of Road Lighting—Lighting of Roads and Public Amenity Areas. Code of Practice: London, UK, 2020.
15. Schivelbusch, W. *Disenchanted Night: The Industrialisation of Light in the Nineteenth Century/Wolfgang Schivelbusch/Translated from the German by Angela Davies Schivelbusch*; University of California Press: Berkeley, CA, USA, 1988.
16. Haans, A.; de Kort, Y.A.W. Light distribution in dynamic street lighting: Two experimental studies on its effects on perceived safety, prospect, concealment, and escape. *J. Environ. Psychol.* **2012**, *32*, 342–352. [CrossRef]
17. Welsh, B.C.; Farrington, D.P. Effects of Improved Street Lighting on Crime. *Campbell Syst. Rev.* **2008**, *4*, 1–51. [CrossRef]
18. Wright, R.; Heilweil, M.; Pelletier, P.; Dickinson, K. *The Impact of Street Lighting on Street Crime*; The University of Michigan: Ann Arbor, MI, USA, 1974.
19. Painter, K.; Gunnell, P.; Fleming, R. *Middlesex Polytechnic Lighting and Crime Prevention: The Edmonton Project*; Middlesex polytechnic: London, UK, 1988.
20. Nair, G.; Ditton, J. "In the Dark, a Taper Is Better than Nothing". A One Year Follow-Up of a Successful Street Lighting and Crime Prevention Experiment. *Light. J.* **1994**, *59*, 25–27.
21. Painter, K. An Evaluation of Public Lighting. *Light. J.* **1991**, *56*, 228–232.
22. Steinbach, R.; Perkins, C.; Tompson, L. The effect of reduced street lighting on road casualties and crime in England and Wales: Controlled interrupted time series analysis. *J. Epidemiol. Community Health* **2015**, *69*, 1118–1124. [CrossRef]
23. Peng, C.; Sun, W.; Zhang, X. Crime under the Light? Examining the Effects of Nighttime Lighting on Crime in China. *Land* **2022**, *11*, 2305. [CrossRef]
24. Unwin, J.; Symonds, P.; Laike, T. Does lighting affect pedestrian flows? A pilot study in Lund, Market Harborough and Dublin. In Proceedings of the Lux Europa 2017 European Lighting Conference-Lighting for Modern Society, Ljubljana, Slovenia, 18–20 September 2017; pp. 1–5.
25. Kids Make Town a "Living Hell". *South Yorksh Times*, 16 February 2001; p. 1.

26. Mansfield, K.; Raynham, P. Urban Lights—Sustainable Urban Lighting for Town Centre Regeneration. In Proceedings of the Lux Europa, Berlin, Germany, 19 September 2005; pp. 491–493.
27. Sullivan, J.M.; Flannagan, M.J. The role of ambient light level in fatal crashes: Inferences from daylight saving time transitions. *Accid. Anal. Prev.* **2002**, *34*, 487–498. [CrossRef]
28. Uttley, J.; Fotios, S. The effect of ambient light condition on road traffic collisions involving pedestrians on pedestrian crossings. *Accid. Anal. Prev.* **2017**, *108*, 189–200. [CrossRef]
29. Ferguson, S.A.; Preusser, D.F.; Lund, A.K.; Zador, P.L.; Ulmer, R.G. Daylight saving time and motor vehicle crashes: The reduction in pedestrian and vehicle occupant fatalities. *Am. J. Public Health* **1995**, *85*, 92–96. [CrossRef]
30. Muneer, T.; Kambezidis, H. *Solar Radiation and Daylight Models for the Energy Efficient Design of Buildings/T. Muneer/with a Chapter on Solar Spectral Radiation by H. Kambezidis*, 1st ed.; Architectural Press: Oxford, UK; Boston, MA, USA, 1997.
31. Raynham, P.; Unwin, J.; Khazova, M.; Tolia, S. The role of lighting in road traffic collisions. *Light. Res. Technol.* **2020**, *52*, 485–494. [CrossRef]
32. Fotios, S.; Robbins, C.J. Incorrect categorisation of ambient light level at the time of a road traffic collision. *Light. Res. Technol.* **2022**, *56*, 87–101. [CrossRef]
33. Fotios, S.A.; Robbins, C.J.; Farrall, S. The effect of lighting on crime counts. *Energies* **2021**, *14*, 4099. [CrossRef]
34. Umbach, R.; Raine, A.; Ridgeway, G. Aggression and sleep: A daylight saving time natural experiment on the effect of mild sleep loss and gain on assaults. *J. Exp. Criminol.* **2017**, *13*, 439–453. [CrossRef]
35. Tealde, E. The unequal impact of natural light on crime. *J. Popul. Econ.* **2021**, *35*, 893–934. [CrossRef]
36. Open Science Framework. Crime Open Database (CODE). 2021. Available online: https://osf.io/zyaqn/ (accessed on 15 June 2022).
37. Metropolitan Police. *All Crimes in London*; Metropolitan Police: London, UK, 2019.
38. Metropolitan Police. Crime Type Definitions. Metropolitan Police. 2022. Available online: https://www.met.police.uk/sd/stats-and-data/met/crime-type-definitions/ (accessed on 14 March 2022).
39. National Oceanic and Atmospheric Administration. Solar Calculation Details. 2005. Available online: https://gml.noaa.gov/grad/solcalc/calcdetails.html (accessed on 28 February 2022).
40. astral 3.2. AnacondaOrg. 2022. Available online: https://anaconda.org/conda-forge/astral (accessed on 12 May 2022).
41. Johansson, Ö.; Wanvik, P.O.; Elvik, R. A new method for assessing the risk of accident associated with darkness. *Accid. Anal. Prev.* **2009**, *41*, 809–815. [CrossRef]
42. Fleiss, J.L.; Levin, B.; Paik, M.C. *Statistical Methods for Rates and Proportions*, 3rd ed.; John Wiley and Sons: Hoboken, NJ, USA, 2003.
43. Shadish, W.R.; Haddock, C.K. Combining Estimates of Effect Size. In *The Handbook of Research Synthesis*; Harris, C., Hedges, L.V., Eds.; Russell Sage Foundation: New York, NY, USA, 1994; pp. 261–280.
44. Tompson, L.; Steinbach, R.; Johnson, S.D.; Teh, C.S.; Perkins, C.; Edwards, P.; Armstrong, B. Absence of Street Lighting May Prevent Vehicle Crime, but Spatial and Temporal Displacement Remains a Concern. *J. Quant. Criminol.* **2022**, *39*, 603–623. [CrossRef]
45. Doleac, J.L.; Sanders, N.J. Under the cover of darkness: How ambient light influences criminal activity. *Rev. Econ. Stat.* **2015**, *97*, 1093–1103. [CrossRef]

International Journal of
Geo-Information

MDPI

Article

AED Inequity among Social Groups in Guangzhou

Feng Gao [1,2,3,*], Siyi Lu [4], Shunyi Liao [1,2,3], Wangyang Chen [1,2,3], Xin Chen [1,2,3], Jiemin Wu [1,2,3], Yunjing Wu [1,2,3], Guanyao Li [1,2,3] and Xu Han [1,2,3]

1. Guangzhou Urban Planning & Design Survey Research Institute Co., Ltd., Guangzhou 510060, China; liaoshunyi@gzsghy.wecom.work (S.L.); e0403826@u.nus.edu (W.C.); chenxin@gzsghy.wecom.work (X.C.); wujm23@mail2.sysu.edu.cn (J.W.); gyli@gzpi.com.cn (G.L.); m202073659@mail.hust.edu.cn (X.H.)
2. Collaborative Innovation Center for Natural Resources Planning and Marine Technology of Guangzhou, Guangzhou 510060, China
3. Guangdong Enterprise Key Laboratory for Urban Sensing, Monitoring and Early Warning, Guangzhou 510060, China
4. Business School, University of Auckland, Auckland 999030, New Zealand; slu791@aucklanduni.ac.nz

* Correspondence: 2111801048@e.gzhu.edu.cn

Abstract: Automated external defibrillators (AEDs) are regarded as the most important public facility after fire extinguishers due to their importance to out-of-hospital cardiac arrest (OHCA) victims. Previous studies focused on the location optimization of the AED, with little attention to inequity among different social groups. To comprehensively investigate the spatial heterogeneity of the AED inequity, we first collected AED data from a WeChat applet. Then, we used the geographically weighted regression (GWR) model to quantify the inequity level and identify the socio-economic status group that faced the worst inequity in each neighborhood. Results showed that immigrants of all ages suffer a more severe AED inequity than residents after controlling population and road density. Immigrants face more severe inequity in downtown, while residents face more severe inequity in the peripheral and outer suburbs. AED inequity among youngsters tends to be concentrated in the center of each district, while inequity among the elderly tends to be distributed at the edge of each district. This study provides a new perspective for investigating the inequity in public facilities, puts forward scientific suggestions for future AED allocation planning, and emphasizes the importance of the equitable access to AED.

Keywords: AED; inequity; spatial disparities; social groups

1. Introduction

Out-of-hospital cardiac arrest (OHCA) is a major cause of mortality worldwide [1,2]. According to the China Cardiovascular Health and Disease Report 2019, it was estimated that there are 544,000 OHCA cases in China annually, equivalent to one person dying of cardiac arrest every minute, but less than 1% survive [3]. A 7–10% decrease in survival has been reported for each minute delay in the treatment of the patients with OHCA [4,5]. The early implementation of cardiopulmonary resuscitation (CPR) and defibrillation has been proven in numerous clinical practices to be an effective measure to improve the survival rate [6]. Thanks to technology, the emergence and application of automated external defibrillators (AEDs) offer a glimmer of hope for OHCA patients [7]. The AED is a portable medical device that can diagnose specific arrhythmias and provide electrical countershock automatically, which can be used by non-specialists to save patients in OHCA [8,9]. It was found that performing first aid with AED within 3 to 5 min improved the survival rate to 50 to 70% [10]. Therefore, AEDs are vital to the life safety and health of urban residents, especially in megacities.

However, due to the insufficient numbers or uneven distribution of AEDs, only a minority of the OHCA cases in public places use AED before the ambulance arrives [7,11–13]. Due to the late start of the implementation and popularization of the AED in China, the number and popularization rate of the existing AED is lower than that of the developed countries. Therefore, relevant research mainly focused on AED site selection or location optimization [8,13–17]. In general, these studies suggested that AEDs should be located in high-risk areas and readily accessible by proposing strategies for location optimization, which can be categorized into 3 types: previous OHCA cases-based strategy, population density-based strategy, and land use-based strategy. The first strategy selects AED locations in high-risk areas, which is extracted by geocoding the historical OHCA cases and mapping their density [4,8,13,18]. The second strategy advocates placing more AEDs in areas with higher population density [13,17,19–21]. The third strategy quantifies the risk of OHCA by assigning weights to various land uses according to their human activity intensity [4,8,22]. These existing studies have well provided various strategies for AED placement, but they remained in the site selection stage where AED started from scratch, and the equity of AED distribution was seldom discussed.

As an emergency medical facility, the equity of AED is critical. Equitable AED distribution helps to promote the health and safety of the residents and mitigates the inequality of emergency medical resources [13,15]. Currently, studies have investigated medical facility equity with different socio-economic levels and household registration or different ages of population distribution [23–25]. They demonstrated that medical facilities are more likely to be constrained in socio-economically disadvantaged areas than in more affluent communities because low-income groups often have less access to medical facilities due to geographic remoteness and the low-cost modes of travel [23,26–30]. Firstly, the local financial input tends to favor the communities of high socio-economic status, maintaining adequate local medical resources. Secondly, neighborhoods with rich medical resources and high accessibility have higher land prices keeping disadvantaged groups away [28,30]. However, as a public emergency medical facility, the equity of AED distribution should prioritize those disadvantaged for benefits, such as the elderly and immigrants [29,31,32]. Some cases illustrated that medical facilities are located disproportionally among different social groups, especially vulnerable such as the poor, immigrant, and elderly populations in both developing and developed countries which are related to the ongoing healthcare system development by high-capital investment [24,33]. Increasing the number of multi-level medical facilities has always been the goal of the healthcare system reform; however, equity is often ignored.

Despite the fact that numerous studies have explored the accessibility of medical facilities and their equity [24–26,29,31,32], most of them made great contributions to the overall association between medical facilities and socio-economic status by using regression models, Gini coefficient method, and Mann–Whitney U test and so on [26,28,29,32]. For example, Rong et al., indicated that the supply of healthcare institutions was balanced with the total population by using the Gini index, ignoring the variation in different social groups [28]. Jin et al. found that high-income groups have better access to medical facilities than low-income groups in a study which compared equities in different social groups [23]. Cheng et al. compared the inequitable distribution of the elderly and three types of geriatric medical facilities by using accessibility analysis and the Gini index and found the distribution of nursing homes is more equitable for the elderly, compared to daycare centers and assisted-dining facilities [32].

However, most of the existing studies seldom considered spatial heterogeneity. That is, the distribution of social groups and the medical facility's equity for them are both spatially varying. Theoretically, ignoring the spatial heterogeneity of the AED equity may result in neutralizing the positive (equitable) and negative (inequitable) relationship between the medical facilities and socio-economic status in different spatial locations. In addition, in the process of allocating emergency medical resources such as AED, it is challenging to consider the degree of population agglomeration and equitable distribution at the urban scale, while achieving this goal at the local scale (such as a region) is relatively more practical and instructive. The inequity of the AED needs to be considered on both urban and local scales. The urban scale gives priority to strategic control, and the local scale centers on implementation. Therefore, it is of practical significance to explore the spatial heterogeneity of the correlation between AED distribution and sociodemographic attributes. As a local regression model, geographically weighted regression (GWR) has advantages in unraveling the spatially varying relationship between AED availability and any neighborhood sociodemographic groups, hence quantifying the AED inequity level in each neighborhood on the urban scale [34,35]. In addition, the AED inequity will be comprehensively measured and the social group facing the worst inequity in each neighborhood will be identified based on the spatially varying coefficients of the GWR model, which yields helpful insights for AED planning and optimization and the mitigation of the AED inequity.

To address the existing limitations above, the GWR model was adopted to explore the association between AED and social groups in each neighborhood in Guangzhou, China. The purpose of this study is twofold: (1) How is the spatial pattern of AED inequity among different social groups? And (2) which groups are undergoing the worst AED inequity?

2. Materials and Methods

2.1. Theoretical Framework

The research object of this study is equity. The correlation between the proportion of various social groups and the availability of the AED in each neighborhood is essential to measuring equity. Figure 1. defines the inequity [35]. The negative correlation indicates the inequity for this social group [35,36]. For instance, the proportion of the elderly immigrants is negatively associated with the available AED, indicating that the elderly immigrants in this neighborhood are unlikely to be covered by more AEDs than the locals.

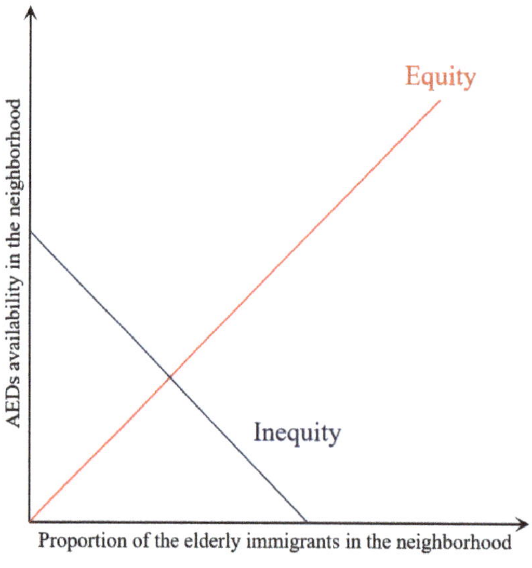

Figure 1. Definition of AED inequity.

Figure 2 displays the theoretical framework of this study. Due to data availability, we take into account the population diversification in terms of age and household registration status. Hence, the social groups included in this study are divided into six categories: young residents, middle-aged residents, elderly residents, young immigrants, middle-aged immigrants, and elderly immigrants. The relationship between neighborhood AED and social groups is established. Given the spatial non-stationarity, the distribution of the AED inequity is examined in multi-social groups. The inequity level and the group facing the worst AED inequity are ascertained by comprehensively measuring the AED inequity across neighborhoods and social groups.

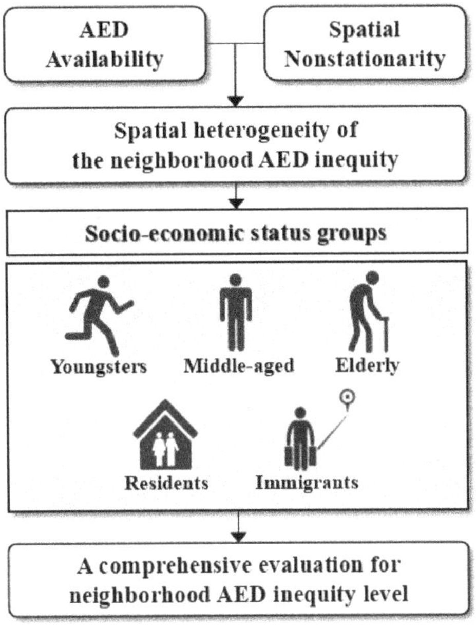

Figure 2. The theoretical framework of the AED inequity.

2.2. Study Area

Guangzhou, China, is a megacity in southern China with a population of more than 18 million [35,37]. This study chooses nine districts of Guangzhou as the study area with 2055 neighborhoods and an area of about 3600 km^2 [38]. The analytics spatial unit is the neighborhood, which is the census unit at the grass-roots level in China. The downtown of Guangzhou comprises the first four districts [39,40]. At present, the total number of AEDs in public has exceeded 1100, among which 16 metro lines and 302 stations have been realizing a complete coverage by AED. In 2021, the Guangzhou Municipal Government promulgated the Work Plan for the Allocation of AEDs in Public Places of Guangzhou (Draft for Comment) [41], planning to fully cover the city's landmark transportation hubs and scenic spots, large sports venues, street offices, community health service centers, and other crowded places by 2025, and to install 4500 AEDs by 2035 (30 per 100,000 population). However, the population structure of Guangzhou is complex, accommodating a large number of vulnerable groups, including the elderly and migrant workers [35]. Therefore, it is very necessary to analyze the equity of emergency medical facilities for various vulnerable groups in Guangzhou.

2.3. AED Data

The AED data in this study were obtained from a WeChat applet named Lifesaving Map via a Python script [42] (Figure 3a). After collecting the text address of the AEDs from an applet, the geo-locations (coordinates) of the AEDs were obtained by using Baidu Map geocoding API. Through manual inspection by overlay geocoding results with online maps, the correct geo-locations of 1006 AEDs were finally obtained and the geocoding hit rate reached 91.5%, which is of high accuracy and can be used for subsequent research.

The measurement of AED availability is shown in Figure 3b. Firstly, the effective rescue time of OHCA patients is between 3 and 5 min [43]. Second, it takes about 1.5 min to set up an AED before use [44], which means only 3.5 min is left for AED delivery. Third, the average running speed is 8 km/h (133 m/min), and the maximum travel distance in which an OHCA eyewitness can successfully deliver an AED (round trip) is about 230 m [15,45]. Therefore, we first generated a point density raster layer with a search radius of 230 m and then calculated the mean of the density raster value of each neighborhood as the AED availability.

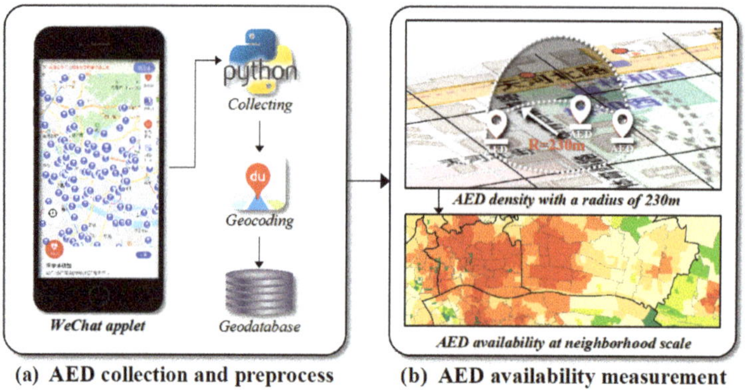

Figure 3. The process of the data collection and availability measurement of the AED.

2.4. Demographic Data

The demographic data at the neighborhood census scale were obtained from the Seventh National Census data. In the current study area, the predominant demographic characteristics were notably marked by high rates of aging and a substantial proportion of immigrants [35,46–48]. Hence, a delineation into three age brackets was conducted, based on the differentiation between the residents and immigrants: the young (ages 19–45), the middle-aged (ages 46–60), and the elderly (over 60 years of age). Specifically, within the study region, the populations of the young residents, young immigrants, middle-aged residents, middle-aged immigrants, elderly residents, and elderly immigrants were quantified at 9.656 million, 6.929 million, 3.358 million, 1.904 million, 1.858 million, and 0.564 million, respectively (Figure 4, Table 1). Given the uneven distribution of the urbanization level and population density in Guangzhou [49], the density of the population and road network were taken as control variables in addition to the above six social group variables.

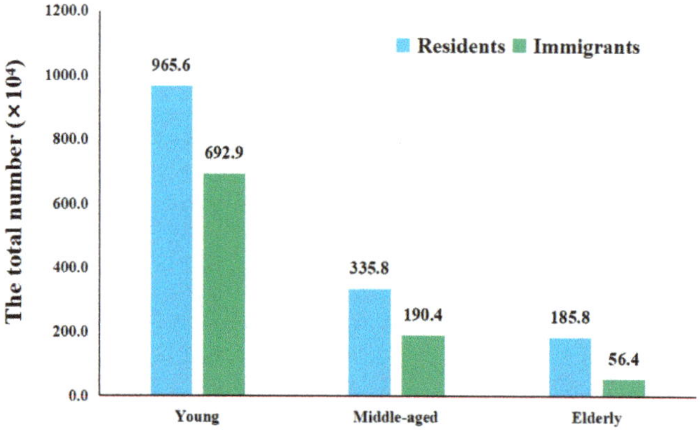

Figure 4. The number of the six social groups in the study area.

First, Pearson's correlation was applied to test potential multicollinearity. If the absolute value of Pearson's coefficient exceeded 0.7, only one of the two variables was retained. Second, the selected variables were standardized so that the mean was 0 and the standard deviation was 1 to identify the most essential determinant [35,36]. The correlation coefficient between MR and ER reached 0.831, which is greater than 0.7. Previous studies have shown that OHCA occurs mainly in the elderly [17,50,51]. Therefore, ER was retained in the model. Finally, the model included YR, ER, YI, MI, and EI as the predictor variables, and POP and RD as control variables.

Table 1. Summary statistics of the variables.

Categories	Variables	Explanation	Mean	SD
Social groups	Young residents (YR)	Proportion of residents aged 19–45 (%)	31.57	0.05
	Middle-aged residents (MR)	Proportion of residents aged 46–60 (%)	14.37	0.04
	Elderly residents (ER)	Proportion of residents aged above 60 (%)	10.25	0.06
	Young immigrants (YI)	Proportion of immigrants aged 19–45 (%)	18.46	0.09
	Middle-aged immigrants (MI)	Proportion of immigrants aged 46–60 (%)	6.31	0.03
	Elderly immigrants (EI)	Proportion of immigrants aged above 60 (%)	2.34	0.02
Control variables	Population density (POP)	Population density (person/km^2)	27,512.36	29,854.67
	Road density (RD)	Road density (km/ km^2)	6.72	7.03

2.5. Geographically Weighted Regression

First, OLS regression was used to model the global association between AED availability and social groups. Multicollinearity was measured by a variance inflation factor (VIF). Jarque–Bera test was used to check the normal distribution of the residual, which determines if the application of the GWR was necessary [52].

However, the OLS regression model is a global model, and its estimated coefficients are constant rather than spatially heterogeneous, ignoring the model coefficients and fitting differences of different geographical units [53]. The GWR model is a regression model considering spatial autocorrelation [54]. Because GWR incorporates spatial variability into the coefficient estimation, it has a better fitting performance in the regression results [55]. To comprehensively quantify the spatially varying association between AED availability and social groups, the inequity was modeled by applying GWR, which can be expressed as follows.

$$y_i = \beta_0(u_i, v_i) + \sum_k \beta_k(u_i, v_i) X_{ik} + \varepsilon_i \tag{1}$$

where y_i is the response variable at neighborhood i; $\beta_0(u_i, v_i)$ is the intercept at position i; $\beta_k(u_i, v_i)$ is the coefficient (weight) of the kth predictor variable estimated for each neighborhood i at location (u_i, v_i); ε_i is a random error. Weights were generated based on bandwidth, which is related to kernel type, bandwidth method, distance, and the number of adjacent points. Using a fixed kernel type, the corrected Akaike Information Criterion (AICc) was applied to calculate the optimal bandwidth. AICc is an indicator to compare the OLS and GWR in terms of the model performance and fitting. When the difference of AICc between models exceeds 3, the lower AICc and higher R-square indicate better goodness of fit [34,54].

To measure the type and level of the AED inequity considering spatial heterogeneity, we further extended the results of the GWR model by overlaying and summarizing the GWR coefficients of the social group variables. The neighborhood where the GWR coefficient of each variable is significantly negative is coded as 1, and the remaining neighborhood is coded as 0 [36]. According to previous studies, the level of inequity is categorized into four types: low (0–1), moderate (1–2), high (2–3), and extreme (3–5) [35]. Moreover, the neighborhood-scale map of the social group facing the worst inequity is visualized based on the standardized negative coefficient of the social groups [35,36].

3. Results

3.1. Spatial Distribution of AED Availability

Figure 5 displays the neighborhood AED availability. High availability areas are concentrated in the downtown, including Yuexiu, western Tianhe, eastern Liwan, northern Haizhu district, and southern Baiyun. In general, the spatial distribution of the AED availability is highly consistent with the pattern of the urban population and economic distribution.

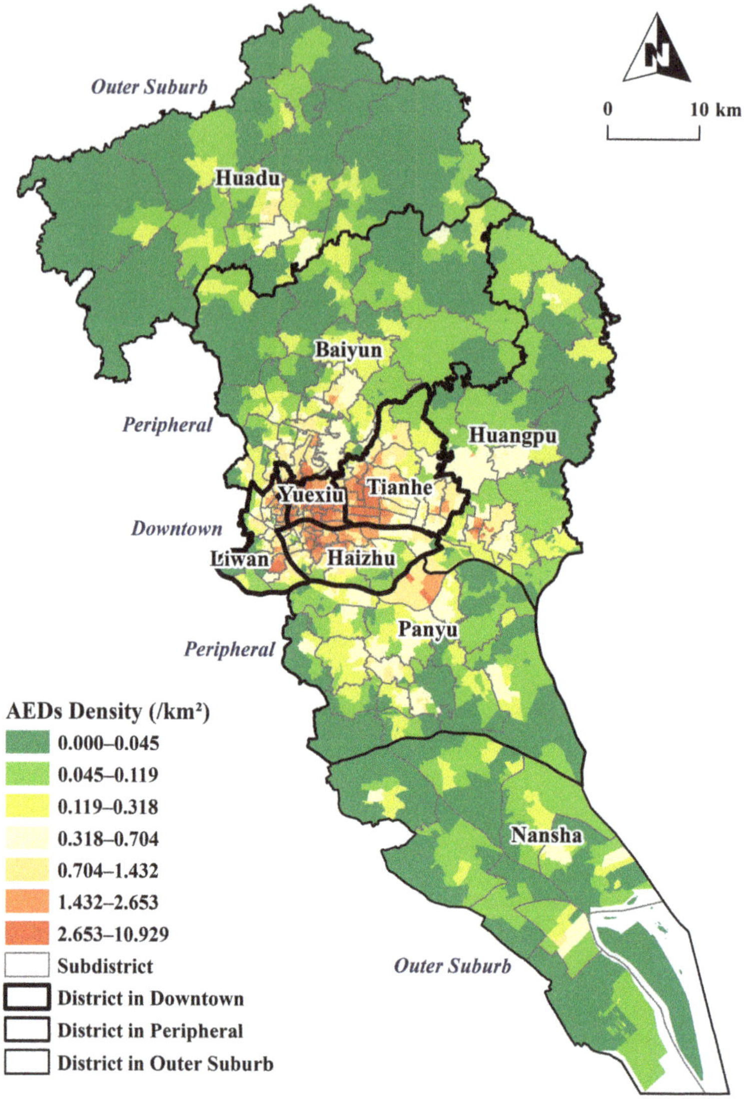

Figure 5. Spatial distribution of AED availability.

3.2. Global AED Inequity

The AED availability was significantly and negatively associated with YR and MI, while ER, YI, EI, POP, and RD were the opposite (Table 2). It indicates that young residents and middle-aged immigrants are suffering AED inequity, while elderly residents, young immigrants, and elderly immigrants tend to be covered by more AEDs on a city-wide level. Among the five social groups, the maximum absolute value of the negative coefficient is 0.303 of MI, which indicates that middle-aged immigrants are the groups facing the worst AED inequity. The high residual autocorrelation was found in the Jarque–Bera statistics and spatial autocorrelation analysis, so a local GWR analysis is necessary.

Table 2. Results of OLS regression model.

Categories	Variables	Coefficient	Robust SE	Robust t	Robust P	VIF
	Intercept	0.979	0.030	32.441	0.000	-
Social groups	YR	−0.122	0.028	−4.369	0.000	1.807
	ER	0.689	0.054	12.832	0.000	2.304
	YI	0.519	0.054	9.572	0.000	2.175
	MI	−0.303	0.033	−9.177	0.000	1.494
	EI	0.205	0.083	2.481	0.013	1.311
Control variables	POP	0.674	0.002	10.689	0.000	1.407
	RD	0.536	0.003	9.974	0.000	1.032
Model diagnostics	R^2: 0.336, adjusted R^2: 0.324, AICc: −3752.491, Koenker (BP): 178.213 **, Jarque–Bera: 402.121 **					

SE = standard error; VIF = variance inflation factor. ** Significant at the 0.01 level.

3.3. Local AED Inequity

Table 3 presents the GWR model results, which quantify the local relationship between the AED availability inequity and the social groups in the neighborhood. Compared with OLS, the lower AICc and higher R-square of the GWR model indicate that GWR was more effective in quantifying the local relationship between the AED availability inequity and social groups. The mean GWR coefficients of YI are the lowest (−0.434), followed by EI (−0.14) and MI (−0.077), indicating that the immigrants of all ages are suffering from a more severe AED inequity than the residents. In addition, the spatial patterns of the AED inequity of the social groups are shown in Figure 6.

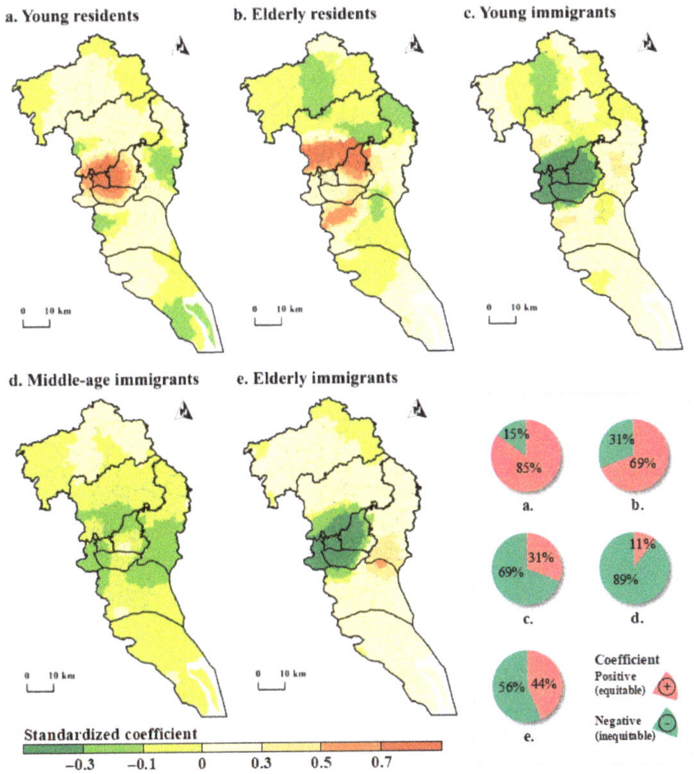

Figure 6. Spatial distribution of the GWR coefficients.

Table 3. Results of GWR regression model.

Categories	Variables	Min	Max	Mean	SD
	Intercept	−0.011	2.511	1.253	0.031
Social groups	YR	−0.279	0.919	0.329	0.067
	ER	−0.196	1.147	0.186	0.290
	YI	−1.294	0.497	−0.434	0.108
	MI	−0.211	0.046	−0.077	0.060
	EI	−0.568	0.520	−0.140	0.054
Control variables	POP	0.105	0.684	0.489	0.347
	RD	0.078	0.541	0.414	0.607
Model diagnostics	R^2: 0.724, adjusted R^2: 0.702, AICc: −3856.174, bandwidth: 24,247.853				

3.3.1. Young Residents

In terms of young residents, the result of the global OLS regression model hints that the proportion of young residents is negatively associated with the neighborhood AED availability (Table 2). However, the local GWR regression model reports that inequity is observed in only 15% of the neighborhoods with the mean GWR coefficients of 0.329, especially in southern Nansha, middle Huangpu, western Panyu, and Huadu districts (Figure 6a). Equity is observed in the downtown, including Yuexiu and western Tianhe district.

3.3.2. Elderly Residents

The global OLS model reports that elderly residents are significantly positively correlated with the neighborhood AED availability with the highest standardized coefficient of 0.689 (Table 2). Moreover, the local GWR model finds more details that the AED equity for elderly residents is observed in 69% of the neighborhoods with the mean GWR coefficients of 0.186, especially in southern Baiyun, northern Tianhe, and north-western Panyu district (Figure 6b). The AED inequity for elderly residents is distributed in northern (including Huadu, northern Baiyun, and northern Huangpu district) and southern Guangzhou (including eastern Panyu and northern Nansha district).

3.3.3. Young Immigrants

Regarding young immigrants, 69% of the neighborhoods are observed with AED inequity with the lowest mean GWR coefficients of −0.434 (Table 3). On the contrary to young residents, the downtown including Yuexiu and western Tianhe district is the area that suffers from the most severe AED inequity for young immigrants, while equity is observed in the peripheral and outer suburbs including southern Huangpu, southern Nansha, western Baiyun, north-western Haizhu district (Figure 6c).

3.3.4. Middle-Aged Immigrants

Both the OLS and GWR models report a significant negative relationship between middle-aged immigrants and AED availability (Table 2). Compared with OLS, GWR results provide more details on the spatial heterogeneity of the AED inequity. The middle-aged immigrants are the group with the largest number of 89% neighborhoods with significant AED inequity, especially in peripheral areas including southern Huangpu, northern Panyu, the middle of Baiyun, and Liwan district (Figure 6d).

3.3.5. Elderly Immigrants

Like young immigrants, downtown is the area with severe inequity for elderly immigrants, especially at the junction of Tianhe, Yuexiu, and Haizhu districts. In contrast, the peripheral and outer suburbs such as eastern Guangzhou including southern Huangpu and northern Panyu district are observed with relative equity. Among the five groups of the population, elderly immigrants are the group with the most balanced number of equitable (44%) and inequitable (56%) neighborhoods.

3.4. Spatial Patterns of AED Inequity Level

Figure 7 displays the spatial distribution of the comprehensive AED inequity level. A high level of AED inequity is mainly distributed in the northern half of Guangzhou, including all over the four districts of downtown, and half of Baiyun and Huadu districts, where most of the neighborhoods suffer from high AED inequity. In addition, a small number of neighborhoods facing extremely high inequity are located in the outer suburbs including the marginal areas of Huadu and Baiyun district. On the contrary, low and moderate levels of comprehensive AED inequity are observed in southern and eastern Guangzhou including most of the Huangpu, Panyu, and Nansha districts.

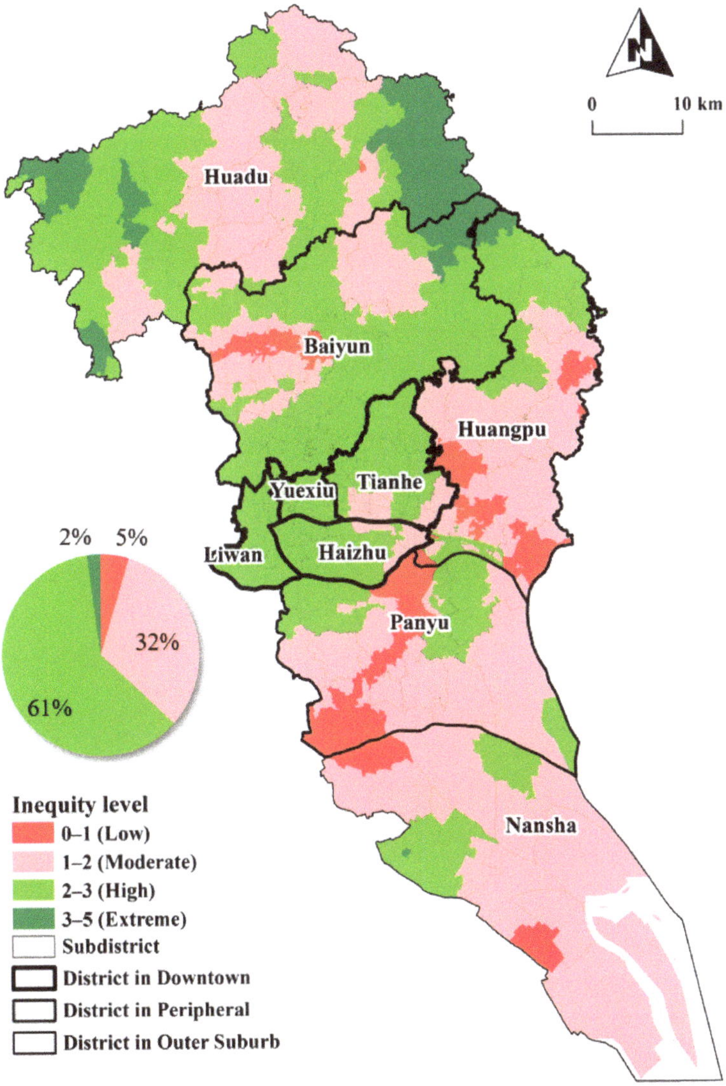

Figure 7. Spatial distribution of AED inequity.

Figure 8 presents the supply map of the social groups facing the worst AED inequity, which is conducive to identifying the AED inequity differences faced by the social groups within each neighborhood. The distribution of the group facing the worst AED inequity is spatially heterogeneous. The downtown including four districts is the area where the immigrants are facing more severe AED inequity than the residents, while the AED inequity of the residents is observed in the peripheral and outer suburbs oppositely. Regardless of being residents or immigrants, the AED inequity among youngsters tends to be concentrated in the center of each district, while the AED inequity among the elderly is distributed in the fringe of each district.

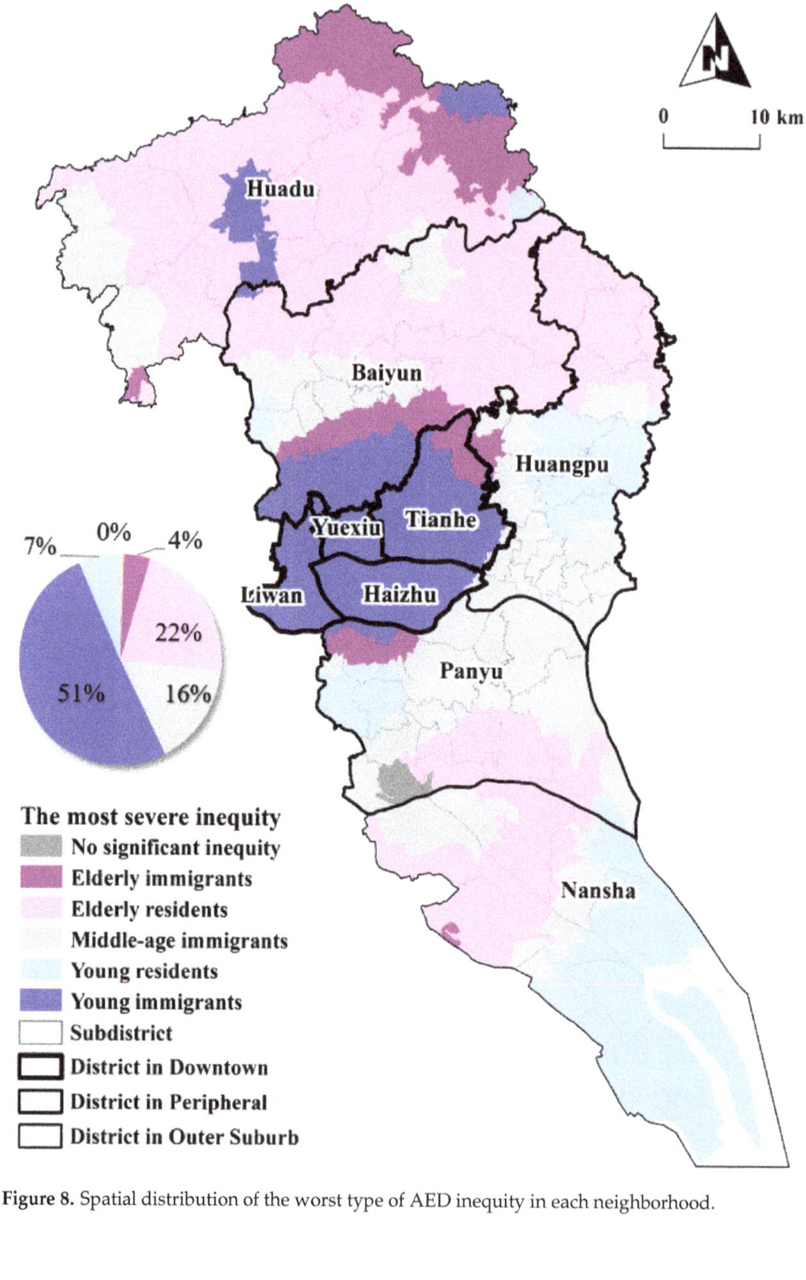

Figure 8. Spatial distribution of the worst type of AED inequity in each neighborhood.

Figure 9 compares the equity of various social groups in each type of neighborhood in Figure 8. Although Figure 8 identifies the social groups facing the most unfair access to AEDs in each neighborhood, it can be observed from Figure 9 that the equity degree of the different social groups in each neighborhood was significantly different. It is worth noting that groups of the same age but different categories in each type of neighborhood in Figure 8 exhibited opposite characteristics. For example, in the Yi-inequity neighborhood, which accounted for 51% of the study area, the YI group had the most severe degree of inequality, with the lowest average standardization coefficient of −0.889. On the contrary, the YR group in this kind of neighborhood had the highest degree of equity, and its average standardized coefficient was the highest, reaching 0.627. Similar patterns had been observed in other types of neighborhoods. This phenomenon reflects the inequity of access to AED facilities among residents and immigrants of the same age group. The relevant reason may be the mismatch between the residence of the various groups and the distribution of AED facilities, which still needs further investigation in future work.

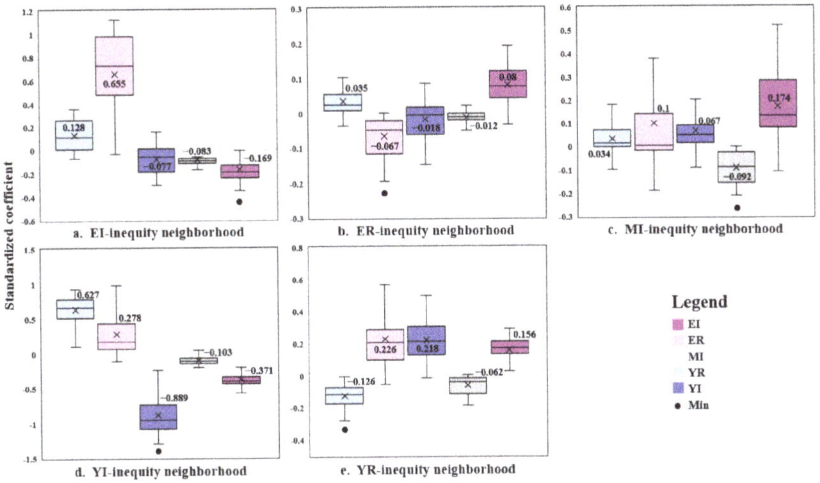

Figure 9. Standardized coefficient statistics for each type of neighborhood.

4. Discussion

4.1. Inequitable Access to AED in Guangzhou

Severe local AED inequity is mainly observed among immigrants including youngsters, middle-aged, and the elderly. From a macro point of view, the spatial distribution of AED equity faced by the five groups of the social groups is significantly heterogeneous. In general, the neighborhoods where immigrants suffer from inequity are concentrated in four districts of downtown and southern Baiyun district. On the contrary, the AED inequity of the residents is mainly distributed in the peripheral and outer suburban neighborhoods. Whether immigrants or residents, the youngsters faced with AED inequity mostly live in the center of Guangzhou or each district, while the AED inequity among the elderly is mostly distributed on the outskirts of downtown and in the outer boroughs of the city. It indicates that the supply and demand relationship between the AED facilities and the social groups is imbalanced. Through the comprehensive evaluation of the AED inequity, it is suggested that policymakers and urban planners should be attentive to the equity between the social groups in the neighborhoods, rather than just the total population when allocating such emergency medical facility resources.

The high aging population is one of the demographic features in Guangzhou [48]. Regarding age, OHCA is most common in the elderly because of the higher rates of cardiovascular disease, compared with the young and middle-aged [17,50,51]. Previous studies have found that the elderly are often at a disadvantage in terms of the access to medical care [32,56,57]. As an emergency medical facility, AED inequity for the elderly is observed in 26% of the neighborhoods, especially in the peripheral and outer suburbs of Guangzhou, which is consistent with previous studies on healthcare inequity. The elderly are the disadvantaged group with particular demands for AED due to their physical condition. The local inequity of the AED availability across the two elderly groups is identified and located by the GWR model, which should be mitigated in future AED allocating.

Excessive immigration is another demographic feature that Guangzhou attracts a large number of young migrant workers every year [47]. Although OHCA rates are lower in younger people, the number of young people is more than six times that of the elderly, especially young immigrants. Existing studies have reported that due to the institutionalized discrimination caused by the Hukou system, immigrants are often excluded from local benefits, including public services and healthcare [58,59]. In this study, AED inequity for young immigrants is observed in 51% of the neighborhoods, especially downtown. Urban villages in downtown are often regarded as immigrant-receiving neighborhoods, because most immigrants live in urban villages in the inner fringe of downtown or the urban and rural fringe of the city, and the number of immigrants living in these places far exceeds the number of residents [60].

On the one hand, due to the lack of economic development and the low socio-economic level of such low-cost neighborhoods, the government's financial investment is usually relatively small, resulting in the inadequate allocation of the public service facilities in various aspects [24,33], including medical facilities such as AED. In addition, most low-cost neighborhoods represented by urban villages and old communities have few public places suitable for AED placement due to disrepair or single functions of buildings and land [61]. On the other hand, current AED facility planning is usually configured according to the population in each neighborhood [15]. However, due to large numbers and high mobility, and the fact that some migrants are not registered, the population statistics are inaccurate but take too long to update. Therefore, it is difficult to allocate a sufficient number of AEDs to residents and immigrants in each neighborhood. In addition to population and land characteristics, low-cost neighborhoods with immigrant concentrations, typically have lower levels of education and income, which may indirectly affect the risk of OHCA in public [15]. Bystanders with lower income and education levels usually have insufficient medical common knowledge and rescue skills, which makes it difficult for them to provide effective first aid to victims and promotes the survivor rate [62,63]. In conclusion, the demographics and geographical location of the neighborhood can influence the inequity in the availability of AED facilities.

4.2. Implications for AED Facility Management and Optimization

The results of this study provide new insights and implications for AED configuration strategies. First, although the current AED facility planning takes into account the local population density, most of them ignore the characteristics of the population structure and socio-economic level, which have significant spatial heterogeneity in the high-density megacity of Guangzhou. As an emergency medical facility for the whole people, the government should intervene in the equity distribution of AED facilities to improve the coverage of the vulnerable groups in the neighborhoods with sufficient AED facilities, instead of focusing on the overall population and continuing to ignore vulnerable groups. This study urges the equity of AEDs as a goal to achieve social equity and basic public service planning. Second, this study provides a technical framework for evaluating the spatial heterogeneity of the inequity in AED facilities, which can provide a comprehensive demographic analysis and visualization of the supply map for AED facility allocation planning and provide a scientific reference for equitable distribution of medical facilities. It should be noted that there are disparities in AED equity among neighborhoods and that neighborhoods with more AED facilities are not necessarily equitable. Therefore, it is necessary to consider the balance between the supply and demand of AED facilities and the spatial disparities of the socio-economic groups, especially in areas with high concentrations of disadvantaged groups. The government should intervene in the redistribution of AED facilities in severely inequitable neighborhoods to ensure vertical equity, giving priority to the interests of the vulnerable groups. Third, the newly released AED resources should be further supplemented to the vulnerable group-gathering neighborhoods, and the local population density, mobility, and structure should be considered. For example, to supplement AEDs in urban villages, 24 h security duty rooms and the largest local wet market can be considered. Finally, it is suggested that the government build an "Internet + First Aid" system, construct an AED network and system, conduct unified management of AED network information, and use information technology to draw an AED public online map. For example, the AED data applied in this study came from the WeChat applet named "AED Lifesaving Map". However, this very powerful applet lacks publicity, which is likely to lead to low usage. Therefore, it is necessary for the government to increase the exposure of this emergency information on social media through online and offline channels.

4.3. Theoretical Implications

Theoretically, the main findings and contributions of this study are to emphasize that the integrated application of the consolidated geospatial modeling technology to other fields will bring new added value. For example, this study applied it to the management and optimization of urban public medical facilities to investigate the equity problem in the distribution of AED facilities. Compared with traditional non-geospatial methods, such as the Gini coefficient and Lorenz curve, the spatial heterogeneity of equity was observed in this study. First, the AED data are obtained through the WeChat applet and Python script, and its neighborhood availability is measured considering the effective rescue time of OHCA and average running speed. Second, given the unique characteristics of population structure in Guangzhou where population aging and mass migration coexist, we focus on the AED inequity instead of the inequality from the perspective of spatial and socio-economic heterogeneity. Third, we investigate the spatially varying AED inequity by the GWR model and identify the severe AED deprivation neighborhoods. The socio-economic status and AED availability of each neighborhood differ greatly. That is, the inequity or equity is only observed in specific neighborhoods, and the global modeling of the whole city will lead to overgeneralization. In this study, AED inequity is comprehensively analyzed for multiple social groups from a micro perspective. The framework of inequity identification using the local regression model in this study can be applied to other social equity issues.

4.4. Limitations

Despite the advantages, there are limitations to be addressed in the future.

- Although this study examines inequity in AED facilities from the perspective of spatial heterogeneity, it could not cover the analysis of the whole social group due to the availability of data, such as for groups with different housing sizes.
- The neighborhood administrative boundary is taken as the spatial unit in this study, and the analysis modeling results may be affected by the modifiable areal unit problem [64].
- Due to data availability, our analysis does not cover the historical OHCA cases. Future studies should obtain more comprehensive variables, AED facility data of more cities, and modeling to consider scale effects.
- This study measured the AED availability based on the maximum rescue time. Further investigation should incorporate both minimum and maximum rescue time ranges for comprehensive understanding.
- Since the collinearity problem needs to be solved before the linear regression model is adopted, one kind of social group was omitted from the model result. In the next step, we will consider other models to avoid this limitation, because inequity is equally important for each social group.

- Although this study identified spatial heterogeneity in the inequality of access to AEDs across social groups, the next step should be to explore the relationship between the equity of various social groups in each neighborhood.

5. Conclusions

The major contribution of this study is to adopt geospatial modeling technology to solve the equity problem in the distribution of medical facilities. The GWR reveals the spatially varying associations between AED and different social groups. Model results show that immigrants of all ages suffer from more severe AED inequity than residents, after controlling the population density and road density. The most significant result of this study, the AED inequity supply map, shows that the distribution of the groups that faced the worst AED inequity has significant spatial heterogeneity. The immigrants downtown face more severe AED inequity than the residents. Conversely, the residents face more severe inequity in peripheral and outer suburbs. Whether resident or immigrant, the AED inequity among youngsters tends to be concentrated in the center of each district, while the AED inequity among the elderly tends to be distributed at the edge of each district. These spatial characteristics of AED supply and demand relations should be emphasized in future AED planning.

The highly aging population and the large number of immigrants are the unique demographic characteristics of Guangzhou. Therefore, when planning and allocating basic medical emergency facilities such as AED, it is particularly important to consider the differences in the population structure and socio-economic status. AEDs are regarded as the most important public facilities after fire extinguishers due to their importance to the lives of citizens. Therefore, for AED planning, it is equally important to improve the number of per capita ownership and promote local equity. This study provides a new perspective for investigating the inequity in public service facilities and emergency medical facilities, puts forward scientific suggestions for future AED distribution planning, and emphasizes the importance of social equity.

Author Contributions: Conceptualization, Feng Gao, Siyi Lu and Shunyi Liao; methodology, Feng Gao, Wangyang Chen and Xin Chen; software, Jiemin Wu and Yunjing Wu; validation, Guanyao Li and Xu Han; formal analysis, Feng Gao and Shunyi Liao; investigation, Feng Gao, Wangyang Chen, and Xin Chen; resources, Shunyi Liao; data curation, Feng Gao; writing—original draft preparation, Feng Gao; writing—review and editing, Feng Gao and Siyi Lu; visualization, Feng Gao; supervision, Wangyang Chen and Xin Chen; project administration, Wangyang Chen and Xin Chen; funding acquisition, Feng Gao and Shunyi Liao. All authors have read and agreed to the published version of the manuscript.

Funding: This research was funded by the Youth Fund Sustentation Project of Guangzhou Urban Planning and Design Survey Research Institute (RDI2230205004), Guangzhou Collaborative Innovation Center of Natural Resources Planning and Marine Technology (No. 2023B04J0301), Key-Area Research and Development Program of Guangdong Province (No. 2020B0101130009), and Guangdong Enterprise Key Laboratory for Urban Sensing, Monitoring and Early Warning (No. 2020B121202019), National Natural Science Foundation of China (No. 42271467).

Data Availability Statement: Data are contained within the article.

Conflicts of Interest: Authors have received part of research grants from Company—Guangzhou Urban Planning & Design Survey Research Institute Co., Ltd.

References

1. Kitamura, T.; Iwami, T.; Kawamura, T.; Nagao, K.; Tanaka, H.; Hiraide, A. Nationwide Public-Access Defibrillation in Japan. *N. Engl. J. Med.* **2010**, *362*, 994–1004. [CrossRef]
2. Zhang, S. Sudden Cardiac Death in China: Current Status and Future Perspectives. *Europace* **2015**, *17*, ii14–ii18. [CrossRef]
3. The Writing Committee of the Report on Cardiovascular Health and Diseases in China. Report on Cardiovascular Health and Diseases in China 2022: An Updated Summary. *Biomed. Environ. Sci.* **2023**, *35*, 669–701. [CrossRef]

4. Brooks, S.C.; Hsu, J.H.; Tang, S.K.; Jeyakumar, R.; Chan, T.C.Y. Determining Risk for Out-of-Hospital Cardiac Arrest by Location Type in a Canadian Urban Setting to Guide Future Public Access Defibrillator Placement. *Ann. Emerg. Med.* **2013**, *61*, 530–538.e2. [CrossRef] [PubMed]
5. Deakin, C.D.; Shewry, E.; Gray, H.H. Public Access Defibrillation Remains out of Reach for Most Victims of Out-of-Hospital Sudden Cardiac Arrest. *Heart* **2014**, *100*, 619–623. [CrossRef]
6. Pulver, A.; Wei, R. Optimizing the Spatial Location of Medical Drones. *Appl. Geogr.* **2018**, *90*, 9–16. [CrossRef]
7. Blom, M.T.; Beesems, S.G.; Homma, P.C.M.; Zijlstra, J.A.; Hulleman, M.; van Hoeijen, D.A.; Bardai, A.; Tijssen, J.G.P.; Tan, H.L.; Koster, R.W. Improved Survival After Out-of-Hospital Cardiac Arrest and Use of Automated External Defibrillators. *Circulation* **2014**, *130*, 1868–1875. [CrossRef] [PubMed]
8. Folke, F.; Lippert, F.K.; Nielsen, S.L.; Gislason, G.H.; Hansen, M.L.; Schramm, T.K.; Sørensen, R.; Fosbøl, E.L.; Andersen, S.S.; Rasmussen, S.; et al. Location of Cardiac Arrest in a City Center: Strategic Placement of Automated External Defibrillators in Public Locations. *Circulation* **2009**, *120*, 510–517. [CrossRef]
9. Lwanga, A.; Garcia-Sayan, E.; Lwanga, S.; Karreman, E.; Mohamed, A. Automated External Defibrillators and Survival After Nonresidential Out of Hospital Cardiac Arrest in a Small North American City. *Am. J. Cardiol.* **2017**, *119*, 1979–1982. [CrossRef]
10. Ringh, M.; Hollenberg, J.; Palsgaard-Moeller, T.; Svensson, L.; Rosenqvist, M.; Lippert, F.K.; Wissenberg, M.; Malta Hansen, C.; Claesson, A.; Viereck, S.; et al. The Challenges and Possibilities of Public Access Defibrillation. *J. Intern. Med.* **2018**, *283*, 238–256. [CrossRef]
11. Fredman, D.; Haas, J.; Ban, Y.; Jonsson, M.; Svensson, L.; Djarv, T.; Hollenberg, J.; Nordberg, P.; Ringh, M.; Claesson, A. Use of a Geographic Information System to Identify Differences in Automated External Defibrillator Installation in Urban Areas with Similar Incidence of Public Out-of-Hospital Cardiac Arrest: A Retrospective Registry-Based Study. *BMJ Open* **2017**, *7*, e014801. [CrossRef] [PubMed]
12. Pollack, R.A.; Brown, S.P.; Rea, T.; Aufderheide, T.; Barbic, D.; Buick, J.E.; Christenson, J.; Idris, A.H.; Jasti, J.; Kampp, M.; et al. Impact of Bystander Automated External Defibrillator Use on Survival and Functional Outcomes in Shockable Observed Public Cardiac Arrests. *Circulation* **2018**, *137*, 2104–2113. [CrossRef]
13. Tsai, Y.-S.; Ko, P.C.-I.; Huang, C.-Y.; Wen, T.-H. Optimizing Locations for the Installation of Automated External Defibrillators (AEDs) in Urban Public Streets through the Use of Spatial and Temporal Weighting Schemes. *Appl. Geogr.* **2012**, *35*, 394–404. [CrossRef]
14. Bonnet, B.; Gama Dessavre, D.; Kraus, K.; Ramirez-Marquez, J.E. Optimal Placement of Public-Access AEDs in Urban Environments. *Comput. Ind. Eng.* **2015**, *90*, 269–280. [CrossRef]
15. Chen, G.; Widener, M.J.; Zhu, M.; Wang, C.C. Identification of Priority Areas for Public-Access Automated External Defibrillators (AEDs) in Metropolitan Areas: A Case Study in Hangzhou, China. *Appl. Geogr.* **2023**, *154*, 102922. [CrossRef]
16. Huang, C.-Y.; Wen, T.-H. Optimal Installation Locations for Automated External Defibrillators in Taipei 7-Eleven Stores: Using GIS and a Genetic Algorithm with a New Stirring Operator. *Comput. Math. Methods Med.* **2014**, *2014*, 241435. [CrossRef] [PubMed]
17. Lin, B.-C.; Chen, C.-W.; Chen, C.-C.; Kuo, C.-L.; Fan, I.; Ho, C.-K.; Liu, I.-C.; Chan, T.-C. Spatial Decision on Allocating Automated External Defibrillators (AED) in Communities by Multi-Criterion Two-Step Floating Catchment Area (MC2SFCA). *Int. J. Health Geogr.* **2016**, *15*, 17. [CrossRef] [PubMed]
18. Aeby, D.; Staeger, P.; Dami, F. How to Improve Automated External Defibrillator Placement for Out-of-Hospital Cardiac Arrests: A Case Study. *PLoS ONE* **2021**, *16*, e0250591. [CrossRef] [PubMed]
19. Rea, T.D.; Olsufka, M.; Bemis, B.; White, L.; Yin, L.; Becker, L.; Copass, M.; Eisenberg, M.; Cobb, L. A Population-Based Investigation of Public Access Defibrillation: Role of Emergency Medical Services Care. *Resuscitation* **2010**, *81*, 163–167. [CrossRef]
20. Yang, L.; Xiong, L.; Yang, W. An Accessibility Spatial Search Algorithm to Optimize Defibrillator Deployment in Indoor Space. *Int. J. Geogr. Inf. Sci.* **2021**, *35*, 1251–1272. [CrossRef]
21. Yasunaga, H.; Miyata, H.; Horiguchi, H.; Tanabe, S.; Akahane, M.; Ogawa, T.; Koike, S.; Imamura, T. Population Density, Call-Response Interval, and Survival of out-of-Hospital Cardiac Arrest. *Int. J. Health Geogr.* **2011**, *10*, 26. [CrossRef] [PubMed]
22. Tsukigase, K.; Tanaka, H.; Takyu, H. Mismatch between Sites of Incidence of Out-of-Hospital Cardiac Arrest and Locations of Installed Automated External Defibrillator in the Tokyo Metropolitan Area. *WJCD* **2017**, *7*, 185–194. [CrossRef]
23. Jin, T.; Cheng, L.; Wang, K.; Cao, J.; Huang, H.; Witlox, F. Examining Equity in Accessibility to Multi-Tier Healthcare Services across Different Income Households Using Estimated Travel Time. *Transp. Policy* **2022**, *121*, 1–13. [CrossRef]
24. Mayaud, J.R.; Tran, M.; Nuttall, R. An Urban Data Framework for Assessing Equity in Cities: Comparing Accessibility to Healthcare Facilities in Cascadia. *Comput. Environ. Urban Syst.* **2019**, *78*, 101401. [CrossRef]
25. Mishra, S.; Sahu, P.K.; Sarkar, A.K.; Mehran, B.; Sharma, S. Geo-Spatial Site Suitability Analysis for Development of Health Care Units in Rural India: Effects on Habitation Accessibility, Facility Utilization and Zonal Equity in Facility Distribution. *J. Transp. Geogr.* **2019**, *78*, 135–149. [CrossRef]
26. Gu, Z.; Luo, X.; Tang, M.; Liu, X. Does the Edge Effect Impact the Healthcare Equity? An Examination of the Equity in Hospitals Accessibility in the Edge City in Multi-Scale. *J. Transp. Geogr.* **2023**, *106*, 103513. [CrossRef]
27. Hare, T.S.; Barcus, H.R. Geographical Accessibility and Kentucky's Heart-Related Hospital Services. *Appl. Geogr.* **2007**, *27*, 181–205. [CrossRef]
28. Rong, P.; Zheng, Z.; Kwan, M.-P.; Qin, Y. Evaluation of the Spatial Equity of Medical Facilities Based on Improved Potential Model and Map Service API: A Case Study in Zhengzhou, China. *Appl. Geogr.* **2020**, *119*, 102192. [CrossRef]

29. Yan, X.; Shan, L.; He, S.; Zhang, J. Cross-City Patient Mobility and Healthcare Equity and Efficiency: Evidence from Hefei, China. *Travel Behav. Soc.* **2022**, *28*, 1–12. [CrossRef]
30. Zhao, P.; Li, S.; Liu, D. Unequable Spatial Accessibility to Hospitals in Developing Megacities: New Evidence from Beijing. *Health Place* **2020**, *65*, 102406. [CrossRef]
31. Chen, Y.; Liu, B.; Shen, Y.; Li, L. Assessing Accessibility to Service Facilities for Older People in Age-Restricted Communities from the Perspective of Equity. *J. Transp. Health* **2022**, *27*, 101515. [CrossRef]
32. Cheng, T.; Liu, C.; Yang, H.; Wang, N.; Liu, Y. From Service Capacity to Spatial Equity: Exploring a Multi-Stage Decision-Making Approach for Optimizing Elderly-Care Facility Distribution in the City Centre of Tianjin, China. *Sustain. Cities Soc.* **2022**, *85*, 104076. [CrossRef]
33. Darcy, S. The Politics of Disability and Access: The Sydney 2000 Games Experience. *Disabil. Soc.* **2003**, *18*, 737–757. [CrossRef]
34. Brunsdon, C.; Fotheringham, A.S.; Charlton, M.E. Geographically Weighted Regression: A Method for Exploring Spatial Nonstationarity. *Geogr. Anal.* **2010**, *28*, 281–298. [CrossRef]
35. Yang, W.; Yang, R.; Zhou, S. The Spatial Heterogeneity of Urban Green Space Inequity from a Perspective of the Vulnerable: A Case Study of Guangzhou, China. *Cities* **2022**, *130*, 103855. [CrossRef]
36. Lin, J.; Wang, Q.; Li, X. Socioeconomic and Spatial Inequalities of Street Tree Abundance, Species Diversity, and Size Structure in New York City. *Landsc. Urban Plan.* **2021**, *206*, 103992. [CrossRef]
37. Shi, H.; Huang, H.; Ma, D.; Chen, L.; Zhao, M. Capturing Urban Recreational Hotspots from GPS Data: A New Framework in the Lens of Spatial Heterogeneity. *Comput. Environ. Urban Syst.* **2023**, *103*, 101972. [CrossRef]
38. Gao, F.; Liao, S.; Wang, Z.; Cai, G.; Feng, L.; Yang, Z.; Chen, W.; Chen, X.; Li, G. Revealing Disparities in Different Types of Park Visits Based on Cellphone Signaling Data in Guangzhou, China. *J. Environ. Manag.* **2024**, *351*, 119969. [CrossRef] [PubMed]
39. Gao, F.; Wu, J.; Xiao, J.; Li, X.; Liao, S.; Chen, W. Spatially Explicit Carbon Emissions by Remote Sensing and Social Sensing. *Environ. Res.* **2023**, *221*, 115257. [CrossRef]
40. Shi, H.; Yu, L.; Xu, Y.; Liu, Y.; Zhao, M. The Impact of the Streetscape Built Environment on Recreation Satisfaction: A Case Study of Guangzhou. *J. Transp. Geogr.* **2023**, *112*, 103702. [CrossRef]
41. Guangzhou Municipal Government. *Work Plan for the Allocation of AED in Public Places of Guangzhou (Draft for Comment)*; Guangzhou Municipal Government: Guangzhou, China, 2021.
42. Liao, S.; Gao, F.; Feng, L.; Wu, J.; Wang, Z.; Chen, W. Observed Equity and Driving Factors of Automated External Defibrillators: A Case Study Using WeChat Applet Data. *ISPRS Int. J. Geo-Inf.* **2023**, *12*, 444. [CrossRef]
43. Valenzuela, T.D.; Roe, D.J.; Nichol, G.; Clark, L.L.; Spaite, D.W.; Hardman, R.G. Outcomes of Rapid Defibrillation by Security Officers after Cardiac Arrest in Casinos. *N. Engl. J. Med.* **2000**, *343*, 1206–1209. [CrossRef] [PubMed]
44. Gundry, J.W.; Comess, K.A.; DeRook, F.A.; Jorgenson, D.; Bardy, G.H. Comparison of Naive Sixth-Grade Children with Trained Professionals in the Use of an Automated External Defibrillator. *Circulation* **1999**, *100*, 1703–1707. [CrossRef] [PubMed]
45. Chan, T.C.Y.; Demirtas, D.; Kwon, R.H. Optimizing the Deployment of Public Access Defibrillators. *Manag. Sci.* **2016**, *62*, 3617–3635. [CrossRef]
46. Jin, X.; Bolt, G.; Hooimeijer, P. Africans in Guangzhou: Is the Ethnic Enclave Model Applicable in the Chinese Context? *Cities* **2021**, *117*, 103320. [CrossRef]
47. Liu, Y.; Li, Z.; Breitung, W. The Social Networks of New-Generation Migrants in China's Urbanized Villages: A Case Study of Guangzhou. *Habitat Int.* **2012**, *36*, 192–200. [CrossRef]
48. Zhou, S.; Xie, M.; Kwan, M.-P. Ageing in Place and Ageing with Migration in the Transitional Context of Urban China: A Case Study of Ageing Communities in Guangzhou. *Habitat Int.* **2015**, *49*, 177–186. [CrossRef]
49. Deng, X.; Liu, Y.; Gao, F.; Liao, S.; Zhou, F.; Cai, G. Spatial Distribution and Mechanism of Urban Occupation Mixture in Guangzhou: An Optimized GeoDetector-Based Index to Compare Individual and Interactive Effects. *IJGI* **2021**, *10*, 659. [CrossRef]
50. Deasy, C.; Bray, J.E.; Smith, K.; Harriss, L.R.; Bernard, S.A.; Cameron, P. Out-of-Hospital Cardiac Arrests in the Older Age Groups in Melbourne, Australia. *Resuscitation* **2011**, *82*, 398–403. [CrossRef]
51. Su, Y.-J.; Lai, Y.-C.; Chen, C.-C.; Chang, W.-H. Out-of-hospital cardiac arrest in the elderly. *Int. J. Gerontol.* **2008**, *2*, 67–71. [CrossRef]
52. Li, S.; Lyu, D.; Huang, G.; Zhang, X.; Gao, F.; Chen, Y.; Liu, X. Spatially Varying Impacts of Built Environment Factors on Rail Transit Ridership at Station Level: A Case Study in Guangzhou, China. *J. Transp. Geogr.* **2020**, *82*, 102631. [CrossRef]
53. Gao, F.; Li, S.; Tan, Z.; Zhang, X.; Lai, Z.; Tan, Z. How Is Urban Greenness Spatially Associated with Dockless Bike Sharing Usage on Weekdays, Weekends, and Holidays? *IJGI* **2021**, *10*, 238. [CrossRef]
54. Fotheringham, A.; Brunsdon, C.F.; Charlton, M. *Geographically Weighted Regression: The Analysis of Spatially Varying Relationships*; John Wiley & Sons: Hoboken, NJ, USA, 2003.
55. Deng, X.; Gao, F.; Liao, S.; Li, S. Unraveling the Association between the Built Environment and Air Pollution from a Geospatial Perspective. *J. Clean. Prod.* **2023**, *386*, 135768. [CrossRef]
56. Chen, G.; Wang, C.C.; Jin, P.; Xia, B.; Xiao, L.; Chen, S.; Luo, J. Evaluation of Healthcare Inequity for Older Adults: A Spatio-Temporal Perspective. *J. Transp. Health* **2020**, *19*, 100911. [CrossRef]
57. Steels, S. Key Characteristics of Age-Friendly Cities and Communities: A Review. *Cities* **2015**, *47*, 45–52. [CrossRef]
58. Liu, L.; Feng, J.; Ren, F.; Xiao, L. Examining the Relationship between Neighborhood Environment and Residential Locations of Juvenile and Adult Migrant Burglars in China. *Cities* **2018**, *82*, 10–18. [CrossRef]

59. Ouyang, W.; Wang, B.; Tian, L.; Niu, X. Spatial Deprivation of Urban Public Services in Migrant Enclaves under the Context of a Rapidly Urbanizing China: An Evaluation Based on Suburban Shanghai. *Cities* **2017**, *60*, 436–445. [CrossRef]
60. Huang, G.; Xue, D.; Guo, Y.; Wang, C. Constrained Voluntary Informalisation: Analysing Motivations of Self-Employed Migrant Workers in an Urban Village, Guangzhou. *Cities* **2020**, *105*, 102760. [CrossRef]
61. Tian, L.; Yao, Z.; Fan, C.; Zhou, L. A Systems Approach to Enabling Affordable Housing for Migrants through Upgrading Chengzhongcun: A Case of Xiamen. *Cities* **2020**, *105*, 102186. [CrossRef]
62. Feero, S.; Hedges, J.R.; Stevens, P. Demographics of Cardiac Arrest: Association with Residence in a Low-Income Area. *Acad. Emerg. Med.* **1995**, *2*, 11–16. [CrossRef]
63. Jonsson, M.; Härkönen, J.; Ljungman, P.; Nordberg, P.; Ringh, M.; Hirlekar, G.; Rawshani, A.; Herlitz, J.; Ljung, R.; Hollenberg, J. Inequalities in Income and Education Are Associated with Survival Differences After Out-of-Hospital Cardiac Arrest: Nationwide Observational Study. *Circulation* **2021**, *144*, 1915–1925. [CrossRef] [PubMed]
64. Gao, F.; Li, S.; Tan, Z.; Wu, Z.; Zhang, X.; Huang, G.; Huang, Z. Understanding the Modifiable Areal Unit Problem in Dockless Bike Sharing Usage and Exploring the Interactive Effects of Built Environment Factors. *Int. J. Geogr. Inf. Sci.* **2021**, *35*, 1905–1925. [CrossRef]

International Journal of
Geo-Information

MDPI

Article

Comparison of Different Green Space Measures and Their Impact on Dementia Cases in South Korea: A Spatial Panel Analysis

Wulan Salle Karurung [1,†], Kangjae Lee [1,†] and Wonhee Lee [2,*]

[1] Department of Convergence and Fusion System Engineering, Kyungpook National University, Sangju 37224, Republic of Korea; wulansalle@knu.ac.kr (W.S.K.); kasbiss@knu.ac.kr (K.L.)
[2] Department of Location-Based Information System, Kyungpook National University, Sangju 37224, Republic of Korea
* Correspondence: wlee33@knu.ac.kr; Tel.: +82-54-530-1492
† These authors contributed equally to this work.

Abstract: Dementia has become a profound public health problem due to the number of patients increasing every year. Previous studies have reported that environmental factors, including greenness, may influence the development and progression of dementia. Studies have found that exposure to green space is associated with a lower incidence of dementia. However, many definitions of green space exist, and the effects of its use may differ with the type of green space. Therefore, two types of green space measures were considered in this study to assess the differences in their impact on the prevalence of dementia among females and males. This study used five years of data (2017–2021) from 235 districts in South Korea. The two green space measures used were open space density and normalized difference vegetation index (NDVI), which were derived from satellite images. The analysis utilized a combination of traditional and spatial panel analyses to account for the spatial and temporal effects of independent variables on dementia prevalence. The spatial autocorrelation results revealed that both measures of greenness were spatially correlated with dementia prevalence. The spatial panel regression results revealed a significant positive association between NDVI and dementia prevalence, and open space had a negative association with dementia prevalence in both genders. The difference in the findings can serve as the basis for further research when choosing a greenspace measure, as it affects the analysis results, depending on the objective of the study. This study adds to the knowledge regarding improving dementia studies and the application of spatial panel analysis in epidemiological studies.

Keywords: dementia; open space; greenness exposure; NDVI; spatial panel analysis; epidemiology

1. Introduction

Aging is universal, and improving healthcare can increase life expectancy and improve the health of older people. Dementia is a cognitive disease that affects older people and leads to memory loss and reduced cognitive abilities. This impairment has a marked effect on the daily lives of patients and physical, psychological, social, and financial impacts on those affected and their families [1]. Additionally, the number of dementia cases in older people is increasing annually and is expected to triple in the next 30 years [2]. The public has limited information on whether dementia risk is clustered geographically [3], how this occurs, and how dementia may be related to sociodemographic and built environment factors [4]. In 2020, it was estimated that 10.25% of people over the age of 65 years have dementia, and this figure is expected to increase to approximately 15.91% by 2050. The rapid pace of aging suggests that the prevalence of dementia will increase significantly in the coming years [5].

Previous studies have demonstrated that environmental factors, such as air pollution and a lack of green spaces, are potential risk factors for cognitive impairment, including dementia [6–8]. Another study emphasized the important role that green space plays in preventing dementia [9]. Green spaces in residential areas can improve individuals' physical health [10,11], reduce stress, and provide clean air [12]. Regarding recreation, green spaces provide space for the community and access to natural landscapes, potentially increasing physical activity and promoting healthy lifestyles to reduce the risk of dementia, brain atrophy, and cognitive decline [1,2,13]. The relationship between the environment and cognitive health is of growing interest, and previous studies have shown that spending time in green space can positively impact cognitive function, as well as reduce the risk of developing dementia [13].

In South Korea, studies on dementia cases have already been conducted to evaluate the association with health status [14], socioeconomic status, and healthcare accessibility [15]; gender-based analyses have also been conducted [16]. In addition, a spatial analysis was conducted to develop a predictive model for regional dementia in South Korea using a geographically weighted regression [3]. Geographic information systems (GISs) have been applied in several studies to investigate the relationship between dementia and the environment [12,17–19]. Another study investigated the insufficiency of assumptions regarding disease occurrence response in conventional spatial models [20]. Temporal and spatial changes in geographic data are essential for inferring the relationships between variables. Spatial panel analysis is recommended because of its ability to examine spatial and temporal effects. Panel and spatial panel regressions can be used to examine how variables, such as the environment, change over time and how they may affect health outcomes [18,21,22], considering the correlation between observations over time [23]. Moreover, panel data allow researchers to substantially increase statistical validity in policy analysis and program evaluation compared to statistical methods using cross-sectional data [24–26].

The normalized difference vegetation index (NDVI) and built green space, such as parks and open spaces, are commonly used as measures of greenness in epidemiology and environmental studies. NDVI data have been used to represent green space exposure [27,28], in combination with land cover data, in several studies on dementia [29]. In these studies, the NDVI values have differed depending on the scale and type of data used, such as buffer or distance data for individual studies, or aggregated NDVI values for population-level studies [30]. Additionally, open space is most commonly used to assess residential green space and its relationship with dementia [13]. Owing to differences in data types, the type of green space data used and how to capture their respective effects by analyzing the combination of green space data should be considered. We hypothesized that the difference in data entry between NDVI and open space density leads to different associations between dementia and green space exposure.

This study aims to compare the influence of two types of green space exposure—NDVI and open space—on the prevalence of dementia among different genders in South Korea from 2017 to 2021. Panel and spatial panel analyses were performed to investigate how green space affects dementia prevalence and reduces the spillover effect in aggregated data [31]. By comparing the impacts of different types of green space from the perspective of different genders, this study provides new insights into the risk factors for dementia and the application of greenness data to the study of cognitive diseases. Additionally, employing conventional panel and spatial panel analyses enhances the novelty of this study. The results of this study can support further research on the use of green space data in advanced dementia health studies.

2. Materials and Methods

2.1. Study Area

This study focused on patients with dementia in South Korea. South Korea consists of eight provinces, seven metropolitan cities (Seoul, Daegu, Busan, Ulsan, Daejeon, Incheon, and Gwangju), two special autonomous cities (Sejong and Jeju), and has a total area of

250 si/gun/gu (http://nationalatlas.ngii.go.kr/, accessed on 7 July 2022) as shown in Figure 1. The metropolitan cities have a population of more than one million, whereas Sejong and Jeju are self-governing entities with populations of less than 500,000. In this study, data were obtained at the si/gun/gu level, which represents the primary administrative division of South Korea. This administrative level consists of municipal subdivisions, including cities (si), counties (gun), and districts (gu).

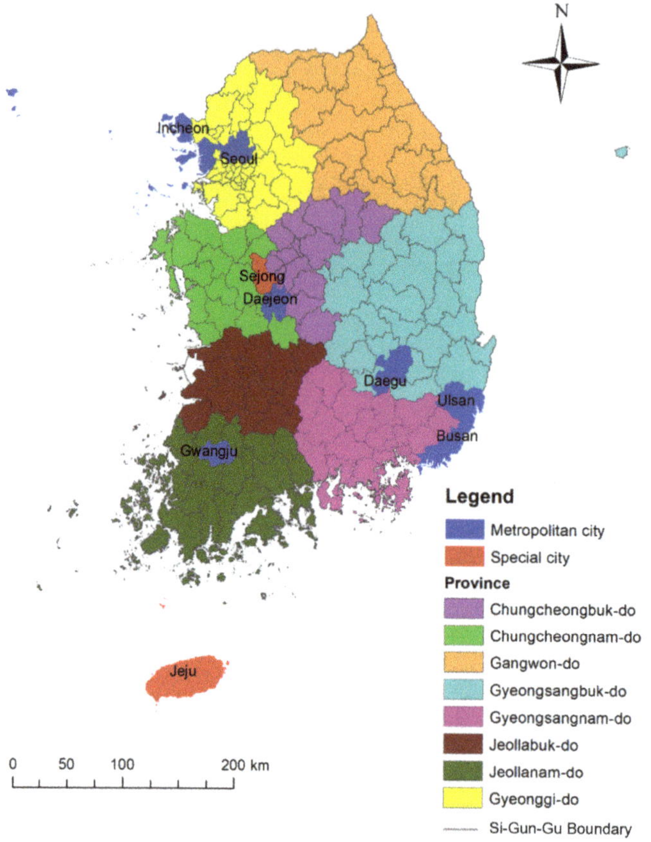

Figure 1. Map of the study area.

2.2. Data Collection

The spatial data in this study were derived from Korean shapefile datasets, which comprise polygon data uniquely identified by a "code" attribute within the dataset to represent each region. Dementia data were collected from the Ministry of Health and Welfare's website (www.data.go.kr, accessed on 7 July 2022). Dementia prevalence was determined using the percentage of male and female patients with dementia aged 65–85 years out of the total population of the same age. Patients with dementia include both populations residing in their homes and those living in hospitals or nursing homes. Demographic information, including age and population, was obtained from the Korean Population and Housing Census data from 2017 to 2020, provided by Statistics Korea (https://sgis.kostat.go.kr/, accessed on 7 July 2022). We substituted the 2021 demographic information with 2020 data, as it was not yet available. The percentage of welfare recipients and their health status was calculated from the Community Health Survey data of the Korea Disease Control and Prevention Agency (https://chs.kdca.go.kr, accessed on 7 July 2022) from 2017 to 2021. Welfare recipients are defined by the Ministry of Health and Welfare and are under the

Korean social welfare program, which provides subsistence support and opportunities for self-sufficiency to people living in extreme poverty [32]. Regarding health status, the lowest score of one indicates "very bad" and the highest value of five denotes "very good".

Greenspace Measures

This study used two different types of green space exposure data sources: NDVI and density of open space from the built environment. Greenness was calculated from the NDVI using the Harmonized Sentinel-2 MSI: Multi-Spectral Instrument, Level-2A image collections. Using the Google Earth Engine, five-year images were collected by running a mosaicking and masking script to reduce cloud coverage from the satellite images. To avoid the change in leaf color during winter and fall, data were collected from May to September. Following the NDVI calculation, the 30 m^2 pixel resolution of the NDVI values was reclassified to filter an area with an NDVI value of 0.3–1, which is defined as a green area. The intersection method was used to extract the NDVI values. Some studies have used this method to obtain a subset of NDVI values within the polygon [33,34]. The green space obtained from NDVI represents the average value at the district level, and its definition of green space is broader. Other measures of green space with specific land uses, such as parks and green spaces or places that the public can visit for physical activity, which are defined as open space in this study, were then used as comparative data. The data for open space were obtained from the spatial facilities website (http://data.nsdi.go.kr/, accessed on 7 July 2022), which provides spatial data for outdoor facilities developed by the government. This shapefile consists of a polygon geometry type. The data were filtered using only the attributes "park" with code "UQT200", and "green space" with code "UQT300", which include parks, recreational forests, and other built green spaces (including the trees along a street) from the dataset attributes. The district boundaries were then intersected to determine the distribution of the open space.

The preprocessed data results were collected and formatted into a comma-separated value table. The descriptive statistics of all variables are listed in Table 1. The dependent variable was the prevalence of female and male patients with dementia, and independent variables included the population of female patients, male patient populations, average age, population density, NDVI, open space, welfare receiver, and health status.

Table 1. Definitions and descriptive statistics of the dependent and independent variables.

Variable	Mean	SD	Min	Max
Prevalence of female patients with dementia over 65 years (%)	6.27	1.12	3.55	9.18
Prevalence of male patients with dementia over 65 years (%)	4.51	0.53	3.03	6.74
Female patient population (%)	50.35	1.39	43.62	53.49
Male patient population (%)	49.65	1.39	46.51	56.38
Age (mean age of population)	45.21	4.95	34.93	57.35
Population density (individuals/km^2)	3666.08	5513.50	17.00	24,588.00
Green-area (NDVI value)	0.47	0.15	0.09	0.75
Open space (%)	4.86	7.71	0.00	58.64
Welfare recipients (%)	3.16	1.55	0.13	10.59
Health status	3.30	0.16	2.85	3.81

2.3. Analysis

2.3.1. Panel Model Estimation

A panel dataset includes information gathered by one uniquely defined "unit" across a predetermined number of periods. Panel data can be regarded as a combination of time-series and cross-sectional data. In cross-sectional data, each line represents different units, each column contains data from one of the variables measured for the unit, and the z-axis includes the order of the period in which the unit has been tracked [26]. This study utilized a balanced panel dataset, in which the total number of observations in the sample is similar across all periods. Panel data combine both qualities into a single model by gathering information from several identical objects over time. The ability to use more observations for analysis makes panel data beneficial. This finding is particularly valid for the pooled ordinary least square (OLS) model. Because observations are repeated over time, we reduced the standard errors compared with those predicted by cross-sectional data analysis. The following is the equation for estimating the OLS regression (pooled OLS):

$$y_{it} = \beta_0 + \beta_1 X_{1it} + \beta_2 X_{2it} + \ldots + \beta_k X_{kit} + \varepsilon_{it} \quad (1)$$

where y_{it} is the response variable, X_{it} is the regression variable, β_0 is the intercept, β_k is the coefficient of the explanatory variable, k is the order of the explanatory variable, and ε is an error term. Compared with that of the cross-sectional OLS, the bias is lower; however, the pooled OLS also includes a consideration of within-variation. Therefore, panel data alone do not address the unobserved heterogeneity problem [24]. One of the assumptions in an OLS regression is that there is no correlation between the independent variables (non-multicollinearity). The OLS regression model utilizes the inflation factor (VIF) variance value to detect non-multicollinearity. If the VIF value for all independent variables is <10, multicollinearity is not recorded in the OLS regression model [35].

In this study, pooled OLS was estimated along with fixed effect (FE). The individual impacts of unobserved independent variables were determined, using the FE model, to be constant over time. The link between endogeneity and unobserved independent variables can exist in the FE model. This approach assumes that the slope value of each variable is fixed; however, the intercept value is different for each cross-sectional dataset and is the same for each time-series dataset [25]. The equation for the FE regression model is as follows.

$$y_{it} = \beta_1 X_{1,it} + \ldots + \beta_k X_{k,it} + \alpha_i + \varepsilon_{it} \quad (2)$$

where $i = 1, \ldots. n$ is the observed entity; $t = 1, \ldots. T$ is the year of the observed data; and α_i is the entity-specific intercept. The next step is to confirm the existence of unobserved effects if the assumption of homogeneity over the coefficients is proven. This is performed by comparing the null of spherical residuals with the alternative group-specific effects in the error term. Thus, in comparing the two estimators under the null hypothesis to determine whether the difference is not substantial, Hausman-type tests are used to decide between fixed and random effects specifications [36], in which FE estimators are used to model the result.

2.3.2. Spatial Autocorrelation

Exploratory spatial data analysis (ESDA) has been used to assess spatial autocorrelation by detecting spatial dependency to determine the spatial properties of a dataset. The Global Moran's I index is one of the most commonly used ESDA indices for determining spatial autocorrelation [37], and it ranges from −1 to 1. Spatial agglomeration is supported if the Global Moran's I value is >0, indicating significant spatial clusters of attribution values with either higher or lower attribute values. Spatial dispersion is supported if the Global Moran's I value is <0, which indicates a sizable spatial variation in the attribution values between the target city and its surroundings. A spatially random pattern is created when the Global Moran's I value is close to 0, indicating that spatial autocorrelation is absent [38]. For comparison, from bivariate Moran's I analysis, we subsequently generated the local patterns of spatial correlation between dementia prevalence and NDVI value using 5-year data. Owing to South Korea's geography, which consists of islands, such as Ulleung-do and Jeju-do, the k-nearest neighbors (kNNs) were used to obtain the spatial weight matrix. The kNN algorithm has been used as a nonparametric method for pattern recognition in statistical predictions. In the context of regression problems, the estimated values are determined by calculating the average or centroid of the kNNs [39].

2.3.3. Spatial Panel Regression

In this study, the spatial data analysis using spatial autocorrelation produced bias owing to the spatial dependence and heterogeneity of geographical data. Previous studies have revealed that the health conditions that occur in an area are not only influenced by local risk factors but also by elements from neighboring areas. Panel data analysis can produce bias, as it does not include the results of the spillover effect [31,40,41]. Accordingly, spatial panel analysis can overcome the bias problem by identifying this effect throughout the region. This can be performed by observing how the relationship between the spatial data and other variables changes over time. The maximum likelihood (ML) estimator applies the fixed effects (FEs) method to the results of panel regression based on the Hausman test, and the FE method is more appropriate for this study. However, because OLS does not work with random effects models, even without spatial components, ML is a different (and better) way to estimate models [36]. The implementation of ML in the FE model only considers the spatial lag and error models.

This study used the spatial lag model (SLM) and spatial error model (SEM) to analyze and quantify potential spatial effects. The SEM process of adding the dependent variable to the spatial association of the covariables may result in the error term of the regression model being missed. Simultaneously, by adding a lagged dependent variable, the SLM combines the spatial dependency regression model [35]. The SLM accounts for spatial autocorrelation by incorporating a lagged version of the dependent variable. Simultaneously, by including a spatial error term in the model, the SEM addresses the dependence between omitted covariates and nearby values.

The following is the equation of the FE SLM:

$$y = \lambda(I_T \otimes W_N)y + (\iota_T \otimes I_N) + X\beta + \varepsilon \quad (3)$$

where λ is the spatial autoregressive coefficient, W_N is a spatial weight matrix, ι_T is a column vector, and I_N is an identity matrix [42].

The following is the equation of the FE SEM:

$$y = (\iota T \otimes IN) + X\beta + uu = \rho(IT \otimes WN)u + \varepsilon \quad (4)$$

where ρ is the coefficient of spatial autocorrelation [43]. Finally, this study produced several results from different, although complementary, analyses, and we obtained results from the OLS regression analysis. By adding spatial aspects, panel regression results for nonspatial data can be used to obtain map results from spatial regression. The global and bivariate Moran's I results were obtained, as map results were used to identify the significant map. Thus, from these results, data interpretation was performed to identify the relationship between the two types of green space and dementia at the regional level and their influence on other data variables. A significant map was obtained for regions with a significant number of dementia cases over five years.

3. Results

Only 235 si/gu/gun districts were considered for spatial panel analysis from a total of 250 districts because the 15 districts containing missing values were removed to avoid singularity errors when running the spatial weighted matrix. The spatial distributions of dementia prevalence from 2017 to 2021 are shown in Figure 2, whereas the spatial distributions of open space prevalence and NDVI values are shown in Figure 3. Table 1 presents the prevalence of dementia among females and males over 65 years, which corresponds to 6.2% and 4.5%, respectively. Meanwhile, differences were observed in the spatial pattern of the green data; a high NDVI value was distributed in the east and south sides of South Korea, mostly in rural areas. The open space prevalence was clustered in urban areas, such as Seoul, the Gyeonggi-do region, Daegu, Busan, Ulsan, Daejeon, Jeonju, and Gwangju.

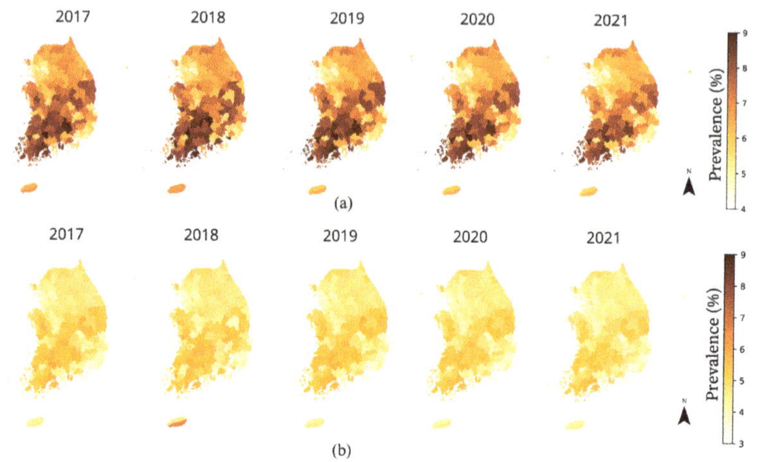

Figure 2. Spatial distribution of prevalence of dementia from 2017 to 2021: (**a**) prevalence of female dementia; (**b**) prevalence of male dementia.

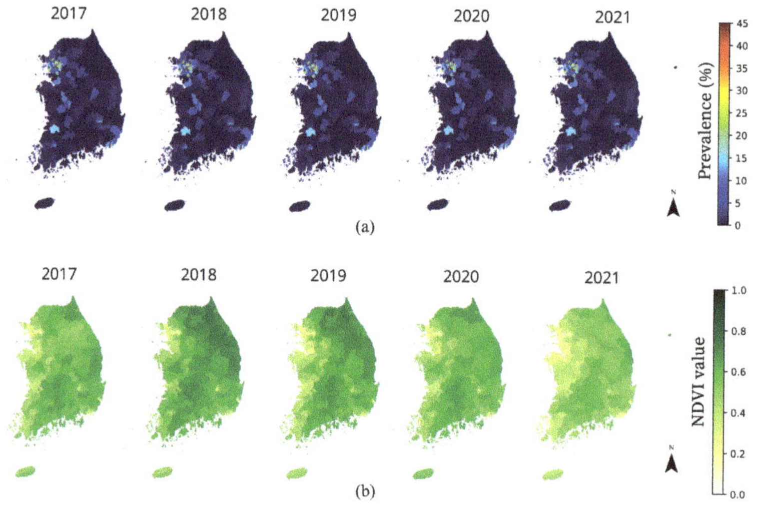

Figure 3. Spatial distribution of NDVI and open space from 2017 to 2021: (**a**) prevalence of open space; (**b**) NDVI value.

Figure 4 compares dementia prevalence between female and male patients from 2017 to 2021. For both female and male patients, the prevalence increased from 2017 to 2018 and decreased from 2018 to 2021. In 2017, 2018, 2019, 2020, and 2021, the prevalence of dementia in females changed by 0.06%, −0.05%, −0.11%, and −0.12%, respectively, and data differences in the median value were observed. Conversely, for males, the prevalence changes were 0.07%, −0.02%, −0.04%, and −0.03%, respectively.

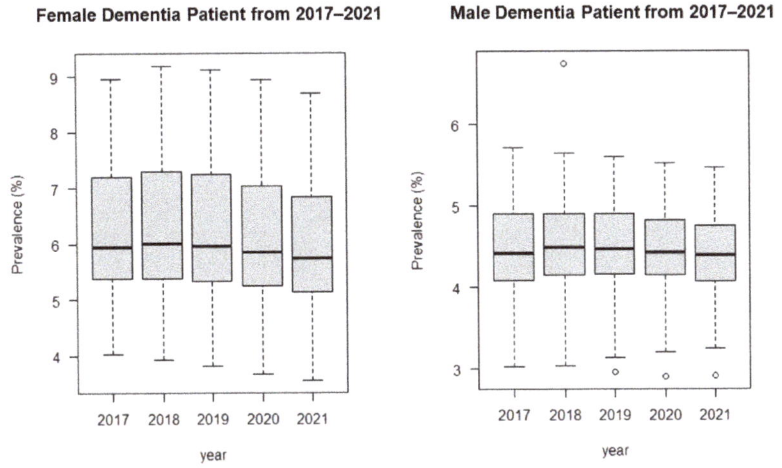

Figure 4. Boxplot of dementia prevalence in females and males from 2017 to 2021.

3.1. Spatial Autocorrelation

The Global Moran's I result for the entire dataset of dementia prevalence in females and males from 2017 to 2021 is presented in Figure 5. The results indicate that all observed values for dementia prevalence in females and males were moderately positively associated based on the statistical range value. This finding suggests that the prevalence of dementia is spatially dependent. Additionally, local indicators of spatial association cluster maps were generated from the prevalence of dementia patients with NDVI and open spaces in each region from 2017 to 2021.

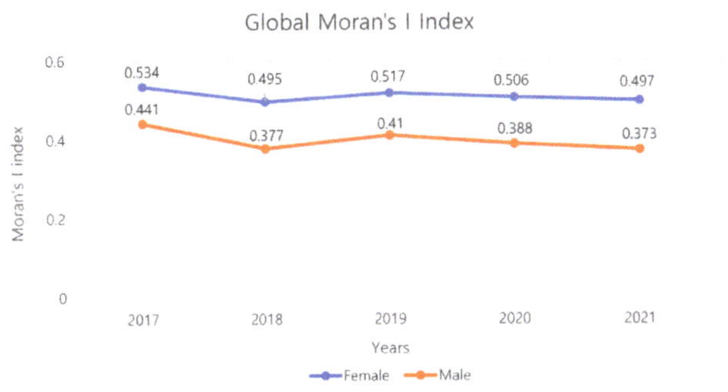

Figure 5. Statistics value of global Moran's I of the dementia prevalence in female and male patients from 2017 to 2021.

Figure 6 shows the spatial associations between the prevalence of dementia in females and males with NDVI from 2017 to 2021. These maps exhibit nearly identical spatial distribution patterns, with high–high (HH) and low–low (LL) patterns being prevalent. The HH patterns, characterized by high dementia prevalence and high NDVI, were clustered from the northeast to the southwest, which comprised almost all areas of Gangwon-do, the north side of Gyeongsangbuk-do, east side of Chungcheongbuk-do, east side of Jeollabuk-do, east side of Gyeongsangnam-do, and northeast of Jeollanam-do. The LL patterns were clustered in the Seoul area, several parts of Gyeonggi-do, and the Incheon area and are located on the south side of South Korea, specifically in the Busan area and several parts of the south side area of Gyeongsangnam-do. This suggests that the two big cities in South Korea have a spatial pattern with low dementia cases and low greenness values.

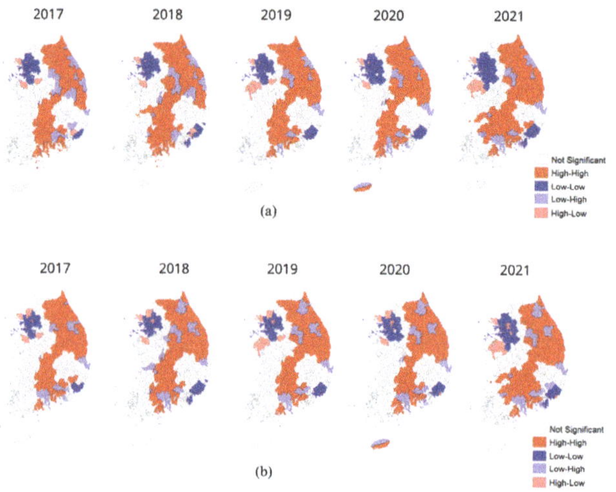

Figure 6. Cluster map of the result of bivariate Moran's I between dementia patients and NDVI from 2017 to 2021: (**a**) female dementia and NDVI; (**b**) male dementia and NDVI.

Figure 7 presents the LISA map of dementia patients and open space from 2017 to 2021. The results reveal spatial clusters between female and male dementia patients with dominant low–high and high–low associations. Specifically, in 2017, a low–high pattern was observed among both male and female patients in the Seoul city area and some parts of Busan. Conversely, a high–low pattern was observed in most areas of Gangwon-do, extending southwards to Gyeongsangnam-do, and clustered in several locations of Chungcheongnam-do. For the 2021 case, the cluster pattern for patients with dementia was almost identical to that observed in 2017. However, the association between male dementia patients and open space in 2021 was high in Busan.

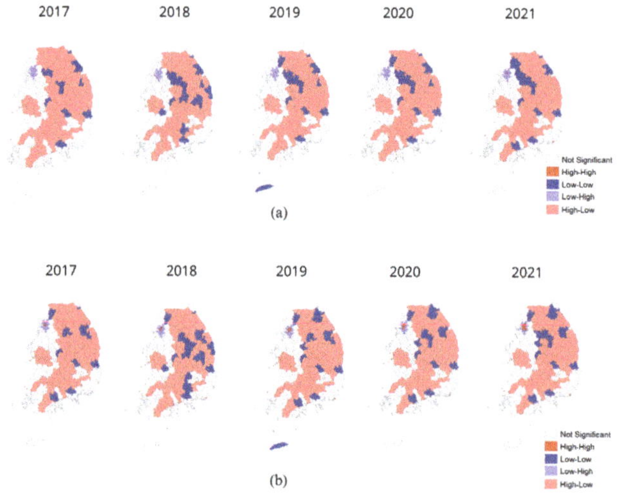

Figure 7. Cluster map of the result of bivariate Moran's I between dementia patients and open space: (**a**) female dementia and open space; (**b**) male dementia and open space.

3.2. Panel Regression

The aforementioned results suggest that this study has significant value in the context of spatial autoregression, and the relationship between dementia prevalence, NDVI, and open space data is substantial. The results of multicollinearity, assessed using VIFs, revealed that all the independent variables, namely, the female and male population, average age, density population, open space, NDVI, welfare recipients, and health condition, had low correlations or low multicollinearity, with the following results: 1.37, 1.37, 2.01, 3.45, 2.19, 2.33, 1.31, and 1.39, respectively. Subsequently, the panel regression methods, which included the common pooled OLS method, random effects model, and fixed effect model, are presented in Table 2.

Table 2. Estimation of the panel model (nonspatial data).

Variables	NDVI				Open Space			
	Pooled OLS		Fixed-Effect		Pooled OLS		Fixed-Effect	
	Female	Male	Female	Male	Female	Male	Female	Male
Female patient pop.	0.107 ***		0.072		0.109 ***		0.045	
Male patient pop.		−0.084 ***		−0.098 ***		−0.084 ***		−0.094 ***
Age	0.129 ***	0.062 ***	−0.069 ***	−0.026 ***	0.134 ***	0.065 ***	0.048	−0.012
Population density	−0.0001 ***	−0.00002 ***	−0.0003 ***	−0.0002 ***	−0.0001 ***	−0.00002 ***	−0.0003 ***	−0.0002 ***
NDVI	0.805 ***	0.300 ***	1.381 ***	0.421 ***				
Open space					−0.003	0.001	−8666.450 ***	−1466.621 *
Welfare recipients	−0.002	0.006	−0.007	0.002	−0.011	0.002	−0.009	0.0003
Health status	−1.035 ***	−0.303 ***	−0.167 *	−0.067	−1.066 ***	−0.322 ***	−0.159 *	−0.065
Con.	−1.650 *	6.766 ***			−1.468	6.886 ***		
N	1175	1175	1175	1175	1175	1175	1175	1175
R^2	0.724	0.635	0.156	0.094	0.721	0.633	0.144	0.084
Adjusted R2	0.723	0.634	−0.061	−0.139	0.719	0.631	−0.076	−0.151
F statistic	511.829 ***	339.336 ***	28.724 ***	16.131 ***	501.847 ***	335.230 ***	26.180 ***	14.328 ***
AIC	2261.532	667.128	167.806	−1134.243	2278.252	676.196	184.132	−1121.845

* $p < 0.05$; *** $p < 0.001$.

According to the Chow and Hausman test in Table 3, the null hypotheses were rejected because the results exhibited autocorrelation and heteroscedasticity. The FE model was the preferable estimator because the *p*-values were smaller than 5%. Furthermore, the Akaike information criterion values of the FE model for females and males were lower than those of the pooled OLS, indicating that the FE model is a better fit. Therefore, based on the supported data, the test results determined that estimation obtained using the FE model is the best model to explain the panel regression results in this study.

Table 3. Test results of the Chow and Hausman test.

Test	F	chisq	Df	*p*-Value	Result
Chow test (NDVI-female)	19.682		235	<0.001	H_0 rejected
Chow test (NDVI-male)	14.467		235	<0.001	H_0 rejected
Chow test (Open space-female)	19.69		235	<0.001	H_0 rejected
Chow test (Open space -male)	14.415		235	<0.001	H_0 rejected
Hausman test (NDVI-female)		188.04	6	<0.001	H_0 rejected
Hausman test (NDVI-male)		94.25	6	<0.001	H_0 rejected
Hausman test (Open space-female)		265.33	6	<0.001	H_0 rejected
Hausman test (Open space-male)		97.681	6	<0.001	H_0 rejected

As listed in Table 2, eight models of panel model estimation using the FE and pooled OLS were considered, and the classifications were based on the model using the NDVI and open space variables and stratified by gender in each specification. The results of NDVI in the fixed effects models revealed that the prevalence of female and male patients with dementia was statistically significant, and the relationship was positive. Comparatively, the results of the open space model in this analysis revealed that the open space density has a significant negative relationship with the prevalence of dementia in both genders in the fixed effect model.

3.3. Spatial Panel Regression

The results of the spatial FE estimations, which utilized maximum likelihood methods to estimate the spatial interactions of explanatory variables, are presented in Table 4. The estimation results for the spatial autoregressive of SLM (SAR-FE) and spatial error within a model (SEM-FE) include the individual and temporal effects in each NDVI and open space model, and the temporal effects are presented in Table 5. The ML estimations of SEM and SAR utilized individual effects in the model, in which individual data were aggregated at the regional level. The results of spatial autoregression in the NDVI model revealed that the NDVI variable had a positive and significant association with dementia prevalence in female and male patients. Next, the SEM results from the NDVI model exhibited a significant positive association between NDVI and dementia prevalence in female and male patients. Furthermore, the results obtained from the open-space model exhibited a contrast between the effect of NDVI and the prevalence of dementia. The results were obtained after conducting the SAR and SEM analyses of this model.

Table 4. Estimation of spatial panel results using maximum likelihood.

Variables	NDVI				Open Space			
	SAR-FE		SEM-FE		SAR-FE		SEM-FE	
	Female	Male	Female	Male	Female	Male	Female	Male
Female patient pop.	0.0451		0.05494		0.0242		0.0251	
Male patient pop.		−0.0730 **		−0.0787 **		−0.0692 **		−0.0744 **
Age	−0.0485 **	−0.0220 *	−0.0674 ***	−0.0314 **	0.0348	−0.0127	0.0221	−0.0236 ***
Population density	−0.0002 ***	−0.0002 ***	−0.0002 ***	−0.0001 ***	−0.0002 **	−0.0002 ***	−0.0002 ***	−0.0002 ***
NDVI	0.9793 ***	0.3136 **	1.3181 ***	0.3844 **				
Open space					−6142.9 **	−1022.9	−7943.2 ***	−1161.7
Welfare recipients	−0.0054	0.0017	−0.0037	0.0032	−0.0065	0.0009	−0.0045	0.0027
Health status	−0.1392	−0.0569	−0.2037 *	−0.074	−0.1309	−0.0553	−0.1563	−0.0692
σ^2			0.6427	0.3208				
Rho	0.0561 ***	0.0511 ***	0.1188 ***	0.1172 ***	0.057	0.051	0.061 ***	0.
AIC	100.305	−1186.981	170.653	−1129.437	106.101	−1180.336	188.781	−1115.99

* $p < 0.05$; ** $p < 0.01$; *** $p < 0.001$.

Table 5. Time-period estimations of the fixed-effect (SEM-FE).

Years	NDVI		Open Space	
	Female	Male	Female	Male
2017	0.1420	0.0591	0.1601	0.0637
2018	0.0764	0.0496	0.1425	0.0675
2019	−0.0352	0.0025	−0.0083	0.0086
2020	−0.0126	−0.0314	−0.0248	−0.0328
2021	−0.1706	−0.0798	−0.2694	−0.1071
p-value		***		***

*** $p < 0.001$.

The results of generating the time effect from the SEM-FE estimators are listed in Table 5. The results were obtained from the estimation of the time effect in the SEM, which explains the changes in the estimation over time and provides information about the relationship between the time-period dummy variables and the dependent variable. The time effect from the NDVI and open space models generated similar estimations, but that from the open space was higher than that from NDVI. The outcome of the time-period estimation revealed that the period from 2017 to 2018 had a positive effect; however, the estimation in 2018 was lower than that in 2017. Subsequently, from 2019 to 2021, a negative influence of the time effect was observed, with the number of time estimations decreasing.

4. Discussion

Recent studies on dementia have reported that no definite factors cause dementia as a cognitive impairment disease [11]. However, dementia has been linked to physical activity, diet, congenital diseases, and environmental influences. Having a good environment and maintaining greenery can improve human quality of life and sustainability [4]. Several researchers have noted that individuals living in green neighborhoods have a lower dementia risk, lower rate of cognitive decline, and better mental health [6,9,21,44]. By utilizing a spatial panel data analysis using 5-year data, this study explained the existing pattern of the spread of dementia spatially and temporally at the district level, and its relationship with greenery exposure, with NDVI and open space serving as representations of green spaces. The spatial panel regression method modeled the variables based on the distance of regions by accounting for spatial dependencies and heterogeneity and spatial and time invariants [31], and controlling the potential confounding factors, such as socioeconomic status and health welfare, at the regional level that vary over time to improve the validity of the findings.

This study demonstrated the differences between NDVI and open space in terms of spatial distribution. The observed pattern indicates that rural areas are dominated by high NDVI values, and most urban areas have high concentrations of open space. Furthermore, a bivariate Moran's I analysis revealed significant spatial autocorrelation between the two green space measures and the prevalence of dementia using five years of data. A previous cross-sectional analysis model of regional dementia in South Korea [3] reported that urban areas had a lower dementia prevalence than rural areas, based on 2020 data. Other studies [27,29] have shown that green spaces in cities improve health and reduce dementia. The different types of green space measures in this study refer to digitized green space areas with specific land use, such as parks and green space facilities, along with NDVI values converted to aggregated data at the regional level. The disadvantage of using aggregated NDVI data for health studies is that they generalize based on the green index for all areas without classifying them based on land use. This inability hinders a detailed explanation of the direct relationship between individuals and all green areas represented in NDVI. Therefore, caution should be exercised in future research when performing analyses of the relationship between green space and dementia at a national level, as such an ecological study relates to health risk factors that are susceptible to ecological fallacy [45].

This study found that the aggregated NDVI values had a positive relationship with the prevalence of dementia in all models. Specifically, in regional-level studies, areas with a high NDVI value have a high prevalence of dementia, and the percentage of open space has a negative relationship with the prevalence of dementia among both genders. This observed pattern indicates that a high NDVI value is associated with a high prevalence of dementia and a high percentage of open space in one area is associated with a low prevalence of dementia in both genders. The spatial distribution of open space areas in South Korea reveals that most cities have a high percentage of open space, and most rural areas have high NDVI values. To strengthen this finding, a study conducted a comparative analysis of dementia incidence rates between Seoul, a major city, and Gangwon-do, which represent city-side to rural areas with high NDVI values [46]. Surprisingly, the incidence of dementia in Gangwon-do was found to be higher than that in Seoul in 2017 and 2018. Following the implementation of dementia care strategies, the incidence rate in Seoul decreased but not in Gangwon-do.

The findings of this study revealed that open space and NDVI results differ from those of the analysis. This difference occurs because of differences in green space measurement, where the NDVI value in this study includes all greenness exposures, including forests, grass, bushes, shrubs, and others, without filtering out differences in land cover types. Meanwhile, the open space data in this study consist of built green space facility data for parks, recreational forests, and other built green spaces. Therefore, researchers who conduct epidemiological studies using green space data need to be cautious about the differences in the definition of green space because each type varies and can affect health differently, especially in ecological studies. This difference is essential because greenness exposure is sensitive to the spatial resolution, area-level data, and green values. Many researchers still use NDVI and open space interchangeably, and the NDVI value has been used as residential green space exposure and converted aggregated data [27,47,48]. In contrast, the findings from the present study demonstrated differences between the two green spaces and their relationship with the prevalence of dementia. Additionally, a systematic review of the association between greenness and dementia revealed that the misclassification of green spaces affects the results [6]. Several studies have also compared the results of comparative analyses using NDVI and built environments and defined them as distinct aspects of green space studies [49,50].

The spread of the coronavirus, which started in early 2020, has extended worldwide. One study found that patients with dementia who were infected with COVID-19 faced double threats [51]. Other studies have explained that lockdown strategies during the COVID-19 pandemic negatively impacted individuals by decreasing physical activity and social interaction, increasing stress, and worsening dementia [52–54]. The present study showed that the prevalence of dementia had decreased in both male and female patients by 2020 (Figure 4). Furthermore, the spatial panel analysis results for the time-period estimations of the relationship between dementia and NDVI and open space are presented in Table 5. The coefficients of time effects for the prevalence of female and male patients have decreased since 2019 and 2020, respectively. There was no strong reason for the decline in the prevalence of dementia during the COVID-19 pandemic. Although the number of patients with dementia has been increasing, the prevalence continues to decrease. Thus, further research is needed to determine the effects of the pandemic on the prevalence of patients with dementia and their interactions with the environment, especially greenness, because of the massive change between individuals and the surrounding environment due to activity restrictions during the pandemic. To explore the reasons behind the decline in dementia cases in 2020, research from South Korea has been conducted to explore steps for preventing and treating dementia patients. This has been conducted in keeping with the national dementia plans program implemented in 2020 based on the WHO action plan for prevention, diagnosis, awareness, health services, and others [55,56]. Thus, this aspect can be used to compare whether the decrease in the prevalence of dementia was due to the spread of COVID-19 or because the national dementia plans have been implemented.

This study has advantages in overcoming biased estimation by conducting two analyses in a traditional panel analysis, which is corroborated by spatial panel analysis because it considers the spillover effect. Subsequently, extensive data that covered five years can be updated throughout the most recent year to further analyze dementia or other health outcomes. Furthermore, the analysis results used two green space measures that could be selectively used in further studies. This study fills gaps in the application of spatial econometrics in health risk factor studies, especially in dementia research. However, this study had several limitations. First, aggregated data were used based on population at the regional level in this ecological study. Therefore, caution should be exercised when inferring a causal relationship between variables and using individual-level data for further studies, to avoid ecological fallacies. Second, in the demographic dataset, only data from 2017 to 2020 were available, and we could not access data for 2021. Therefore, we only used the same 2020 data in 2021. Therefore, we may have missed any changes in population trends or specific demographics in 2021 caused by the COVID-19 pandemic, which started in 2020. Third, because data collection in this study started in 2020 when the COVID-19 outbreak occurred worldwide, patients' behavior and activity changes can affect the prevalence of dementia. However, this study did not add variables related to changes in activity during the pandemic, which may affect its conclusions. Therefore, future research should examine whether changes in regulations during a pandemic influence the prevalence of dementia and the environment. Moreover, to obtain more generalizable results and more complete models, data covering longer time spans, such as 10-year data, should be used, and additional environmental variables, such as air quality and noise pollution, which may be used as confounding factors, should be added.

5. Conclusions

Spatial panel regression can explain the relationship between dementia and greenness, demographic factors, and healthcare both spatially and temporally. The prevalence of dementia in South Korea had a statistically positive relationship with NDVI and a statistically negative relationship with open space data. The results for the greenness models were different because the green data had different types and sources. In future research, care will be needed when choosing the type of green space data in the analysis of studies on dementia or other epidemiological studies. This study emphasizes the importance of considering green space as a potential risk factor for dementia because the difference in green space data affects the estimation results. The findings of this study contribute to the existing literature on the relationship between green spaces and dementia using statistical techniques and longitudinal data. By highlighting the potential impact of green spaces on dementia, this study provides important insights into the prevention and management of the disease, particularly in urban and rural areas. Further research in this area could help in developing targeted interventions and policies to promote green spaces as a potential means to reduce the risk of developing dementia.

Author Contributions: Conceptualization, Wulan Salle Karurung and Kangjae Lee; methodology, Wulan Salle Karurung and Kangjae Lee; software, Wulan Salle Karurung; validation, Wulan Salle Karurung, Kangjae Lee and Wonhee Lee; formal analysis, Wulan Salle Karurung; data curation, Wulan Salle Karurung and Kangjae Lee; writing—original draft, Wulan Salle Karurung; writing—review and editing, Kangjae Lee; visualization, Wulan Salle Karurung; supervision, Kangjae Lee and Wonhee Lee; funding acquisition, Wonhee Lee. All authors have read and agreed to the published version of the manuscript.

Funding: This research was supported by the Basic Science Research Program through the National Research Foundation of Korea (NRF) funded by the Ministry of Education (NRF-2020R1I1A3061750), and a National Research Foundation of Korea (NRF) grant funded by the Korean government (MSIT) (no. NRF-2021R1A5A8033165).

Institutional Review Board Statement: Not applicable.

Informed Consent Statement: Not applicable.

Data Availability Statement: This can be provided upon request.

Conflicts of Interest: The authors declare no conflicts of interest.

References

1. Van Der Flier, W.M.; Scheltens, P. Epidemiology and Risk Factors of Dementia. *J. Neurol. Neurosurg. Psychiatry* **2005**, *76*, V2–V7. [CrossRef] [PubMed]
2. Dhana, K.; Evans, D.A.; Rajan, K.B.; Bennett, D.A.; Morris, M.C. Healthy Lifestyle and the Risk of Alzheimer Dementia: Findings from 2 Longitudinal Studies. *Neurology* **2020**, *95*, e374–e383. [CrossRef] [PubMed]
3. Lim, J.; Park, J.-H. Predictive Model of Regional Dementia Prevalence Using Geographic Weighted Regression Analysis. *J. Pers. Med.* **2022**, *12*, 1388. [CrossRef] [PubMed]
4. Besser, L. Outdoor Green Space Exposure and Brain Health Measures Related to Alzheimer's Disease: A Rapid Review. *BMJ Open* **2021**, *11*, e043456. [CrossRef] [PubMed]
5. Shon, C.; Yoon, H. Health-Economic Burden of Dementia in South Korea. *BMC Geriatr.* **2021**, *21*, 54. [CrossRef] [PubMed]
6. Zagnoli, F.; Filippini, T.; Jimenez, M.P.; Wise, L.A.; Hatch, E.E.; Vinceti, M. Is Greenness Associated with Dementia? A Systematic Review and Dose–Response Meta-Analysis. *Curr. Environ. Health Rep.* **2022**, *9*, 574–590. [CrossRef] [PubMed]
7. Astell-Burt, T.; Navakatikyan, M.A.; Feng, X. Urban Green Space, Tree Canopy and 11-Year Risk of Dementia in a Cohort of 109,688 Australians. *Environ. Int.* **2020**, *145*, 106102. [CrossRef]
8. Rodriguez-Loureiro, L.; Gadeyne, S.; Bauwelinck, M.; Lefebvre, W.; Vanpoucke, C.; Casas, L. Long-Term Exposure to Residential Greenness and Neurodegenerative Disease Mortality among Older Adults: A 13-Year Follow-up Cohort Study. *Environ. Health A Glob. Access Sci. Source* **2022**, *21*, 49. [CrossRef]

9. Hu, H.Y.; Ma, Y.H.; Deng, Y.T.; Ou, Y.N.; Cheng, W.; Feng, J.F.; Tan, L.; Yu, J.T. Residential Greenness and Risk of Incident Dementia: A Prospective Study of 375,342 Participants. *Environ. Res.* **2023**, *216*, 114703. [CrossRef]
10. Browning, M.; Lee, K. Within What Distance Does "Greenness" Best Predict Physical Health? A Systematic Review of Articles with Gis Buffer Analyses across the Lifespan. *Int. J. Environ. Res. Public Health* **2017**, *14*, 675. [CrossRef]
11. Dhana, K.; Franco, O.H.; Ritz, E.M.; Ford, C.N.; Desai, P.; Krueger, K.R.; Holland, T.M.; Dhana, A.; Liu, X.; Aggarwal, N.T.; et al. Healthy Lifestyle and Life Expectancy with and without Alzheimer's Dementia: Population Based Cohort Study. *BMJ* **2022**, *377*, e068390. [CrossRef] [PubMed]
12. Younan, D.; Wang, X.; Millstein, J.; Petkus, A.J.; Beavers, D.P.; Espeland, M.A.; Chui, H.C.; Resnick, S.M.; Gatz, M.; Kaufman, J.D.; et al. Air Quality Improvement and Cognitive Decline in Community-Dwelling Older Women in the United States: A Longitudinal Cohort Study. *PLoS Med.* **2022**, *19*, e1003893. [CrossRef] [PubMed]
13. Mmako, N.J.; Courtney-Pratt, H.; Marsh, P. Green Spaces, Dementia and a Meaningful Life in the Community: A Mixed Studies Review. *Health Place* **2020**, *63*, 102344. [CrossRef]
14. Choi, H.G.; Kim, J.H.; Kim, J.H.; Kim, E.S.; Park, H.Y.; Min, K.W.; Kwon, M.J. Associations between Proton Pump Inhibitors and Alzheimer's Disease: A Nested Case–Control Study Using a Korean Nationwide Health Screening Cohort. *Alzheimer's Res. Ther.* **2022**, *14*, 1–11. [CrossRef] [PubMed]
15. Lee, S. Spatial and Socioeconomic Inequalities in Accessibility to Healthcare Services in South Korea. *Healthcare* **2022**, *10*, 2049. [CrossRef] [PubMed]
16. Choi, J.; Kwon, L.; Lim, H.; Chun, H. Gender-Based Analysis of Risk Factors for Dementia Using Senior Cohort. *Int. J. Environ. Res. Public Health* **2020**, *17*, 7274. [CrossRef]
17. Sun, H.; Wang, A.; He, S. Temporal and Spatial Analysis of Alzheimer's Disease Based on an Improved Convolutional Neural Network and a Resting-State FMRI Brain Functional Network. *Int. J. Environ. Res. Public Health* **2022**, *19*, 4508. [CrossRef] [PubMed]
18. Firouraghi, N.; Kiani, B.; Jafari, H.T.; Learnihan, V.; Salinas-Perez, J.A.; Raeesi, A.; Furst, M.A.; Salvador-Carulla, L.; Bagheri, N. The Role of Geographic Information System and Global Positioning System in Dementia Care and Research: A Scoping Review. *Int. J. Health Geogr.* **2022**, *21*, 8. [CrossRef] [PubMed]
19. Scerpella, D.L.; Adam, A.; Marx, K.; Gitlin, L.N. Implications of Geographic Information Systems (GIS) for Targeted Recruitment of Older Adults with Dementia and Their Caregivers in the Community: A Retrospective Analysis. *Contemp. Clin. Trials Commun.* **2019**, *14*, 100338. [CrossRef]
20. Su, C.; Lee, K.; Yen, C.; Wu, L.; Huang, C.; Lu, M. Use of Spatial Panel-Data Models to Investigate Factors Related to Incidence of End-Stage Renal Disease: A Nationwide Longitudinal Study in Taiwan. *BMC Public Health.* **2023**, *23*, 247. [CrossRef]
21. Lee, K.; Browning, M.H.E.M.; Park, Y.M. Spatiotemporal Non-Stationarity in Green Space and Stress Relationships: Recent Evidence from South Korea. *Environ. Res.* **2023**, *220*, 115214. [CrossRef] [PubMed]
22. Hirsch, J.A.; Michael, Y.L.; Moore, K.A.; Melly, S.; Hughes, T.M.; Hayden, K.; Luchsinger, J.A.; Jimenez, M.P.; James, P.; Besser, L.M.; et al. Longitudinal Neighbourhood Determinants with Cognitive Health and Dementia Disparities: Protocol of the Multi-Ethnic Study of Atherosclerosis Neighborhoods and Aging Prospective Cohort Study. *BMJ Open* **2022**, *12*, e066971. [CrossRef] [PubMed]
23. Glaser, S.; Jung, R.C.; Schweikert, K. Spatial Panel Count Data: Modeling and Forecasting of Urban Crimes. *J. Spat. Econom.* **2022**, *3*, 2. [CrossRef]
24. Eom, T.H.; Lee, S.H.; Xu, H. Introduction to Panel Data Analysis. In *Handbook of Research Methods in Public Administration*, 2nd ed.; Miller, G.J., Brandler, S., Roman, C.P., Yang, K., Eds.; CRC Press: Boca Raton, FL, USA, 2007; pp. 571–590; ISBN 978-042-924-549-7.
25. Greene, W.H. *Econometric Analysis*, 4th ed.; Prentice Hall: New York, NY, USA, 2000.
26. Salima, B.A.; Julie, L.G.; Lionel, V. Spatial Econometrics on Panel Data. In *Handbook of Spatial Analysis: Theory and Practical Application with R*; Institut National de la Statistique et des Études Économiques: Paris, France, 2018; pp. 179–203.
27. Paul, L.A.; Hystad, P.; Burnett, R.T.; Kwong, J.C.; Crouse, D.L.; van Donkelaar, A.; Tu, K.; Lavigne, E.; Copes, R.; Martin, R.V.; et al. Urban Green Space and the Risks of Dementia and Stroke. *Environ. Res.* **2020**, *186*, 109520. [CrossRef]
28. Bagheri, N.; Wangdi, K.; Cherbuin, N.; Anstey, K.J. Combining Geospatial Analysis With Dementia Risk Utilising General Practice Data: A Systematic Review. *J. Prev. Alzheimer's Dis.* **2017**, *5*, 71–77. [CrossRef]
29. Slawsky, E.D.; Hajat, A.; Rhew, I.C.; Russette, H.; Semmens, E.O.; Kaufman, J.D.; Leary, C.S.; Fitzpatrick, A.L. Neighborhood Greenspace Exposure as a Protective Factor in Dementia Risk among US Adults 75 Years or Older: A Cohort Study. *Environ. Health* **2022**, *21*, 14. [CrossRef] [PubMed]
30. de la Iglesia Martinez, A.; Labib, S.M. Demystifying Normalized Difference Vegetation Index (NDVI) for Greenness Exposure Assessments and Policy Interventions in Urban Greening. *Environ. Res.* **2023**, *220*, 115155. [CrossRef]
31. Elhorst, J.P. The Dynamic General Nesting Spatial Econometric Model for Spatial Panels with Common Factors: Further Raising the Bar. *Rev. Reg. Res.* **2022**, *42*, 249–267. [CrossRef]
32. Jung, I. Explaining the Development and Adoption of Social Policy in Korea: The Case of the National Basic Livelihood Security Act. *Heal. Soc. Welf. Rev.* **2009**, *29*, 44–68. [CrossRef]
33. Lu, M.; Chen, J.; Tang, H.; Rao, Y.; Yang, P.; Wu, W. Land Cover Change Detection by Integrating Object-Based Data Blending Model of Landsat and MODIS. *Remote Sens. Environ.* **2016**, *184*, 374–386. [CrossRef]
34. Wang, Y.; Liu, Z.; Liao, H.; Li, C. Improving the Performance of GIS Polygon Overlay Computation with MapReduce for Spatial Big Data Processing. *Clust. Comput.* **2015**, *18*, 507–516. [CrossRef]

35. Copeland, K.A.F. Applied Linear Statistical Models. *J. Qual. Technol.* **1997**, *29*, 233. [CrossRef]
36. Croissant, Y.; Millo, G. Panel Data Econometrics in R: The Plm Package. *J. Stat. Softw.* **2008**, *27*, 1–43. [CrossRef]
37. Feng, Y.; Wang, X.; Du, W.; Wu, H.; Wang, J. Effects of Environmental Regulation and FDI on Urban Innovation in China: A Spatial Durbin Econometric Analysis. *J. Clean. Prod.* **2019**, *235*, 210–224. [CrossRef]
38. Liu, Q.; Wang, S.; Zhang, W.; Zhan, D.; Li, J. Does Foreign Direct Investment Affect Environmental Pollution in China's Cities? A Spatial Econometric Perspective. *Sci. Total Environ.* **2018**, *613*, 521–529. [CrossRef] [PubMed]
39. Tamamadin, M.; Lee, C.; Kee, S.H.; Yee, J.J. Regional Typhoon Track Prediction Using Ensemble K-Nearest Neighbor Machine Learning in the GIS Environment. *Remote Sens.* **2022**, *14*, 5292. [CrossRef]
40. Xu, P.; Zhao, X.; Li, H.; Guo, S. Spatial Effect Analysis of Health Expenditure and Health Output in China From 2011 to 2018. *Front. Public Health* **2022**, *10*, 794177. [CrossRef] [PubMed]
41. Chen, X.; Shao, S.; Tian, Z.; Xie, Z.; Yin, P. Impacts of Air Pollution and Its Spatial Spillover Effect on Public Health Based on China's Big Data Sample. *J. Clean. Prod.* **2017**, *142*, 915–925. [CrossRef]
42. Elhorst, J.P. Specification and Estimation of Spatial Panel Data Models. *Int. Reg. Sci. Rev.* **2003**, *26*, 244–268. [CrossRef]
43. Millo, G.; Piras, G. Splm: Spatial Panel Data Models in R. *J. Stat. Softw.* **2012**, *47*, 1–38. [CrossRef]
44. Lee, K. Association between depression and green space before and after the COVID-19: Panel data evidence in South Korea. *J. Korean Soc. Surv. Geod. Photogramm. Cartogr.* **2022**, *40*, 459–467. [CrossRef]
45. Wakefield, J.; Lyons, H. Spatial Aggregation and the Ecological Fallacy. In *Handbook of Spatial Statistics*, 1st ed.; Gelfand, A.E., Diggle, P., Guttorp, P., Fuentes, M., Eds.; CRC Press: Boca Raton, FL, USA, 2010; pp. 541–558; ISBN 978-042-913-650-4.
46. Byeon, G.; Kwon, S.O.; Jhoo, J.; Jang, J.-W.; Kim, Y. Dementia Incidence Rate Before and After Implementing the National Responsibility Policy for Dementia Care in Patients With Vascular Risk Factors in Korea. *Dement. Neurocognitive Disord.* **2023**, *22*, 49. [CrossRef] [PubMed]
47. Gascon, M.; Cirach, M.; Martínez, D.; Dadvand, P.; Valentín, A.; Plasència, A.; Nieuwenhuijsen, M.J. Normalized Difference Vegetation Index (NDVI) as a Marker of Surrounding Greenness in Epidemiological Studies: The Case of Barcelona City. *Urban For. Urban Green.* **2016**, *19*, 88–94. [CrossRef]
48. Barboza, E.P.; Cirach, M.; Khomenko, S.; Iungman, T.; Mueller, N.; Barrera-Gómez, J.; Rojas-Rueda, D.; Kondo, M.; Nieuwenhuijsen, M. Green Space and Mortality in European Cities: A Health Impact Assessment Study. *Lancet Planet. Health* **2021**, *5*, e718–e730. [CrossRef]
49. Jimenez, R.B.; Lane, K.J.; Hutyra, L.R.; Fabian, M.P. Spatial Resolution of Normalized Difference Vegetation Index and Greenness Exposure Misclassification in an Urban Cohort. *J. Expo. Sci. Environ. Epidemiol.* **2022**, *32*, 213–222. [CrossRef] [PubMed]
50. Vilcins, D.; Sly, P.D.; Scarth, P.; Mavoa, S. Green Space in Health Research: An Overview of Common Indicators of Greenness. *Rev. Environ. Health* **2022**. [CrossRef] [PubMed]
51. Kyoung, D.-S.; Lee, J.; Nam, H.; Park, M.H. Dementia and COVID-19 Mortality in South Korea. *Dement. Neurocognitive Disord.* **2021**, *20*, 38. [CrossRef]
52. Chen, Z.C.; Liu, S.; Gan, J.; Ma, L.; Du, X.; Zhu, H.; Han, J.; Xu, J.; Wu, H.; Fei, M.; et al. The Impact of the COVID-19 Pandemic and Lockdown on Mild Cognitive Impairment, Alzheimer's Disease and Dementia With Lewy Bodies in China: A 1-Year Follow-Up Study. *Front. Psychiatry* **2021**, *12*, 711658. [CrossRef]
53. Axenhus, M.; Schedin-Weiss, S.; Tjernberg, L.; Wimo, A.; Eriksdotter, M.; Bucht, G.; Winblad, B. Changes in Dementia Diagnoses in Sweden during the COVID-19 Pandemic. *BMC Geriatr.* **2022**, *22*, 365. [CrossRef]
54. Gaigher, J.M.; Lacerda, I.B.; Dourado, M.C.N. Dementia and Mental Health During the COVID-19 Pandemic: A Systematic Review. *Front. Psychiatry* **2022**, *13*, 879598. [CrossRef]
55. Choi, Y.J.; Kim, S.; Hwang, Y.J.; Kim, C. Prevalence of Dementia in Korea Based on Hospital Utilization Data from 2008 to 2016. *Yonsei Med. J.* **2021**, *62*, 948–953. [CrossRef] [PubMed]
56. Seong, S.J.; Kim, B.N.; Kim, K.W. Comparative Analysis on the Policy Approaches in the National Dementia Plans of G7 Countries and Korea and Their Implementation. *J. Korean Med. Sci.* **2023**, *38*, e227. [CrossRef] [PubMed]

International Journal of
Geo-Information

Article

Hourly PM2.5 Concentration Prediction Based on Empirical Mode Decomposition and Geographically Weighted Neural Network

Yan Chen and Chunchun Hu *

School of Geodesy and Geomatics, Wuhan University, Wuhan 430079, China
* Correspondence: chchhu@sgg.whu.edu.cn

Abstract: Accurate prediction of fine particulate matter (PM2.5) concentration is crucial for improving environmental conditions and effectively controlling air pollution. However, some existing studies could ignore the nonlinearity and spatial correlation of time series data observed from stations, and it is difficult to avoid the redundancy between features during feature selection. To further improve the accuracy, this study proposes a hybrid model based on empirical mode decomposition (EMD), minimal-redundancy-maximal-relevance (mRMR), and geographically weighted neural network (GWNN) for hourly PM2.5 concentration prediction, named EMD-mRMR-GWNN. Firstly, the original PM2.5 concentration sequence with distinct nonlinearity and non-stationarity is decomposed into multiple intrinsic mode functions (IMFs) and a residual component using EMD. IMFs are further classified and reconstructed into high-frequency and low-frequency components using the one-sample *t*-test. Secondly, the optimal feature subset is selected from high-frequency and low-frequency components with mRMR for the prediction model, thus holding the correlation between features and the target variable and reducing the redundancy among features. Thirdly, the residual component is predicted with the simple moving average (SMA) due to its strong trend and autocorrelation, and GWNN is used to predict the high-frequency and low-frequency components. The final prediction of the PM2.5 concentration value is calculated by an artificial neural network (ANN) composed of the predictive values of each component. PM2.5 concentration prediction experiments in three representational cities, such as Beijing, Wuhan, and Kunming were carried out. The proposed model achieved high accuracy with a coefficient of determination greater than 0.92 in forecasting PM2.5 concentration for the next 1 h. We compared this model with four baseline models in forecasting PM2.5 concentration for the next few hours and found it performed the best in PM2.5 concentration prediction. The experimental results indicated the proposed model can improve prediction accuracy.

Keywords: PM2.5 concentration prediction; empirical mode decomposition; minimal-redundancy-maximal-relevance; geographically weighted neural network

1. Introduction

The United Nations Sustainable Development Goals (SDGs) are a set of 17 social, economic and environmental goals set by the United Nations in 2015 to address global challenges and achieve sustainable development [1]. One of them is to build inclusive, safe, resilient, and sustainable cities and human settlements. However, amid the expeditious economic and societal advancement, the worldwide ecological milieu has suffered tremendous harm, precipitating a notable catalyst in compromising human well-being—air quality degradation [2,3]. The deleterious impacts of air pollution on human health are unequivocal [4]. The main culprit is fine particulate matter (PM2.5) [5], with ramifications extending beyond its adverse effects on air quality and visibility. PM2.5 harbors toxic and detrimental substances that permeate deep within the lungs, heart, and bloodstream, exerting a pernicious influence on vital organs such as the heart and brain, which poses a grave menace to human health [5–7]. The precise forecasting of PM2.5 concentration is crucial to ameliorating environmental conditions, effectively managing air pollution, and proactively averting the myriad health afflictions triggered by atmospheric contamination [8–10].

Recent research methodologies employed for PM2.5 concentration prediction can be broadly classified into three main categories: mechanistic, statistical, and artificial intelligence models [11,12]. Mechanistic models leverage meteorological principles and mathematical techniques to simulate air quality at specific scales [9,12]. Typical mechanistic models include the Community Multiscale Air Quality (CMAQ) model [13,14] and the Weather Research and Forecasting (WRF) model [15,16]. High computational requirements and complex modeling processes are among the factors that impede the broader utilization of mechanistic models [12–17]. Statistical models explore the dynamics of PM2.5 using statistical analysis techniques, which are devoid of modeling intricacies, yet display superior performances [18,19]. Statistical models primarily include the autoregressive moving average model (ARMA) [20,21] and the autoregressive integrated moving average model (ARIMA) [22]. The reliance of statistical models on historical PM2.5 concentration data poses a challenge when incorporating external factors into the analysis [23]. Additionally, statistical models struggle to capture the nonlinear characteristics present in PM2.5 concentration effectively [12]. Artificial intelligence models mainly include machine learning and deep learning [23]. For instance, He et al. [24] employed an artificial neural network (ANN) to forecast PM2.5 concentration. Experiments indicated that the ANN successfully captured the nonlinear relationship between PM2.5 and the input variables.

The rapid advancement of deep learning technology has garnered significant scholarly acclaim while simultaneously being used for air quality forecasting [12]. Long short-term memory neural networks (LSTMs) [25,26] and convolutional neural networks (CNNs) [27] represent two extensively utilized deep learning architectures within the domain of air quality prediction. Li et al. [8] introduced a hybrid model that combined CNN and LSTM to predict the 24-h PM2.5 concentration in Beijing. Previous research [25–27] has demonstrated the commendable predictive capabilities of deep learning in discerning PM2.5 concentration with the utmost precision. Nonetheless, most existing deep learning models have struggled to advance beyond their current performance, primarily due to their inadvertent disregard for the non-stationarity inherent in time series [28]. Considering the detailed nature of PM2.5 sequences, delving into data preprocessing techniques for PM2.5 prediction has become imperative. These approaches have exhibited promising achievements, contributing to a discernible enhancement in prediction accuracy [29]. The adoption of data decomposition techniques is effective for preprocessing PM2.5 time series data, with the potential to advance the accuracy of PM2.5 concentration prediction significantly [30]. Most data decomposition techniques are based on empirical mode decomposition (EMD) [28,31]. For instance, Huang et al. [28] demonstrated the efficacy of employing EMD to decompose the initial PM2.5 sequence into multiple subsequences. Subsequently, they applied a well-constructed gated recurrent unit (GRU) to forecast each subsequence. The predicted value of each subsequence was aggregated to yield the final predicted value of PM2.5 concentration. Numerous previous studies [28–31] have confirmed the efficacy of data decomposition techniques in enhancing the accuracy of air quality predictions. Hence, the model proposed in this study employs EMD to preprocess the original PM2.5 sequence into multiple intrinsic mode functions (IMFs). Subsequently, the IMFs are reconstructed based on the one-sample *t*-test. This approach reduces the model's complexity and runtime while maintaining prediction accuracy.

Feature selection contributes to improved model performance and reduced model complexity [32]. For PM2.5 concentration prediction, several common feature selection criteria were utilized, including the Pearson correlation coefficient [33], Kendall's tau coefficient [34], causality [32], and mutual information [35]. While these feature selection methods perform well in selecting features that are highly relevant to the target variable, they may still face challenges in avoiding redundancy between the selected features. The minimal-redundancy-maximal-relevance (mRMR) algorithm considers both the redundancy between features and their relevance to the target variable [36]. Consequently, the model proposed in this study utilizes the mRMR algorithm for feature selection.

Considering the data from neighboring stations surrounding the target station can further improve the prediction accuracy [18]. Geographically weighted regression (GWR) is a spatial statistical analysis method for exploring spatial non-stationarity and spatial relationships in geographic data [37]. Combining the idea of GWR and ANN, this study proposes the novel geographically weighted neural network (GWNN) model for predicting PM2.5 concentration. GWNN model leverages the capabilities of ANN to determine the coefficients of GWR, thereby eliminating the issue of traditional methods for tedious kernel function and bandwidth selection.

Combining data decomposition, data reconstruction, feature selection, and considering the spatial relationship of PM2.5 monitoring stations, this study proposes a hybrid model called EMD-mRMR-GWNN for PM2.5 concentration prediction. The main contributions of this study are as follows:

- The analysis of PM2.5 concentration in three representative cities, such as Beijing, Wuhan, and Kunming, reveals that the PM2.5 concentration has distinct nonlinearity as well as the diversity of seasonal patterns.
- The EMD-mRMR-GWNN model was developed for PM2.5 concentration prediction. This model effectively integrates the advantages of data decomposition, data reconstruction, and feature selection techniques while considering the spatial relationship of PM2.5 monitoring stations. Experimental results on datasets from three cities in China (Beijing, Wuhan, and Kunming) indicate that the proposed hybrid model performed well.
- The original PM2.5 sequence is adaptively decomposed into multiple IMFs and a residual component using EMD and classified into high-frequency and low-frequency components by the one-sample *t*-test, significantly reducing the prediction difficulty and model complexity.
- For prediction accuracy, considering the correlation between features and the target variable, as well as the redundancy among features, we utilize the mRMR to select the optimal feature subset. By leveraging the nonlinear modeling capability of ANN and the spatial correlation capturing ability of GWR, we build a GWNN model to predict the high-frequency and low-frequency components, which significantly improves the accuracy of PM2.5 prediction.

This study is structured as follows: Section 2 introduces the material of this study and presents the modeling framework. Section 3 analyzes the performance of the EMD-mRMR-GWNN model and compares it with LSTM, GRU, GWNN, and mRMR-GWNN models. Finally, a conclusion is provided in Section 4.

2. Materials and Methods

2.1. Data Description

Three Chinese cities were selected as the study areas: Beijing, Wuhan, and Kunming. Beijing has 12 air quality monitoring stations (1001A–1012A), Wuhan has 9 (1325A–1334A, of which 1332A was excluded due to too many missing values), and Kunming has 6 (1450A–1455A). These cities were chosen to represent different geographical regions and varying levels of air pollution. Thus, the study provided a more comprehensive understanding of PM2.5 concentration prediction in diverse urban environments. The distribution of air quality monitoring stations in these three cities is shown in Figure 1.

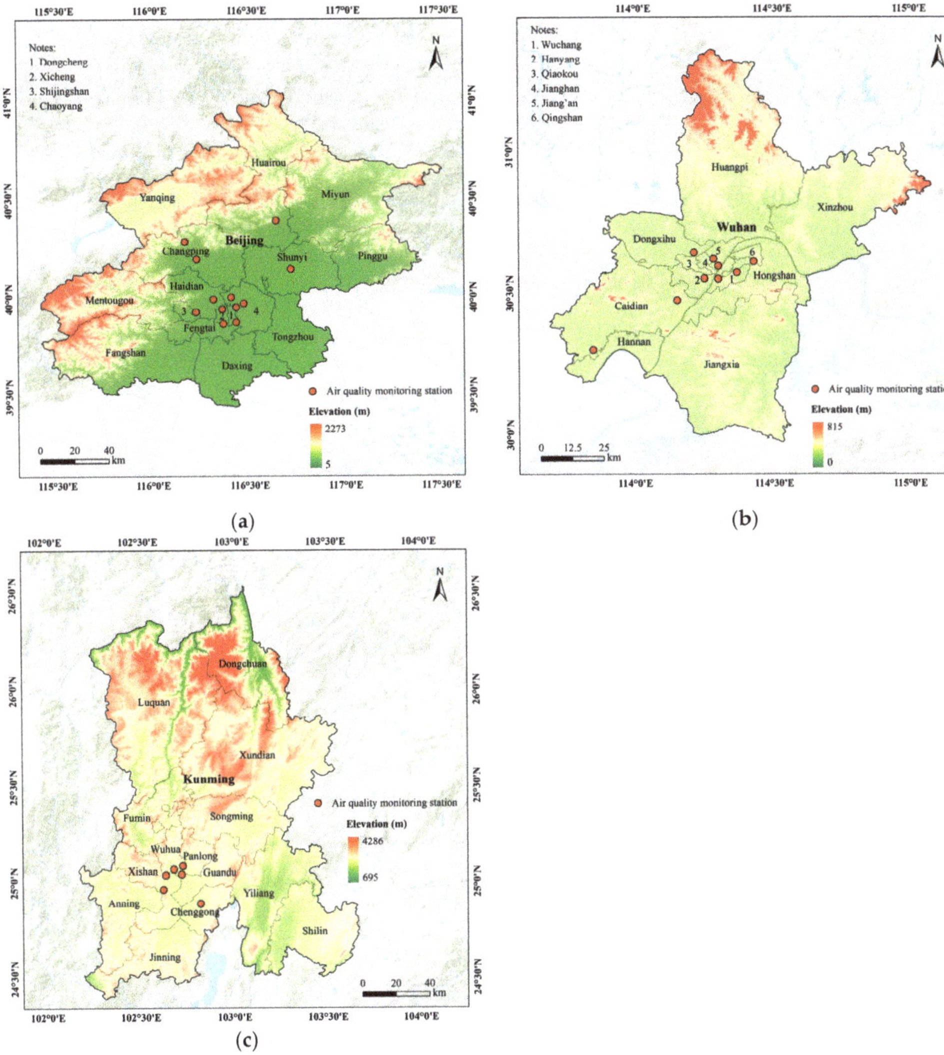

Figure 1. The distribution of air quality monitoring stations: (**a**) The distribution of air quality monitoring stations in Beijing; (**b**) The distribution of air quality monitoring stations in Wuhan; (**c**) The distribution of air quality monitoring stations in Kunming.

The air quality data were obtained from the China National Environmental Monitoring Centre (CNEMC). Hourly pollutant concentration data, including PM2.5, PM10, SO_2, NO_2, O_3, and CO, were collected from air quality monitoring stations in Beijing, Wuhan, and Kunming. The data collection period spanned from 1 January 2016, to 31 December 2020.

Figure S1 shows the PM2.5 concentration sequences of Beijing, Wuhan, and Kunming (one station is shown per city). Table S1 shows the statistical data of PM2.5 concentrations. The PM2.5 concentrations in all three cities exhibited volatility and had significantly different characteristics. The average PM2.5 concentration in Beijing was high and very volatile. In contrast, Kunming maintained a low average PM2.5 concentration with little volatility, resulting in stable air quality. Wuhan's air quality was intermediate between the first two cities, with moderate PM2.5 concentration and volatility. Overall, these three cities displayed a declining trend in PM2.5 concentration, indicating an improvement in air quality. One possible reason was that the Chinese government has made significant efforts to adjust the energy structure, industrial structure, and transportation structure. In recent years, the Chinese Government has taken positive action on many fronts to achieve the goal of sustainable development. First, it has promoted energy transformation, limiting the use of highly polluting coal energy and encouraging clean energy alternatives [38]. Second, the Chinese government has actively promoted industrial upgrading and transformation to reduce dependence on resource-intensive and highly polluting industries. Finally, the Chinese government focuses on public transport in urban planning, building convenient public transport systems such as subways and light railways, and supporting the development of new energy vehicles through policies such as subsidies for car purchases [39]. Figure S2 shows the PM2.5 concentration for each season from December 2019 to November 2020 at the three stations. For Beijing and Wuhan, the highest PM2.5 concentrations were in winter, and the lowest were in summer. Heating is one of the major reasons for the high PM2.5 concentration during winter in Beijing. Wuhan has predominantly northerly winds in winter, thus the transmission of pollutants from centralized heating in the north may contribute to air pollution in Wuhan. The seasonal characteristics of PM2.5 in Kunming were different from those in Wuhan and Beijing. The PM2.5 concentration in Kunming was greatest during spring. Possible causes were spring drought, large temperature differences between day and night, scarce rainfall, and being prone to inversions and fog, which affected the dispersion of PM2.5. In this study, the three cities were considered representative as they corresponded to regions with high, moderate, and low PM2.5 concentrations, respectively. The proposed model's stability was verified using different PM2.5 concentration datasets.

2.2. Empirical Mode Decomposition

EMD is a data analysis method used to decompose a nonstationary signal into a set of IMFs and a residual component. Each IMF has a specific frequency range. EMD is an adaptive data decomposition method that does not require predefined basis functions or filters [40]. The EMD implementation process is as follows:

1. Detect and extract the local maximum and local minimum in the signal $x(t)$ and set the initial index $i = 1$.
2. The upper envelope $u(t)$ and lower envelope $l(t)$ of the signal are obtained by cubic spline interpolation of the envelope between the extreme points.
3. Calculate the mean value $m(t)$ of the upper and lower envelope.

$$m(t) = \frac{u(t) + l(t)}{2} \tag{1}$$

4. The mean value $m(t)$ of the upper and lower envelope is removed from the original signal $x(t)$ to obtain a new sequence $h(t)$.

$$h(t) = x(t) - m(t) \tag{2}$$

5. A judgment is made on the new sequence $h(t)$. If $h(t)$ satisfies the following two conditions: the number of extreme points and the number of points crossing the zero point are equal or differ by no more than one, and the average value of the upper envelope formed by the local extreme points and the lower envelope formed by the local extreme points is zero, then $h(t)$ is considered to be an IMF, $IMF_i(t) = h(t)$. If $h(t)$ does not satisfy the above conditions, $h(t)$ is considered the original signal for the next round of iterations until the conditions are satisfied.
6. The above steps are repeated until no more new IMFs can be decomposed, and the remaining signal is regarded as the residual component $Res(t)$.

7. Finally, the original signal is decomposed into multiple IMFs and a residual component.

$$x(t) = \sum_{n=1}^{i} IMF_i(t) + Res(t) \quad (3)$$

2.3. *Minimal-Redundancy-Maximal-Relevance*

The mRMR (minimal-redundancy-maximal-relevance) is a feature selection method used to select the most representative subset of features from a given feature set that is highly correlated with the target variable and has less redundancy [36]. The mRMR algorithm evaluated the importance of each feature by measuring its relevance and redundancy. The goal of the mRMR algorithm was to reduce redundancy in the subset of features while maintaining high correlation.

2.3.1. Maximal Relevance

According to mRMR, maximal relevance is achieved by finding a subset of features that satisfies Equation (4), maximizing the average of the mutual information between the features in the subset of features and the target variable.

$$\max D = \frac{1}{|K|} \sum_{x_i \in K} I(x_i; y) \quad (4)$$

where K is the subset of features, x_i is the feature, and y is the target variable. I is the mutual information between the feature x_i and the target variable y, and D is the average of the mutual information between the features and the target variable in the subset of features.

Mutual information is a concept used to measure the correlation between two random variables [36] to capture and assess the interdependence between these variables by evaluating the amount of information one variable provides about another variable [41]. Specifically, for two discrete random variables x and y, their mutual information is defined as:

$$I(x; y) = \iint p(x,y) log \frac{p(x,y)}{p(x)p(y)} dxdy \quad (5)$$

where $p(x,y)$ denotes the joint probability distribution of x and y, and $p(x)$ and $p(y)$ denote the marginal probability distribution of x and y, respectively. A larger value of mutual information indicates a stronger correlation between the two variables. A value of 0 indicates that the two variables are independent.

2.3.2. Minimal Redundancy

When selecting a subset of features based on the maximal relevance criterion, a significant amount of redundant information may be generated within the chosen features. This redundancy can adversely affect the computational effort required by the model and potentially decrease the prediction accuracy [36]. Consequently, eliminating the redundant information to optimize the selected subset of features becomes necessary. According to the mRMR, minimal redundancy is achieved by minimizing the mutual information between features in the subset as follows:

$$\min R = \frac{1}{|K|^2} \sum_{x_i, x_j \in K} I(x_i; x_j) \quad (6)$$

where K is the subset of features, x_i and x_j are the features in the subset, and I is the mutual information between the features. Redundant information is removed by minimizing mutual information between features.

Ultimately, considering both the relevance between the features and the target variable, and the redundancy between the features, the goal of the mRMR is to satisfy Equation (7).

$$\max\Phi = D - R \tag{7}$$

Φ denotes the difference between the relevance and the redundancy. By maximizing the difference between relevance and redundancy, the mRMR can reduce redundancy in the subset of features while maintaining high relevance. The mRMR finds a subset of features through an incremental search. Suppose that the $n-1$ features were selected from the original feature set X, constituting the subset of features K_{n-1}, then the selection of the nth feature x_n needs to satisfy Equation (8).

$$\max_{x_n \in X - K_{n-1}} \left\{ I(x_n; y) - \frac{1}{n-1} \sum_{x_i \in K_{n-1}} I(x_n; x_i) \right\} \tag{8}$$

According to Equation (8), the mRMR successively selects features from the remaining set of features $X - K$ and adds them to the subset of features K. Finally, the subset of features with the largest mRMR value is selected as the model input.

2.4. Geographically Weighted Neural Network

The PM2.5 concentration sequence is nonstationary and a nonlinear relationship exists between PM2.5 and the dependent variables. However, the GWR model is a linear model that does not address the nonlinear relationship inherent in the data. Furthermore, the GWR model relies solely on the spatial distance and the spatial weight matrix generated by the kernel function to calculate the model, which is insufficient for capturing and explaining the intricate relationship between the dependent variable and the independent variables [37]. In addition, the selection of an appropriate kernel function posed a challenge. Therefore, when it comes to predicting PM2.5 concentration, relying solely on the GWR model was unreliable. ANN possessed a more robust capability for nonlinear modeling compared to traditional linear models. By incorporating a hierarchical structure and activation functions, ANN effectively captured and represented intricate nonlinear relationships among input features [42]. Furthermore, ANN learned from extensive amounts of data and dynamically adjusted model parameters to suit various problems. To exploit the benefits of both ANN and GWR, we proposed the GWNN model for predicting PM2.5 concentration. The GWNN model integrated the geographically weighted conception into ANN to enhance the accuracy of PM2.5 concentration prediction. By combining the robust nonlinear modeling capabilities of ANN with the spatial correlation capturing abilities of GWR, GWNN aimed to improve the accuracy and reliability of PM2.5 concentration prediction. The structure of GWNN is shown in Figure 2.

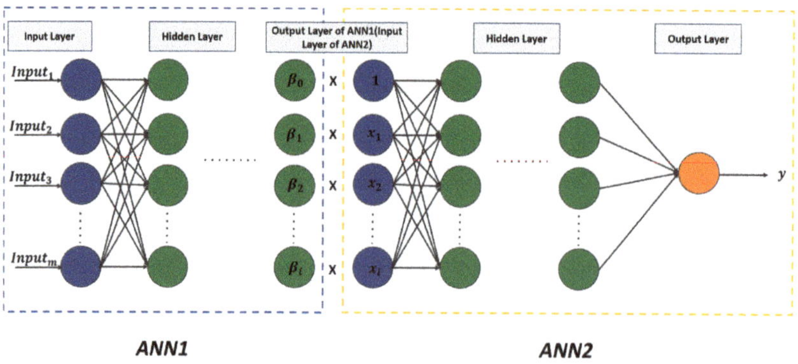

Figure 2. Structure of GWNN.

GWNN consisted of two ANNs with different roles. The ANN1 is a coefficient estimation neural network used to learn the coefficients β in GWR. Any reasonably defined distance metric can be used for GWR model solving [43]. Simple spatial distances could not express the complex spatial relationships between stations. Consequently, we designated the PM2.5 concentration data from neighboring stations surrounding the target station within the previous 24 h of the prediction time as the ANN1 input. This was used to capture the spatial relationship of PM2.5 concentration among different stations. The ANN1 output was the regression coefficient β. The product of the regression coefficient β (learned by ANN1) and the dependent variable x was employed as input to the second neural network, ANN2. The independent variable x contained the constant 1 and the features selected by the mRMR. Through the nonlinear transformation, ANN2 provided the predicted output value, y. Both ANN1 and ANN2 consisted of an input layer, multiple hidden layers, and an output layer.

2.5. Proposed Model

Based on data decomposition, mRMR, and GWNN, this study proposed a hybrid model EMD-mRMR-GWNN for PM2.5 concentration prediction, as shown in Figure 3. The EMD reduced the non-stationarity of the original PM2.5 sequence by decomposing it into a set of subsequences. Additionally, the one-sample *t*-test was introduced to classify and reconstruct the subsequences into high-frequency component and low-frequency components. The mRMR was used to select features that were highly correlated with the target variable and had less redundancy. This approach aimed to reduce model complexity while improving prediction accuracy. GWNN was used for predicting high-frequency and low-frequency components. GWNN integrated the geographically weighted idea into ANN, leveraging the nonlinear modeling capabilities of ANN and the spatial correlation capturing ability of GWR to improve prediction accuracy. The model was implemented as follows:

1. Firstly, the original PM2.5 sequence was decomposed into multiple IMFs and a residual component using EMD.
2. To reduce the complexity, the running time, and the cumulative error of the model, the IMFs were classified and reconstructed into high-frequency component and low-frequency components using the one-sample *t*-test.
3. SMA was employed to predict the residual component with a strong trend and autocorrelation, which avoids overfitting while ensuring prediction accuracy.
4. GWNN was employed to predict the high-frequency and low-frequency components. The input of ANN1 in GWNN was the PM2.5 concentration data in the past 24 h at the stations surrounding the target station. The product of the regression coefficient β learned by ANN1 and the dependent variable x, was the input of ANN2 in GWNN. The features selected by the mRMR and the constant 1 constitute the independent variable x.
5. Finally, the predicted value of each component was input into an ANN to predict the PM2.5 concentration.

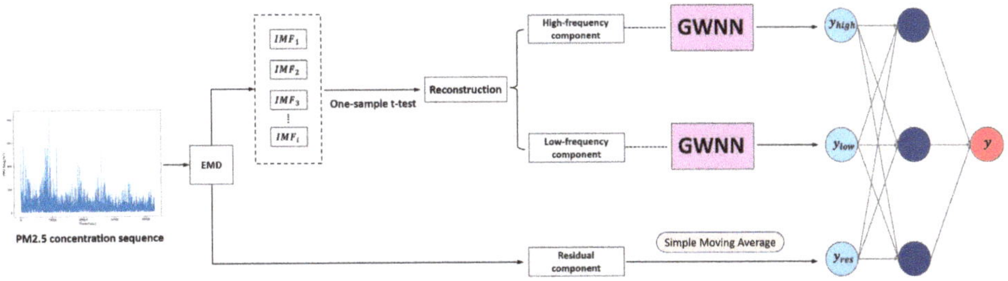

Figure 3. Structure of EMD-mRMR-GWNN.

2.6. Prediction Performance Evaluation Metrics

To evaluate the model prediction results objectively and intuitively and compare the prediction performance of different models, this study utilizes three classical metrics: root mean square error (RMSE), mean absolute error (MAE) and coefficient of determination (R^2), as the prediction performance evaluation metrics.

$$RMSE = \sqrt{\frac{1}{N}\sum_{i=1}^{N}(y_i - \hat{y}_i)^2} \quad (9)$$

$$MAE = \frac{1}{N}\sum_{i=1}^{N}|y_i - \hat{y}_i| \quad (10)$$

$$R^2 = 1 - \frac{\sum_{i=1}^{N}(y_i - \hat{y}_i)^2}{\sum_{i=1}^{N}(y_i - \overline{y})} \quad (11)$$

where N is the number of data, y_i denotes the true value, $\hat{y}_i$ denotes the predicted value, and $\overline{y}$ denotes the average of the true values. Smaller values of RMSE and MAE indicate a more accurate model, as they reflect a smaller difference between the predicted values and the true values. The value of R^2 ranges from 0 to 1. A higher value of R^2 indicates that the independent variables are more capable of explaining the dependent variable, demonstrating the better performance of the model.

3. Results and Discussion

3.1. Decomposition and Reconstruction of PM2.5 Sequence

3.1.1. Decomposition with EMD

Due to the highly nonlinear and nonstationary nature of the PM2.5 sequence, improving the accuracy of direct prediction of the original PM2.5 concentration becomes challenging. Therefore, we have employed EMD to decompose the original PM2.5 sequence into a set of IMFs and a residual component. Taking the Beijing 1005A, Wuhan 1328A, and Kunming 1454A stations as examples, the results of decomposing the original PM2.5 sequence using EMD are shown in Figures S3–S5. The PM2.5 sequences at the three stations were decomposed into multiple IMFs at different frequencies and a residual component. The PM2.5 sequence at the Beijing 1005A Station was decomposed into 15 IMFs, while the PM2.5 sequence at the Wuhan 1328A and Kunming 1454A stations were decomposed into 13 IMFs each. The decomposition results illustrated the strong volatility of the PM2.5 concentration in Beijing.

3.1.2. Reconstruction of IMFs with the One-Sample t-Test

Directly predicting the IMFs decomposed from the PM2.5 sequence increased the complexity of the model significantly. To address this issue and reduce computational time, we employed the one-sample t-test to reconstruct these IMFs. According to the EMD algorithm, the IMFs must satisfy the local symmetry of the upper and lower envelope relative to the time axis. In the initial stages of the EMD process, the first few IMFs generated tend to be high frequencies. The upper and lower envelopes of these IMFs were obtained by connecting numerous peaks in the signal. As a result, these IMFs were essentially symmetric, and the mean value of the data approached zero. However, the latter IMFs were produced by EMD with low frequency. The upper and lower envelopes were derived by interpolating a limited number of peaks, which resulted in significant deviations from the original signal's trend. This led to an asymmetric signal; thus, maintaining a mean value of zero for the data became challenging. Consequently, we used the one-sample t-test to determine whether the IMFs were significantly different from zero, thus dividing the IMFs into high-frequency and low-frequency components.

The results of the one-sample t-test for each IMF of PM2.5 at the Beijing 1005A, Wuhan 1328A, and Kunming 1454A stations are shown in Table S2. We set the significance level at

0.05. When the p-value was less than 0.05, the null hypothesis was rejected, and the mean of the IMF was considered significantly different from 0, and the IMF was categorized as a low-frequency component. When the p-value was greater than 0.05, the null hypothesis could not be rejected, and the mean of the IMF was considered not significantly different from 0 and the IMF was categorized as a high-frequency component. According to the results of the one-sample t-test, the classification of each IMF of PM2.5 at Beijing 1005A, Wuhan 1328A, and Kunming 1454A stations is shown in Table S3. The IMFs classified as high-frequency components were combined and reconstructed into a new high-frequency component. The IMFs classified as low-frequency components were combined and reconstructed into a new low-frequency component. The reconstruction results are shown in Figure 4. After reconstruction, the original PM2.5 sequence was finally decomposed into three components: a high-frequency component, a low-frequency component, and a residual component. The high-frequency component was characterized by pronounced volatility, exhibiting substantial fluctuations. In contrast, the volatility of the low-frequency component was weak and demonstrated periodic patterns. The residual components exhibited a distinct trend.

3.2. Feature Selection with mRMR

After decomposing and reconstructing the original PM2.5 sequence into high-frequency, low-frequency, and residual components, the subsequent work was to predict each of these three components separately. The residual component, which exhibited a distinct trend, was predicted using SMA. The high-frequency and low-frequency components were predicted using the proposed GWNN model. The mRMR algorithm was employed to perform feature selection for the input of ANN2 in the GWNN model. The original features were the PM2.5, PM10, SO_2, NO_2, O_3, and CO concentration data and the high-frequency and low-frequency components of the target station within the previous 24 h at the prediction time. The mRMR was utilized to select the optimal features from the original features. The original features are shown in Table 1. The features selected by the mRMR at Beijing 1005A, Wuhan 1328A, and Kunming 1454A stations, are listed in Table S4, Table S5, and Table S6, respectively.

3.3. Prediction Results of EMD-mRMR-GWNN

The high-frequency, low-frequency, and residual components, the previous 24 h of PM2.5 concentration data from neighboring stations surrounding the target station, and the features selected by mRMR, were input to the EMD-mRMR-GWNN model to predict the PM2.5 concentration of the target station at the prediction time. The PM2.5 concentration data from neighboring stations surrounding the target station within the previous 24 h was the input to ANN1 in the GWNN model. The product of the independent variables and the output of ANN1 was the input to ANN2 in the GWNN model. The independent variables consisted of the constant value 1 and features selected by mRMR. The EMD-mRMR-GWNN model parameters were set as follows: the number of ANN1 hidden layers was 2, the number of ANN2 hidden layers was 5, the training batch size was 128, the learning rate was 0.001, and the maximum number of iterations was 100. Every air quality monitoring station had 42,803 data points. These data points were divided into training, validation, and test sets according to the ratio of 6:2:2. To prevent overfitting, an early stopping strategy was implemented during the training of the EMD-mRMR-GWNN model. This strategy involved monitoring the validation set loss during training. If the validation set loss increased continuously for three consecutive times, the training process was stopped. The prediction results of EMD-mRMR-GWNN in forecasting PM2.5 concentration for the next 1 h, as illustrated at the Beijing 1005A, Wuhan 1328A, and Kunming 1454A stations, are shown in Figure 5.

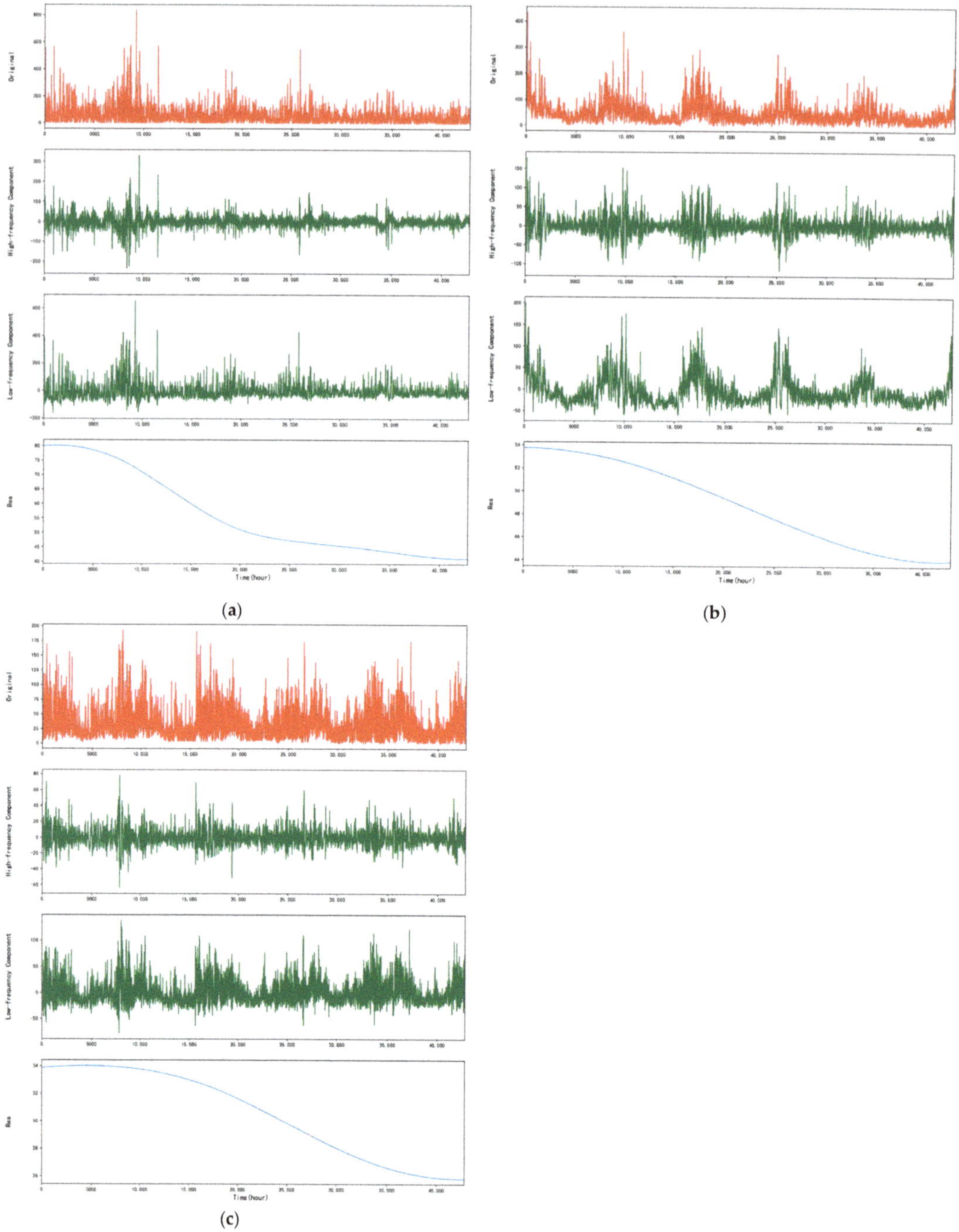

Figure 4. Reconstruction result of PM2.5 IMFs: (**a**) Reconstruction result of PM2.5 IMFs of Beijing 1005A Station; (**b**) Reconstruction result of PM2.5 IMFs of Wuhan 1328A Station; (**c**) Reconstruction result of PM2.5 IMFs of Kunming 1454A Station.

Table 1. Original features.

Feature	Description
$PM2.5_{t-n}$	PM2.5 concentration at the time t − n (previous nth hour to time t)
$PM10_{t-n}$	PM10 concentration at the time t − n
$SO2_{t-n}$	SO_2 concentration at the time t − n
$NO2_{t-n}$	NO_2 concentration at the time t − n
$O3_{t-n}$	O_3 concentration at the time t − n
CO_{t-n}	CO concentration at the time t − n
$High_{t-n}$	High-frequency component value at the time t − n
Low_{t-n}	Low-frequency component value at the time t − n

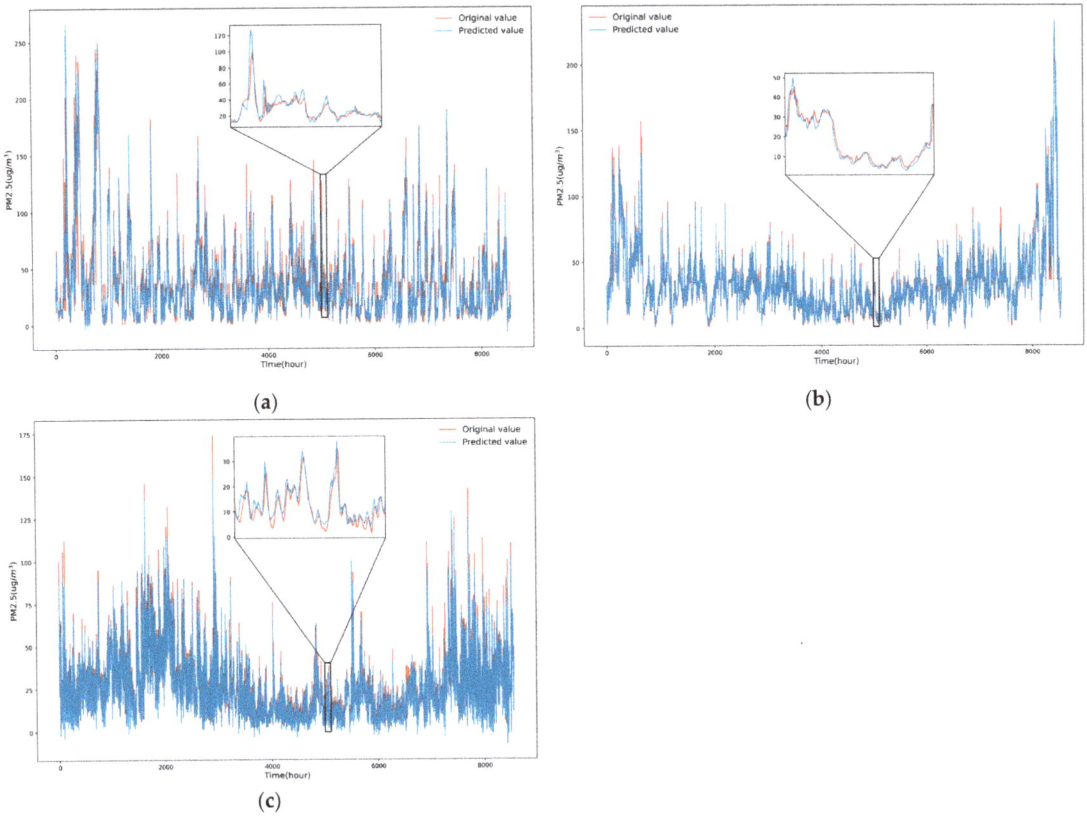

Figure 5. Prediction results of EMD-mRMR-GWNN in forecasting PM2.5 concentration for the next 1 h: (**a**) Prediction results of EMD-mRMR-GWNN at Beijing 1005A Station; (**b**) Prediction results of EMD-mRMR-GWNN at Wuhan 1328A Station; (**c**) Prediction results of EMD-mRMR-GWNN at Kunming 1454A Station.

As shown in Figure 5, the prediction performance of EMD-mRMR-GWNN was excellent at the Beijing 1005A, Wuhan 1328A, and Kunming 1454A stations. Based on the consistent predicted and actual values of PM2.5 across all three stations, the EMD-mRMR-GWNN model provided high-precision predictions for PM2.5 concentration. Table 2 demonstrates the prediction performance evaluation metrics of the EMD-mRMR-GWNN model at these three stations in forecasting PM2.5 concentration for the next 1 h. The RMSE and MAE at the Beijing 1005A Station were significantly larger than those at the Wuhan 1328A and Kunming 1454A stations, which may be attributed to the high PM2.5

concentration and greater volatility in Beijing than in Wuhan and Kunming. RMSE at Kunming 1454A Station was the smallest. The proposed model performed best at Wuhan 1328A Station, with the smallest MAE and the largest R^2 value. The R^2 values at all three stations were close to 1 and greater than 0.92, showing the stabilizing performance of the proposed model when predicting PM2.5 concentration at different levels. In particular, the R^2 at Wuhan 1454A Station was greater than 0.95. Table S7 demonstrates the prediction performance evaluation metrics of the EMD-mRMR-GWNN model at these three stations in forecasting PM2.5 concentration for the next few hours. The prediction accuracy of the proposed model decreased with the increase in prediction hours. Taking the results of the Beijing1005A Station as an example, R^2 value dropped from 0.9435 in forecasting PM2.5 concentration for the next 1 h to 0.8941 in forecasting PM2.5 concentration for the next 12 h.

Table 2. Prediction performance evaluation metrics in forecasting PM2.5 concentration for the next 1 h.

Station	Prediction Performance Evaluation Metric		
	RMSE	MAE	R^2
Beijing 1005A Station	8.9714	5.4614	0.9435
Wuhan 1328A Station	5.7730	3.2199	0.9514
Kunming 1454A Station	5.3323	3.6039	0.9286

3.4. Prediction Performance Comparison of Different Models

To validate the superiority of the proposed EMD-mRMR-GWNN model in predicting PM2.5 concentration, four benchmark models were employed for comparison: LSTM, GRU, GWNN, and mRMR-GWNN. The prediction results of comparative models at the Beijing 1005A, Wuhan 1328A, and Kunming 1454A stations in forecasting PM2.5 concentration for the next 1 h are shown in Figure 6. As two variants of the recurrent neural network, LSTM and GRU have high prediction accuracy. GRU achieves comparable predictive performance to the LSTM with fewer parameters. Therefore, it can be considered that GRU is superior to LSTM in this experiment. The other three models showed higher prediction accuracy than LSTM and GRU. Our method proved to be highly effective in enhancing the accuracy of PM2.5 concentration prediction, as evidenced by the proximity between the predicted values of the GWNN, mRMR-GWNN, and EMD-mRMR-GWNN models and the true values. Compared to the benchmark models, the proposed model exhibited the closest proximity between the predicted values and the true values, thereby demonstrating the highest level of prediction accuracy. This strongly indicated that the proposed model was superior to the other models under consideration. The prediction accuracy of the models was ranked from low to high as follows: LSTM, GRU, GWNN, mRMR-GWNN, and EMD-mRMR-GWNN. The mRMR effectively reduced the complexity of the model by selecting a smaller set of input features, which not only decreased redundancy between features but also enhanced prediction accuracy. By employing the EMD, the original PM2.5 concentration sequence was decomposed into components characterized by smaller volatility. This decomposition process effectively reduced the difficulty and improved the accuracy of prediction. The application of EMD facilitated a more refined analysis of the data, leading to improved forecasting outcomes.

Table 3 shows prediction performance evaluation metrics of the comparative models at the Beijing 1005A, Wuhan 1328A, and Kunming 1454A stations in forecasting PM2.5 concentration for the next 1 h. The table indicated that, considering RMSE, MAE, and R^2, the proposed model is optimal with the smallest RMSE and MAE, and the largest R^2. This indicated that the proposed model had the highest prediction accuracy. At the Beijing 1005A Station, the RMSE, MAE, and R^2 of the proposed model were 8.9714, 5.4614, and 0.9435, respectively. At the Wuhan 1328A Station, the RMSE, MAE, and R^2 of the proposed model are 5.7730, 3.2199, and 0.9514, respectively. At the Kunming 1454A Station, the RMSE, MAE, and R^2 of the proposed model are 5.3323, 3.6039, and 0.9286, respectively.

The predicted values of the proposed model were the closest to the true values at all three stations. Tables S8–S10 show prediction performance evaluation metrics of the comparative models at the Beijing 1005A, Wuhan 1328A, and Kunming 1454A stations in forecasting PM2.5 concentration for the next few hours. The prediction accuracy of all the models declined with the increase in prediction hours. It should be noted that the proposed model still performed best in all the experiments, demonstrating its stability and superiority.

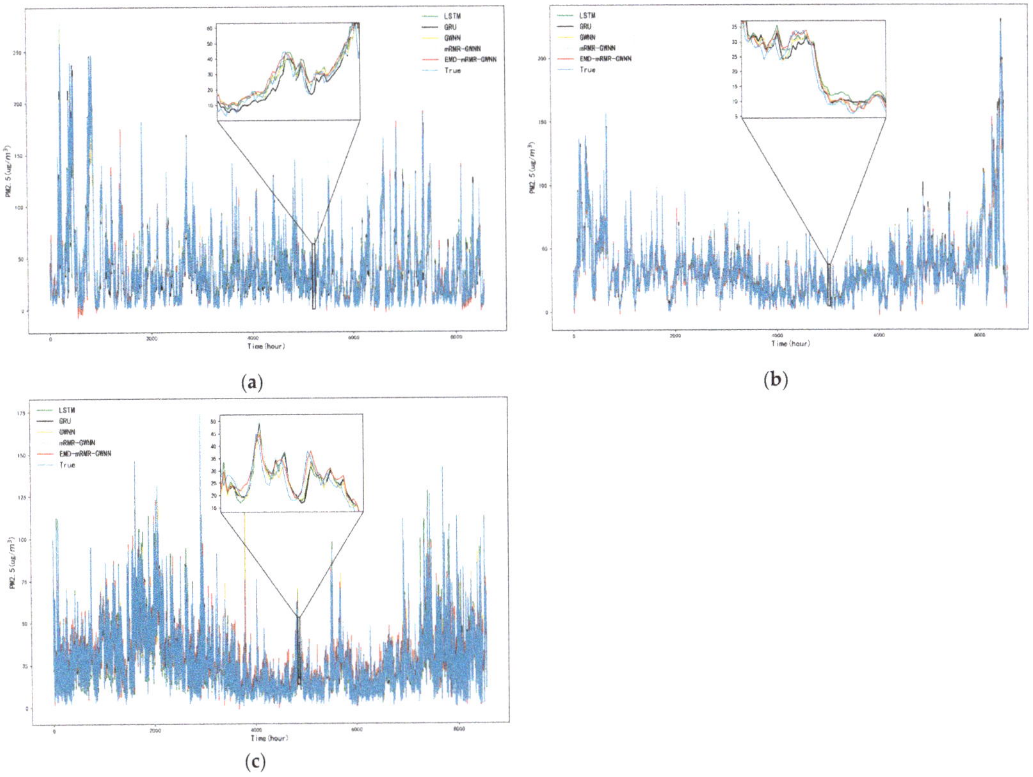

Figure 6. Prediction results of comparative models in forecasting PM2.5 concentration for the next 1 h: (**a**) Prediction results of comparative models at Beijing 1005A Station; (**b**) Prediction results of comparative models at Wuhan 1328A Station; (**c**) Prediction results of comparative models at Kunming 1454A Station.

To quantify prediction accuracy improvement in the proposed model, we calculated the percentage of improvement in prediction evaluation metrics. We abbreviated LSTM, GRU, GWNN, mRMR-GWNN, and EMD-mRMR-GWNN as M1, M2, M3, M4, and M5, respectively. Table 4 shows the percentage of improvement in the prediction evaluation metrics of different models at the Beijing 1005A, Wuhan 1328A, and Kunming 1454A stations in forecasting PM2.5 concentration for the next 1 h. Considering RMSE, MAE, and R^2 comprehensively, models M1 and M2 were comparable and performed the worst and model M5 was optimal. Compared to M1 and M2 at these three stations, the M5 RMSE decreased by a maximum of 29.18%, MAE decreased by a maximum of 19.85%, and R^2 increased by a maximum of 8.28%. Compared to M1 and M2, the M3 RMSE decreased by a maximum of 7.05%, MAE decreased by a maximum of 10.56%, and R^2 increased by a maximum of 2.19%, indicating the superior performance of GWNN in predicting PM2.5 concentration. The prediction accuracy was significantly improved by GWNN due to its utilization of two key capabilities: the powerful nonlinear modeling capability of

ANN and the spatial correlation capturing capability of GWR. Compared to M3, the M4 RMSE decreased by a maximum of 3.38%, MAE decreased by a maximum of 8.52%, and R^2 increased by a maximum of 0.94%, demonstrating the effectiveness of mRMR in improving model prediction accuracy. The mRMR integrated the relevance between features and the target variable and the redundancy between features to improve the predictive ability of the model while reducing the model complexity. In addition, compared to M4, the M5 RMSE decreased by a maximum of 21.33%, MAE decreased by a maximum of 14.01% and R^2 increased by a maximum of 4.97%. The use of EMD reduced the complexity of the original PM2.5 sequence and improved the prediction accuracy of the model.

Table 3. Prediction performance evaluation metrics of comparative models at Beijing 1005A Station, Wuhan 1328A Station, and Kunming 1454A Station in forecasting PM2.5 concentration for the next 1 h.

Station	Comparative Models	Prediction Performance Evaluation Metric		
		RMSE	MAE	R²
Beijing 1005A Station	LSTM	10.4934	6.2824	0.9227
	GRU	10.5864	6.2223	0.9213
	GWNN	9.8403	6.2026	0.9320
	mRMR-GWNN	9.5402	5.6744	0.9361
	EMD-mRMR-GWNN	8.9714	5.4614	0.9435
Wuhan 1328A Station	LSTM	6.5348	3.9133	0.9377
	GRU	6.4942	3.7342	0.9384
	GWNN	6.4606	3.5002	0.9391
	mRMR-GWNN	6.2692	3.3808	0.9426
	EMD-mRMR-GWNN	5.7730	3.2199	0.9514
Kunming 1454A Station	LSTM	7.5294	4.4959	0.8576
	GRU	7.0243	4.4414	0.8761
	GWNN	7.0149	4.3063	0.8764
	mRMR-GWNN	6.7782	4.1910	0.8846
	EMD-mRMR-GWNN	5.3323	3.6039	0.9286

Table 4. Improvement percentage of prediction performance evaluation metrics of different models in forecasting PM2.5 concentration for the next 1 h.

Station	Model	Improvement Percentage of Prediction Performance Evaluation Metric		
		RMSE	MAE	R²
Beijing 1005A Station	M3 vs. M1	6.22%	1.27%	1.00%
	M3 vs. M2	7.05%	0.32%	1.16%
	M4 vs. M3	3.05%	8.52%	0.44%
	M5 vs. M4	5.96%	3.75%	0.79%
	M5 vs. M1	14.50%	13.07%	2.25%
	M5 vs. M2	15.26%	12.23%	2.41%
Wuhan 1328A Station	M3 vs. M1	1.14%	10.56%	0.15%
	M3 vs. M2	0.52%	6.27%	0.07%
	M4 vs. M3	2.96%	3.41%	0.38%
	M5 vs. M4	7.91%	4.76%	0.93%
	M5 vs. M1	11.66%	17.72%	1.46%
	M5 vs. M2	11.11%	13.77%	1.39%
Kunming 1454A Station	M3 vs. M1	6.83%	4.22%	2.19%
	M3 vs. M2	0.13%	3.04%	0.03%
	M4 vs. M3	3.38%	2.68%	0.94%
	M5 vs. M4	21.33%	14.01%	4.97%
	M5 vs. M1	29.18%	19.85%	8.28%
	M5 vs. M2	24.09%	18.86%	5.99%

M1:LSTM, M2:GRU, M3:GWNN, M4:mRMR-GWNN, M5: mRMR-GWNN-EMD.

4. Conclusions

This study introduces a novel hybrid model combining three distinct techniques called EMD-mRMR-GWNN, designed specifically for predicting hourly PM2.5 concentration. Extensive experiments conducted in three different study areas, Beijing, Wuhan, and Kunming, validate the stability and superior performance of this hybrid model for accurate prediction. The results obtained present the efficacy and reliability of the EMD-mRMR-GWNN model for dealing with PM2.5 concentration prediction challenges. The primary conclusions are as follows:

1. The analysis of the PM2.5 concentration of Beijing, Wuhan, and Kunming reveals that Beijing had the highest and most volatile PM2.5 concentration, while Kunming had the lowest and least volatile PM2.5 concentration. The three cities have shown a declining trend in PM2.5 concentration, indicating air quality improvement. Beijing and Wuhan showed similar seasonal patterns, with the highest PM2.5 concentrations in winter and the lowest in summer. However, Kunming had its peak PM2.5 concentration during spring, showing a different seasonal pattern from Beijing and Wuhan.
2. We propose a model called GWNN that combines ANN and GWR. Experiments to forecast PM2.5 concentration for the next 1 h at the Beijing 1005A, Wuhan 1328A, and Kunming 1454A stations show that GWNN RMSE decreases by a maximum of 7.05%, MAE decreases by a maximum of 10.56%, and R^2 increases by a maximum of 2.19%, compared to LSTM and GRU.
3. For feature selection, the mRMR is introduced, which considers the relevance between features and the target variable as well as the redundancy between features. Compared to GWNN, at the Beijing 1005A, Wuhan 1328A, and Kunming 1454A stations, mRMR-GWNN RMSE decreases by a maximum of 3.38%, MAE decreases by a maximum of 8.52%, and R^2 increases by a maximum of 0.94%. The mRMR-GWNN model achieves higher prediction accuracy with fewer input features.
4. The complexity of the original PM2.5 sequence is reduced by decomposing the original PM2.5 sequence into a set of IMFs and a residual component through EMD. Meanwhile, the one-sample *t*-test is introduced to reconstruct the IMFs into high-frequency and low-frequency components.
5. The high-frequency and low-frequency components are predicted using mRMR-GWNN. The residual component is predicted using SMA. The predicted value of each component is input to an ANN for predicting PM2.5 concentration. Experiments at the Beijing 1005A, Wuhan 1328A, and Kunming 1454A stations, show that the EMD-mRMR-GWNN model outperforms baseline models. Compared to mRMR-GWNN, the RMSE of the EMD-mRMR-GWNN model decreases by a maximum of 21.33%, MAE decreases by a maximum of 14.01%, and R^2 increases by a maximum of 4.97%. Compared to LSTM and GRU, the RMSE of the EMD-mRMR-GWNN model decreases by a maximum of 29.18%, MAE decreases by a maximum of 19.85%, and R^2 increases by a maximum of 8.28%.
6. Experiments to forecast PM25 concentration for the next 4, 8, and 12 h verified the stability and superiority of the EMD-mRMR-GWNN model, compared with baseline models.

This study presents an effective tool for the short-term prediction of PM2.5 concentration. At the theoretical level, this study incorporates data decomposition and GWNN into the task of predicting PM2.5 concentration. The proposed model demonstrates promising outcomes and offers a novel perspective on PM2.5 concentration prediction. At the practical application level, the enhanced accuracy in predicting PM2.5 concentration can greatly assist in assessing the exposure to air pollutants for people [44]. Additionally, it can support the formation of environmental policies related to traffic management to mitigate air pollution resulting from vehicles, as vehicles contribute to air pollution to a significant extent [45]. However, the model proposed in this study solely focuses on short-term PM2.5 concentration prediction and does not consider long-term scenarios. Furthermore, meteorological factors are not incorporated within the proposed model in this study. Meteorological factors, including wind speed, wind direction, temperature, and humidity have a discernible impact on PM2.5 concentration. Consequently, subsequent studies should consider the influence of meteorological factors on air quality to improve the prediction accuracy and to achieve the long-term prediction of PM2.5 concentration.

Supplementary Materials: The following supporting information can be downloaded at: https://www.mdpi.com/article/10.3390/ijgi13030079/s1, Figure S1: PM2.5 concentration sequences; Figure S2: PM2.5 concentrations for different seasons; Figure S3: EMD decomposition of the PM2.5 sequence of Beijing 1005A Station; Figure S4: EMD decomposition of the PM2.5 sequence of Wuhan 1328A Station; Figure S5: EMD decomposition of the PM2.5 sequence of Kunming 1454A Station; Table S1: Statistical analysis of PM2.5 dataset; Table S2: Results of the one sample *t*-test; Table S3: Classification of IMFs; Table S4: Features selected by mRMR at Beijing 1005A station; Table S5: Features selected by mRMR at Wuhan 1328A station; Table S6: Features selected by mRMR at Kunming 1454A station. Table S7: Prediction performance evaluation metrics in forecasting PM2.5 concentration for the next few hours; Table S8: prediction performance evaluation metrics of the comparative models at the Beijing 1005A Station in forecasting PM2.5 concentration for the next few hours; Table S9: prediction performance evaluation metrics of the comparative models at the Wuhan 1328A Station in forecasting PM2.5 concentration for the next few hours; Table S10: prediction performance evaluation metrics of the comparative models at the Kunming 1454A Station in forecasting PM2.5 concentration for the next few hours.

Author Contributions: Conceptualization, Yan Chen; methodology, Yan Chen; data curation, Yan Chen; writing—original draft preparation, Yan Chen; writing—review and editing, Yan Chen and Chunchun Hu; visualization, Yan Chen; project administration, Chuchun Hu; funding acquisition, Chunchun Hu. All authors have read and agreed to the published version of the manuscript.

Funding: This research was funded by the Natural Science Foundation of Hubei Province of China under grant number 2022CFB194.

Data Availability Statement: The data of this work can be shared to the readers depending on the request.

Conflicts of Interest: The authors declare no conflict of interest.

References

1. Pradhan, P.; Costa, L.; Rybski, D.; Lucht, W.; Kropp, J.P. A Systematic study of Sustainable Development Goal (SDG) interactions. *Earth's Future* **2017**, *5*, 1169–1179. [CrossRef]
2. Lu, J.G. Air pollution: A systematic review of its psychological, economic, and social effects. *Curr. Opin. Psychol.* **2020**, *32*, 52–65. [CrossRef]
3. Yang, T.; Zhou, K.; Yang, Y. Air pollution impacts on public health: Evidence from 110 cities in Yangtze River Economic Belt of China. *Sci. Total Environ.* **2022**, *851*, 158125. [CrossRef]
4. Zu, D.; Zhai, K.; Qiu, Y.; Pei, P.; Zhu, X.; Han, D. The Impacts of Air Pollution on Mental Health: Evidence from the Chinese University Students. *Int. J. Environ. Res. Public Health* **2020**, *17*, 6734. [CrossRef] [PubMed]
5. Li, X.; Jin, L.; Kan, H. Air pollution: A global problem needs local fixes. *Nature* **2019**, *570*, 437–439. [CrossRef] [PubMed]
6. Xu, G.; Ren, X.; Xiong, K.; Li, L.; Bi, X.; Wu, Q. Analysis of the driving factors of PM2.5 concentration in the air: A case study of the Yangtze River Delta, China. *Ecol. Indic.* **2020**, *110*, 105889. [CrossRef]
7. Jin, H.; Chen, X.; Zhong, R.; Liu, M. Influence and prediction of PM2.5 through multiple environmental variables in China. *Sci. Total Environ.* **2022**, *849*, 157910. [CrossRef]
8. Li, T.; Hua, M.; Wu, X. A Hybrid CNN-LSTM Model for Forecasting Particulate Matter (PM2.5). *IEEE Access* **2020**, *8*, 26933–26940. [CrossRef]
9. Gao, X.; Li, W. A graph-based LSTM model for PM2.5 forecasting. *Atmos. Pollut. Res.* **2021**, *12*, 101150. [CrossRef]
10. Nguyen, M.T.; Nguyen, P.L.; Nguyen, K.; Le, V.B.; Ji, Y. PM2.5 Prediction Using Genetic Algorithm-Based Feature Selection and Encoder-Decoder Model. *IEEE Access* **2021**, *9*, 57338–57350. [CrossRef]
11. Qiao, W.; Tian, W.; Tian, Y.; Yang, Q.; Wang, Y.; Zhang, J. The Forecasting of PM2.5 Using a Hybrid Model Based on Wavelet Transform and an Improved Deep Learning Algorithm. *IEEE Access* **2019**, *7*, 142814–142825. [CrossRef]
12. Li, Y.; Peng, T.; Hua, L.; Ji, C.; Ma, H.; Nazir, M.S.; Zhang, C. Research and application of an evolutionary deep learning model based on improved grey wolf optimization algorithm and DBN-ELM for AQI prediction. *Sustain. Cities Soc.* **2022**, *87*, 104209. [CrossRef]
13. Djalalova, I.; Monache, L.D.; Wilczak, J.M. PM2.5 analog forecast and Kalman filter post-processing for the Community Multiscale Air Quality (CMAQ) model. *Atmos. Environ.* **2015**, *108*, 76–87. [CrossRef]

14. Lightstone, S.D.; Moshary, F.; Gross, B. Comparing CMAQ Forecasts with a Neural Network Forecast Model for PM2.5 in New York. *Atmosphere* **2017**, *8*, 161. [CrossRef]
15. Thongthammachart, T.; Araki, S.; Shimadera, H.; Eto, S.; Matsuo, T.; Kondo, A. An integrated model combining random forests and WRF/CMAQ model for high accuracy spatiotemporal PM2.5 predictions in the Kansai region of Japan. *Atmos. Environ.* **2021**, *262*, 118620. [CrossRef]
16. Cheng, F.; Feng, C.W.; Yang, Z.M.; Hsu, C.; Chan, K.W.; Lee, C.; Chang, S.C. Evaluation of real-time PM2.5 forecasts with the WRF-CMAQ modeling system and weather-pattern-dependent bias-adjusted PM2.5 forecasts in Taiwan. *Atmos. Environ.* **2021**, *244*, 117909. [CrossRef]
17. Xu, Y.; Chen, Y. Short-term PM2.5 prediction based on variational mode decomposition and machine learning methods. In Proceedings of the 2022 International Conference on Machine Learning and Knowledge Engineering (MLKE), Guilin, China, 25–27 February 2022.
18. Pak, U.; Ma, J.; Wang, J.; Ryom, K.; Juhyok, U.; Pak, K.; Pak, C. Deep learning-based PM2.5 prediction considering the spatiotemporal correlations: A case study of Beijing, China. *Sci. Total Environ.* **2020**, *699*, 133561. [CrossRef] [PubMed]
19. Yeo, I.; Choi, Y.; Lops, Y.; Sayeed, A. Efficient PM2.5 forecasting using geographical correlation based on integrated deep learning algorithms. *Neural Comput. Appl.* **2021**, *33*, 15073–15089. [CrossRef]
20. Zhu, H.; Lu, X. The Prediction of PM2.5 Value Based on ARMA and Improved BP Neural Network Model. In Proceedings of the 2016 International Conference on Intelligent Networking and Collaborative Systems (INCoS), Ostrava, Czech Republic, 7–9 September 2016.
21. Yang, J.; Zhou, X. Prediction of PM2.5 Concentration Based on ARMA Model Based on Wavelet Transform. In Proceedings of the 2020 12th International Conference on Intelligent Human-Machine Systems and Cybernetics (IHMSC), Hangzhou, China, 22–23 August 2020.
22. Wang, P.; Zhang, H.; Qin, Z.; Zhang, G. A novel hybrid-Garch model based on ARIMA and SVM for PM 2.5 concentrations forecasting. *Atmos. Pollut. Res.* **2017**, *8*, 850–860. [CrossRef]
23. Wu, C.; He, H.; Song, R.; Zhu, X.; Peng, Z.; Fu, Q.; Pan, J. A hybrid deep learning model for regional O_3 and NO_2 concentrations prediction based on spatiotemporal dependencies in air quality monitoring network. *Environ. Pollut.* **2023**, *320*, 121075. [CrossRef]
24. He, Z.; Guo, Q.; Wang, Z.; Li, X. Prediction of Monthly PM2.5 Concentration in Liaocheng in China Employing Artificial Neural Network. *Atmosphere* **2022**, *13*, 1221. [CrossRef]
25. Zhang, B.; Zhang, H.; Zhao, G.; Lian, J. Constructing a PM2.5 concentration prediction model by combining auto-encoder with Bi-LSTM neural networks. *Environ. Model. Softw.* **2020**, *124*, 104600. [CrossRef]
26. Kristiani, E.; Lin, H.; Lin, J.; Chuang, Y.; Huang, C.; Yang, C. Short-Term Prediction of PM2.5 Using LSTM Deep Learning Methods. *Sustainability* **2022**, *14*, 2068. [CrossRef]
27. Chae, S.; Shin, J.; Kwon, S.; Lee, S.; Kang, S.; Lee, D.H. PM10 and PM2.5 real-time prediction models using an interpolated convolutional neural network. *Sci. Rep.* **2021**, *11*, 11952. [CrossRef]
28. Huang, G.; Li, X.; Zhang, B.; Ren, J. PM2.5 concentration forecasting at surface monitoring sites using GRU neural network based on empirical mode decomposition. *Sci. Total Environ.* **2021**, *768*, 144516. [CrossRef]
29. Wang, W.; Tang, Q. Combined model of air quality index forecasting based on the combination of complementary empirical mode decomposition and sequence reconstruction. *Environ. Pollut.* **2023**, *316*, 120628. [CrossRef] [PubMed]
30. Chen, S.; Zheng, L. Complementary ensemble empirical mode decomposition and independent recurrent neural network model for predicting air quality index. *Appl. Soft Comput.* **2022**, *131*, 109757. [CrossRef]
31. Wang, Z.; Chen, L.; Ding, Z.; Chen, H. An enhanced interval PM2.5 concentration forecasting model based on BEMD and MLPI with influencing factors. *Atmos. Environ.* **2020**, *223*, 117200. [CrossRef]
32. Lai, X.; Li, H.; Pan, Y. A combined model based on feature selection and support vector machine for PM2.5 prediction. *J. Intell. Fuzzy Syst.* **2021**, *40*, 10099–10113. [CrossRef]
33. Lin, L.; Liang, Y.; Liu, L.; Zhang, Y.; Xie, D.; Yin, F.; Ashraf, T. Estimating PM2.5 Concentrations Using the Machine Learning RF-XGBoost Model in Guanzhong Urban Agglomeration, China. *Remote Sens.* **2022**, *14*, 5239. [CrossRef]
34. Zhou, Y.; Chang, F.; Chang, L.; Kao, I.; Wang, Y.; Kang, C. Multi-output support vector machine for regional multi-step-ahead PM2.5 forecasting. *Sci. Total Environ.* **2019**, *651*, 230–240. [CrossRef]
35. Wang, P.; Zhang, G.; Chen, F.; He, Y. A hybrid-wavelet model applied for forecasting PM2.5 concentrations in Taiyuan city, China. *Atmos. Pollut. Res.* **2019**, *10*, 1884–1894. [CrossRef]
36. Peng, H.; Long, F.; Ding, C. Feature selection based on mutual information criteria of max-dependency, max-relevance, and min-redundancy. *IEEE Trans. Pattern Anal. Mach. Intell.* **2005**, *27*, 1226–1238. [CrossRef]
37. Feng, L.; Wang, Y.; Zhang, Z.; Du, Q. Geographically and temporally weighted neural network for winter wheat yield prediction. *Remote Sens. Environ.* **2021**, *262*, 112514. [CrossRef]
38. Zhao, C.; Ju, S.; Xue, Y.; Ren, T.; Ji, Y.; Xue, C. China's energy transitions for carbon neutrality: Challenges and opportunities. *Carbon Neutrality* **2022**, *1*, 7. [CrossRef]
39. Yuan, X.L.; Liu, X.; Zuo, J. The development of new energy vehicles for a sustainable future: A review. *Renew. Sustain. Energy Rev.* **2015**, *42*, 298–305. [CrossRef]

40. Huang, N.E.; Shen, Z.; Long, S.R.; Wu, M.; Shih, H.H.; Zheng, Q.; Yen, N.; Tung, C.C.; Liu, H.X. The empirical mode decomposition and the Hilbert spectrum for nonlinear and non-stationary time series analysis. *Proc. R. Soc. A Math. Phys. Eng. Sci.* **1998**, *454*, 903–995. [CrossRef]
41. Liang, Y.; Niu, D.; Hong, W. Short term load forecasting based on feature extraction and improved general regression neural network model. *Energy* **2019**, *166*, 653–663. [CrossRef]
42. Huh, J.; Youn, J.; Park, P.; Jeon, K.; Park, S. Development of a Prediction Model for Daily PM2.5 in Republic of Korea by Using an Artificial Neutral Network. *Appl. Sci.* **2023**, *13*, 3575. [CrossRef]
43. Lu, B.; Ge, Y.; Qin, K.; Zheng, J.H. A Review on Geographically Weighted Regression. *Geomat. Inf. Sci. Wuhan Univ.* **2020**, *45*, 1356–1366.
44. Tang, M.; Acharya, T.D.; Niemeier, D. Black Carbon Concentration Estimation with Mobile-Based Measurements in a Complex Urban Environment. *ISPRS Int. J. Geo-Inf.* **2023**, *12*, 290. [CrossRef]
45. Guo, M.; Miao, N.; Sun, S.; Xu, C.; Zhang, G.M.; Zhang, L.; Zhang, R.; Zheng, J.; Chen, C.; Jia, Z.; et al. Estimation and Analysis of Air Pollutant Emissions from On-Road Vehicles in Changzhou, China. *Atmosphere* **2024**, *15*, 192. [CrossRef]

International Journal of
Geo-Information

MDPI

Review

Assessing Contamination in Transitional Waters Using Geospatial Technologies: A Review

Itzel Arroyo-Ortega [1], Yaselda Chavarin-Pineda [2] and Eduardo Torres [3,*]

[1] Instituto de Ecología, A.C.-, Antigua Carretera a Coatepec No. 351, Xalapa 91073, VC, Mexico; itzel.arroyo@inecol.mx

[2] Centro de Investigación en Ciencias Agrícolas, Instituto de Ciencias, Benemérita Universidad Autónoma de Puebla, Puebla 72570, PU, Mexico; yaselda.chavarinp@correo.buap.mx

[3] Centro de Química, Instituto de Ciencias, Benemérita Universidad Autónoma de Puebla, Puebla 72570, PU, Mexico

* Correspondence: eduardo.torres@correo.buap.mx

Abstract: Transitional waters (TWs) are relevant ecological and economical ecosystems that include estuaries, deltas, bays, wetlands, marshes, coastal lakes, and coastal lagoons and play a central role in providing food, protecting coastal environments, and regulating nutrients. However, human activities such as industrialization, urbanization, tourism, and agriculture are threatening these ecosystems, which results in contamination and habitat degradation. Therefore, it is essential to evaluate contamination in TW to develop effective management and protection strategies. This study analyses the application of geospatial technologies (GTS) for monitoring and predicting contaminant distribution in TW. Cartography, interpolation, complex spatial methods, and remote sensing were applied to assess contamination profiles by heavy metals, and persistent organic compounds, and analyze contamination indices or some physicochemical water parameters. It is concluded that integrating environmental and demographic data with GTS would help to identify critical points of contamination and promote ecosystem resilience to ensure long-term health and human well-being. This review comprehensively analyzes the methods, indicators, and indices used to assess contamination in transitional waters in conjunction with GTS. It offers a valuable foundation for planning future research on pollution in these types of waters or other similar water bodies worldwide.

Keywords: environmental pollution; health risk; water quality parameters; heavy metals; anthropogenic activities; cartography; remote sensing; interpolation techniques

1. Introduction

Due to their unique and dynamic nature, transitional waters (TWs) are considered one of the world's most important ecological and economic ecosystems [1,2]. Historically, they have been the focus of human settlements, being the sites of major cities and ports [3]. These water bodies are the interphase between land and sea and comprehend estuaries, deltas, coastal lagoons, wetlands, marshes, and fjords [4–6]. Their connectivity and interaction between fresh and saline waters characterize them as complex, highly diverse, and highly productive environments [7], so a wide range of goods and services are associated with these water bodies [8]. The goods and services from TW include providing food such as fish, crustaceans, and mollusks; protecting coastal environments from floods, storms, and chemical disturbance from pollution; protecting biodiversity; cycling and transforming elements and nutrients; and wastewater treatment, among others [9].

However, TWs are frequently affected by increased industrialization, urbanization, tourism, livestock, and agricultural and aquaculture activities [8], by which [9] physical and chemical transformation, habitat destruction, and changes in the biodiversity, composition, and ecological structure could be experienced [7,10]. Figure 1 displays some of the anthropogenic activities and processes that alter the natural condition of TW. Pollutants can enter TW through atmospheric deposition, runoff, sewage, drainage, or effluents from municipal or industrial wastewater [1,9]. After contaminants have entered the water, the water column promotes their dispersion and distribution to other environmental compartments; in some cases, the pollutants are transported to open waters, while others are accumulated in the sediments, though there is some partial degradation of pollutants by the native microorganism and other physicochemical processes [1,11]. Depending on the nature of pollutants, aquatic organisms may experience adverse effects in the short, medium, or long term. Bioaccumulation and biomagnification can also impact the entire food chain [12]. In addition, the increasing levels of nutrients can lead to water pollution through eutrophication, which is one of the most common pollution problems in coastal lagoons and estuaries worldwide [13]. Additionally, the unsustainable exploitation of resources (mangrove deforestation, extraction of aquatic organisms), unmanaged tourism, the introduction of invasive species, and climate change may change transitional waters into very fragile systems [10].

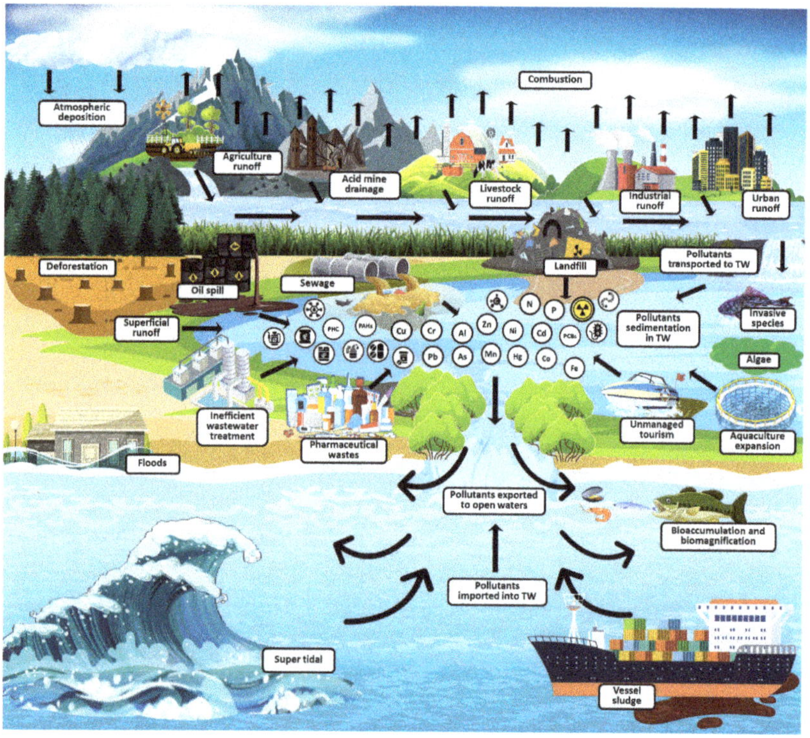

Figure 1. Overview of source and dispersion of pollutants in transitional waters (TWs).

Therefore, there is an urgent need to develop and apply tools and methods to assess the status of pollution in TW to develop effective management strategies for their restoration, use, and protection. To this end, several parameters and indices have been reported over time to assess the quality level of water. Some of them are oriented to determine the concentration of chemical pollutants in different environmental compartments, while others evaluate the toxicity and environmental or human health risks. However, most of these indices can only be applied by determining pollutant concentrations through in situ measurements, which may limit their application due to the high cost and time-consuming nature of some analytical techniques, especially when a large area is under study [14]; therefore, a partial spatial and temporal condition of the water quality is obtained.

Geospatial technologies (GTS), such as cartography, global positioning systems (GPSs), remote sensing (RS), and Geographic Information Systems (GISs), have proven to be essential tools for studies of water quality, monitoring, and pollution assessment [15–17]. GIS is specially used to predict water quality and map spatial distribution patterns of pollutants on the water surface and in depths [18,19]. Also, GIS has been used to map the degrees, toxicity, and risk of pollutant concentrations by integrating chemometric methods and interpolation techniques [20]. On the other hand, RS provides valuable real-time spatial information on natural resources, physical terrain parameters, and anthropogenic processes [21]. This information helps to assess the pressures and impacts, identify potential pollutant sources, and relate them to environmental parameters [22–24]. In any case, the most significant benefit of GIS-based techniques and remote sensing is the visualization of specific and contextualized environmental problems, which, coupled with the integration of in situ measurements and statistical methods, can result in a comprehensive assessment of the pollution condition in transitional waters [18,20].

This review aims to provide a general and current overview of the tools and methods for assessing pollution in transitional waters by combining parameters, indices, and models, as well as remote sensing, and Geographic Information Systems as the leading geospatial technologies. To this end, studies concerning the topic were searched by evaluating keywords, titles, and abstracts. Studies that did not assess TW pollution/quality and GIS or Remote Systems were excluded. We considered articles published in English with full text available from the past decade (2012–2023). This review highlights the potential for a more comprehensive and cost-effective assessment of water quality in transitional waters, serving as a foundation for future studies.

2. Materials and Methods

The search was performed using the following components for the SCOPUS database:

- Search component 1 (SC1) combines one of the following keywords: transitional water OR coastal lagoon OR coastal lake OR coastal wetland OR marsh OR estuary OR bay with pollution OR contamination.
- Search component 2 (SC2), including the following key terms: transitional water OR coastal lagoon OR coastal lake OR coastal wetland OR marsh OR estuary OR bay with GIS OR Geographic Information System OR remote sensing.

The following data were extracted and captured in an Excel spreadsheet containing the article title, authors, index description and application, type of TW, type of pollutants, and type of pollution index. As mentioned, for the inclusion of the studies, titles and abstracts were independently analyzed by two reviewers; when those were not clear enough to accomplish inclusion criteria, the full-text articles were read. The exclusion criteria include at least one of the following criteria: the full text was written in a different language to English, GIS and/or remote sensing techniques were applied in water studies different to pollution issues, and abstract-only papers as proceeding papers, conference papers, editorials, and author response theses and books. Finally, index development or water applications without GIS or remote sensing were also excluded.

3. Results

3.1. *Transitional Waters Worldwide*

Broadly speaking, TW are those ecosystems located between riverine ecosystems and coastal marine ecosystems [7]. However, worldwide, there is no unified term and definition to refer to these water bodies, probably because there is a wide variety of characteristics that make them unique and distinct from each other. For example, according to Chapman et al. [1], TWs are not entirely saline or utterly fresh water, can be both large and small geographic areas, and can be vertically stratified or homogeneous, shallow, or very deep, with greater or lesser fluvial dominance or with greater or lesser tidal influence; also, they can present seasonal variation. Therefore, transitional waters present heterogeneous and complex conditions that complicate their characterization.

The term transitional waters was introduced in 2000 by the Water Framework Directive (WFD) [25], and it was rapidly consolidated as a scientific term [4]. The WFD defined TW as "surface water bodies in the vicinity of river mouths that have a partially saline character due to their proximity to coastal waters but are substantially influenced by freshwater flows" [25], being the most widespread definition. However, this term and its definition are generally coined for European member countries. On the other side, the U.S. legislation (Code of Federal Regulations) includes the definition of TW in the term "coastal waters" as "all U.S. waters subject to the tide, U.S. waters of the Great Lakes, specified ports and harbors on the inland rivers, waters of the contiguous zone, or other waters of the high seas subject to discharges in connection with activities [. . .] which may affect natural resources belonging to, appertaining to, or under the exclusive management authority of the United States [. . .]". As can be seen, rather than a definition, the water bodies considered as coastal waters are those along the coastal line. For its part, the U.S. Environmental Protection Agency (EPA) refers to coastal waters "As the interface between terrestrial environments and open oceans", which include estuaries, coastal wetlands, seagrass meadows, coral reefs, mangrove forests, kelp forests, and upwelling areas [26].

This difference in terminology can also be observed in Latin America. In Mexico, the equivalent term for TW is "coastal aquatic ecosystems", defined as those water bodies found in the coastal zone, maintaining permanent or temporary communication with the sea and which may or may not be connected to freshwater aquaculture systems [27]. The coastal aquatic ecosystems include coastal lagoons, marshes, estuaries, swamps, and bays, leaving out the reefs as they are considered marine aquatic ecosystems. Meanwhile, Brazil's legislation only provides classification and environmental guidelines for surface water bodies and exoreic basins [28,29]. In Colombia, the term used is coastal marine ecosystems and englobing coastal lagoons and estuaries, coral reefs, mangroves, seagrass beds, sandy beaches, and rocky shorelines, among others [30]. Generally, the waters referred to in this research as TW are classified in most countries as coastal lagoons or estuaries.

This absence of characterizing associated with the geographic diversity, high spatio-temporal variability, and complexity of this type of ecosystem promotes complications in their identification and visualization of their importance at a global level, which in turn causes a delay in the application of adequate directives for their assessment, management, and conservation. Although transitional waters is accepted as a scientific term [3,4], only seven studies included it; the rest used one or more equivalent terms. This review identified 55 papers that met the search criteria.

3.2. General Description of Data Collection

Figures 2–4 provide a general overview of the information. Figure 2 focuses explicitly on the geographical distribution of the studies. It reveals that research on this topic has been reported in six distinct international regions, with Europe and Central Asia having the highest number of studies.

The Vos Viewer keyword analysis unveiled a notable network of interactions comprising 58 interconnected keywords, each appearing at least five times, linked by 1344 interactions, and a cumulative link strength of 5546 (Figure 3). These keywords were classified into four distinct clusters. The first cluster, labeled "GIS", consists of 23 keywords, with the term "GIS" appearing 46 times, accompanied by 55 links and a total link strength of 609. The second cluster, categorized as "environmental," comprises 18 items, with "environmental monitoring" being the predominant term, occurring 33 times and boasting 56 links, resulting in a total link strength of 510. Lastly, the third cluster, "pollutants", encompasses 16 items, with "heavy metals" emerging as the most prevalent term. It appeared 18 times, with 53 links, yielding a total link strength of 340. Finally, the fourth cluster, with just one term, "geographical distribution", is connected to the other clusters by 25 links.

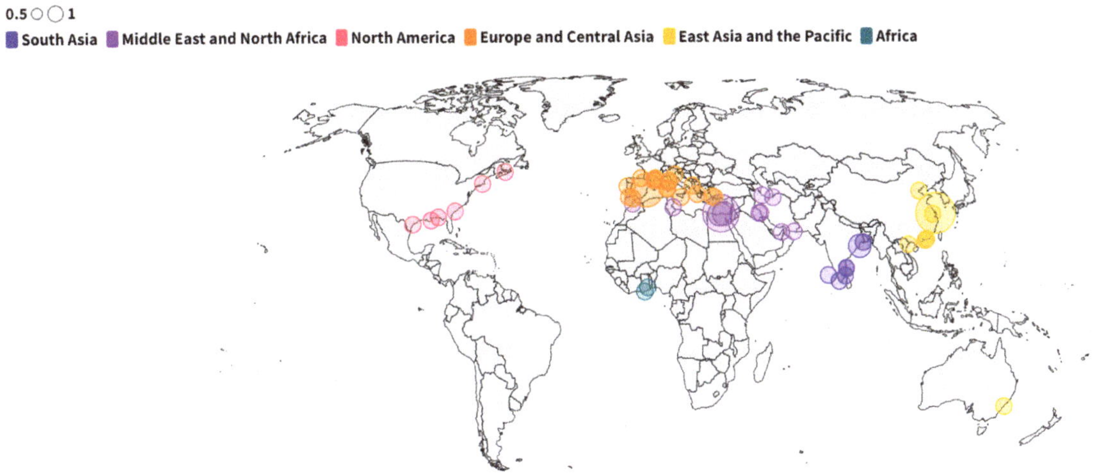

Figure 2. The global distribution of evaluated transitional water bodies in this research. The size of the circle indicates the number of papers. Created with flourish.studio.

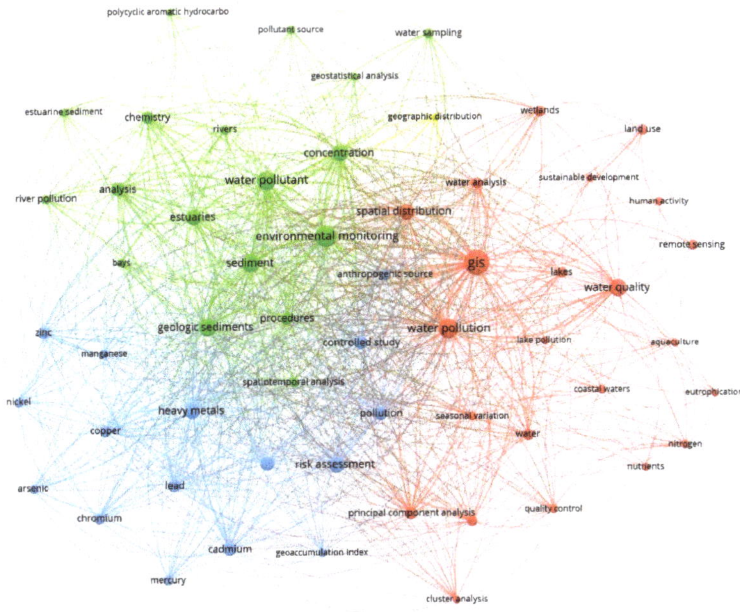

Figure 3. VOSviewer network visualization map of keyword co-occurrence. VOSviewer version 1.6.20. Copyright 2009–2023 Nees and Jan van Eck and Ludo Waltman [31].

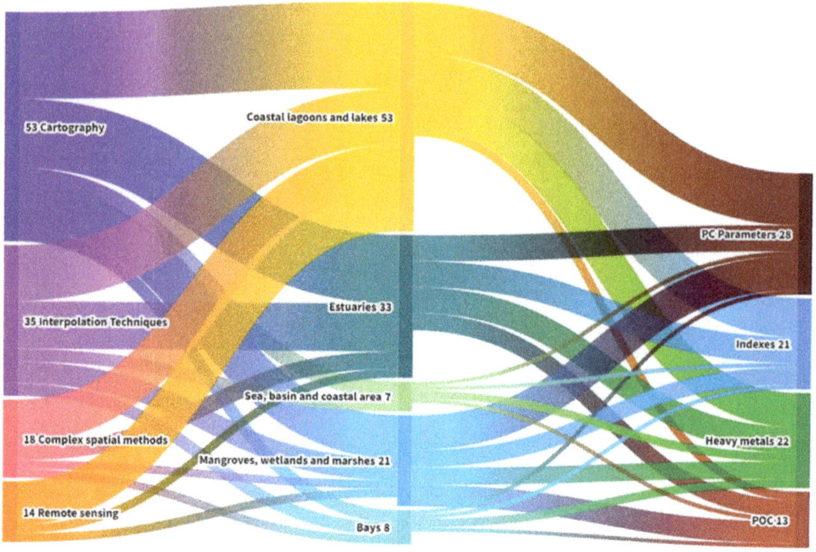

Figure 4. Applications of GTS in the study of polluted transitional waters from 2012 to 2023. POC: Persistent organic compounds (including polycyclic aromatic hydrocarbons, pesticides, and pharmaceutical compounds) and PC parameters, such as physicochemical parameters. The term "index" integrates several quantitative values (pollutant concentration and/or PC parameters). The numbers indicate the number of total papers. Created with flourish.studio.

Figure 4 shows a Sankey diagram to illustrate the categories of GTS used in the study of polluted TW. Fifty-five papers reported applying four types of GTS, cartography, interpolation methods, complex spatial methods, and remote sensing, for studying several polluted tidal waters. Most papers (98%) used cartography combined with one or two other GTS. The most studied polluted TWs were coastal lagoons and lakes. Pollution was determined by quantifying different physicochemical parameters (PC parameters: temperature, salinity, pH, etc.), heavy metals, and persistent organic compounds (POCs: polycyclic aromatic hydrocarbons, pesticides, and pharmaceutical compounds); in some cases, the pollution level was calculated by integrating the above parameters into pollution or water quality indices.

Tables 1 and 2 provide more detailed information about study areas, the type of TW, monitored pollution parameters (Table 1), and the specific geospatial technologies (Table 2) for the identified studies. The tables show that most studies combined geospatial technologies to achieve their goals. This highlights the multifaceted nature of environmental research and the need for integrating various spatial analysis techniques. Interestingly, the studies also included the analysis of pollutants of high concern directly relevant to both environmental and health research, such as polycyclic aromatic hydrocarbons (PAHs) and pharmaceutical products, here both integrated as persistent organic compounds (POCs). These findings emphasize the growing focus on understanding the complex interactions between anthropogenic activities, environmental pollution, and public health.

Table 1. Studies about Transitional Waters and monitoring of pollution.

Reference	Study Area	Type of TW	Parameter or Pollutant Assessed
Assessment of sediment quality in the Mediterranean Sea-Boughrara lagoon exchange areas (southeastern Tunisia): GIS approach-based chemometric methods [32]	Boughrara lagoon, Tunisia	Coastal lagoon	Cd, Pb, Zn, Cu, Mn, and Fe in sediments
Assessing a bioremediation strategy in a shallow coastal system affected by a fish farm culture—Application of GIS and shellfish dynamic models in the Rio San Pedro, SW Spain [33]	Rio San Pedro, Spain	Estuary	Water quality parameters
An assessment of landscape characteristics affecting estuarine nitrogen loading in an urban watershed [34]	Pensacola estuarine, USA	Estuary	Nitrogen loading in water
Evaluation of the anthropogenic influx of metal and metalloid contaminants into the Moulay Bousselham lagoon, Morocco, using chemometric methods coupled to geographical information systems [35]	Moulay Bousselham Lagoon, Morocco	Coastal lagoon	Al, Fe, Cu, Zn, Pb, Mn, Ni, Cr, As, Hg, and Cd in sediments
Source characterization and spatio-temporal evolution of the metal pollution in the sediments of the Basque estuaries (Bay of Biscay) [36]	Basque Estuaries, Spain	Estuaries	Cd, Cr, Cu, Hg, Ni, Pb, and Zn in sediments
Spatial distribution and pollution assessment of mercury in sediments of Lake Taihu, China [37]	Lake Taihu, China	Coastal lake	Total mercury in sediments
Optimization of marine environmental monitoring sites in the Yangtze River estuary and its adjacent sea, China [38]	Yangtze River estuary, China	Estuary	Dissolved inorganic nitrogen (DIN), oil, PO_4-P, COD, OD, pH, Cu, Hg, Pb, and Cd in water
Assessment and monitoring of nutrient loading in the sediments of tidal creeks receiving shrimp farm effluent in Quang Ninh, Vietnam [39]	Quang Ninh, Vietnam	Estuary	Total nitrogen, total phosphorus, and total organic carbon in sediments
Spatial distribution of cadmium and lead in the sediments of the western Anzali wetlands on the coast of the Caspian Sea (Iran) [40]	Anzali Wetlands, Iran	Coastal wetland	Cd, Pb, and total organic matter in sediments
TMDL balance: A model for coastal water pollutant loadings [41]	Copano Bay, USA	Coastal basin	Fecal coliform loading in water
Spatio-Temporal Variations in Water Quality of Muttukadu Backwaters, Tamilnadu, India [42]	Muttukadu Backwaters, India	Estuary	Temperature, pH, salinity, DO, total nitrogen, total PO_4, silicate, and chlorophyll-a (Chl-ß) in water

Table 1. *Cont.*

Reference	Study Area	Type of TW	Parameter or Pollutant Assessed
An environmental forensic procedure to analyse anthropogenic pressures of urban origin on surface water of protected coastal agro-environmental wetlands (L'Albufera de Valencia Natural Park, Spain) [43]	L'Albufera de Valencia Natural Park, Spain	Coastal wetland	Drugs of abuse and pharmaceuticals in water: Cocainics, amphetamine, cannabinoids, opiates, oxytetracycline, tetracycline, ofloxacin, fenofibrate, ciprofloxacin, norfloxacin, codeine, trimethoprim, diazepam, metoprolol, propranolol, ibuprofen, sulfamethoxazole, carbamazepine, acetaminophen, clofibric acid, and diclofenac
An interactive WebGIS observatory platform for enhanced support of integrated coastal management [44]	Aveiro lagoon, Portugal	Coastal lagoon	Oil spill
Dispersion pattern of petroleum hydrocarbon in coastal water of Bay of Bengal along Odisha and West Bengal, India using geospatial approach [45]	Odisha and West Bengal, India	Estuaries, ports, and coastal area	Petroleum hydrocarbons
Heavy metals risk assessment in water and bottom sediments of the eastern part of Lake Manzala, Egypt, based on remote sensing and GIS [15]	Lake Manzala, Egypt	Coastal lake	Zn, Cd, Cu, Mn, and Pb in water and bottom sediments
Source apportionment of PAHs in surface sediments using positive matrix factorization combined with GIS for the estuarine area of the Yangtze River, China [46]	Yangtze River estuary, China	Estuary	PAHs in sediments: Nap, Ace, Flu, Phe, Ant, Fla, Pyr, BaA, Chr, BbF, BkF, BaP, DahA, BgP, InP, Acy
Spatial variation, environmental risk and biological hazard assessment of heavy metals in surface sediments of the Yangtze River estuary [47]	Yangtze River estuary, China	Estuary	As, Cd, Cr, Cu, Mn, Ni, Pb, and Zn in sediments
Spatio-temporal distribution of major and trace metals in estuarine sediments of Dhamra, Bay of Bengal, India—its environmental significance [48]	Dhamra Estuary, India	Estuary	Cu, Ni, Co, Pb, Zn, Cr, Cd, Fe, Mn, Ca, Mg, Na, and K in sediments
A spatial assessment of baseline nutrient and water quality values in the Ashepoo–Combahee–Edisto (ACE) Basin, South Carolina, USA [49]	Ashepoo–Combahee–Edisto (ACE) Basin, USA	Estuaries	Temperature, salinity, chlorophyll-a, total nitrogen, total phosphorus, DO, DOC, TSS, and VSS
Current anthropogenic pressures on agro-ecological protected coastal wetlands [23]	L'Albufera de Valencia Natural Park, Spain	Coastal wetland	Pharmaceutical compounds: Oxytetracycline, tetracycline, ofloxacin, fenofibrate, ciprofloxacin, norfloxacin, codeine, trimethoprim, diazepam, metoprolol, propranolol, sulfamethoxazole, carbamazepine, acetaminophen, ibuprofen, clofibric acid, and diclofenac

Table 1. *Cont.*

Reference	Study Area	Type of TW	Parameter or Pollutant Assessed
Prioritization of pollution potential zones for conservation activities of a lake system [50]	Akkulam–Veli Lake, India	Coastal lake	pH, DO, BOD, and fecal coliform in water
Spatial distribution and pollution evaluation of heavy metals in Yangtze estuary sediment [51]	Yangtze River estuary, China	Estuary	Al, As, Cd, Cr, Cu, Fe, Hg, Mn, Ni, Pb, Sb, and Zn in sediments
Risk assessment and uncertainty analysis of PAHs in the sediments of the Yangtze River Estuary, China [52]	Yangtze River estuary, China	Estuary	PAHs in sediments: Baa, Chr, Bbf, Bkf, Bap, Daa, Bgp, Nap, Any, Ane, Fle, Phe, Ant, Fla, Pyr, Ilp
Assessment of water pollution induced by human activities in Burullus Lake using Landsat 8 operational land imager and GIS [53]	Lake Burullus, Egypt	Coastal lake	BOD, total nitrogen, and total PO_4
Multivariate statistical and GIS-based approaches for toxic metals in tropical mangrove ecosystem, southeast coast of India [54]	Muthupet mangrove ecosystem, India	Coastal lagoon, river mouth, and wetlands	Temperature, pH, salinity of NO_2, NO_3, phosphate, ammonia, and heavy metals: Cd, Cu, and Zn in water and sediment
A water quality management strategy for regionally protected water through health risk assessment and spatial distribution of heavy metal pollution in 3 marine reserves [55]	Tianjin Ancient Coast and Wetlands National Nature Reserve, China	Coastal wetlands and sea	Pb, As, Cd, Hg, and Cr in water samples
Spatiotemporal assessment (quarter century) of pulp mill metal (loid) contaminated sediment to inform remediation decisions [56]	Boat Harbour, Canada	Coastal lagoon	As, Cd, Cr, Cu, Pb, Hg, and Zn in sediments
Oiling accelerates loss of salt marshes, southeastern Louisiana [57]	Louisiana, USA	Marsh	Oil spill
Baseline physio-chemical characteristics of Sydney estuary water under quiescent conditions [58]	Sydney, Australia	Estuary	Secchi depth transparency, turbidity, salinity, and TSS
Biological risk assessment of heavy metals in sediments and health risk assessment in bivalve mollusks from Kaozhouyang Bay, South China [12]	Kaozhouyang Bay, China	Bay	Cd, Pb, Cr, Ni, Cu, Zn, Hg, and As in surface sediments and bivalve mollusks
Detection of Isotope Stable Radioactive in Soil and Water Marshes of Southern Iraq [59]	Maysan Governorate Marshes, Iraq	Marsh	Isotope Stable Radioactivity in water: Th-138, CS-137, AG-110M, ZR-97, Fe-59, Pb-138, Pb-212, Pb-214, AS-76, W-187
The Tale of a Disappearing Lagoon: A Habitat Mapping and Ecological Assessment of Fosu Lagoon, Ghana [60]	Fosu Lagoon, Ghana	Coastal lagoon	NA

Table 1. *Cont.*

Reference	Study Area	Type of TW	Parameter or Pollutant Assessed
Spatial and temporal variations of water quality in Pallikaranai wetland, Chennai, India [61]	Pallikaranai wetland, India	Coastal wetland	pH, salinity, dissolved oxygen, NO_3, PO_4, DOC, suspended particulate matter, dissolved inorganic carbon, particulate organic carbon, dissolved CO_2, dissolved CH_4, and heavy metals: Fe, Mn, Ni, Co, Cd, Cr, Zn, Cu, and Pb
Spatial-temporal variation of heavy metals' sources in the surface sediments of the Yangtze River Estuary [11]	Yangtze River estuary, China	Estuary	Cd, Cr, Cu, Mn, Ni, Pb, and Zn in surface sediments
Holocene background concentrations and actual enrichment factors of metals in sediments from Ria Formosa, Portugal [62]	Ria Formosa, Portugal	Coastal lagoon	Granulometric characteristics and heavy metals: Al, Fe, As, Co, Cr, Cu, Ni, Pb, and Zn in sediment cores
Towards monitoring of nutrient pollution in coastal lake using remote sensing and regression analysis [63]	Dubai Creek, United Arab Emirates	Coastal lagoon	Chlorophyll-a, NO_3, orthophosphates, DO, turbidity, pH, and salinity in water
Evaluation of water quality parameters in marshes zone southern of Iraq based on remote sensing and GIS techniques [21]	Al-Hawizeh marsh, Iraq	Marsh	Salinity, silicates, and $CaCO_3$
An investigation into the impacts of climate change on anthropogenic polluted coastal lagoons in Ghana [64]	Coastal Lagoons, Ghana	Coastal lagoons	NO_2, NO_3, PO_4, total ammonia, DO, dissolved nitrogen, FC, temperature, salinity, pH, and turbidity in water
Prediction of future situation of land use/cover change and modeling sensitivity to pollution in Edku Lake, Egypt based on geospatial analyses [65]	Edku Lake, Egypt	Coastal lake	Pollution sources
GIS-Based Study on the Environmental Sensitivity to Pollution and Susceptibility to Eutrophication in Burullus Lake, Egypt [13]	Lake Burullus, Egypt	Coastal lake	Temperature, pH, EC, salinity, TDS, DO, NH_4, NO_2, PO_4, silicates, chlorophyll-a, and organic matter in water
Assessment of the pressure level over lentic waterbodies through the estimation of land uses in the catchment and hydro-morphological Alterations: The LUPLES method [16]	Mediterranean coastal lagoons	Coastal lagoons	Contribution of pressures such as eutrophication, organic enrichment, acidification, and specific pollutants associated with each land use
Pharmaceuticals and personal care products in a Mediterranean coastal wetland: Impact of anthropogenic and spatial factors and environmental risk assessment [66]	L'Albufera de Valencia Natural Park, Spain	Coastal wetland	Temperature, pH, total soluble salts, DO and redox potential, and pharmaceuticals and personal care products in water and sediment
Heavy metals in coral reef sediments of Kavaratti Island, India: An integrated quality assessment using GIS and pollution indicators [24]	Kavaratti Island, India	Coastal lagoon	Al, Pb, Cd, Cu, Cr, Mn, Ni, and Zn in sediments

Table 1. *Cont.*

Reference	Study Area	Type of TW	Parameter or Pollutant Assessed
How agriculture, connectivity and water management can affect water quality of a Mediterranean coastal wetland [67]	L'Albufera de Valencia Natural Park, Spain	Coastal wetland	Turbidity, pH, conductivity, organic matter, dissolved inorganic nitrogen, phosphorus concentrations, total inorganic carbon, total organic carbon, and total nitrogen in water
Elucidation of the Phytoplankton Distribution at an Egyptian Ramsar Site (Burullus Lake, Egypt) using Alpha Diversity Indices Supported with RS and GIS Maps [68]	Lake Burullus, Egypt	Coastal lake	Temperature, TDS, NH_4, NO_2, NO_3, PO_4, silicate DO, pH, chlorophyll-a, and total count of phytoplankton species in water
Polluted waters of the reclaimed islands of Indian Sundarban promote more greenhouse gas emissions from mangrove ecosystem [69]	Sundarban Mangrove, India	Mangrove	In water: pH, DO, BOD, TSS, ammonia, nitrate, total phosphorous, chlorophyll-a, and fecal coliform In soil: Litterfall biomass, soil organic carbon, soil pH, soil salinity, soil temperature, oxygen reduction potential In gas: Nitrate, CH_4, CO_2, and NO
Legacy halogenated organic contaminants in urban-influenced waters using passive polyethylene samplers: Emerging evidence of anthropogenic land-use-based sources and ecological risks [70]	Narragansett Bay, USA	Estuary	Organochlorine pesticides and polychlorinated biphenyls in water samples
Coastal sediment heavy metal (loid) pollution under multifaceted anthropogenic stress: Insights based on geochemical baselines and source-related risks [71]	Daya Bay, China	Bay	Cd, Cu, Cr, Pb, Zn, Hg, As, and total organic carbon in water and sediment
Impact Assessment of the Land Use Dynamics and Water Pollution on Ecosystem Service Value of the Nile Delta Coastal Lakes, Egypt [72]	Nile Delta Coastal Lakes, Egypt	Coastal lakes	Volatile phenol (V-phenol), DO, and NH_4-N in water
GIS-based approach and multivariate statistical analysis for identifying sources of heavy metals in marine sediments from the coast of Hong Kong [73]	Hong Kong, China	Coastal areas	Cd, Hg, Cu, Pb, Ni, Cr, As, Zn, Fe, and V in sediment
A comparative assessment of the lagoons with water quality indices and based on GIS: A study on the Aegean Sea and Mediterranean Sea [74]	Gulluk Lagoon and Koycegiz–Dalyan Lagoon, Turquía	Coastal lagoons	Temperature, pH, DO, BOD, SSM, total phosphorus, NO_2-N, NO_3-N, and ammonium nitrogen in water
Analysis of water quality, heavy metals and nutrient of Karavasta Lagoon using GIS Assessment of Ecological Risk [75]	Karavasta Lagoon, Albany	Coastal lagoon	pH, temperature, conductivity, salinity, DO, chlorophyll-a, total nitrogen, NO_3-N, total phosphorus, and heavy metals: Cd, Cr, Cu, Pb, and Hg in surface water and bottom sediment

Table 1. *Cont.*

Reference	Study Area	Type of TW	Parameter or Pollutant Assessed
Water quality assessment of Lake Burullus, Egypt, utilizing statistical and GIS modeling as environmental hydrology applications [76]	Lake Burullus, Egypt	Coastal lake	DO, temperature, salinity, Total-Nitrogen-to-Total-Phosphorus ratio, orthophosphate, nitrate, chlorophyll-a, COD, pH, turbidity, and electrical conductivity in water
Occurrence and source of PAHs in Miankaleh International Wetland in Iran [77]	Miankaleh wetland, Iran	Coastal wetland	pH, temperature, electrical conductivity, redox potential, DO, and PAHs: Nap Flu, Phe, Ant, Fl, Pyr, and Chr in water, and Nap Flu, Phe, Ant, Fl, Pyr, BaA, Chr, BbF, BkF, BaP, InP, and BghiP in sediments
Combining theoretical concepts and Geographic Information System (GIS) to highlight source, risk, and hotspots of sedimentary PAHs: A case study of Chabahar Bay [78]	Chabahar Bay, Iran	Bay	PAHs in sediment samples: Nap, 1*m*-Nap, 2*m*-Nap, Acy, Ace, Flu, Phe, Ant, 3*m*-Phe, 2*m*-Phe, 9*m*-Phe, 1*m*-Phe, Fluo, Py, B(a)A, Chr, B(b)F, B(k)F, B(a)P, I(c,d)P, DB(a,h)A, B(g,h,i)P

Table 2. Specific GTS methods for the identified studies.

Principle/Description	General Term	Technique or Method	References
Geospatial data representation involves the spatial location of sampling points, information integration at sampling points, spatial delineation, distance determination, temporal–spatial analysis, and analytical processes.	Cartography	Geolocation Punctual distributions Spatial delineation Temporal point variability Spatial analytical process	[11–13,15,21,23,24,32–43,45,47–56,58,59,61–63,66–71,73–78] [12,23,39,43,67,68,70] [16,32–34,50,57,58,60,64,65,72] [56] [23,33,43,49,66,78]
Estimation of unknown values at locations within a geographic area based on known values at nearby locations.	Interpolation techniques	Inverse distance weighted (IDW) Kriging, ordinary kriging, or kriging variance analysis Kernel Interpolation with Barrier's geoprocessing tool	[12,13,24,35,36,42,54,55,58,61,69,71–74,76,78] [15,33,34,37,38,40,45–48,51,52,75] [62]
Development of mathematical or computational representations that attempt to capture and explain spatial relationships and patterns in geographic datasets using geostatistics.	Complex spatial models	Prediction/simulation models Land use dynamics models Sensitivity, contamination risk models	[34,41,53,64,65,68,69,72,77] [16,65,70] [11,13,15,44,46,50,65,71,77,78]
Information from the Earth is acquired by sensors mounted on airborne or satellite platforms.	Remote sensing	Band value extraction and spatial distribution Land cover, land loss, and land conversion Oil fraction cover maps	[21,63,68,72] [13,15,16,34–36,53,57,60,65,72] [57]

3.3. Pollutants in Transitional Waters

Due to their shallow depth, direct connection to open seas, and inherent origins, TWs are highly vulnerable ecosystems prone to contamination by a diverse array of pollutants [24]. Human activities have notably contributed to introducing substantial volumes of toxic substances into these fragile environments [51].

Water quality assessment encompasses various methods, including evaluating pollutant concentrations, which may consist of chemicals with similar or distinct properties. Additionally, physicochemical parameters such as temperature, pH, turbidity, and dissolved or suspended solids levels are employed for assessment. Global indicators like chemical or biochemical oxygen demand are also utilized in legislative frameworks to gauge water quality levels. Among the most alarming contaminants are heavy metals, pharmaceutical residues, and excessive nutrients like nitrates, phosphates, and silicates, alongside total suspended solids. Furthermore, persistent organic compounds (POCs) such as polycyclic aromatic hydrocarbons (PAHs), pesticides, and some pharmaceutical compounds have emerged as significant concerns in contamination issues [24,43,46,52,68,70]. This amalgamation of pollutants substantially threatens TW ecosystems' ecological integrity and, consequently, jeopardizes the quality of life for human communities reliant on these aquatic resources.

3.3.1. Heavy Metals

During the period under analysis, heavy metals emerged as the focal point in studying pollutants within TW, with 21 papers dedicated to their investigation. These metals find their way into TW through myriad pathways, originating from both natural phenomena and human activities. Volcanic eruptions and the gradual weathering of geological formations release metals into the environment, where they disperse across various ecological compartments, including seawater aerosols and forest fire residues. However, human actions significantly exacerbate this natural process. Anthropogenic sources, such as power plants, biomedical waste disposal, industrial discharge, mining operations, electronic waste disposal, and agricultural practices, all contribute to the influx of heavy metals into TW [79]. The escalation of heavy metal concentrations can be chiefly attributed to the expansion of industrial sectors and urban landscapes, which, through runoff mechanisms, introduce pollutants into water bodies [80].

Heavy metals present in coastal lagoons pose a significant concern due to their high phytotoxicity, potentially disrupting the primary productivity of these vital coastal ecosystems [32]. Understanding the sediment enrichment factor in TW is crucial for identifying the origins of heavy metal emissions; for instance, in Jakarta Bay, Indonesia, the prevalence of elements such as Cu, Cr, and As is primarily influenced by natural factors stemming from the composition of volcanic rocks. Conversely, elements like Zn, Ni, Pb, and Cu are predominantly sourced from anthropogenic activities such as metal processing industries, fertilizer use, and the discharge of untreated animal waste [81].

3.3.2. Persistent Organic Compounds (POCs)

Persistent organic compounds (POCs) are substances characterized by their chemical and biological degradation resistance, resulting in extended half-lives in the environment, predominantly comprising xenobiotic compounds. These compounds exhibit key traits such as persistence, bioaccumulation, toxicity, and mobility [82]. POCs include plastics and plastic-derived chemicals, pesticides, polychlorinated biphenyls (PCBs), and polycyclic aromatic hydrocarbons (PAHs). Certain pharmaceutical compounds also share similar attributes of persistence and bioaccumulation, qualifying them as POCs [83,84]. For this study, polycyclic aromatic hydrocarbons (PAHs), pesticides, and pharmaceutical compounds were collectively categorized as POC. The investigation identified eight relevant papers addressing GTS and POC contamination in TW, mainly found in estuaries (Figure 4).

PAHs are a large group of ubiquitous substances primarily introduced into the environment through industrial and urban waste, petroleum hydrocarbon production, and transportation activities [85–87]. Nonetheless, it is worth noting that natural occurrences, such as forest and brush fires, can also contribute to the contamination of TW by PAH [88]. PAH pollution remains severe in coastal regions worldwide, with areas of elevated anthropogenic activity exhibiting heightened contamination levels, particularly by high-molecular-weight PAHs [88]. These large molecular-size PAHs have demonstrated significant genotoxic, mutagenic, and carcinogenic effects [89]. In regions characterized by commercial ports, oil, and gas exploration, there is a prevalence of low molecular weight (LMW) PAHs such as fluorene, naphthalene, anthracene, and phenanthrene, which are comparatively less toxic. This predominance of LMW PAHs is attributed to fuel leakage [88].

Pharmaceutical compounds constitute various chemical substances extensively used in promoting human, animal, and plant health. The presence of these compounds in environmental settings reflects deficiencies in disposal and treatment measures, stemming from both the chemical and pharmaceutical industries as well as household waste and agro-industrial activities. Because they are designed to have specific biological effects, their presence in environmental settings is likely to negatively affect ecosystem health, as documented in numerous studies [90–92]. Given the large number of pharmaceutical compounds in circulation, significant effort is required to properly assess and diagnose the level of environmental contamination, the fate, and the potential harm caused by these compounds in various environments, including TW. During the investigation period, only two studies were published regarding GTS and the contamination of marshes by pharmaceutical compounds.

Pesticides constitute another category of compounds with diverse chemical compositions, extensively utilized to enhance crop production. Engineered to be lethal to pests, their non-selective nature often harms non-target organisms, reinforced by their dispersion throughout environmental compartments due to application methods and prevailing environmental conditions [93,94]. Despite well-documented damage to ecosystems and human health over the years, global application rates have not diminished [95–97]. Remarkably, only one paper addressing the contamination of water bodies with pesticides and the utilization of GTS was identified in this review.

3.3.3. PC Parameters

Pollution in water bodies is typically assessed by measuring various physicochemical parameters (PC parameters) such as nutrient concentration, pH, temperature, and conductivity, among others [98]. Water quality is then commonly evaluated by comparing these parameters to reference values, which vary depending on regional regulations. Nutrient pollution, for instance, arises from the excessive use of fertilizers in agriculture, wastewater discharge, and stormwater runoff. Elevated nutrient levels lead to harmful algal blooms and oxygen depletion. Coastal farms, like shrimp farms, serve as significant sources of nutrients. In these areas, high nitrogen, phosphorus, and organic carbon levels near production sites are attributed to inputs like shrimp feed, feces, and decomposing organisms [39]. Other parameters are affected by anthropogenic activities: temperature is influenced by the discharge of industrial or cooling wastewater, pH levels are altered by the release of acidic or alkaline compounds, and turbidity is heightened by the influx of fine sediments originating from soil erosion caused by deforestation or construction activities. A total of 21 works were identified using GTS and PC parameters in TW for pollution determination.

3.3.4. Indices

In addition, pollution is usually expressed using various indices that combine several parameters or measurements to reflect the quality or pollution of water bodies more comprehensively. These indices consider other biotic and abiotic components with which the water interacts. Indices are usually described according to the following classification [99–101]:

Water Quality Indices: a comprehensive index integrating multiple water quality parameters into a single value, providing an overall quality assessment. Parameters considered often include pH, dissolved oxygen (DO), biochemical oxygen demand (BOD), chemical oxygen demand (COD), total suspended solids (TSSs), nutrients (nitrogen and phosphorus), heavy metals, and fecal coliform bacteria. The calculated index value categorizes water quality into different classes (e.g., excellent, good, fair, poor, and very poor).

Pollution Indices: focus specifically on assessing the pollution level in water bodies. These indices consider parameters such as levels of various pollutants, including heavy metals, pesticides, industrial chemicals, and organic compounds.

Eutrophication Indices: evaluate the degree of nutrient enrichment in water bodies, particularly nitrogen and phosphorus. Parameters such as total nitrogen, total phosphorus, chlorophyll-a concentration, and algal biomass are often used. Eutrophication indices help identify water bodies susceptible to excessive algal growth and hypoxia (low oxygen levels) due to nutrient pollution.

Sediment Quality Indices: consider parameters such as sediment texture, organic matter content, heavy metal concentrations, and toxicity. These indices help in evaluating the potential risks associated with contaminated sediments, such as the bioaccumulation of pollutants and adverse effects on benthic organisms.

Biotic Indices: assess water quality based on the composition and abundance of aquatic organisms. These indices utilize metrics such as species diversity, the presence of indicator species (e.g., mayflies, stoneflies, and caddisflies), and organisms' tolerance levels to pollution. Biotic indices provide insights into the ecological health of water bodies and can indicate long-term trends in water quality.

Human Health Indices: assess and quantify various potential impacts on human health within populations or specific communities when exposed to pollution. These indices typically incorporate multiple health-related parameters to comprehensively evaluate health status, healthcare access, and health outcomes. When these indices and parameters are integrated with GTS, it may offer a more comprehensive insight into water quality and pollution levels. In this review, 21 studies were identified that utilized indices and GTS for assessing pollution in water bodies, employing 30 different indices (Table S1).

3.4. *Analyses of GTS in TW Studies*

Geospatial technologies, with Geographic Information Systems (GISs) at their core, integrate remote sensing, GPS, mapping, and surveying data to generate valuable geographic information [17,102,103]. This synergistic approach using a combination of GIS tools has been demonstrably successful in comprehensively studying transitional waters (TWs). While the following sections will describe specific techniques employed environmentally for TW analyses, it is crucial to emphasize that these techniques are used in collaboration with others. The complexity and heterogeneity of spatial data, the diverse research goals, and the interplay of multiple variables within TW research necessitate a combined approach (Table 2).

3.4.1. Cartography

Cartography transforms spatial data into meaningful information using visual representations [104]. As a GIS tool, it is highly effective for visualizing and communicating geospatial data, highlighting the distribution patterns of data points based on location [105]. This facilitates the integration of spatial data from diverse sources, enabling the exploration of research questions [104].

In most of the articles reviewed, the spatial distribution of contaminants and their concentrations are presented using the vector data model, which employs points for the location of sampling points and shows the concentration and number of pollutants. This constitutes a simple and easy way to elaborate a spatial analysis distribution of data that helps identify sectors with contaminants and favors the understanding of connectivity patterns between environments [43].

In three similar studies [23,43,66], environmental analyses were conducted on various pharmaceuticals, personal care products, and illicit drugs in an agro-environmental wetland in L'Albufera Natural Park, Valencia, Spain. They quantified between 13 and 32 pharmaceutical and personal care products as well as nine illicit drugs to assess their prevalence and distribution in the area. Cartographic techniques such as geolocation, punctual distributions, and spatial analytical processes were employed. The integration of total numbers and concentrations of pharmaceuticals, personal care products, and illicit drugs in sampling points, along with the punctual distribution of risk indices and additional layers of data, including soil sealing, municipal population density, and locations of sewage water treatment plants (SWTPs), facilitated the identification of connectivity patterns within the park. Higher pollutant concentrations were observed near ditches linked to SWTP outflows or in areas with denser populations, highlighting anthropogenic origins. Conversely, areas without detected compounds were typically located away from urban water sources or the natural park. The persistent presence of these compounds in the environment poses significant risks to terrestrial and aquatic organisms, with potential impacts on wildlife and human health.

Bui et al. [39] assessed and monitored nutrient loading in tidal creek sediments at two sites in Quang Ninh, northern Vietnam, where intense and semi-intense shrimp farms are present. The evaluation involved measuring total nitrogen, phosphorus, and organic carbon and then calculating a sediment nutrient index (SNI) using a factor analysis. Spatial variation was studied through sampling at three locations: inside effluent channels (IEC), outside effluent channels (OEC), and away from shrimp farms (ASF). Temporal impacts were evaluated by collecting samples in three seasons: before shrimp growing (T0), after the first harvest (T1), and during the second harvest of shrimp (T2). Data obtained from the sediment analysis were incorporated at the monitoring points to examine the spatial and temporal punctual distribution of nutrients in sediments. The results indicated that spatial variation exists in the nutrient load in sediment and SNI values (Figure 5), which decrease as the distance to the shrimp farms increases. However, temporal variation showed no patterns across sites. It was concluded that GIS tools helped represent a punctual distribution of the SNI patterns along the study location to manage the aquatic ecosystem health around farming areas.

A similar approach with geolocation and punctual distributions was adopted by Vera et al. [67], who integrated physicochemical data into GIS vector layers to map the most problematic pollution hotspots, considering the agricultural types associated with each sampling point (Figure 6). Subsequently, the point spatial distribution maps for water indices were developed to evaluate environmental pollution and environmental risk through the Trophic State Index and ecological potential. Their findings revealed that the wetland exhibited overall eutrophication and had limited ecological potential. Other studies have applied cartography tools to perform the punctual distribution of indicators [70], diversity indices [68], or sediment indices to evaluate biological hazards and toxicity and human health risk assessment [12].

In another study [49], land use at sampling points was analyzed to identify correlations between water quality parameters and the total percentage of land occupancy. Specifically, elevated concentrations of total nitrogen, total phosphorus, chlorophyll, and dissolved organic carbon (DOC) were found to be associated with higher proportions of tidal creek sites compared to open water sites, indicating that, in addition to land use, the dilution and flushing capacity of the system have a significant impact on water quality in the Ashepoo–Combahee–Edisto (ACE) Basin, USA.

Under these scenarios, using cartographic tools has played a crucial role. These tools have facilitated the identification of environmental risks, connectivity patterns, and spatial variations in pollutant concentrations.

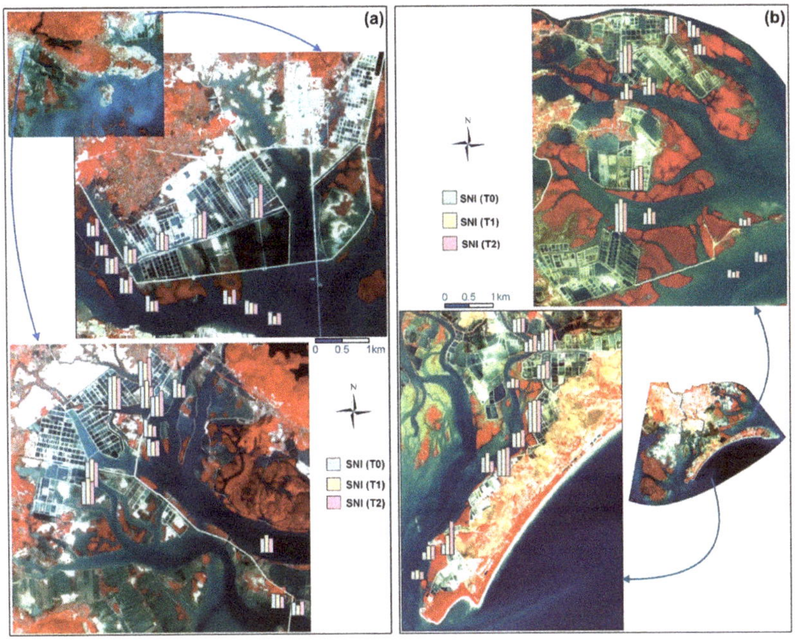

Figure 5. (**a**) The punctual spatial distribution of a sediment nutrient index (SNI) at sampling sites in Ha Long, Quang Ninh, Vietnam. (**b**) Punctual spatial distribution of patterns of SNI at sampling sites in Mong Cai, Quang Ninh, Vietnam. Adapted from Bui et al. [39]. Copyright © 2013, Springer Nature.

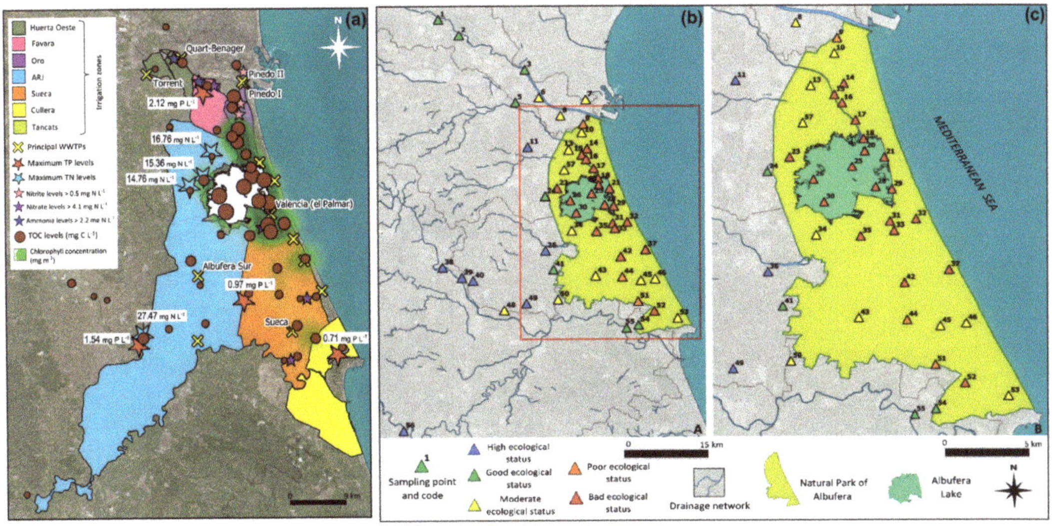

Figure 6. Natural Park of Albufera in Valencia, Spain. (**a**) Irrigation zones, urban contextualization, and point spatial distribution of the maximum levels of TP, TN, nitrite, nitrate, ammonium nitrogen, average concentrations of TOC, and phytoplanktonic chlorophyll. (**b**) The ecological potential point spatial distribution limit of the Natural Park of Albufera. (**c**) Ecological potential point spatial distribution in Albufera Lake. Adapted from Vera et al. [67]. Copyright © 2022 MDPI, Basel.

3.4.2. Interpolation Techniques

The use of the interpolation technique has increased in environmental pollution studies [42]. Interpolation, also known as gridding, involves estimating the values of unknown points based on known points [105]. Inverse distance weighting (IDW) is a widely used deterministic interpolation technique known for its simplicity and effectiveness in spatial analyses [42]. This method relies on the relationship between attribute values of pairs of points, where similarity decreases as the distance between locations increases [106]. The accuracy of the interpolated surfaces depends on the weighting power used, which in turn is associated with the samples' local coefficient of variation (CV) [36].

Some studies have employed this interpolation method to generate spatial mapping distributions of PC parameters [13,42,58,69,74], heavy metals [12,24,35,36,73], or both [24,54,61,71] and to discern spatial patterns and variations in water quality. A significant finding from these studies is the recognition of variations across seasons on water quality parameters and pollutants, influenced by natural factors such as high precipitation, seasonal runoff, and anthropogenic factors like shipping, fishing, tourism activities, and idol immersion activities. Similarly, PC values and POC concentrations have been jointly assessed [72,78] to determine the significance of ongoing development in TW areas, aiming to enhance diagnoses and identify critical hazard points stemming from these compounds.

On the other hand, some studies evaluate indicators and combine the IDW interpolation technique with a multivariate statistical analysis to identify sources of contamination and assess the ecological and health risks associated with various pollutants. An example is the study of Wang et al. [12] on Kaozhouyang Bay in Guangdong Province, China, where the bay receives discharges and runoff from seven rivers. Using the IDW technique, the distribution patterns of heavy metals in surface sediments were determined. The maps revealed similar distribution patterns for Cd, Ni, Zn, Hg, and As, suggesting a potential common source. The elevated Pb, Cr, and Cu concentrations could be attributed to the downstream movement and deposition of suspended sediments containing heavy metals compounded by local pollution sources. Two principal components (PCs) were identified, explaining 81.63% of the total variance. PC1, accounting for 53.50% of the variance, primarily consisted of Cd, Pb, Ni, Zn, Hg, and As, while PC2, explaining 28.13% of the variance, mainly comprised Cr, Ni, and Cu. Also, the spatial distribution of these components was analyzed using the IDW technique, revealing that regions impacted by PC1 were near urban areas, indicating anthropogenic influence. In contrast, PC2 impacts were observed near farm areas, suggesting contamination from agronomic practices (Figure 7). Concerningly, heavy metals from nearby industrial and agricultural areas can accumulate in bivalve species, posing risks to human consumers through food contamination. Although the heavy metal concentrations were lower than the allowable limits for human consumption, a 21% chance of toxicity incidence was identified by the spatial distribution map of the indicated mean PEL (probable effect level) quotient, an index to evaluate biological hazard and toxicity in sediments. Subsequently, the target hazard quotient (THQ) was calculated to assess non-carcinogenic health risks from exposure to toxic elements, with higher THQ and total THQ (TTHQ) values observed in residential areas compared to rural areas, indicating elevated health risks from bivalve consumption among exposed populations due to the levels exceeding safe thresholds.

In addition to the IDW interpolation method, kriging is another commonly used method in water quality assessment. The kriging method is used to interpolate the value of a random field at an unobserved location from observations at nearby locations [107]. Ordinary kriging also uses a semivariogram to quantify the spatial variability of regionalized variables [40], a measure of the spatial correlation between two points. It also provides a measure of the error or uncertainty so that the weights vary according to their spatial extent [45]. If kriging should be used and the data are not normally distributed, they must be transformed, for example, to a logarithmic scale [40]. Kriging is a moderately fast interpolator that can be accurate or smooth depending on the measurement model; it also uses statistical models that generate a wide variety of results, such as predictions, standard errors of prediction, and probability [37,45]. In kriging interpolation, the absolute value of the mean standard error (MSE) should be close to 0; minimize the root mean square error of prediction (RMSE), which should be close to the thematic standard error (TME); and the root mean square standard error (RMSS) should be close to 1 [37]. In the kriging analysis of variance, the semivariogram is a function of distance, and the method puts more emphasis on the distance of the monitoring sites than on the values of the monitoring sites. This means that a kriging variance analysis is a good option for improving the selection of the optimal sites for monitoring and management [38].

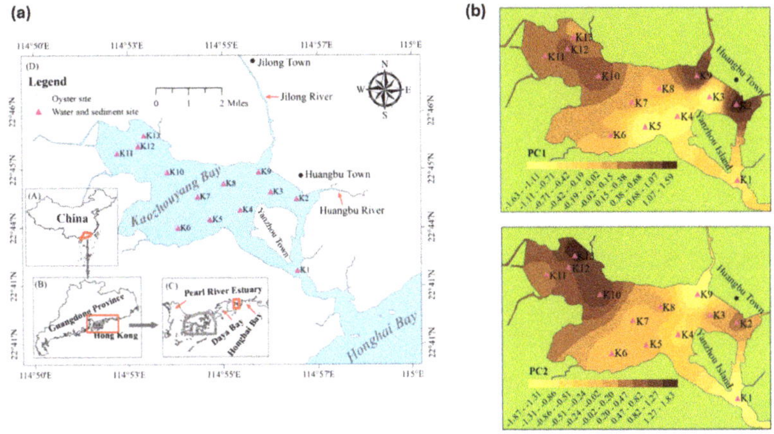

Figure 7. (**a**) Map of study area indicating location of Kaozhouyang Bay in China (A–C) and sampling sites in Kaozhouyang Bay. (**b**) Spatial distribution of factor scores of PC1 and PC2 using inverse distance weighting (IDW) technique in GIS. Taken from Wang et al. [12]. © 2018 Elsevier Ltd.

A series of studies [38,46,47,51,52] carried out in the Yangtze River estuary, China, employed the kriging interpolation method to predict the values of attributes at unsampled locations and to optimize monitoring networks. In the investigation by Shen et al. [38], PC parameters and heavy metals were evaluated at predefined control points. These variables were then used to establish a Seawater Environmental Quality Index (SEQI) and devise an optimal environmental monitoring network design. This method emphasizes the importance of the distance between monitoring sites, with more minor variances indicating better monitoring network quality and more abundant information about the marine environment. As a result, the authors expanded the number of monitoring locations from 42 to 59, concluding that this expansion enhanced the quality of the marine monitoring network.

In another application of the kriging method, Liu et al. [52] examined the distribution of polycyclic aromatic hydrocarbons (PAHs) within the same estuary, alongside their environmental repercussions, using various indices. The TEQBap index is commonly employed to assess the toxicity of PAHs, while the SQGQ index determines the potential impact of sediment-associated contaminants on aquatic organisms; both are utilized to evaluate biological hazards and toxicity. Additionally, a human health risk assessment was employed to calculate the risk, aiming to assess the potential biological effects of contaminant exposure. Subsequently, the obtained values for each index were interpolated using ordinary kriging. The results revealed a gradual decrease in TEQBap values from the inner estuary towards the adjacent sea, with elevated concentrations noted in the estuary's northern region during winter, attributable to heightened coal and gasoline combustion. The SQGQ method results indicated minimal adverse effects from pollutants, although the spatial distribution showed elevated values at the bay's bifurcations, but gradually diminishing towards the estuary's mouth. Furthermore, cancer risk (CR) and non-cancer hazard index (HI) values were interpolated using ordinary kriging in ArcGIS 10.0 software to extrapolate values for unsampled locations (Figure 8). The spatial distribution showed that the highest levels of cancer risk were detected in the area adjacent to the maritime area, which threatens the inhabitants of the near-shore area. Conversely, the non-cancer risk index exhibited relatively low levels, suggesting limited or no adverse health risks for local inhabitants. The spatial analysis of this work made it possible to assess the risks of PAHs to the environment and human health.

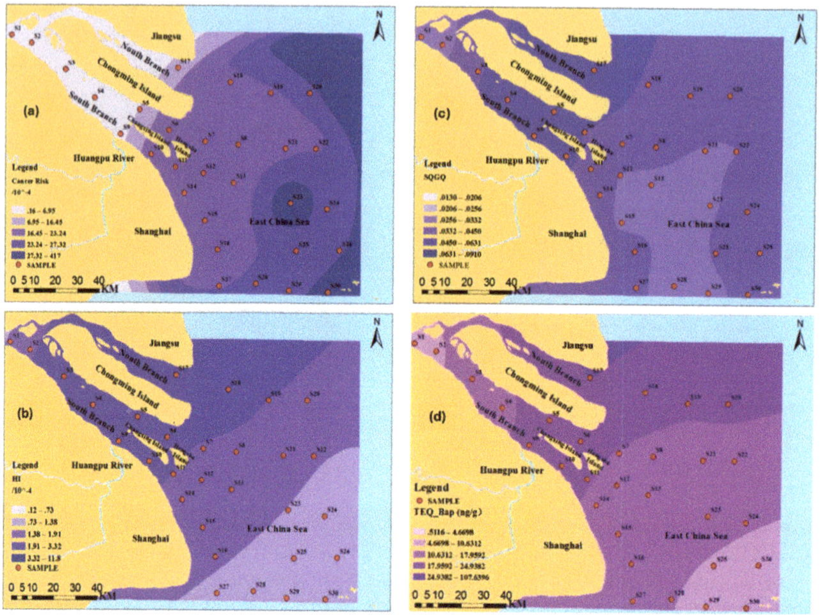

Figure 8. The spatial distribution of cancer risk (**a**), non-cancer hazard index (HI) (**b**), SQGQ index (c), and TEQBaP index (**d**) in the Yangtze River estuary, China. Adapted from Liu et al. [52]. © 2016 Elsevier Ltd.

Kriging has played a significant role in various studies focusing on environmental factors. It has been utilized to estimate sites of heavy metal pollution, highlighting sediment and water as primary sinks for these pollutants [15]. Moreover, it aided in identifying suitable areas for aquaculture by interpolating water quality parameters [33]. Yang investigated the relationship between landscape characteristics and estuarine nitrogen loading and illustrated the impact of urban sprawl on Pensacola Bay, USA [34]. Additionally, kriging was central in evaluating mercury concentrations in Lake Taihu, revealing their distribution patterns and indicating elevated concentrations in enclosed and semi-enclosed water bodies compared to open areas, suggesting anthropogenic influences [37]. Furthermore, it facilitated the assessment of cadmium, lead [40], and petroleum hydrocarbon spatial concentrations [45] in the analysis of major and trace metal variations in marine sediments [48]. Kriging enabled the determination of ecological risk by interpolating heavy metals and PC parameters in the Karavasta Lagoon [75].

Finally, another interpolation method utilized is Kernel Interpolation with Barrier. This method enables the estimation of values between known points on a map. Using information from scattered points, the method employs a moving window to calculate the shortest distance between two points and connects them with straight lines, creating a smooth surface between known points [108]. In other words, it estimates regression coefficients to prevent instability in the calculation process. This method is employed in areas where the landscape or geographic conditions change abruptly, which may influence the interpolation [109].

This method was employed to determine the pollution history in Ria Formosa, Portugal [62], by analyzing heavy metals in sediments, interpolating their concentration, and estimating the enrichment factor (EF). The analysis showed that while the system appears largely undisturbed, surface sediments exhibit significant contamination, with high EF observed for As, Cu, Pb, and Zn. Moreover, the interpolation of the enrichment index also pointed to diffuse contamination, primarily originating from stormwater drains near major urban areas, as the most significant contributor of metals to the system.

Expanding on investigations utilizing indices, numerous studies have interpolated a wide range of indices related to pollution, potential ecological risk, ecosystem health, and health risk to assess, monitor, and detect sources of contamination [13,24,35,55,69,72–74,76]. Among the identified pollution sources for TW are aquaculture and agricultural practices, disposal of municipal waste, discharge of untreated agricultural sewage, industry, and urbanization.

As can be seen, interpolation techniques have played a role in the study of TW pollution by providing valuable insights into spatial patterns and variations in key parameters such as water quality indicators, heavy metal concentrations, and ecological risk assessments. Such interpolation techniques serve as essential tools for environmental status determination, as a starting point for future management processes to protect these ecosystems and safeguard human health.

3.4.3. Complex Spatial Models

Complex models and GIS are complementary tools that, when working in tandem, offer a comprehensive and robust approach to ecosystem management. Additionally, the integration of complex models and GIS data provides the ability to assess the impact of environmental changes on human health. The analyzed studies primarily employed models that utilize indices. These indices calculate a single value for each spatial unit (e.g., pixel, grid cell) and subsequently generate a classified map based on the calculated values.

In the realm of prediction/simulation models, Yang's study [34] utilized a multivariate statistical analysis and regression modeling to simulate nitrogen loading based on landscape characteristics. The results showed that landscape features predominantly explained nitrogen variability, although the impact of urban expansion also contributes to this variability. In a similar work, Johnson et al. [41] developed a Total Maximum Daily Load (TMDL) model to simulate the loads and concentrations of coliform bacteria in coastal systems. Employing equations from continuously stirred tank reactors and plug-flow reactors, this model routes loads from spatially distributed point and nonpoint sources through a watershed, degrading via first-order kinetics. They simulated bacterial loads in the Copano Bay watershed in Southeast Texas by incorporating bacterial load data and hydrological characteristics. The study revealed spatial variations in decay values, suggesting potential regrowth and resuspension in specific areas.

El-Zeiny and El-Kafrawy [53] utilized empirical models for PC parameters (BOD, TN, and TP) in conjunction with a GIS model to pinpoint areas with high pollution levels categorized into three classes: high (class 1), moderate (class 2), and low (class 3) (Figure 9). Their results revealed that Lake Burullus faces contamination from diverse sources, predominantly domestic and agricultural runoff. Furthermore, shallow waters influenced by human activities exhibited heightened levels of the analyzed contaminants.

Boateng et al. [64] described a study on eight coastal lagoons in Tema and Winneba along the Ghanaian coast to evaluate the potential impact of climate change-induced inundation on various land uses in the region. They analyzed 2100 scenarios to predict sea-level rise and determined vulnerability assessments. Maps illustrating sea-level rise (SLR) and rainfall inundation scenarios were created to identify flood-prone areas. High-resolution georeferenced panchromatic bands from the Shuttle Radar Topographic Mission (SRTM) for Ghana were used to assess flood extent and associated uncertainty. These data, obtained from the Global Land Cover Facility, were integrated into ERDAS Imagine and overlaid on the 2002 topographic map of Ghana at a 1:50,000 scale. Coordinates and point heights were validated using data from the topographic map. Subsequently, using ERDAS Virtual GIS, three inundation layers were superimposed on the image to represent sea level rises of 1 m (mean projection for 2100), 2 m (upper limit projection), and 5 m (long-term scenario involving the West Antarctic Ice Sheet melting). The study highlighted the significant impact of a 2 m sea level rise on lagoons and surrounding land, with levels below 2 m causing minimal flooding. Storm surges could exacerbate the erosion of barriers, potentially leading to breaches and coastal flooding. Moreover, the study emphasized the greater risk of inland flooding from rainfall compared to seafront flooding, with increased rainfall runoff posing a threat of carrying pollutants into the lagoons. These findings highlight the importance of measures to address future climate change scenarios and inform the development of adaptation strategies and implementation recommendations.

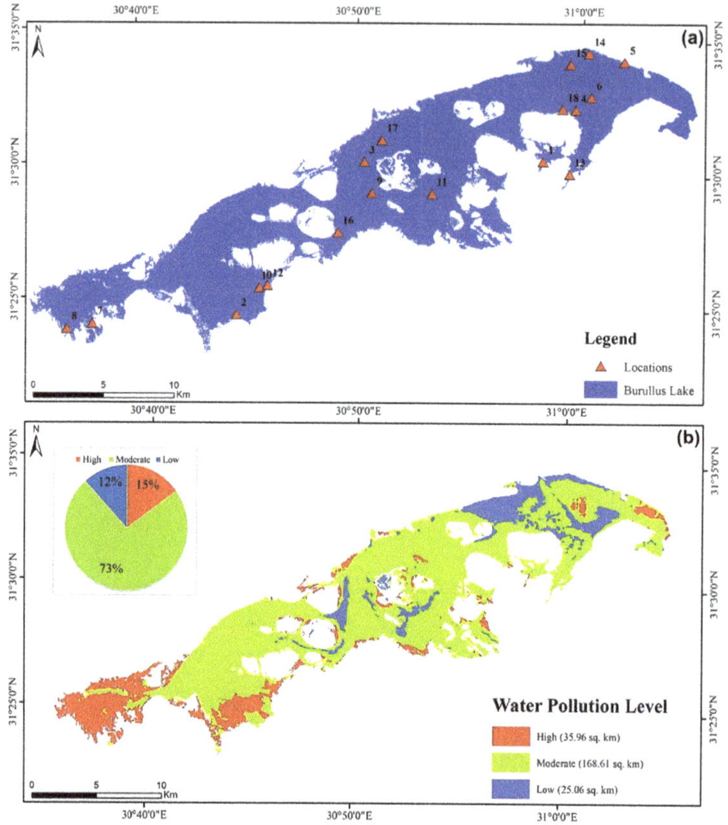

Figure 9. (**a**) Spatial distribution of eighteen sampling points, Lake Burullus, Egypt. (**b**) Prediction of water pollution level in Lake Burullus, applying empirical complex models. Adapted from El-Zeiny and El-Kafrawy [53], with permission from authors.

Land use dynamics models are useful for understanding and predicting how changes in land occupation affect natural resources, the environment, and society, providing information for land management planning. In the study by Abd El-Hamid et al. [65], a simulation model combining cellular automata and Markov chains was developed to analyze land use changes in three wetlands of Egypt. The aim was to explore how these changes in land use and land cover (LULC) affect the water quality of the lakes. After assessing land use patterns from 2011 and 2021, the model was capable of predicting land use for 2031 (Figure 10). This result, along with data on PC parameter concentrations for 2011 and 2021 and an assessment of ecosystem services, allowed the identification of urgent intervention regarding changes in land use and vegetation classes.

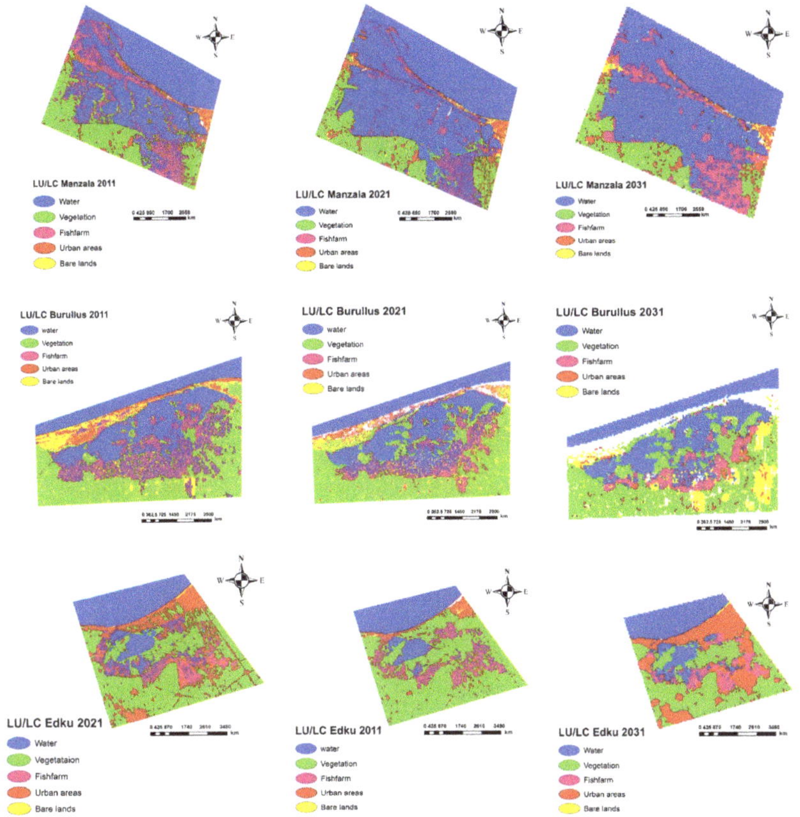

Figure 10. Land use and land cover (LULC) of the Nile Delta wetlands for 2011 and 2021, along with their simulation for 2031. Taken from Abd El-Hamid et al. [65]. © 2020 Elsevier Ltd.

Another example is the one of Zhao et al. [70], where the influence of land use patterns on the spatial distribution of dissolved PCBs and organochlorine pesticides (OCPs) was examined using Land Use Regression (LUR) in the Narragansett watershed–coastal area. This model established relationships between concentrations of the pollutants of concern and key descriptive variables such as population density, building density, road networks, sewer areas, impervious surface coverage, and land use classes. The findings indicated that contaminant levels in urban and built-up regions were higher than in other areas, with changes in land use being the primary drivers of this distribution pattern. Furthermore, it was suggested that historical levels of PCBs in surface water could be linked to PCBs present in construction materials and equipment, such as sealants, paints, and adhesives, which may continue to be released as buildings age. A similar approach was adopted by Morant et al. [16], who developed a land use model to quantify the primary pressures on water bodies, predicting the potential impacts of these pressures on their ecological status in Mediterranean lentic ecosystems.

Sensitivity and contamination risk models offer crucial frameworks for assessing environmental vulnerability and predicting the likelihood of contamination events, facilitating proactive risk management and mitigation strategies. An example is the study by El-Alfy et al. [13], who developed a model to investigate the susceptibility to contamination and the probability of eutrophication in Lake Burullus. Multivariate statistical analyses and proximity analyses were employed for this purpose. The study considered water quality parameters that could influence the likelihood of eutrophication in the former case. Meanwhile, in the latter case, proximity factors of anthropogenic activities, such as drains; industrial, agricultural, and urban areas; and fish farms, were considered by assigning weights based on their distance to Lake Burullus. As expected, the results identified that the most susceptible regions to contamination are those where industrial activities are located and drain outlets are concentrated.

Several other research studies have been carried out using complex spatial models to improve the understanding of pollution risks in coastal areas. The aforementioned studies include the development of a novel WebGIS observatory platform dedicated to risk assessment, emergency preparedness, and response [44]. Additionally, efforts have been made to pinpoint hotspots of PAH pollution using Voronoi maps and Fuzzy Membership Functions [78], conduct source–ecological risk assessments by establishing geochemical baseline values for metalloids [71], and assess heavy metal contamination in water and sediment through a cluster analysis, correlation coefficients, and a factor analysis [15]. Furthermore, a multi-thematic overlay analysis has identified priority pollution zones for protection [50]. A notable approach involved the integration of positive matrix factorization (PMF) and GIS, enabling the identification of PAH occurrence and their contamination sources [46,77].

3.4.4. Remote Sensing

Remote sensing is a powerful tool for acquiring and analyzing information about specific characteristics of phenomena, objects, or materials without direct contact. Typically, this involves measuring the electromagnetic properties of objects using sensors mounted on aircraft or satellites orbiting the Earth. Integrated within the GIS framework, remote sensing facilitates the collection and management of both field and remotely sensed data [110]. It also offers an alternative approach to increase spatial and temporal coverage, complementing traditional techniques for water quality monitoring [111]. This capability is particularly advantageous in inland and near-coastal transitional waters, where remote sensing can accurately measure water quality parameters such as chlorophyll-a, suspended sediments, and other pollutants [112].

In the reviewed articles, authors employed remote sensing techniques utilizing digital image processing algorithms and various methods for image visualization, enhancement, and interpretation. Through these approaches, it has been possible to identify the distribution of water quality parameters [21,65], as well as levels of chlorophyll-a [63] and phytoplankton distribution [68]. Specifically, Landsat-8 data were employed to predict and assess the spatial variation and distribution of salinity, SO_4, and $CaCO_3$ in the Al-Hawizeh marsh in southern Iraq during winter and autumn in 2017 [21]. In the process, band value extraction and spatial distribution techniques were employed to derive quantitative information from specific bands of the Landsat-8 imagery. Surface water samples from the marsh underwent a chemical analysis to determine the levels of these parameters, and subsequently, water quality equations were developed to evaluate, monitor, and map their distribution. For salinity assessment, the salinity index based on Bands 6 (Shortwave Infrared—SWIR, 1.57–1.65 μm) and 11 (Thermal Infrared—TIRS2, 11.5–12.51 μm) from Landsat-8 was employed. An equation derived from Landsat-8 salinity output data and field measurements of SO_4 and $CaCO_3$ was used to estimate mineral values. Results indicated lower salinity, SO_4, and $CaCO_3$ levels during winter, with higher concentrations observed in autumn, particularly notable in the eastern and southeastern regions of the marsh. The images' spectral, spatial, and temporal resolution facilitated a precise assessment of spatial and temporal variations in these parameters.

In the study by Mortula et al. [63], they employed a WorldView-2 satellite image to investigate chlorophyll-a levels in Dubai Creek, USA. A band ratio model derived from satellite imagery to estimate chlorophyll-a concentration was applied. Additionally, a regression model incorporating eutrophication parameters, such as the total nitrogen–orthophosphate (TN/P) ratio, was developed. The regression analysis revealed a strong correlation between TN/P and chlorophyll-a, highlighting the significant impact of nutrients on eutrophication. The study emphasizes the importance of considering the spectral characteristics of the water column for accurate chlorophyll-a estimation and its association with nutrient content. Moreover, the model was validated using in situ data and correlated with eutrophication indicators. The analysis identified chlorophyll-a concentrations exceeding local limits, particularly in the lagoon area (Figure 11), attributed to anthropogenic activities and sewage discharge.

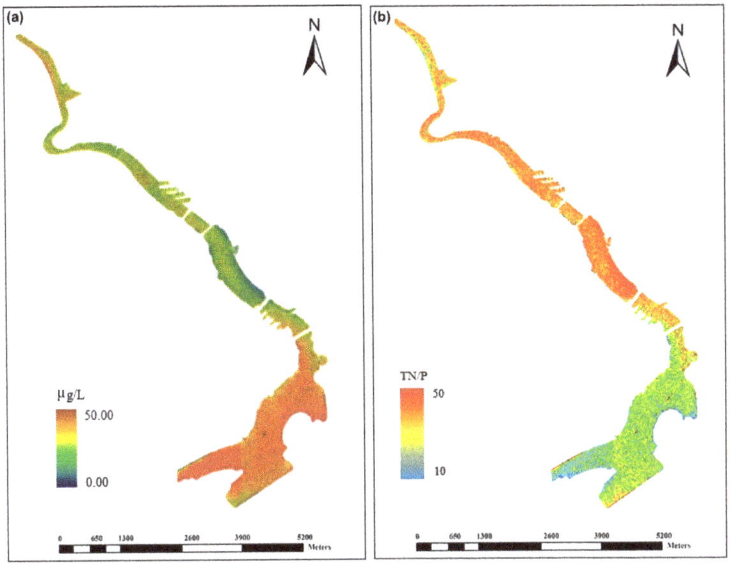

Figure 11. (**a**) Chlorophyll-a map extracted from WorldView-2 imagery of Dubai Creek. (**b**) Total nitrogen to phosphorus (TN/P) ratio (mass/mass). Taken from Mortula et al. [63]. Copyright © 2020 MDPI, Basel.

Various studies have employed diverse techniques and satellite imagery types to identify land cover, land loss, and landscape changes to assess pollution in coastal water bodies [13,15,16,34–36,53,57,60,65,72]. These analyses have utilized Google Earth Pro images [16], high-resolution aerial photos [60], SPOT-5 satellite images [35], Landsat images [13,15,34,53,65,72], and Airborne Visible/Infrared (AVIRIS) imagery [57]. For instance, a land use/land cover change analysis has been described by comparing satellite images from different periods to identify alterations in land cover [15,36,72]. Moreover, specific studies have been undertaken to analyze land loss, such as segmenting marsh shorelines into oil-affected and non-affected areas and calculating land loss rates [57]. These remote sensing approaches have been essential for understanding land dynamics and their effects on coastal water bodies.

Specifically, Essel et al. [60] published a study to map and evaluate the habitat of Fosu Lagoon, located in Cape Coast, southeastern Ghana, using GIS and remote sensing. One high-resolution aerial photograph for each study year (2009 and 2017) was acquired from the Ghana Town and Country Planning Department, with a ground sampling distance (GSD or pixel size) of 0.39 m, to map the study area. An object-based classification technique was then applied using eCognition software version 9.5, identifying classes such as standing water, mangrove vegetation, semi-natural mangrove, coastal marsh, semi-natural marsh, scrub, and induced shrub. To ensure classification accuracy, field verification was conducted at 20 randomly selected points, and the ArcGIS confusion matrix calculation tool was utilized to determine overall accuracy and the Kappa coefficient, providing an assessment of classification accuracy. The accuracy for the 2009 map was 92% with a Kappa coefficient of 0.8599, and for the 2017 map, the accuracy was 90% with a Kappa coefficient of 0.8251, both considered satisfactory. The 2009 and 2017 habitat maps of the lagoon identified a significant decline in habitat size, a considerable fragmentation of ecosystems, and significant changes in land use and land cover, significantly impacting local populations.

Advanced remote sensing techniques were utilized to assess the impact of marsh contamination on landscape degradation and land loss in three time periods resulting from the 2010 BP oil spill on the Deepwater Horizon (DWH) platform in Barataria Bay, USA [57]. This included the production of oil maps through Airborne Visible/Infrared Imaging Spectrometer (AVIRIS) imagery and the development of a Multiple Endmember Spectral Mixture Analysis (MESMA) model to identify various vegetation and soil types, including areas covered by oil in marshlands. Additionally, changes in coastlines were mapped using QuickBird-2 and WorldView images. The marsh coastlines were divided into segments with and without oil, and land loss rates were computed to determine significant differences between affected and unaffected regions. Moreover, land loss rates attributed to oil were estimated by adjusting background rates before and after the spill. To validate these findings, binary classification maps of marsh and open water coverage were generated for each image using the Normalized Difference Vegetation Index (NDVI). Results indicated that the oil spill led to a land loss increase of over 50%, but land loss rates reverted to background levels within 3 to 6 years post-spill (Figure 12).

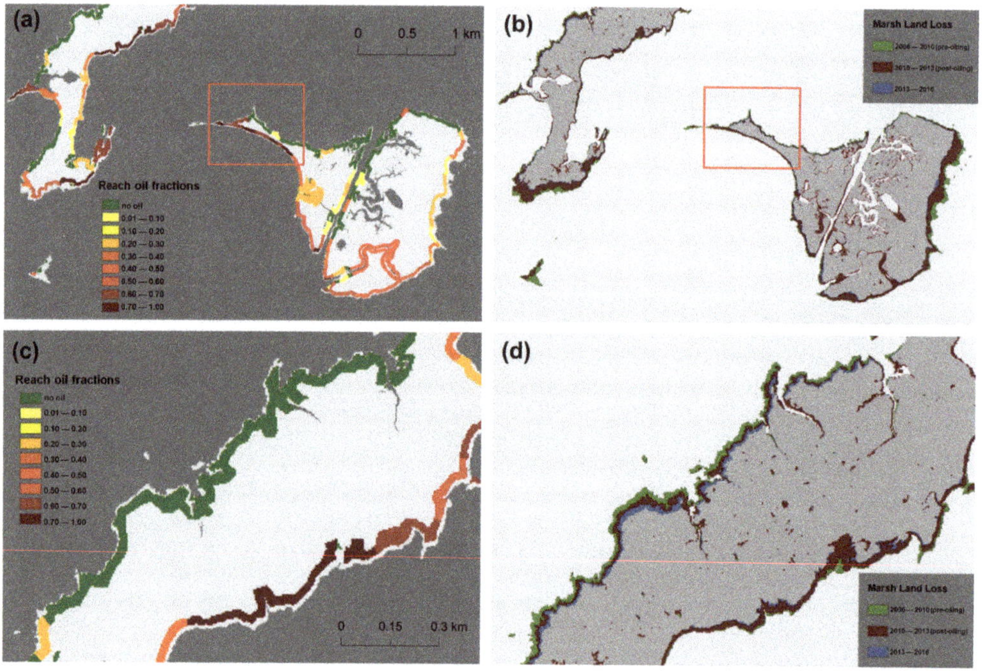

Figure 12. (**a**,**c**) Distribution of mean oil fractions in different shoreline zones in Barataria Bay, USA. (**b**,**d**) Marshland loss along same reaches over three periods. Adapted from Beland et al. [57]. Copyright © 2017 PLOS.

Remote sensing has been employed for a diverse range of analyses, including identifying pollutant distribution and changes in land cover, which are often linked to pollution in transitional or coastal waters. Compared to conventional in situ measurements, remote sensing provides a comprehensive view of the water body, allowing for a more cost-effective and reliable monitoring of quantitative parameters. When combined with in situ measurements for validation purposes, remote sensing and GIS techniques effectively monitor water quality across various water bodies [14].

4. Perspective

As can be seen, the diversity of geospatial technologies and their combination facilitates spatial monitoring of water quality parameters, pollutant concentrations, and ecological indicators, enabling real-time assessment of the environmental status of TWs, which are susceptible to pollution from various anthropogenic sources, including industrial discharge, agricultural runoff, and urban sewage. The contamination of these ecosystems poses substantial risks to human health through direct exposure to polluted water and consuming contaminated seafood. Exposure to polluted TW can adversely affect human health, ranging from acute illnesses to chronic diseases. Contaminants such as heavy metals and persistent organic pollutants (POPs) have been associated with neurological disorders, developmental abnormalities, reproductive impairments, and carcinogenic effects. Furthermore, microbial pollution from sewage discharge and agricultural runoff can lead to waterborne diseases such as gastroenteritis, hepatitis, and cholera, posing significant public health concerns, particularly in communities reliant on these waters for drinking, bathing, and recreational activities. Vulnerable populations, such as children, pregnant women, and indigenous communities, are disproportionately affected by pollution-related health disparities. Subsistence fishermen and indigenous communities relying on traditional fishing practices are at heightened risk of exposure to contaminated seafood, exacerbating health disparities among vulnerable populations.

Although it was not detected in the studies analyzed, GIS-based exposure modeling may allow quantifying human exposure to these contaminants, identifying vulnerable populations and assessing health risks associated with different pollution levels. Integrating environmental data, population demographics, and health outcomes with GIS tools and other geospatial technologies facilitates the identification of pollution "hotspots" where interventions are most urgently needed to prevent adverse health effects. In addition, incorporating GTS into pollution management strategies would allow decision-makers to promote equity, justice, and public health for all communities affected by pollution in TW.

Future research in these areas should increase remote sensing studies to gain insights into environmental factors that influence disease outbreaks, distribution, and risk. This information is vital for disease surveillance, risk mapping, and informing public health interventions [113,114]. As sensor technology advances and integrates with other geospatial information, remote sensing would support the development of more comprehensive and predictive public health strategies for TW. Additionally, studies monitoring the pollutants such as micropollutants, emerging pollutants, or antibiotic-resistant microorganisms are needed.

5. Conclusions

Transitional waters are relevant ecosystems due to the different roles and services they provide, playing a central role in environmental sustainability and human well-being. However, they are facing increasing threats, particularly from anthropogenic pollution. To diagnose the environmental state of TW, GTS have become increasingly valuable for mapping pollution in TW. These technologies effectively characterize the spatial distribution of pollutants, mainly from anthropogenic point sources. Integrating the diversity of geospatial technologies would help to better understand pollution patterns within these dynamic ecosystems. Future research should advance our understanding of TW's interactions between pollutants, ecosystems, and human health. Long-term monitoring programs, epidemiological studies, and risk assessments are essential for identifying emerging contaminants, assessing their health impacts, and informing evidence-based management strategies. Additionally, community-based approaches, citizen science initiatives, and environmental education efforts can promote community participation in pollution monitoring and mitigation efforts.

Supplementary Materials: The following supporting information can be downloaded at: https://www.mdpi.com/article/10.3390/ijgi13060196/s1, Table S1: Pollution indices applied in the Transitional Waters studies. References [115–143] are cited in the Supplementary Materials.

Author Contributions: Conceptualization, Itzel Arroyo-Ortega and Eduardo Torres; methodology, Itzel Arroyo-Ortega and Yaselda Chavarin-Pineda; formal analysis, Itzel Arroyo-Ortega and Eduardo Torres; investigation, Itzel Arroyo-Ortega; writing—original draft preparation, Itzel Arroyo-Ortega and Yaselda Chavarin-Pineda; writing—review and editing, Eduardo Torres. All authors have read and agreed to the published version of the manuscript.

Funding: This research received no external funding.

Data Availability Statement: No new data were created or analyzed in this study. Data sharing is not applicable to this article.

Acknowledgments: Itzel Arroyo-Ortega wants to express her gratitude to the Consejo Nacional de Humanidades, Ciencias y Tecnologías (CONAHCYT) and its program "Investigadoras e Investigadores por México".

Conflicts of Interest: The authors declare no conflicts of interest.

References

1. Chapman, P.M.; Wang, F.; Caeiro, S.S. Assessing and Managing Sediment Contamination in Transitional Waters. *Environ. Int.* **2013**, *55*, 71–91. [CrossRef]
2. Zaldívar, J.; Cardoso, A.C.; Viaroli, P.; De Wit, R.; Ibañez, C.; Reizopoulou, S.; Razinkovas, A.; Basset, A.; Holmer, M.; Murray, N. Eutrophication in Transitional Waters: An Overview. *TWM Transit. Waters Monogr.* **2008**, *1*, 1–78. [CrossRef]
3. Facca, C. Ecological Status Assessment of Transitional Waters. *Water* **2020**, *12*, 3159. [CrossRef]
4. Tagliapietra, D.; Sigovini, M.; Ghirardini, A.V. A Review of Terms and Definitions to Categorise Estuaries, Lagoons and Associated Environments. *Mar. Freshw. Res.* **2009**, *60*, 497–509. [CrossRef]
5. Feola, A.; Ponis, E.; Cornello, M.; Busà, R.B.; Cacciatore, F.; Oselladore, F.; Matticchio, B.; Canesso, D.; Sponga, S.; Peretti, P.; et al. An Integrated Approach for Evaluating the Restoration of the Salinity Gradient in Transitional Waters: Monitoring and Numerical Modeling in the Life Lagoon Refresh Case Study. *Environments* **2022**, *9*, 31. [CrossRef]
6. O'Brien, P.A.J.; Asteman, I.P.; Bouchet, V.M.P. Benthic Foraminiferal Indices and Environmental Quality Assessment of Transitional Waters: A Review of Current Challenges and Future Research Perspectives. *Water* **2021**, *13*, 1898. [CrossRef]
7. Elliott, M.; Day, J.W.; Ramachandran, R.; Wolanski, E.; Fang, Q.; Sheehan, M.R.; Seen, A.J.; Ellison, J.C. A Synthesis: What Is the Future for Coasts, Estuaries, Deltas and Other Transitional Habitats in 2050 and Beyond? In *Coasts and Estuaries: The Future*; Elsevier Inc.: Amsterdam, The Netherlands, 2019; pp. 1–28, ISBN 9780128140048.
8. Pérez-Ruzafa, A.; Pérez-Ruzafa, I.M.; Newton, A.; Marcos, C. Coastal Lagoons: Environmental Variability, Ecosystem Complexity, and Goods and Services Uniformity. In *Coasts and Estuaries: The Future*; Elsevier Inc.: Amsterdam, The Netherlands, 2019; pp. 253–276, ISBN 9780128140048.
9. Nilsson, H.; Povilanskas, R.; Stybel, N. (Eds.) *Transboundary Management of Transitional Waters—Code of Conduct and Good Practice Examples*; The Coastal Union Germany: Rostock, Germany, 2012; ISBN 9783939206040.
10. Borja, A.; Basset, A.; Bricker, S.; Dauvin, J.C.; Elliott, M.; Harrison, T.; Marques, J.C.; Weisberg, S.B.; West, R. Classifying Ecological Quality and Integrity of Estuaries. In *Treatise on Estuarine and Coastal Science*; Academic Press: Cambridge, MA, USA, 2012; Volume 1, pp. 125–162, ISBN 9780080878850.
11. Liu, R.; Guo, L.; Men, C.; Wang, Q.; Miao, Y.; Shen, Z. Spatial-Temporal Variation of Heavy Metals' Sources in the Surface Sediments of the Yangtze River Estuary. *Mar. Pollut. Bull.* **2019**, *138*, 526–533. [CrossRef]
12. Wang, X.-N.; Gu, Y.-G.; Wang, Z.-H.; Ke, C.-L.; Mo, M.-S. Biological Risk Assessment of Heavy Metals in Sediments and Health Risk Assessment in Bivalve Mollusks from Kaozhouyang Bay, South China. *Mar. Pollut. Bull.* **2018**, *133*, 312–319. [CrossRef] [PubMed]
13. El-Alfy, M.A.; Darwish, D.H.; Basiony, A.I.; Elnaggar, A.A. GIS-Based Study on the Environmental Sensitivity to Pollution and Susceptibility to Eutrophication in Burullus Lake, Egypt. *Mar. Geod.* **2021**, *44*, 554–572. [CrossRef]
14. Vallidevi, K.; Gopinath, K.P.; Nagarajan, K.K.; Prakash, D.G.; Sudhamsu, G.; Sudhish, S.; Al-Zahrani, S.A. Water Pollution Monitoring through Remote Sensing. *Curr. Anal. Chem.* **2020**, *17*, 802–814. [CrossRef]

15. Arnous, M.O.; Hassan, M.A.A. Heavy Metals Risk Assessment in Water and Bottom Sediments of the Eastern Part of Lake Manzala, Egypt, Based on Remote Sensing and GIS. *Arab. J. Geosci.* **2015**, *8*, 7899–7918. [CrossRef]
16. Morant, D.; Perennou, C.; Camacho, A. Assessment of the Pressure Level over Lentic Waterbodies through the Estimation of Land Uses in the Catchment and Hydro-Morphological Alterations: The Luples Method. *Appl. Sci.* **2021**, *11*, 1633. [CrossRef]
17. Reddy, G.P.O. Geospatial Technologies in Land Resources Mapping, Monitoring, and Management: An Overview. In *Geospatial Technologies in Land Resources Mapping, Monitoring and Management*; Reddy, G.P.O., Singh, S.K., Eds.; Springer International Publishing: Cham, Switzerland, 2018; Volume 21, pp. 1–18.
18. Masood, A.; Aslam, M.; Pham, Q.B.; Khan, W.; Masood, S. Integrating Water Quality Index, GIS and Multivariate Statistical Techniques towards a Better Understanding of Drinking Water Quality. *Environ. Sci. Pollut. Res.* **2022**, *29*, 26860–26876. [CrossRef] [PubMed]
19. Lateef, Z.Q.; Al-Madhhachi, A.S.T.; Sachit, D.E. Evaluation of Water Quality Parameters in Shatt Al-Arab, Southern Iraq, Using Spatial Analysis. *Hydrology* **2020**, *7*, 79. [CrossRef]
20. Yan, C.A.; Zhang, W.; Zhang, Z.; Liu, Y.; Deng, C.; Nie, N. Assessment of Water Quality and Identification of Polluted Risky Regions Based on Field Observations & GIS in the Honghe River Watershed, China. *PLoS ONE* **2015**, *10*, e0119130. [CrossRef]
21. Hasab, H.A.; Jawad, H.A.; Dibs, H.; Hussain, H.M.; Al-Ansari, N. Evaluation of Water Quality Parameters in Marshes Zone Southern of Iraq Based on Remote Sensing and GIS Techniques. *Water Air Soil. Pollut.* **2020**, *231*, 183. [CrossRef]
22. Malcangio, D.; Manella, N.; Ungaro, N. Environmental Quality Characteristics of the Apulian Transitional Waters. Case Study: Lagoons of Lesina and Varano (Italy). *Aquat. Ecosyst. Health Manag.* **2020**, *23*, 427–435. [CrossRef]
23. Pascual-Aguilar, J.; Andreu, V.; Gimeno-García, E.; Picó, Y. Current Anthropogenic Pressures on Agro-Ecological Protected Coastal Wetlands. *Sci. Total Environ.* **2015**, *503–504*, 190–199. [CrossRef]
24. Antony, S.; Unnikrishnan, K.; Aswin, S.; Dev, V.V.; Arun, V.; Krishnan, K.A. Heavy Metals in Coral Reef Sediments of Kavaratti Island, India: An Integrated Quality Assessment Using GIS and Pollution Indicators. *Mar. Pollut. Bull.* **2022**, *180*, 113721. [CrossRef]
25. European Commission Directive 2000/60/EC of the European Parliament and of the Council of 23 October 2000 Establishing a Framework for Community Action in the Field of Water Policy. *Off. J. Eur. Communities* **2000**, *72*.
26. Environmental Protection Agency Coastal Waters. Available online: https://www.epa.gov/report-environment/coastal-waters (accessed on 8 February 2023).
27. Cervantes, M. Conceptos Fundamentales Sobre Ecosistemas Acuáticos y Su Estado En México. In *Perspectivas Sobre Conservación de Ecosistemas Acuáticos en México*; Instituto Nacional de Ecología y Cambio Climático (INECC): Mexico City, Mexico, 2007; pp. 37–67.
28. Dos Santos Sá, A.K.D.; Cutrim, M.V.J.; do Nascimento Feitosa, F.A.; de Jesus Flores-Montes, M.; Cavalcanti, L.F.; dos Santos Costa, D.; da Cruz, Q.S. Multiple Stressors Influencing the General Eutrophication Status of Transitional Waters of the Brazilian Tropical Coast: An Approach Utilizing the Pressure, State, and Response (PSR) Framework. *J. Sea Res.* **2022**, *189*, 102282. [CrossRef]
29. Zamboni, A.; Nicolodi, J.L.; Fonseca Barroso, G.; Serrano Léllis, F.; Nunes Garcia, A. La gestión integrada de zonas costeras y cuencas hidrográficas en Brasil. In Proceedings of the Libro del II Congreso Andaluz de Desarrollo Sostenible: "Una Mirada desde las Ciencias Ambientales a Nuestra Costas", Cadiz, Spain, 12–14 April 2007; pp. 65–86.
30. Avella, F.; Osorio, A.; Parra, E.; Burgos, S.; Vilardy, S.; Botero, C.; Ramos, A.; Mendoza, J.; Sierra, P.; López, Á.; et al. Gestión Del Litoral En Colombia. Reto de Un País Con Tres Costas. *Manejo Costero Integrado Política Pública Iberoamérica Diagnóstico Necesidad Cambio* **2010**, *26*, 175–209.
31. Van Eck, N.J.; Waltman, L. *VOSviewer Manual*; Leiden University: Leiden, The Netherlands, 2012.
32. Kharroubi, A.; Gargouri, D.; Baati, H.; Azri, C. Assessment of Sediment Quality in the Mediterranean Sea-Boughrara Lagoon Exchange Areas (Southeastern Tunisia): GIS Approach-Based Chemometric Methods. *Environ. Monit. Assess.* **2012**, *184*, 4001–4014. [CrossRef]
33. Silva, C.; Yáñez, E.; Martín-Díaz, M.L.; DelValls, T.A. Assessing a Bioremediation Strategy in a Shallow Coastal System Affected by a Fish Farm Culture—Application of GIS and Shellfish Dynamic Models in the Rio San Pedro, SW Spain. *Mar. Pollut. Bull.* **2012**, *64*, 751–765. [CrossRef] [PubMed]
34. Yang, X. An Assessment of Landscape Characteristics Affecting Estuarine Nitrogen Loading in an Urban Watershed. *J. Environ. Manag.* **2012**, *94*, 50–60. [CrossRef]
35. Maanan, M.; Landesman, C.; Maanan, M.; Zourarah, B.; Fattal, P.; Sahabi, M. Evaluation of the Anthropogenic Influx of Metal and Metalloid Contaminants into the Moulay Bousselham Lagoon, Morocco, Using Chemometric Methods Coupled to Geographical Information Systems. *Environ. Sci. Pollut. Res.* **2013**, *20*, 4729–4741. [CrossRef] [PubMed]
36. Legorburu, I.; Rodríguez, J.G.; Borja, Á.; Menchaca, I.; Solaun, O.; Valencia, V.; Galparsoro, I.; Larreta, J. Source Characterization and Spatio-Temporal Evolution of the Metal Pollution in the Sediments of the Basque Estuaries (Bay of Biscay). *Mar. Pollut. Bull.* **2013**, *66*, 25–38. [CrossRef] [PubMed]
37. Chen, C.; Zheng, B.; Jiang, X.; Zhao, Z.; Zhan, Y.; Yi, F.; Ren, J. Spatial Distribution and Pollution Assessment of Mercury in Sediments of Lake Taihu, China. *J. Environ. Sci.* **2013**, *25*, 316–325. [CrossRef] [PubMed]
38. Shen, Y.; Wu, Y. Optimization of Marine Environmental Monitoring Sites in the Yangtze River Estuary and Its Adjacent Sea, China. *Ocean. Coast. Manag.* **2013**, *73*, 92–100. [CrossRef]

39. Bui, T.D.; Luong-Van, J.; Maier, S.W.; Austin, C.M. Assessment and Monitoring of Nutrient Loading in the Sediments of Tidal Creeks Receiving Shrimp Farm Effluent in Quang Ninh, Vietnam. *Environ. Monit. Assess.* **2013**, *185*, 8715–8731. [CrossRef]
40. Zamani-Ahmadmahmoodi, R.; Esmaili-Sari, A.; Mohammadi, J.; Bakhtiari, A.R.; Savabieasfahani, M. Spatial Distribution of Cadmium and Lead in the Sediments of the Western Anzali Wetlands on the Coast of the Caspian Sea (Iran). *Mar. Pollut. Bull.* **2013**, *74*, 464–470. [CrossRef] [PubMed]
41. Johnson, S.L.; Maidment, D.R.; Kirisits, M.J. TMDL Balance: A Model for Coastal Water Pollutant Loadings. *J. Am. Water Resour. Assoc.* **2013**, *49*, 838–850. [CrossRef]
42. Srinivasan, K.; Natesan, U. Spatio-Temporal Variations in Water Quality of Muttukadu Backwaters, Tamilnadu, India. *Water Environ. Res.* **2013**, *85*, 587–595. [CrossRef] [PubMed]
43. Pascual-Aguilar, J.; Andreu, V.; Picó, Y. An Environmental Forensic Procedure to Analyse Anthropogenic Pressures of Urban Origin on Surface Water of Protected Coastal Agro-Environmental Wetlands (L'Albufera de Valencia Natural Park, Spain). *J. Hazard. Mater.* **2013**, *263*, 214–223. [CrossRef] [PubMed]
44. Oliveira, A.; Jesus, G.; Gomes, J.L.; Rogeiro, J.; Azevedo, A.; Rodrigues, M.; Fortunato, A.B.; Dias, J.M.; Tomas, L.M.; Vaz, L.; et al. An Interactive WebGIS Observatory Platform for Enhanced Support of Integrated Coastal Management. *J. Coast. Res.* **2014**, *SI70*, 507–512. [CrossRef]
45. Panigrahy, P.K.; Satapathy, D.R.; Panda, C.R.; Kar, R.N. Dispersion Pattern of Petroleum Hydrocarbon in Coastal Water of Bay of Bengal along Odisha and West Bengal, India Using Geospatial Approach. *Environ. Monit. Assess.* **2014**, *186*, 8303–8315. [CrossRef] [PubMed]
46. Yu, W.; Liu, R.; Wang, J.; Xu, F.; Shen, Z. Source Apportionment of PAHs in Surface Sediments Using Positive Matrix Factorization Combined with GIS for the Estuarine Area of the Yangtze River, China. *Chemosphere* **2015**, *134*, 263–271. [CrossRef]
47. Wang, H.; Wang, J.; Liu, R.; Yu, W.; Shen, Z. Spatial Variation, Environmental Risk and Biological Hazard Assessment of Heavy Metals in Surface Sediments of the Yangtze River Estuary. *Mar. Pollut. Bull.* **2015**, *93*, 250–258. [CrossRef]
48. Satapathy, D.R.; Panda, C.R. Spatio-Temporal Distribution of Major and Trace Metals in Estuarine Sediments of Dhamra, Bay of Bengal, India—Its Environmental Significance. *Environ. Monit. Assess.* **2015**, *187*, 4133. [CrossRef]
49. Keppler, C.J.; Bergquist, D.C.; Brock, L.M.; Felber, J.; Greenfield, D.I. A Spatial Assessment of Baseline Nutrient and Water Quality Values in the Ashepoo-Combahee-Edisto (ACE) Basin, South Carolina, USA. *Mar. Pollut. Bull.* **2015**, *99*, 332–337. [CrossRef]
50. Moses, S.A.; Janaki, L.; Joseph, S.; Joseph, J.; Thomas, J.; Lal, P. Prioritization of Pollution Potential Zones for Conservation Activities of a Lake System. *Lakes Reserv.* **2016**, *21*, 188–205. [CrossRef]
51. Liu, R.; Men, C.; Liu, Y.; Yu, W.; Xu, F.; Shen, Z. Spatial Distribution and Pollution Evaluation of Heavy Metals in Yangtze Estuary Sediment. *Mar. Pollut. Bull.* **2016**, *110*, 564–571. [CrossRef]
52. Liu, L.; Liu, R.; Yu, W.; Xu, F.; Men, C.; Wang, Q.; Shen, Z. Risk Assessment and Uncertainty Analysis of PAHs in the Sediments of the Yangtze River Estuary, China. *Mar. Pollut. Bull.* **2016**, *112*, 380–388. [CrossRef]
53. El-Zeiny, A.; El-Kafrawy, S. Assessment of Water Pollution Induced by Human Activities in Burullus Lake Using Landsat 8 Operational Land Imager and GIS. *Egypt. J. Remote Sens. Space Sci.* **2017**, *20*, S49–S56. [CrossRef]
54. Rajaram, R.; Ganeshkumar, A.; Vinothkumar, S.; Rameshkumar, S. Multivariate Statistical and GIS-Based Approaches for Toxic Metals in Tropical Mangrove Ecosystem, Southeast Coast of India. *Environ. Monit. Assess.* **2017**, *189*, 288. [CrossRef]
55. Zhang, Y.; Chu, C.; Li, T.; Xu, S.; Liu, L.; Ju, M. A Water Quality Management Strategy for Regionally Protected Water through Health Risk Assessment and Spatial Distribution of Heavy Metal Pollution in 3 Marine Reserves. *Sci. Total Environ.* **2017**, *599–600*, 721–731. [CrossRef] [PubMed]
56. Hoffman, E.; Lyons, J.; Boxall, J.; Robertson, C.; Lake, C.B.; Walker, T.R. Spatiotemporal Assessment (Quarter Century) of Pulp Mill Metal(Loid) Contaminated Sediment to Inform Remediation Decisions. *Environ. Monit. Assess.* **2017**, *189*, 257. [CrossRef] [PubMed]
57. Beland, M.; Biggs, T.W.; Roberts, D.A.; Peterson, S.H.; Kokaly, R.F.; Piazza, S. Oiling Accelerates Loss of Salt Marshes, Southeastern Louisiana. *PLoS ONE* **2017**, *12*, e0181197. [CrossRef]
58. Birch, G.F.; Lee, S.B. Baseline Physio-Chemical Characteristics of Sydney Estuary Water under Quiescent Conditions. *Mar. Pollut. Bull.* **2018**, *137*, 370–381. [CrossRef] [PubMed]
59. Ajmi, R.N.; Lami, A.; Ati, E.M.; Ali, N.S.M.; Latif, A.S. Detection of Isotope Stable Radioactive in Soil and Water Marshes of Southern Iraq. *J. Glob. Pharma Technol.* **2018**, *10*, 160–171.
60. Essel, B.; Gyesi, J.K.; Addo, R.K.; Galley, W.; MacCarthy, G. The Tale of a Disappearing Lagoon: A Habitat Mapping and Ecological Assessment of Fosu Lagoon, Ghana. *Int. J. Ecol.* **2019**, *2019*, 6931329. [CrossRef]
61. Sridevi Karpagavalli, M.; Ramachandran, A.; Palanivelu, K. Spatial and Temporal Variations of Water Quality in Pallikaranai Wetland, Chennai, India. *Int. J. Glob. Environ. Issues* **2019**, *18*, 86–106. [CrossRef]
62. Sousa, C.A.M.; Delgado, J.; Szalaj, D.; Boski, T. Holocene Background Concentrations and Actual Enrichment Factors of Metals in Sediments from Ria Formosa, Portugal. *Mar. Pollut. Bull.* **2019**, *149*, 110533. [CrossRef] [PubMed]
63. Mortula, M.; Ali, T.; Bachir, A.; Elaksher, A.; Abouleish, M. Towards Monitoring of Nutrient Pollution in Coastal Lake Using Remote Sensing and Regression Analysis. *Water* **2020**, *12*, 1954. [CrossRef]
64. Boateng, I.; Mitchell, S.; Couceiro, F.; Failler, P. An Investigation into the Impacts of Climate Change on Anthropogenic Polluted Coastal Lagoons in Ghana. *Coast. Manag.* **2020**, *48*, 601–622. [CrossRef]

65. Abd El-Hamid, H.T.; El-Alfy, M.A.; Elnaggar, A.A. Prediction of Future Situation of Land Use/Cover Change and Modeling Sensitivity to Pollution in Edku Lake, Egypt Based on Geospatial Analyses. *GeoJournal* **2021**, *86*, 1895–1913. [CrossRef]
66. Sadutto, D.; Andreu, V.; Ilo, T.; Akkanen, J.; Picó, Y. Pharmaceuticals and Personal Care Products in a Mediterranean Coastal Wetland: Impact of Anthropogenic and Spatial Factors and Environmental Risk Assessment. *Environ. Pollut.* **2021**, *271*, 116353. [CrossRef] [PubMed]
67. Vera-Herrera, L.; Romo, S.; Soria, J. How Agriculture, Connectivity and Water Management Can Affect Water Quality of a Mediterranean Coastal Wetland. *Agronomy* **2022**, *12*, 486. [CrossRef]
68. Radwan, A.-A.M.; Abdelmoneim, M.A.; Darwish, D.H.; El-Alfy, M.A.; Basiony, A.I. Elucidation of the Phytoplankton Distribution at an Egyptian Ramsar Site (Burullus Lake, Egypt) Using Alpha Diversity Indices Supported with RS and GIS Maps. *Egypt. J. Aquat. Biol. Fish.* **2022**, *26*, 595–612. [CrossRef]
69. Das, N.; Mondal, A.; Mandal, S. Polluted Waters of the Reclaimed Islands of Indian Sundarban Promote More Greenhouse Gas Emissions from Mangrove Ecosystem. *Stoch. Environ. Res. Risk Assess.* **2022**, *36*, 1277–1288. [CrossRef]
70. Zhao, W.; Cai, M.; Adelman, D.; Khairy, M.; Lin, Y.; Li, Z.; Liu, H.; Lohmann, R. Legacy Halogenated Organic Contaminants in Urban-Influenced Waters Using Passive Polyethylene Samplers: Emerging Evidence of Anthropogenic Land-Use-Based Sources and Ecological Risks. *Environ. Pollut.* **2022**, *298*, 118854. [CrossRef] [PubMed]
71. Kuang, Z.; Wang, H.; Han, B.; Rao, Y.; Gong, H.; Zhang, W.; Gu, Y.; Fan, Z.; Wang, S.; Huang, H. Coastal Sediment Heavy Metal(Loid) Pollution under Multifaceted Anthropogenic Stress: Insights Based on Geochemical Baselines and Source-Related Risks. *Chemosphere* **2023**, *339*, 139653. [CrossRef]
72. Abdel-Hamid, H.T.; R.Kaloop, M.; Elbeltagi, E.; Hu, J.W. Impact Assessment of the Land Use Dynamics and Water Pollution on Ecosystem Service Value of the Nile Delta Coastal Lakes, Egypt. *J. Indian Soc. Remote Sens.* **2023**, *51*, 963–981. [CrossRef]
73. Huang, F.; Chen, C. GIS-Based Approach and Multivariate Statistical Analysis for Identifying Sources of Heavy Metals in Marine Sediments from the Coast of Hong Kong. *Environ. Monit. Assess.* **2023**, *195*, 518. [CrossRef] [PubMed]
74. Özdemir, N.; Dokuyucu, A.; Ceviz, N.A.; Döndü, M.; Demirak, A.; Keskin, F. A Comparative Assessment of the Lagoons with Water Quality Indexes and Based on GIS: A Study on the Aegean Sea and Mediterranean Sea. *Environ. Forensics* **2023**, 1–23. [CrossRef]
75. Koto, R.; Hoxha, L.; Bani, A. Analysis of Water Quality, Heavy Metals and Nutrient of Karavasta Lagoon Using Gis Assessment of Ecological Risk. *J. Hyg. Eng. Des.* **2023**, *41*, 162–169.
76. Mohsen, A.; Zeidan, B.; Elshemy, M. Water Quality Assessment of Lake Burullus, Egypt, Utilizing Statistical and GIS Modeling as Environmental Hydrology Applications. *Environ. Monit. Assess.* **2023**, *195*, 93. [CrossRef] [PubMed]
77. Rokhbar, M.; Keshavarzi, B.; Moore, F.; Zarei, M.; Hooda, P.S.; Risk, M.J. Occurrence and Source of PAHs in Miankaleh International Wetland in Iran. *Chemosphere* **2023**, *321*, 138140. [CrossRef] [PubMed]
78. Seyed Hashtroudi, M.; Aghadadashi, V.; Mehdinia, A.; Sheijooni Fumani, N. Combining Theoretical Concepts and Geographic Information System (GIS) to Highlight Source, Risk, and Hotspots of Sedimentary PAHs: A Case Study of Chabahar Bay. *Environ. Res.* **2023**, *216*, 114540. [CrossRef]
79. Kumar, R.; Sankhla, M.S.; Kumar, R.; Sonone, S.S. Impact of Pesticide Toxicity in Aquatic Environment. *Biointerface Res. Appl. Chem.* **2021**, *11*, 10131–10140. [CrossRef]
80. Kapoor, D.; Singh, M.P. Heavy Metal Contamination in Water and Its Possible Sources. In *Heavy Metals in the Environment*; Elsevier: Amsterdam, The Netherldans, 2021; pp. 179–189. [CrossRef]
81. Sindern, S.; Tremöhlen, M.; Dsikowitzky, L.; Gronen, L.; Schwarzbauer, J.; Siregar, T.H.; Ariyani, F.; Irianto, H.E. Heavy Metals in River and Coast Sediments of the Jakarta Bay Region (Indonesia)—Geogenic versus Anthropogenic Sources. *Mar. Pollut. Bull.* **2016**, *110*, 624–633. [CrossRef] [PubMed]
82. Vagi, M.C.; Petsas, A.S.; Kostopoulou, M.N. Potential Effects of Persistent Organic Contaminants on Marine Biota: A Review on Recent Research. *Water* **2021**, *13*, 2488. [CrossRef]
83. Patel, M.; Kumar, R.; Kishor, K.; Mlsna, T.; Pittman, C.U.; Mohan, D. Pharmaceuticals of Emerging Concern in Aquatic Systems: Chemistry, Occurrence, Effects, and Removal Methods. *Chem. Rev.* **2019**, *119*, 3510–3673. [CrossRef] [PubMed]
84. González-González, R.B.; Sharma, P.; Singh, S.P.; Américo-Pinheiro, J.H.P.; Parra-Saldívar, R.; Bilal, M.; Iqbal, H.M.N. Persistence, Environmental Hazards, and Mitigation of Pharmaceutically Active Residual Contaminants from Water Matrices. *Sci. Total Environ.* **2022**, *821*, 153329. [CrossRef] [PubMed]
85. Janarthanam, V.A.; Issac, P.K.; Guru, A.; Arockiaraj, J. Hazards of Polycyclic Aromatic Hydrocarbons: A Review on Occurrence, Detection, and Role of Green Nanomaterials on the Removal of PAH from the Water Environment. *Environ. Monit. Assess.* **2023**, *195*, 1531. [CrossRef] [PubMed]
86. Lin, A.M.; Timshina, A.S.; Magnuson, J.K.; Bowden, J.A.; Townsend, T.G. Emerging Polycyclic Aromatic Hydrocarbon (PAH) and Trace Metal Leachability from Reclaimed Asphalt Pavement (RAP). *Chemosphere* **2023**, *333*, 138937. [CrossRef] [PubMed]
87. Soclo, H.H.; Garrigues, P.; Ewald, M. Origin of Polycyclic Aromatic Hydrocarbons (PAHs) in Coastal Marine Sediments: Case Studies in Cotonou (Benin) and Aquitaine (France) Areas. *Mar. Pollut. Bull.* **2000**, *40*, 387–396. [CrossRef]
88. Dai, C.; Han, Y.; Duan, Y.; Lai, X.; Fu, R.; Liu, S.; Leong, K.H.; Tu, Y.; Zhou, L. Review on the Contamination and Remediation of Polycyclic Aromatic Hydrocarbons (PAHs) in Coastal Soil and Sediments. *Environ. Res.* **2022**, *205*, 112423. [CrossRef] [PubMed]

89. Da Silva Junior, F.C.; Felipe, M.B.M.C.; de Castro, D.E.F.; Araújo, S.C.d.S.; Sisenando, H.C.N.; Batistuzzo de Medeiros, S.R. A Look beyond the Priority: A Systematic Review of the Genotoxic, Mutagenic, and Carcinogenic Endpoints of Non-Priority PAHs. *Environ. Pollut.* **2021**, *278*, 116838. [CrossRef]
90. De Rezende, A.T.; Mounteer, A.H. Ecological Risk Assessment of Pharmaceuticals and Endocrine Disrupting Compounds in Brazilian Surface Waters. *Environ. Pollut.* **2023**, *338*, 122628. [CrossRef]
91. Ben Chabchoubi, I.; Lam, S.S.; Pane, S.E.; Ksibi, M.; Guerriero, G.; Hentati, O. Hazard and Health Risk Assessment of Exposure to Pharmaceutical Active Compounds via Toxicological Evaluation by Zebrafish. *Environ. Pollut.* **2023**, *324*, 120698. [CrossRef] [PubMed]
92. Gómez-Regalado, M.d.C.; Martín, J.; Santos, J.L.; Aparicio, I.; Alonso, E.; Zafra-Gómez, A. Bioaccumulation/Bioconcentration of Pharmaceutical Active Compounds in Aquatic Organisms: Assessment and Factors Database. *Sci. Total Environ.* **2023**, *861*, 160638. [CrossRef]
93. Rajput, S.; Sharma, R.; Kumari, A.; Kaur, R.; Sharma, G.; Arora, S.; Kaur, R. Pesticide Residues in Various Environmental and Biological Matrices: Distribution, Extraction, and Analytical Procedures. *Environ. Dev. Sustain.* **2022**, *24*, 6032–6052. [CrossRef]
94. Navarro, I.; de la Torre, A.; Sanz, P.; Baldi, I.; Harkes, P.; Huerta-Lwanga, E.; Nørgaard, T.; Glavan, M.; Pasković, I.; Pasković, M.P.; et al. Occurrence of Pesticide Residues in Indoor Dust of Farmworker Households across Europe and Argentina. *Sci. Total Environ.* **2023**, *905*, 167797. [CrossRef] [PubMed]
95. Raj, A.; Dubey, A.; Malla, M.A.; Kumar, A. Pesticide Pestilence: Global Scenario and Recent Advances in Detection and Degradation Methods. *J. Environ. Manag.* **2023**, *338*, 117680. [CrossRef]
96. Daraban, G.M.; Hlihor, R.M.; Suteu, D. Pesticides vs. Biopesticides: From Pest Management to Toxicity and Impacts on the Environment and Human Health. *Toxics* **2023**, *11*, 983. [CrossRef]
97. Khatun, P.; Islam, A.; Sachi, S.; Islam, M.Z.; Islam, P. Pesticides in Vegetable Production in Bangladesh: A Systemic Review of Contamination Levels and Associated Health Risks in the Last Decade. *Toxicol. Rep.* **2023**, *11*, 199–211. [CrossRef] [PubMed]
98. Fida, M.; Li, P.; Wang, Y.; Alam, S.M.K.; Nsabimana, A. Water Contamination and Human Health Risks in Pakistan: A Review. *Expo Health* **2023**, *15*, 619–639. [CrossRef]
99. Bellan, G. Pollution Indices. In *Encyclopedia of Ecology*; Elsevier: Amsterdam, The Netherlands, 2008; pp. 2861–2868.
100. Prasad Ahirvar, B.; Das, P.; Srivastava, V.; Kumar, M. Perspectives of Heavy Metal Pollution Indices for Soil, Sediment, and Water Pollution Evaluation: An Insight. *Total Environ. Res. Themes* **2023**, *6*, 100039. [CrossRef]
101. Kumar, D.; Khan, E.A. Remediation and Detection Techniques for Heavy Metals in the Environment. In *Heavy Metals in the Environment: Impact, Assessment, and Remediation*; Elsevier: Amsterdam, The Netherlands, 2020; pp. 205–222, ISBN 9780128216569.
102. Hoalst-Pullen, N.; Patterson, M.W. (Eds.) *Geospatial Technologies in Environmental Management*; Springer: Dordrecht, The Netherlands, 2010; ISBN 978-90-481-9524-4.
103. Baker, T.R.; Battersby, S.; Bednarz, S.W.; Bodzin, A.M.; Kolvoord, B.; Moore, S.; Sinton, D.; Uttal, D. A Research Agenda for Geospatial Technologies and Learning. *J. Geogr.* **2015**, *114*, 118–130. [CrossRef]
104. Kraak, M.J.; Ormeling, F.J.; Ormeling, F. *Cartography: Visualization of Spatial Data*; Longman: London, UK, 1996; ISBN 9780582259539.
105. Chang, K.-T. *Introduction to Geographic Information Systems*; McGraw-Hill: New York, NY, USA, 2018; ISBN 9781259929649.
106. Lu, G.Y.; Wong, D.W. An Adaptive Inverse-Distance Weighting Spatial Interpolation Technique. *Comput. Geosci.* **2008**, *34*, 1044–1055. [CrossRef]
107. Dhar, A.; Datta, B. Global Optimal Design of Ground Water Monitoring Network Using Embedded Kriging. *Ground Water* **2009**, *47*, 806–815. [CrossRef] [PubMed]
108. Yang, R.; Xing, B. A Comparison of the Performance of Different Interpolation Methods in Replicating Rainfall Magnitudes under Different Climatic Conditions in Chongqing Province (China). *Atmosphere* **2021**, *12*, 1318. [CrossRef]
109. Kim, J.J.; Delisle, K.; Brown, T.M.; Bishay, F.; Ross, P.S.; Noël, M. Characterization and Interpolation of Sediment Polychlorinated Biphenyls and Polybrominated Diphenyl Ethers in Resident Killer Whale Habitat along the Coast of British Columbia, Canada. *Environ. Toxicol. Chem.* **2022**, *41*, 2139–2151. [CrossRef] [PubMed]
110. Khorram, S.; Nelson, S.A.C.; Koch, F.H.; van der Wiele, C.F. *Remote Sensing*; Pelton, J.N., Ed.; Springer: Berlin, Germany, 2012; ISBN 978-1-4614-3103-9.
111. Arias-Rodriguez, L.F.; Duan, Z.; Díaz-Torres, J.d.J.; Basilio Hazas, M.; Huang, J.; Kumar, B.U.; Tuo, Y.; Disse, M. Integration of Remote Sensing and Mexican Water Quality Monitoring System Using an Extreme Learning Machine. *Sensors* **2021**, *21*, 4118. [CrossRef] [PubMed]
112. Matthews, M.W. A Current Review of Empirical Procedures of Remote Sensing in Inland and Near-Coastal Transitional Waters. *Int. J. Remote Sens.* **2011**, *32*, 6855–6899. [CrossRef]
113. Laureano-Rosario, A.E.; Duncan, A.P.; Symonds, E.M.; Savic, D.A.; Muller-Karger, F.E. Predicting Culturable Enterococci Exceedances at Escambron Beach, San Juan, Puerto Rico Using Satellite Remote Sensing and Artificial Neural Networks. *J. Water Health* **2018**, *17*, 137–148. [CrossRef] [PubMed]
114. Wu, J.; Hilborn, E.D.; Schaeffer, B.A.; Urquhart, E.; Coffer, M.M.; Lin, C.J.; Egorov, A.I. Acute Health Effects Associated with Satellite-Determined Cyanobacterial Blooms in a Drinking Water Source in Massachusetts. *Environ. Health* **2021**, *20*, 83. [CrossRef]
115. Nolting, R.F.; Ramkema, A.; Everaarts, J.M. The Geochemistry of Cu, Cd, Zn, Ni and Pb in Sediment Cores from the Continental Slope of the Banc d'Arguin (Mauritania). *Cont. Shelf Res.* **1999**, *19*, 665–691. [CrossRef]

116. Muller, G. Index of Geoaccumulation in Sediments of the Rhine River. *GeoJournal* **1969**, *2*, 108–118.
117. Hakanson, L. An Ecological Risk Index for Aquatic Pollution Control. A Sedimentological Approach. *Water Res.* **1980**, *14*, 975–1001. [CrossRef]
118. Tomlinson, D.L.; Wilson, J.G.; Harris, C.R.; Jeffrey, D.W. Problems in the Assessment of Heavy-Metal Levels in Estuaries and the Formation of a Pollution Index. *Helgoländer Meeresunters.* **1980**, *33*, 566–575. [CrossRef]
119. Abrahim, G.M.S.; Parker, R.J. Assessment of Heavy Metal Enrichment Factors and the Degree of Contamination in Marine Sediments from Tamaki Estuary, Auckland, New Zealand. *Environ. Monit. Assess.* **2008**, *136*, 227–238. [CrossRef] [PubMed]
120. Primpas, I.; Tsirtsis, G.; Karydis, M.; Kokkoris, G.D. Principal Component Analysis: Development of a Multivariate Index for Assessing Eutrophication According to the European Water Framework Directive. *Ecol. Indic.* **2010**, *10*, 178–183. [CrossRef]
121. Aghadadashi, V.; Mehdinia, A.; Molaei, S. Origin, Toxicological and Narcotic Potential of Sedimentary PAHs and Remarkable Even/Odd n-Alkane Predominance in Bushehr Peninsula, the Persian Gulf. *Mar. Pollut. Bull.* **2017**, *114*, 494–504. [CrossRef]
122. Long, E.R.; Macdonald, D.D.; Smith, S.L.; Calder, F.D. Incidence of Adverse Biological Effects within Ranges of Chemical Concentrations in Marine and Estuarine Sediments. *Environ. Manag.* **1995**, *19*, 81–97. [CrossRef]
123. Long, E.R.; Ingersoll, C.G.; MacDonald, D.D. Calculation and Uses of Mean Sediment Quality Guideline Quotients: A Critical Review. *Environ. Sci. Technol.* **2006**, *40*, 1726–1736. [CrossRef] [PubMed]
124. Carr, R.S.; Long, E.R.; Windom, H.L.; Chapman, D.C.; Thursby, G.; Sloane, G.M.; Wolfe, D.A. Sediment Quality Assessment Studies of Tampa Bay, Florida. *Environ. Toxicol. Chem.* **1996**, *15*, 1218. [CrossRef]
125. MacDonald, D.D.; Carr, R.S.; Eckenrod, D.; Greening, H.; Grabe, S.; Ingersoll, C.G.; Janicki, S.; Janicki, T.; Lindskoog, R.A.; Long, E.R.; et al. Development, Evaluation, and Application of Sediment Quality Targets for Assessing and Managing Contaminated Sediments in Tampa Bay, Florida. *Arch. Environ. Contam. Toxicol.* **2004**, *46*, 147–161. [CrossRef]
126. Van Den Berg, M.; Birnbaum, L.; Bosveld, A.T.C.; Brunström, B.; Cook, P.; Feeley, M.; Giesy, J.P.; Hanberg, A.; Hasegawa, R.; Kennedy, S.W.; et al. Toxic Equivalency Factors (TEFs) for PCBs, PCDDs, PCDFs for Humans and Wildlife. *Environ. Health Perspect.* **1998**, *106*, 775–792. [CrossRef]
127. Feng, H.; Jiang, H.; Gao, W.; Weinstein, M.P.; Zhang, Q.; Zhang, W.; Yu, L.; Yuan, D.; Tao, J. Metal Contamination in Sediments of the Western Bohai Bay and Adjacent Estuaries, China. *J. Environ. Manag.* **2011**, *92*, 1185–1197. [CrossRef] [PubMed]
128. Urban, D.L.; Cook, N.J. *Hazard Evaluation, Standard Evaluation Procedure, Ecological Risk Assessment*; Agency EP: Washington, DC, USA, 1986.
129. Hansen, D.J.; Ditoro, D.M.; Mcgrath, J.A.; Swartz, R.C.; Mount, D.R.; Spehar, R.L.; Burgess, R.M.; Ozretich, R.J.; Bell, H.E.; Reiley, M.C.; et al. *Procedures for the Derivation of Equilibrium Partitioning Sediment. Benchmarks (ESBs) for the Protection of Benthic Organisms: PAH Mixtures*; Environmental Protection Agency: Washington, DC, USA, 2003.
130. Carlson, R.E. A Trophic State Index for Lakes. *Limnol. Oceanogr.* **1977**, *22*, 361–369. [CrossRef]
131. Carlson, R.E.; Simpson, J. A Coordinator's Guide to Volunteer Lake Monitoring Methods. *N. Am. Lake Manag. Soc.* **1996**, *96*, 305.
132. Vollenweider, R.A.; Giovanardi, F.; Montanari, G.; Rinaldi, A.A. Characterization of the Trophic Conditions of Marine Coastal Waters with Special Reference to the NW Adriatic Sea: Proposal for a Trophic Scale, Turbidity and Generalized Water Quality Index. *Envirometrics* **1998**, *9*, 329–357. [CrossRef]
133. Uddin, M.G.; Nash, S.; Olbert, A.I. A Review of Water Quality Index Models and Their Use for Assessing Surface Water Quality. *Ecol. Indic.* **2021**, *122*, 107218. [CrossRef]
134. Lumb, A.; Sharma, T.C.; Bibeault, J.-F. A Review of Genesis and Evolution of Water Quality Index (WQI) and Some Future Directions. *Water Qual. Expo. Health* **2011**, *3*, 11–24. [CrossRef]
135. Nemerow, N.L. *Scientifc Stream Pollution Analysis*; Scripta Book Co.: Gaithersburg, GD, USA, 1974.
136. Nemerow, N.L.; Sumitomo, H. *Benefits of Water Quality Enhancement (Part. A: Pollution Index. for Benefits Analysis) Water Pollution Control Research Series N. 16110 DAJ 12/70*; Environmental Protection Agency, Water Quality Office: New York, NY, USA, 1970.
137. Zhao, Y.; Xia, X.H.; Yang, Z.F.; Wang, F. Assessment of Water Quality in Baiyangdian Lake Using Multivariate Statistical Techniques. *Procedia Environ. Sci.* **2012**, *13*, 1213–1226. [CrossRef]
138. *European Commission Document on Risk Assessment*; Technical Guidance Document on Risk Assessment Part II; European Commission: Brussels, Belgium, 2003; p. 337.
139. Szefer, P.; Ali, A.A.; Ba-haroon, A.A.; Rajeh, A.A.; Ge, J.; Nabrzyski, M. Distribution and Relationships of Selected Trace Metals in Molluscs and Associated Sediments from the Gulf of Aden, Yemen. *Environ. Pollut.* **1999**, *106*, 299–314. [CrossRef]
140. USEPA. *Risk Assessment Guidance for Superfund. Volume I Human Health Evaluation Manual (Part A)*; USEPA: Washington, DC, USA, 1989; Volume 1.
141. USEPA. *Supplemental Guidance for Developing Soil Screening Levels for Superfund Sites*; USEPA: Washington, DC, USA, 2002.
142. Smith, R. *EPA Region III Risk-Based Concentration Table*; Environmental Protection Agency: Washington, DC, USA, 1996.
143. Johnbull, O.; Abbassi, B.; Zytner, R.G. Risk Assessment of Heavy Metals in Soil Based on the Geographic Information System-Kriging Technique in Anka, Nigeria. *Environ. Eng. Res.* **2019**, *24*, 150–158. [CrossRef]

MDPI AG
Grosspeteranlage 5
4052 Basel
Switzerland
Tel.: +41 61 683 77 34

ISPRS International Journal of Geo-Information Editorial Office
E-mail: ijgi@mdpi.com
www.mdpi.com/journal/ijgi

www.ingramcontent.com/pod-product-compliance
Lightning Source LLC
LaVergne TN
LVHW070502061126
851858LV00011B/281